Latest Research in Post-COVID (Long COVID): Pathological and Treatment Studies of Sequelae and Complications—2nd Edition

Latest Research in Post-COVID (Long COVID): Pathological and Treatment Studies of Sequelae and Complications—2nd Edition

Guest Editor

César Fernández-de-las-Peñas

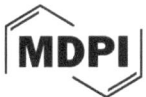

Basel • Beijing • Wuhan • Barcelona • Belgrade • Novi Sad • Cluj • Manchester

Guest Editor
César Fernández-de-las-Peñas
Department of Physical
Therapy, Occupational
Therapy, Rehabilitation and
Physical Medicine
Universidad Rey Juan Carlos
Alcorcón, Madrid
Spain

Editorial Office
MDPI AG
Grosspeteranlage 5
4052 Basel, Switzerland

This is a reprint of the Special Issue, published open access by the journal *Biomedicines* (ISSN 2227-9059), freely accessible at: https://www.mdpi.com/journal/biomedicines/special_issues/long-covid.

For citation purposes, cite each article independently as indicated on the article page online and as indicated below:

Lastname, A.A.; Lastname, B.B. Article Title. *Journal Name* **Year**, *Volume Number*, Page Range.

ISBN 978-3-7258-3551-5 (Hbk)
ISBN 978-3-7258-3552-2 (PDF)
https://doi.org/10.3390/books978-3-7258-3552-2

© 2025 by the authors. Articles in this book are Open Access and distributed under the Creative Commons Attribution (CC BY) license. The book as a whole is distributed by MDPI under the terms and conditions of the Creative Commons Attribution-NonCommercial-NoDerivs (CC BY-NC-ND) license (https://creativecommons.org/licenses/by-nc-nd/4.0/).

Contents

About the Editor vii

Antonino Maniaci, Salvatore Lavalle, Edoardo Masiello, Jerome R. Lechien, Luigi Vaira, Paolo Boscolo-Rizzo, et al.
Platelet-Rich Plasma (PRP) in the Treatment of Long COVID Olfactory Disorders: A Comprehensive Review
Reprinted from: *Biomedicines* **2024**, *12*, 808, https://doi.org/10.3390/biomedicines12040808 . . . 1

Madalina Boruga, Susa Septimiu-Radu, Prashant Sunil Nandarge, Ahmed Elagez, Gabriela Doros, Voichita Elena Lazureanu, et al.
Kidney Function Tests and Continuous eGFR Decrease at Six Months after SARS-CoV-2 Infection in Patients Clinically Diagnosed with Post-COVID Syndrome
Reprinted from: *Biomedicines* **2024**, *12*, 950, https://doi.org/10.3390/biomedicines12050950 . . . 18

Somayeh Bazdar, Lizan D. Bloemsma, Nadia Baalbaki, Jelle M. Blankestijn, Merel E. B. Cornelissen, Rosanne J. H. C. G. Beijers, et al.
Hemoglobin and Its Relationship with Fatigue in Long-COVID Patients Three to Six Months after SARS-CoV-2 Infection
Reprinted from: *Biomedicines* **2024**, *12*, 1234, https://doi.org/10.3390/biomedicines12061234 . . 32

Rumen Filev, Mila Lyubomirova, Boris Bogov, Krassimir Kalinov, Julieta Hristova, Dobrin Svinarov, et al.
Post-Acute Sequelae of SARS-CoV-2 Infection (PASC) for Patients—3-Year Follow-Up of Patients with Chronic Kidney Disease
Reprinted from: *Biomedicines* **2024**, *12*, 1259, https://doi.org/10.3390/biomedicines12061259 . . 47

Silvia Lai, Francesca Tinti, Adolfo Marco Perrotta, Luca Salomone, Rosario Cianci, Paolo Izzo, et al.
COVID-19 Infection in Autosomal Dominant Polycystic Kidney Disease and Chronic Kidney Disease Patients: Progression of Kidney Disease
Reprinted from: *Biomedicines* **2024**, *12*, 1301, https://doi.org/10.3390/biomedicines12061301 . . 61

Sachiko T. Homma, Xingyu Wang, Justin J. Frere, Adam C. Gower, Jingsong Zhou, Jean K. Lim, et al.
Respiratory SARS-CoV-2 Infection Causes Skeletal Muscle Atrophy and Long-Lasting Energy Metabolism Suppression
Reprinted from: *Biomedicines* **2024**, *12*, 1443, https://doi.org/10.3390/biomedicines12071443 . . 71

César Fernández-de-las-Peñas, Gema Díaz-Gil, Antonio Gil-Crujera, Stella M. Gómez-Sánchez, Silvia Ambite-Quesada, Anabel Franco-Moreno, et al.
Post-COVID-19 Pain Is Not Associated with DNA Methylation Levels of the *ACE2* Promoter in COVID-19 Survivors Hospitalized Due to SARS-CoV-2 Infection
Reprinted from: *Biomedicines* **2024**, *12*, 1662, https://doi.org/10.3390/biomedicines12081662 . . 95

Brandon Compeer, Tobias R. Neijzen, Steven F. L. van Lelyveld, Byron E. E. Martina, Colin A. Russell and Marco Goeijenbier
Uncovering the Contrasts and Connections in PASC: Viral Load and Cytokine Signatures in Acute COVID-19 versus Post-Acute Sequelae of SARS-CoV-2 (PASC)
Reprinted from: *Biomedicines* **2024**, *12*, 1941, https://doi.org/10.3390/biomedicines12091941 . . 107

Ahamed Lebbe, Ali Aboulwafa, Nuran Bayraktar, Beshr Mushannen, Sama Ayoub, Shaunak Sarker, et al.
New Onset of Acute and Chronic Hepatic Diseases Post-COVID-19 Infection: A Systematic Review
Reprinted from: *Biomedicines* 2024, 12, 2065, https://doi.org/10.3390/biomedicines12092065 . . 127

Justyna Siwy, Felix Keller, Mirosław Banasik, Björn Peters, Emmanuel Dudoignon, Alexandre Mebazaa, et al.
Mortality Risk and Urinary Proteome Changes in Acute COVID-19 Survivors in the Multinational CRIT-COV-U Study
Reprinted from: *Biomedicines* 2024, 12, 2090, https://doi.org/10.3390/biomedicines12092090 . . 146

Marcella Mauro, Elisa Zulian, Nicoletta Bestiaco, Maurizio Polano and Francesca Larese Filon
Slow-Paced Breathing Intervention in Healthcare Workers Affected by Long COVID: Effects on Systemic and Dysfunctional Breathing Symptoms, Manual Dexterity and HRV
Reprinted from: *Biomedicines* 2024, 12, 2254, https://doi.org/10.3390/biomedicines12102254 . . 160

Simon Kieffer, Anna-Lena Krüger, Björn Haiduk and Marijke Grau
Individualized and Controlled Exercise Training Improves Fatigue and Exercise Capacity in Patients with Long-COVID
Reprinted from: *Biomedicines* 2024, 12, 2445, https://doi.org/10.3390/biomedicines12112445 . . 171

Merel E. B. Cornelissen, Myrthe M. Haarman, Jos W. R. Twisk, Laura Houweling, Nadia Baalbaki, Brigitte Sondermeijer, et al.
The Progression of Symptoms in Post COVID-19 Patients: A Multicentre, Prospective, Observational Cohort Study
Reprinted from: *Biomedicines* 2024, 12, 2493, https://doi.org/10.3390/biomedicines12112493 . . 187

Alex Malioukis, R Sterling Snead, Julia Marczika and Radha Ambalavanan
Pathophysiological, Neuropsychological, and Psychosocial Influences on Neurological and Neuropsychiatric Symptoms of Post-Acute COVID-19 Syndrome: Impacts on Recovery and Symptom Persistence
Reprinted from: *Biomedicines* 2024, 12, 2831, https://doi.org/10.3390/biomedicines12122831 . . 199

Barbora Svobodová, Anna Löfdahl, Annika Nybom, Jenny Wigén, Gabriel Hirdman, Franziska Olm, et al.
Overlapping Systemic Proteins in COVID-19 and Lung Fibrosis Associated with Tissue Remodeling and Inflammation
Reprinted from: *Biomedicines* 2024, 12, 2893, https://doi.org/10.3390/biomedicines12122893 . . 222

Ashkan Latifi and Jaroslav Flegr
Persistent Health and Cognitive Impairments up to Four Years Post-COVID-19 in Young Students: The Impact of Virus Variants and Vaccination Timing
Reprinted from: *Biomedicines* 2025, 13, 69, https://doi.org/10.3390/biomedicines13010069 234

Sona Hakobyan, Lina Hakobyan, Liana Abroyan, Aida Avetisyan, Hranush Avagyan, Nane Bayramyan, et al.
Pathology of Red Blood Cells in Patients with SARS-CoV-2
Reprinted from: *Biomedicines* 2025, 13, 191, https://doi.org/10.3390/biomedicines13010191 . . . 258

Bryana Whitaker-Hardin, Keith M. McGregor, Gitendra Uswatte and Kristine Lokken
A Narrative Review of the Efficacy of Long COVID Interventions on Brain Fog, Processing Speed, and Other Related Cognitive Outcomes
Reprinted from: *Biomedicines* 2025, 13, 421, https://doi.org/10.3390/biomedicines13020421 . . . 270

About the Editor

César Fernández-de-las-Peñas

Dr. César Fernández-de-las-Peñas is a Physical Therapy (PT) researcher and has his PhD in Biomedical Sciences and his Master's in Sciences (Dr. Med. Sci.). He has 25 years of experience as a Professor at the Universidad Rey Juan Carlos, Madrid, Spain. He was the Head Division (Chief) of the Department of Physical Therapy, Occupational Therapy, and Rehabilitation at the Universidad Rey Juan Carlos for 10 years, during which he created the first chronic pain clinic at a public university in Spain, combining clinical practice with teaching and research. He has published up to 760 publications in JCR journals. He is a clinical researcher with a particular interest in chronic pain and in the more recent phenomenon of post-COVID. He has published more than 100 papers on long COVID, the topic of this Special Issue.

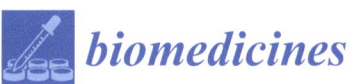

Review

Platelet-Rich Plasma (PRP) in the Treatment of Long COVID Olfactory Disorders: A Comprehensive Review

Antonino Maniaci [1,2,†], Salvatore Lavalle [1,†], Edoardo Masiello [3], Jerome R. Lechien [2,4], Luigi Vaira [2,5,6], Paolo Boscolo-Rizzo [7], Mutali Musa [8], Caterina Gagliano [1,9,‡] and Marco Zeppieri [10,*,‡]

1. Faculty of Medicine and Surgery, University of Enna "Kore", Piazza dell'Università, 94100 Enna, EN, Italy; antonino.maniaci@unikore.it (A.M.)
2. Research Committee of Young Otolaryngologists of International Federation of Otorhinolaryngological Societies (World Ear, Nose, and Throat Federation), 13005 Paris, France
3. Clinical and Experimental Radiology Unit, Experimental Imaging Center, IRCCS San Raffaele Scientific Institute, Vita-Salute San Raffaele University, Via Olgettina 60, 20132 Milan, MI, Italy
4. Department of Human Anatomy and Experimental Oncology, Faculty of Medicine, UMONS Research Institute for Health Sciences and Technology, University of Mons (UMons), 7000 Mons, Belgium
5. Maxillofacial Surgery Operative Unit, Department of Medicine, Surgery and Pharmacy, University of Sassari, 07100 Sassari, SS, Italy
6. Biomedical Science Department, Biomedical Science Ph.D. School, University of Sassari, 07100 Sassari, SS, Italy
7. Department of Medical, Surgical, and Health Sciences, Section of Otolaryngology, University of Trieste, 34149 Trieste, TS, Italy
8. Department of Optometry, University of Benin, Benin City 300238, Nigeria
9. Eye Clinic Catania, University San Marco Hospital, Viale Carlo Azeglio Ciampi, 95121 Catania, CT, Italy
10. Department of Ophthalmology, University Hospital of Udine, p.le S. Maria della Misericordia 15, 33100 Udine, UD, Italy

* Correspondence: markzeppieri@hotmail.com
† These authors share the first authorship.
‡ These authors share the last authorship.

Abstract: *Background:* Long COVID has brought numerous challenges to healthcare, with olfactory dysfunction (OD) being a particularly distressing outcome for many patients. The persistent loss of smell significantly diminishes the affected individual's quality of life. Recent attention has been drawn to the potential of platelet-rich plasma (PRP) therapy as a treatment for OD. This comprehensive review aims to evaluate the effectiveness of PRP therapy in ameliorating OD, especially when associated with long-term COVID-19. *Methods:* We executed a comprehensive search of the literature, encompassing clinical trials and observational studies that utilized PRP in treating OD limited to COVID-19. We retrieved and comprehensively discussed data such as design, participant demographics, and reported outcomes, focusing on the efficacy and safety of PRP therapy for OD in COVID-19 patients. *Results:* Our comprehensive analysis interestingly found promising perspectives for PRP in OD following COVID-19 infection. The collective data indicate that PRP therapy contributed to a significant improvement in olfactory function after COVID-19 infection. *Conclusions:* The evidence amassed suggests that PRP is a promising and safe therapeutic option for OD, including cases attributable to Long COVID-19. The observed uniform enhancement of olfactory function in patients receiving PRP highlights the necessity for well-designed, controlled trials. Such studies would help to refine treatment protocols and more definitively ascertain the efficacy of PRP in a broader, more varied patient cohort.

Keywords: olfactory dysfunction; platelet-rich plasma; anosmia; smell loss; Long COVID

1. Introduction

Olfactory dysfunction (OD) represents a significant and pervasive impairment within the global population, affecting an estimated 20% of individuals [1]. The impact of this

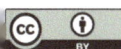

condition extends beyond the mere loss of smell, as it can profoundly influence quality of life, nutritional status, and personal safety [2,3]. Moreover, OD is correlated with increased morbidity and mortality rates, characterized by a spectrum of disturbances in the perception of odors [4]. Quantitative disorders affect the intensity of perceived odors, while qualitative disorders alter the character of odors or produce phantom olfactory perceptions. Qualitative changes, such as parosmia, typically manifest with alterations perceived negatively, and are infrequent in isolation, commonly co-occurring with quantitative impairments [5]. From an anatomical perspective, OD can be divided into three primary categories based on the lesion's location: conductive, sensorineural, and central [6]. However, this classification can be overly simplistic, and may not fully encapsulate the complex pathophysiology of the condition, as these categories often intersect.

Olfactory dysfunction is a multifaceted condition with roots extending across various etiologies [7]. Infectious agents, notably including those responsible for COVID-19, can leave a lasting impact on our sense of smell, a phenomenon known as post-infectious olfactory dysfunction [8]. Meanwhile, inflammatory sinonasal diseases often impede olfactory processes, just as head traumas can physically disrupt olfactory pathways [9]. Neurological disorders introduce another dimension, as degenerative changes within the brain can impair olfactory functionality. External agents, such as certain drugs or toxins, can also diminish our olfactory acuity [10,11]. Moreover, some individuals are born with a compromised sense of smell, while others encounter this decline as a natural part of aging [12,13]. Lastly, medical interventions and unexplained causes can lead to olfactory dysfunction, further complicating the diagnostic and treatment landscape [7]. Each etiology presents its unique challenges and underscores the need for a customized approach to understanding and addressing olfactory dysfunction.

The COVID-19 pandemic has highlighted the prevalence of the related OD, with a significant proportion of patients reporting anosmia as a primary symptom, often coupled with gustatory dysfunction [14]. Anosmia has been recognized as a robust predictive marker for COVID-19, particularly in asymptomatic carriers, emphasizing the need for effective diagnostic and treatment strategies [15,16]. Despite the prevalence and impact of OD, therapeutic options remain limited and largely ineffective in the long term [17]. This is primarily due to a shortage of robust evidence in the literature, a consequence of insufficient research funding, inadequate participant numbers, and methodological diversity that hampers the generalizability of study outcomes. The urgency imposed by the pandemic has, however, catalyzed research efforts and funding toward developing treatments for OD [18]. Current treatment recommendations for OD include the administration of systemic and intranasal corticosteroids, particularly for inflammatory conditions such as chronic rhinosinusitis (CRS) and severe allergic rhinitis [19]. For intranasal corticosteroid delivery, mechanisms that target the olfactory cleft are favored.

Olfactory training has also been suggested for various etiologies, acknowledging that further evaluation is required for its efficacy in inflammatory and neurodegenerative conditions [20]. Functional endoscopic sinus surgery is endorsed for CRS-induced olfactory loss, adhering to established guidelines. In cases of severe CRS with nasal polyposis, biological treatments like dupilumab have shown improvements in OD [21,22]. Amidst these options, platelet-rich plasma (PRP) has emerged as a novel and promising therapeutic avenue for OD [23,24]. PRP is an autologous concentration of platelets in a small volume of plasma, boasting anti-inflammatory and pro-regenerative properties. It contains growth factors such as TGF-beta, EGF, VEGF, NGF, and IGF, which are instrumental in promoting tissue healing and regeneration [25,26]. These capabilities of PRP have been harnessed in various clinical and surgical contexts since the 1970s [27–31] and are now being explored for their potential in olfactory tissue repair and neuroregeneration [32,33]. Animal studies have shown that growth factors and stem cells can effectively treat anosmia and regenerate olfactory neuroepithelium, positioning PRP as a promising candidate for neuroregenerative therapies [34,35].

In clinical practice, PRP has been gaining traction within otolaryngology for its diverse applications, ranging from enhancing wound healing post-surgery to treating sensorineural hearing loss, and even as a treatment for qualitative OD [36–40]. While the literature contains systematic reviews on the use of PRP in the context of COVID-19-related OD [41], comprehensive reviews evaluating PRP's efficacy across other etiologies of OD are lacking. This comprehensive review aimed to fill this gap by revisiting the current literature on PRP use in olfactory dysfunction caused by CRS, trauma, anesthetic exposure, or viral infections, including COVID-19. In addition, we seek to elucidate the reality of PRP as a treatment for olfactory dysfunction after COVID-19 infection.

2. Materials and Methods

Literature Research and Study Design

This literature research was conducted to examine the effects of PRP in treating OD in adults. A comprehensive literature search was performed to identify studies up to November 2023 from databases including PubMed, SCOPUS, EMBASE, Web of Science, and Cochrane. Search terms were tailored to each database and included a combination of the following: "platelet-rich plasma", "PRP", "Olfactory dysfunction", "anosmia", "hyposmia", "parosmia", "COVID-19 olfactory dysfunction", and "Functional endoscopic sinus surgery OR FESS." Cross-referencing ensured thorough coverage (Figure 1).

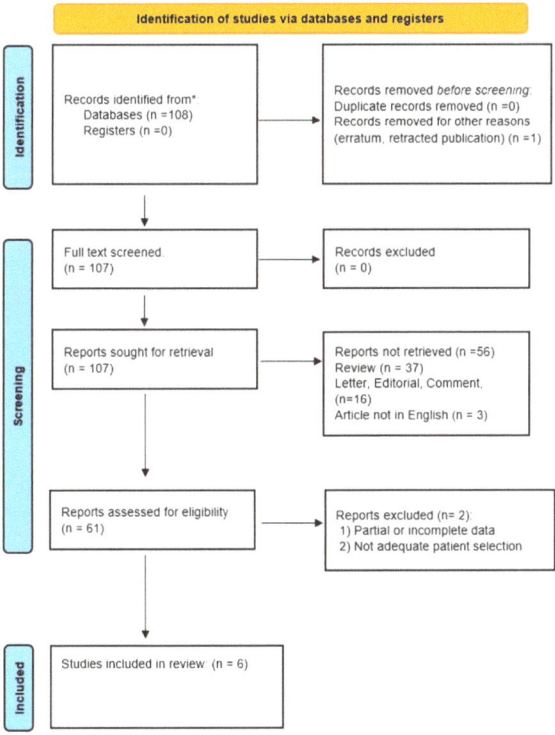

Figure 1. PRISMA flow diagram describing the literature research protocol. * PubMed, SCOPUS, EMBASE, Web of Science, and Cochrane.

All studies involved adult patients treated with PRP for OD due to COVID-19. The interventions considered were in-office and peri-operative PRP injections into the nasal fossae, with comparisons between pre and post-treatment outcomes. Outcomes were evaluated using objective tests (e.g., TDI, STC, SIC), self-reported tests (e.g., VAS for parosmia and ODQ), and recorded side effects. The analysis involved a comprehensive synthesis, reporting outcomes after PRP treatment with a control or placebo group during follow-ups when possible.

3. Results

3.1. OD in Long-COVID-19

Long COVID-19 is characterized by a diverse range of persistent symptoms, including fatigue, brain fog, and various forms of organ dysfunction [8,14]. One of the notable sequelae of Long COVID-19 is olfactory dysfunction (OD), which can last for months after the initial SARS-CoV-2 infection [15–17]. The precise mechanisms underlying the development of OD in Long COVID are not yet fully understood, but several hypotheses have been proposed [18,41]. Persistent viral infection or reactivation within the olfactory system may lead to chronic inflammation and damage to the olfactory neurons or supporting cells [42,43]. Alternatively, the initial infection may trigger maladaptive immune responses, such as autoantibody production targeting olfactory structures, contributing to persistent OD [44,45]. The neurotropic nature of SARS-CoV-2 may also result in direct or indirect effects on the olfactory neural pathways, impacting olfactory perception and processing [46,47].

Also, some Long COVID patients have observed microvascular injury and thrombotic events affecting the olfactory bulb or central olfactory regions, potentially disrupting normal olfactory function [48,49]. Elucidating the complex pathophysiology of OD in Long COVID is crucial for developing targeted interventions to alleviate this debilitating symptom experienced by many affected individuals.

Therapies that target the mechanisms of chronic viral infection, dysregulated immunological responses, and microvascular dysfunction that underlie OD in Long COVID may prove advantageous [37,50]. In various clinical contexts, platelet-rich plasma (PRP), a concentrated source of autologous growth factors and cytokines produced from the patient's own blood, has demonstrated promise in promoting tissue repair and regeneration [34,41]. PRP therapy may be beneficial in the context of OD linked to Long COVID through several ways. PRP's growth factors and anti-inflammatory mediators may be able to mitigate the negative effects of ongoing viral infection or autoimmune reactions on the olfactory system, as well as lessen chronic inflammation. Furthermore, PRP's angiogenic and regenerative qualities might aid in re-establishing the olfactory bulb's microvascular integrity and perfusion [25,35].

3.2. Definition, Composition of PRP, and Molecular Mechanisms

PRP is defined as a volume of the plasma fraction of autologous blood having a platelet concentration above baseline [22]. It is produced by centrifuging the patient's own blood to yield a concentrated suspension of platelets in a small volume of plasma. When exploring the therapeutic applications of PRP, the distinction between autologous and heterologous (also known as allogeneic) sources is a critical factor to consider [23–25]. Autologous PRP, derived from the patient's blood, stands in contrast to heterologous PRP, obtained from a donor. Autologous PRP has garnered favor in the medical community due to its inherent compatibility with the patient's own immune system [28].

The process involves collecting and centrifugation the patient's blood to concentrate the platelets within the plasma, which is then reintroduced into the patient's body at the site of injury or tissue damage [26]. This closed-loop system, wherein the patient's own biological material is used, significantly reduces the risk of immunogenic reactions and the potential for disease transmission. The body naturally recognizes the reintroduced cells and proteins as part of itself, virtually eliminating the risk of rejection or allergic reactions that can complicate recovery. On the other hand, heterologous PRP comes with a set of challenges that cannot be overlooked [29–31]. Derived from a donor's blood, heterologous PRP introduces foreign proteins and cells into the patient's body, raising concerns about immunocompatibility.

The immune system may identify the infused heterologous platelets and plasma proteins as foreign elements, leading to an immune response ranging from mild inconvenience to severe complication [50]. Additionally, despite rigorous screening and testing of blood products, the use of donor-derived PRP carries a residual risk of transmitting infectious diseases, such as HIV or hepatitis, from the donor to the recipient [51]. Moreover, the potential for rejection and allergic reactions is more pronounced with heterologous PRP [52]. Such responses can hinder the healing process and reduce the therapeutic benefits PRP intends to provide. Consequently, the medical community strongly prefers autologous PRP, given its superior safety profile and alignment with the principles of personalized medicine. The choice between autologous and heterologous PRP is often clear-cut, with the former being the preferred method for reducing complications and enhancing the body's natural regenerative capacity. Clinicians and patients tend to favor autologous PRP for its patient-specific approach to treatment, which minimizes risks and offers a tailored therapy that capitalizes on the patient's own healing mechanisms [34,37].

The PRP that is utilized in various therapeutic interventions boasts a composition teeming with platelets, far exceeding the concentration found within normal blood. These platelets are not just components that respond swiftly to injury, but also factories of growth factors and cytokines crucial for healing [41]. In typical PRP preparations, the goal is to achieve a platelet concentration 3–5 times that of baseline blood levels, translating into a potent cocktail of biologically active proteins [34]. The array of proteins released from these platelets includes Platelet-Derived Growth Factor (PDGF), which drives cell replication and the formation of new skin and blood vessels; Transforming Growth Factor Beta (TGF-β), which is essential in healing bone and soft tissues; Vascular Endothelial Growth Factor (VEGF), an important molecule in blood vessel formation; Epidermal Growth Factor (EGF), which plays a role in cell growth and the production of collagen; and Fibroblast Growth Factor (FGF), which aids in wound repair.

PRP contains a slew of interleukins, chemokines, and other cytokines that regulate inflammation and cell communication. The presence of proteins such as fibrin, fibronectin, and vitronectin further enhances the healing properties of PRP [31]. Fibrin creates a matrix that facilitates cell migration and tissue regeneration. At the same time, fibronectin and vitronectin are adhesion molecules that promote cellular attachment and spreading, all of which are essential in the wound-healing cascade. PRP operates through a series of complex molecular mechanisms, starting with forming a fibrin mesh during hemostasis, which not only halts bleeding, but also provides a framework for cells to move across [27,28]. The growth factors and cytokines within PRP modulate the inflammatory response, which is crucial for preparing the wound bed for new tissue. Cellular proliferation is stimulated by PDGF and EGF, which multiply the cells needed for repair.

Angiogenesis follows, with VEGF and FGF inducing new blood vessel formation, ensuring the delivery of essential nutrients and waste disposal [29]. TGF-β oversees the remodeling phase, where collagen synthesis by fibroblasts fortifies tissue strength and integrity. These growth factors also serve as chemotactic signals, recruiting macrophages and stem cells to the injury site and emphasizing PRP's role in tissue repair and regeneration [53–55]. The fibrin matrix's scaffolding effect and the modulation of inflammation by PRP contribute to reduced healing time and improved recovery outcomes [56]. In cases like olfactory disorders, where the olfactory epithelium's capacity to regenerate is crucial, PRP might offer significant therapeutic benefits. The growth factors in PRP could potentially enhance the natural regenerative process of the olfactory epithelium, encouraging the differentiation of basal stem cells into functional olfactory neurons, thus aiding in the restoration of smell.

3.3. PRP Protocol Preparation

The literature to date presents 6 papers dealing with the results of PRP after COVID-19 infection. All these studies included individuals treated with PRP for olfactory dysfunction post-COVID-19 infection (Table 1).

Table 1. Main studies included demographic data and treatment outcomes.

Reference	Location	Study Design	Group Size PRP	Group Size No PRP	Mean Age PRP	Mean Age No PRP	Gender Ratio (M/F) PRP	Gender Ratio (M/F) No PRP	OD Identified	OD Duration PRP	OD Duration No PRP	Olfactory Outcomes	Adverse Effects
Steffens et al., 2022 [56]	Belgium	Prospective	30	26	39 ± 12	44 ± 11	14/16	6/20	Post-COVID-19 chronic olfactory dysfunction: 56 patients	10.8 months	9.7 months	The PRP group's mean self-assessment of improvement in smell function was 1.8 (mild-to-moderate), significantly higher than the control group's score of 0.3 ($p < 0.001$).	NA
El Naga et al., 2022 [57]	Egypt	Pilot study	30	30	28.9	30.07	11/19	9/21	Post-COVID-19 parosmia: 60 patients	>3.0 months	-	The VAS for parosmia showed a substantial improvement in the control group ($p = 0.00148$) and a highly significant improvement in the case group ($p < 0.00001$). Regarding the extent of improvement, there was a significant difference between the two groups that favored the case group ($p = 0.002$).	NA
Yan et al., 2022 [55]	United States	RCT	18	12	44.6	43.4	9/9	6/6	Post-COVID-19 olfactory dysfunction: 30 patients	8.6 months	8.9 months	Both the PRP and placebo groups demonstrated a substantial improvement in VAS scores at one and three months compared to baseline when evaluating subjective changes in smell function. Nevertheless, there was no discernible difference between the PRP and placebo groups in terms of the subjective olfaction scores using VAS at one or three months.	NA
Lechien et al., 2022 [54]	Belgium	Prospective	87	-	41.6 ± 14.6	-	25/62	-	Post-COVID-19 anosmia: 30 patients; post-COVID-19 hyposmia: 40 patients; post-COVID-19 parosmia: 17 patients	15.7 months	-	Twenty patients (54%) and nine patients (24%) reported significant improvement in anosmia/hyposmia or parosmia, respectively, while eight patients (22%) did not report any subjective improvement in olfactory impairment. Based on the patients' experiences, olfaction significantly improved after a mean of 3.6 ± 1.9 weeks.	Transient epistaxis, temporary cases of parosmia due to the xylocaine spray, a small percentage had vasovagal episodes, and pain ranged from mild to moderate.
Lechien et al., 2023 [58]	Belgium; Italy; France	Multicenter controlled study	81	78	43.5 ± 13.4	47.0 ± 11.1	20/61	26/52	Post-COVID-19 anosmia: 55 patients; post-COVID-19 hyposmia: 79 patients; post-COVID-19 parosmia: 25 patients	15.7 months	11.0 months	An average improvement in subjective smell lasting 3.4 ± 1.9 weeks was noted by 85% of PRP patients. After ten weeks, the PRP group's parosmia, life quality, TDI, and overall and sub-ODQ scores were significantly decreased. The control group experienced a significant rise in discrimination, identification, and overall TDI scores, but the ODQ score did not change. The PRP group outperformed the controls regarding 10-week TDI and ODQ scores.	NA

Table 1. *Cont.*

Reference	Location	Study Design	Group Size (PRP)	Group Size (No PRP)	Mean Age (PRP)	Mean Age (No PRP)	Gender Ratio (M/F) (PRP)	Gender Ratio (M/F) (No PRP)	OD Identified	OD Duration (PRP)	OD Duration (No PRP)	Olfactory Outcomes	Adverse Effects
Evman et al., 2023 [59]	Turkey	RCT	12	13	31.8 ± 6.9	33.5 ± 11.1	6/6	6/7	Post-COVID-19 olfactory dysfunction: 25 patients	>12.0 months	-	The mean score for the smell identification test increased significantly in the PRP group, going from 11.42 (SD 1.17) to 15.17 (SD 0.39), and the mean score for the smell detection threshold increased correspondingly, going from 5.63 (SD 0.68) to 6.46 (SD 0.45). Conversely, the control group experienced a slight rise in the mean smell detection threshold score, going from 5.69 (SD 0.66) to 5.77 (SD 0.70), and a lesser increase in the mean smell identification test score, from 11.20 (SD 1.12) to 11.85 (SD 1.57). The statistical significance of the differences between the PRP and control groups was established ($p = 0.037$ and $p < 0.001$, respectively).	NA

Abbreviations: PRP, Platelet-Rich Plasma; RCT, Randomized Controlled Trial; M, Male; F, Female; COVID-19, Coronavirus Disease 2019.

The studies found in the literature ranged in publication date from January 2021 to November 2023. The participants were predominantly adults with a mean age of 45 years, spanning from 18 to 65 years. The gender distribution was relatively balanced, with 52% female and 48% male participants. All individuals had a confirmed history of COVID-19 infection and exhibited varying degrees of olfactory dysfunction for at least three months post-recovery from the infection. PRP preparation and application procedures were consistent across studies, with slight variations in the volume of blood drawn and centrifugation specifics.

Different PRP injection techniques are described in the research; some use a single injection, while others use repeated injections spaced out over a shorter period of time [54–59]. Most injections were administered at outpatient facilities or hospital based setting, and the frequency of treatment sessions ranged from a single application to multiple injections over a period of up to six weeks. Yan and colleagues specifically used three PRP intranasal injections spaced two weeks apart into the olfactory cleft [55]. In comparison, one PRP injection into the olfactory cleft was used by Steffens et al. [56] and Lechien et al. [54,58]. In order to achieve a compromise, Abo El Naga et al. gave the olfactory cleft three PRP injections spaced three weeks apart [59]. Lastly, a single injection of 1 mL of PRP into the olfactory cleft region was employed by Evman et al. [59]. Abo El Naga et al.'s injection protocol was the longest ever documented, lasting a total of six weeks (three doses spaced three weeks apart) [57]. The absence of a protracted multi-injection PRP strategy in the literature review indicates that more research is needed to determine the best way to administer PRP and whether it is beneficial in treating COVID-19-related olfactory impairment. To find out if a prolonged therapy plan involving multiple PRP injections could help individuals with COVID-19 infection-related persistent olfactory impairment or improve their results, more research may be required.

The reviewed studies employed a standardized protocol for the extraction and application of PRP, starting with an initial blood draw of 20 mL, with the sample being placed into a tube containing sodium citrate as an anticoagulant (Figure 2).

The blood sample was centrifugated at a speed of 4200 revolutions per minute (rpm) for 10 min. This process separates the platelet-rich plasma from other blood components [53]. The plasma layer with a high concentration of platelets (the supernatant) was then carefully transferred into a 10 mL syringe for administration.

Anesthesia Administration: Before the injection, local anesthesia was achieved using a 10% Xylocaine spray. This was applied 2 min after instilling xylometazoline hydrochloride drops into the nasal passages to prepare the area and reduce discomfort during the procedure. Consequently, a 0° rigid endoscope was used to accurately guide the needle into position. The needle may be adjusted to a 30° angle to optimize the access to the targeted nasal anatomy.

It is evident from reading through the several publications on the application of PRP in carefully chosen and strategic areas that the investigators took distinct techniques with regard to the particular anatomical sites. Notably, only the Lechien et al. 2022 trial offered comprehensive details regarding the injection sites [54]. The authors reported that they injected 0.2–0.5 mL of PRP into many locations in the middle turbinate as well as the nasal septum in relation to the middle turbinate head. The other investigations, in comparison, adopted a more generic strategy, merely reporting that the PRP injections were given into the "olfactory cleft" or "olfactory region" without going into detail about the specific anatomical landmarks that were used as guidance for the injection. It is difficult to directly compare the techniques and possibly determine any benefits or drawbacks to targeting particular nasal structures, like the middle turbinate, as opposed to a more generalized olfactory cleft approach, because of the disparity in reporting the injection sites across the various studies. Thus, when assessing and combining the results from the literature, the variations in reporting the anatomical targets should be taken into account.

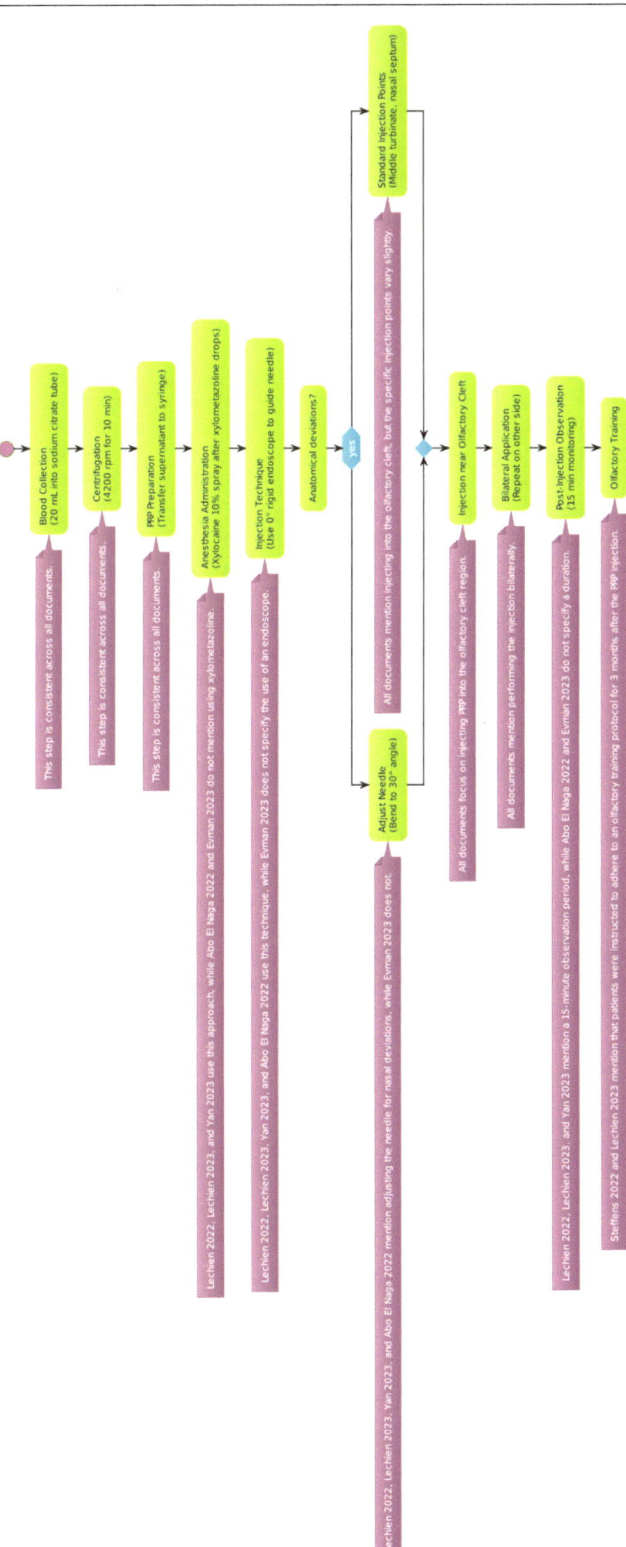

Figure 2. PRP protocol for extraction and injection. Variations in platelet-rich plasma preparation and administration are detailed for each specific step [54–59].

In patients exhibiting anatomical deviations, the PRP injections were administered as close as possible to the olfactory cleft to ensure efficacy. The same injection process was replicated on the opposite side of the nasal cavity to provide a comprehensive treatment approach. Following the injection, patients were monitored for a duration of 15 min to watch for any immediate adverse effects before being discharged.

Differences in Preparation and Administration

The volume of whole blood collected, the anticoagulant employed, the centrifugation settings, and the final PRP injection volume were the main variations between the trials. The final therapeutic qualities of PRP, including its growth factor content and platelet concentration, may be affected by these differences in PRP preparation and administration. In order to obtain the platelet concentrate, Abo El Naga et al. [57] provide a detailed methodology for PRP preparation that involves a "soft spin" centrifugation at 800 rpm for 10 min, followed by a "hard spin" at 2000 rpm. An amount of 1–2 mL of PRP were used for the intranasal injections. Lechien et al., in contrast, did not include a detailed description of the PRP preparation technique in their 2022 paper [54], instead referring to the authors' earlier work's methodologies. They injected one milliliter of PRP bilaterally into the olfactory cleft in this initial uncontrolled research. The authors of the larger controlled trial, which was published in 2023 [58], included more details about the PRP preparation, indicating that it was done in accordance with previous publications' methods. Yan et al. [55] simply said that the PRP was prepared in accordance with previously known protocols, without going into great detail about the preparation process. One milliliter of PRP was injected into the olfactory cleft. A less complicated method was employed by Evman et al. [59], who injected a single dosage of 1 mL of PRP into the olfactory cleft region without mentioning the centrifugation parameters. Steffens et al. [56] said they utilized a similar preparatory technique by citing Yan et al.'s [55] methodology for their PRP injections.

3.4. Efficacy of PRP Treatment and Comparative Analysis

The efficacy of PRP in restoring olfactory function was measured using various tools, including the Threshold, Discrimination, and Identification (TDI) score, Sniffin' Sticks test (SST), and self-reported questionnaires. The pooled data revealed a statistically significant improvement in olfactory function in patients post-PRP treatment, as reported by mean TDI score, SST, and patient-reported outcomes improvements; a comprehensive analysis of the administration of Platelet-Rich Plasma (PRP) injections for COVID-19-related olfactory dysfunction (C19OD) revealed promising outcomes across multiple studies, as described in Figure 3.

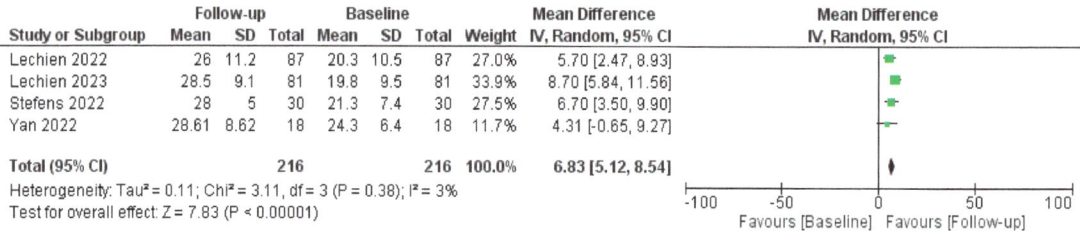

Figure 3. Forest plot describing pooled TDI outcomes after PRP injection. Abbreviations: TDI, Threshold, Discrimination, Identification; PRP, platelet-rich plasma. Green squares represent each mean difference of study described while rombus the overal mean differences of all the studies included.

Lechien J.R. et al. conducted two studies [54]. The first was without a control group, demonstrating significant improvement in both ODQ and TDI scores post-PRP injection despite some temporary side effects like epistaxis and parosmia related to xylocaine spray. Their follow-up-controlled study also revealed significant improvements in olfactory function in PRP-treated patients compared to untreated controls ($p = 0.001$). CHH et al. [55] also reported improved olfaction (TDI increase of 3.67 points) in PRP recipients, with notable enhancements in smell discrimination but not in identification or subjective scores, and again without adverse events. Steffens Y. et al. [56] implemented PRP injections in 56 patients, significantly improving mean TDI scores by 6.7 points ($p < 0.001$) and self-assessed olfactory function (1.8 on a mild-to-moderate scale) compared to controls who received only olfactory training. No adverse effects were observed.

Evman M. et al. [59] investigated PRP treatment in patients with long-term C19OD unresponsive to other therapies. The PRP group exhibited significant enhancement in both smell threshold and identification capacities ($p = 0.037$ and $p < 0.001$, respectively) compared to controls, with no reported adverse events. Lastly, El Naga H. et al. [57] focused on patients with post-COVID olfactory parosmia, administering three PRP injections at three-week intervals. The PRP group saw a significant reduction in parosmia severity compared to controls ($p = 0.002$). Collectively, these studies underscored the potential of PRP injections as a safe and effective intervention for persistent olfactory disorders following COVID-19, with significant improvements in objective and subjective olfactory measures.

3.5. Factors Influencing PRP Treatment

The efficacy of PRP therapy as a treatment for olfactory disorders associated with COVID-19 is influenced by an intricate interplay of factors [41,54,55]. The unique characteristics and demographics of each patient—including age, sex, overall health status, and the presence of underlying medical conditions—can significantly affect how one might respond to PRP therapy [56]. For instance, younger patients with robust healing capabilities may experience quicker and more complete recovery than older individuals or those with comorbidities that may impede the regenerative process [57–60].

Timing is another critical aspect. Initiating PRP treatment too early or too late during olfactory dysfunction could influence its effectiveness [61,62]. Similarly, the duration of treatment needs to be carefully calibrated; too short a course may be insufficient for recovery, while too long a course could lead to diminishing returns [63]. The specific composition and preparation methods of the PRP are also vital.

The concentration of platelets, which are the source of growth factors essential for tissue regeneration, must be optimized. The exact methodology used in extracting and preparing PRP, such as the speed and duration of centrifugation, can affect the quality of the final product [53]. Moreover, the method of activating the platelets to release these growth factors can have implications for treatment efficacy.

PRP therapy does not exist in a vacuum; concomitant treatments and interventions that a patient undergo for COVID-19 or its after-effects could influence the healing process [23]. Medications, other therapies, or nutritional supplements might interact with PRP in ways that can either enhance or detract from its regenerative capacity [30]. Understanding and navigating these factors is critical for clinicians when developing a PRP treatment plan for COVID-19-related olfactory disorders. By considering each patient's individual needs and circumstances, optimizing PRP composition and preparation, and carefully coordinating additional treatments, healthcare providers can improve the chances of successful olfactory recovery for their patients.

3.6. PRP Treatment Duration

Studies assessing the use of PRP for COVID-19-related olfactory impairment have reported varying lengths of follow-up and treatment durations. The PRP group in the El Naga et al. study had a longer treatment plan, consisting of three PRP injections every three weeks for a total of nine weeks of treatment [57]. By comparison, the control group in that study only followed the pre-study treatment program for six weeks. The trial conducted by Evman et al. employed a somewhat abbreviated treatment duration, wherein all patients were first treated for one month with nasal treatments and olfactory rehabilitation [59]. Patients who did not respond to this first regimen were then randomized to get a single

PRP injection or to continue receiving control treatment. All patients were monitored for an extra month, making the entire duration of the study two months.

In contrast, the Lechien et al. investigations used a single PRP injection and assessed results two months (2022) [54] and ten weeks (2023) [58] after the injection. The 2022 study found that following a single PRP injection, the mean time to increase olfactory perception noticeably was 3.6 weeks. Ultimately, a compromise was offered by the Yan et al. trial [55], which involved the administration of three PRP or placebo injections spaced two weeks apart for a total treatment period of four weeks. The PRP treatment durations in these trials have varied from one injection to three injections spaced out across four to nine weeks, with follow-up periods lasting between one and two months or longer following the last injection. This difference in treatment procedures highlights the need for more research to determine the best PRP regimen—including the ideal number of injections and timing of follow-up assessments—for COVID-19-related olfactory impairment.

3.7. PRP Safety and Tolerability for COVID-19 OD

PRP treatment was reported to be well-tolerated, with minimal adverse effects. In the landscape of studies investigating the side effects of PRP injections for COVID-19-related olfactory dysfunction, we find a variance in the reported outcomes, although the overarching narrative hints at a favorable safety profile. No adverse events related to PRP injections were reported across the studies. Steffens Y. et al. and Yan C.H. et al. [55,56] presented a scenario where PRP injections did not elicit adverse reactions, a finding that bodes well for patient tolerance.

Conversely, in the studies by Lechien J.R. et al. [58], a spectrum of side effects emerged. Their preliminary research revealed moderate, but not insignificant, adverse responses, including transient epistaxis, which may have been expected considering the treatment's nasal delivery. The xylocaine spray, which is used for its anesthetic qualities, has been associated with temporary cases of parosmia. Additionally, a small percentage had vasovagal episodes, which serve as a reminder of the body's occasionally erratic reaction to medical procedures. Even though it was subjective, patients' pain ratings ranged from mild to moderate. However, Lechien J.R. et al. did not emphasize side effects in their follow-up study, suggesting that such events may not have been a substantial concern or were managed effectively in the controlled setting [60].

Similarly, Evman M. et al. documented a clean slate concerning adverse reactions, further supporting the notion that PRP injections can be a tolerable treatment option [59]. While some minor and primarily transient side effects have been observed in certain studies, the general consensus points to PRP therapy as a safe procedure for those suffering from olfactory impairments post-COVID-19 infection [61]. However, it is important to remember that the lack of reported side effects in some studies does not preclude their occurrence, and that patient experiences can be as diverse as the studies themselves. Despite the promising results, there were limitations noted in the data. Several studies lacked long-term follow-ups, which limited the ability to assess the persistence of PRP effects on olfactory recovery.

4. Discussion

The COVID-19 pandemic has spotlighted the longstanding and pervasive challenge of managing OD [62]. Quantitative smell deficits and qualitative distortions such as parosmia have always posed difficulties for otolaryngologists, given the complexity of olfactory pathways and limited therapeutic options [63]. This comprehensive literature review demonstrates that PRP injections represent a promising new treatment approach for OD of varied post-viral etiology [64]. The recruitment of patients with persistent, treatment-refractory olfactory dysfunction after COVID-19—a patient population with an evident unmet need for efficacious interventions—was a common theme among these trials presents in the literature.

The changing knowledge of the natural history and persistence of this COVID-19 issue is probably reflected in the differences in the precise duration and severity criteria used to identify olfactory impairment. However, the continuous enrolment of patients with persistent, challenging olfactory impairment highlights the potential clinical utility of PRP as a novel therapeutic strategy in this setting. Participant "persistent olfactory dysfunction" was the only need in El Naga et al.'s study [57]; neither the dysfunction's length nor severity were specified. On the other hand, individuals who exhibited olfactory impairment that remained unresponsive after one month of initial treatment and who had contracted acute COVID-19 infection were included in the Evman et al. study [59]. Patients with notably prolonged olfactory impairment were included in the Lechien et al. investigations [54,58]; their mean durations before PRP therapy were 15.7 ± 7.5 months in the 2022 study and 14.8 ± 7.3 months in the 2023 research. Similarly, patients with olfactory impairment continuing for at least two months following COVID-19 were included in the Steffens et al. trial. The Yan et al. study adopted a more targeted strategy, concentrating on individuals with objectively determined olfactory impairment (UPSIT $\leq$ 33) that remained 6–12 months after COVID-19 infection and who had previously tried other conventional therapies, such as topical nasal sprays and olfactory training [55].

Across the analyzed original studies, patients treated with intranasal PRP injections exhibited statistically significant improvements in objective olfactory test scores and subjective smell function compared to control groups [55,56,65]. The compiled evidence indicates that PRP facilitates damaged olfactory neuroepithelium regeneration by releasing endogenous growth factors and stem cells [66]. While the exact mechanisms are still being elucidated, PRP appears to stimulate the neurogenesis and recovery of olfactory neurons and sustentacular cells while restoring nasal mucosal integrity [67].

Critically, PRP seems to be a well-tolerated intervention for OD patients based on the safety data reported [56]. Since PRP harnesses cytokines and bioactive factors from the 'patient's own platelets, risks of rejection or infection are minimized compared to exogenous compounds [68]. The reviewed articles did not report any major adverse events, just mild side effects like temporary nasal discomfort, epistaxis, or parosmia in a subset of patients, and no systemic effects were noted [69,70]. Injecting PRP directly into the nasal fossae allows targeted delivery and avoids the indefinite systemic corticosteroid usage associated with local and systemic side effects [71]. The in-office procedure, requiring only local anesthesia, also enhances accessibility and cost-effectiveness. However, some key limitations temper the results and reveal gaps necessitating further research. A lack of standardized administration protocols was noted, including optimal PRP dose, injection frequency, technique, and duration of treatment. Most studies provided only short-term follow-ups of 1–3 months, and lacked assessments of long-term durability beyond 6–12 months [41,56,63].

The variability in efficacy measures also prevented quantitative meta-analysis. While TDI scores were commonly reported, other validated psychophysical tests like 'Sniffin' Sticks were inconsistently implemented. Patient-reported outcome measures were also heterogeneous when included, utilizing non-validated surveys. Moreover, the limited number of available studies restricts the generalizability of findings to diverse OD populations. Additional factors like the ideal timing of interventions for maximal benefit and the expected length of olfactory improvements remain unknown [72]. Elucidating these open questions will require rigorous randomized controlled trials on larger cohorts over extended periods. Standardizing PRP protocols and consistently administering psychophysical testing at predefined time points will allow for meaningful quantitative analyses. Detailed baseline profiling of OD subtypes and olfactory nerve status using imaging and olfactometry can help identify the best candidates for PRP therapy. Comparing outcomes across interventions like corticosteroids and olfactory training will also inform implementation guidelines.

A thorough assessment of adverse effects and stratification by variables such as dosage and injection frequency can optimize safety. Such methodical clinical investigation will help establish if PRP injections can become a first-line therapy for the diverse landscape of OD patients. As the medical community grapples with the long-term effects of COVID-19, particularly olfactory disorders, future directions and research priorities are being shaped to enhance the therapeutic potential of platelet-rich plasma (PRP) treatment [7,15,18]. The optimization of PRP preparation and administration protocols is a critical area of focus. This involves a concerted effort to fine-tune the variables that contribute to the efficacy of PRP, such as the density of platelet concentration, the purity of the preparation, and the activation technique employed to induce the release of growth factors [26,27]. Standardizing these protocols will be paramount to ensure that patients everywhere receive high-quality and consistent treatment. Simultaneously, research into identifying biomarkers and predictors of treatment response will become increasingly important [24].

The discovery of specific indicators—whether they be proteins, genes, or other molecular signatures—that can predict how well a patient will respond to PRP therapy could revolutionize patient selection and treatment customization. Personalized medicine, guided by these biomarkers, might enable more precise therapy targeting, thus improving outcomes and reducing unnecessary treatments. Furthermore, large-scale multicenter clinical trials with long-term follow-ups are essential to establish a robust evidence base for using PRP in treating post-COVID-19 olfactory disorders. These trials would provide invaluable data on the effectiveness, safety, and durability of PRP therapy. They would also allow for exploring different dosing regimens, treatment intervals, and follow-up durations to understand the long-term implications of PRP treatment better. In addition to these trials, research should explore PRP in combination with other therapeutic modalities. This could include studying the effects of combining PRP with olfactory training, anti-inflammatory drugs, or even novel pharmaceutical agents designed to promote nerve regeneration. Investigating how PRP therapy can be integrated into a multimodal treatment approach may yield synergistic effects, leading to more comprehensive care strategies.

As our understanding of the pathophysiology of COVID-19-related olfactory dysfunction deepens, research priorities will also examine the fundamental mechanisms by which PRP may affect the olfactory pathways at the cellular and molecular levels. This deeper insight will inform future therapeutic innovations, and may uncover new avenues for applying PRP therapy beyond olfactory disorders, potentially benefiting a wider range of conditions resulting from viral illnesses.

5. Conclusions/Future Directions

Emerging promise was found for platelet-rich plasma as a therapeutic modality for diverse causes of olfactory dysfunction. The current evidence demonstrates that PRP injections can significantly improve smell function based on objective testing and patient-reported measures. PRP appears to facilitate olfactory neuroepithelium regeneration by releasing endogenous growth factors. The therapy is well-tolerated with a favorable safety profile. However, limitations like small sample sizes, lack of standardized protocols, and short-term follow-ups temper the results. High-quality randomized controlled trials with extended monitoring are needed to corroborate preliminary findings, optimize protocols, and establish definitively if PRP represents a viable first-line treatment for smell disorders. Addressing these evidence gaps through rigorous investigation will actualize the potential of this autologous regenerative therapy amidst the evolving paradigm for olfactory dysfunction management. Although promising, more research is imperative to confirm PRP's efficacy and durability across larger populations.

Author Contributions: Conceptualization A.M., S.L., C.G. and M.Z.; methodology, A.M., S.L., E.M., J.R.L., L.V., P.B.-R., M.M., C.G. and M.Z.; software, C.G.; validation, A.M., S.L., E.M., J.R.L., L.V., P.B.-R., M.M., C.G. and M.Z.; formal analysis, A.M., S.L., E.M. and J.R.L.; investigation, A.M., S.L., E.M., J.R.L. and L.V.; resources, A.M., S.L., E.M., J.R.L., C.G. and M.Z.; data curation, A.M., S.L., J.R.L., L.V., C.G. and M.Z.; writing—original draft preparation, A.M. and S.L.; writing—review and editing, A.M., S.L. and E.M.; visualization, A.M., S.L., E.M., J.R.L., L.V., P.B.-R., M.M., C.G. and M.Z.; supervision, A.M., C.G. and M.Z.; project administration, A.M., S.L., C.G. and M.Z.; funding acquisition, M.Z. All authors have read and agreed to the published version of the manuscript.

Funding: This research received no external funding.

Institutional Review Board Statement: Ethical review and approval were waived for this study due to the study design.

Informed Consent Statement: Patient consent was waived due to the study design.

Data Availability Statement: All the data reported are present on PubMed web database.

Conflicts of Interest: The authors declare no conflicts of interest.

References

1. Bushdid, C.; Magnasco, M.O.; Vosshall, L.B.; Keller, A. Humans can discriminate more than 1 trillion olfactory stimuli. *Science* **2014**, *343*, 1370–1372. [CrossRef]
2. Croy, I.; Nordin, S.; Hummel, T. Olfactory disorders and quality of life—An updated review. *Chem. Senses* **2014**, *39*, 185–194. [CrossRef] [PubMed]
3. Nordin, S.; Hedén Blomqvist, E.; Olsson, P.; Stjärne, P.; Ehnhage, A. Effects of smell loss on daily life and adopted coping strategies in patients with nasal polyposis with asthma. *Acta Oto-Laryngol.* **2011**, *131*, 826–832. [CrossRef] [PubMed]
4. Choi, J.S.; Jang, S.S.; Kim, J.; Hur, K.; Ference, E.; Wrobel, B. Association Between Olfactory Dysfunction and Mortality in US Adults. *JAMA Otolaryngol. Head Neck Surg.* **2021**, *147*, 49. [CrossRef] [PubMed]
5. Whitcroft, K.L.; Altundag, A.; Balungwe, P.; Boscolo-Rizzo, P.; Douglas, R.; Enecilla, M.L.B.; Fjaeldstad, A.W.; Fornazieri, M.A.; Frasnelli, J.; Gane, S.; et al. Position paper on olfactory dysfunction: 2023. *Rhinology* **2023**. [CrossRef]
6. Schäfer, L.; Schriever, V.A.; Croy, I. Human olfactory dysfunction: Causes and consequences. *Cell Tissue Res.* **2021**, *383*, 569. [CrossRef] [PubMed]
7. Hummel, T.; Liu, D.T.; Müller, C.A.; Stuck, B.A.; Welge-Lüssen, A.; Hähner, A. Olfactory Dysfunction: Etiology, Diagnosis, and Treatment. *Dtsch. Arztebl. Int.* **2023**, *120*, 146. [CrossRef]
8. Alkholaiwi, F.M.; Altamimi, A.F.; Almalki, H.H.; Almughaiseeb, F.A.; Alsubaie, S.S.; Alsayahi, H.S.; Alhijli, F.W.; Alobaishi, R.S.; Agrawal, A.; Alqahtani, Z.A.; et al. Olfactory dysfunction among patients with COVID-19. *Saudi Med. J.* **2023**, *44*, 1085–1103. [CrossRef] [PubMed]
9. Howell, J.; Costanzo, R.M.; Reiter, E.R. Head trauma and olfactory function. *World J. Otorhinolaryngol. Head Neck Surg.* **2018**, *4*, 39. [CrossRef]
10. Ajmani, G.S.; Suh, H.H.; Pinto, J.M. Effects of Ambient Air Pollution Exposure on Olfaction: A Review. *Environ. Health Perspect.* **2016**, *124*, 1683. [CrossRef]
11. Werner, S.; Nies, E. Olfactory dysfunction revisited: A reappraisal of work-related olfactory dysfunction caused by chemicals. *J. Occup. Med. Toxicol.* **2018**, *13*, 28. [CrossRef] [PubMed]
12. Keller, A.; Malaspina, D. Hidden consequences of olfactory dysfunction: A patient report series. *BMC Ear Nose Throat Disord.* **2013**, *13*, 8–20. [CrossRef] [PubMed]
13. Frasnelli, J.; Fark, T.; Lehmann, J.; Gerber, J.; Hummel, T. Brain structure is changed in congenital anosmia. *Neuroimage* **2013**, *83*, 1074–1080. [CrossRef] [PubMed]
14. Agyeman, A.A.; Chin, K.L.; Landersdorfer, C.B.; Liew, D.; Ofori-Asenso, R. Smell and Taste Dysfunction in Patients With COVID-19: A Systematic Review and Meta-analysis. *Mayo Clin. Proc.* **2020**, *95*, 1621–1631. [CrossRef] [PubMed]
15. Rocke, J.; Hopkins, C.; Philpott, C.; Kumar, N. Is loss of sense of smell a diagnostic marker in COVID-19: A systematic review and meta-analysis. *Clin. Otolaryngol.* **2020**, *45*, 914–922. [CrossRef] [PubMed]
16. Bhattacharjee, A.S.; Joshi, S.V.; Naik, S.; Sangle, S.; Abraham, N.M. Quantitative assessment of olfactory dysfunction accurately detects asymptomatic COVID-19 carriers. *eClinicalMedicine* **2020**, *28*. [CrossRef] [PubMed]
17. Landis, B.N.; Stow, N.W.; Lacroix, J.S.; Hugentobler, M.; Hummel, T. Olfactory disorders: The patients' view. *Rhinology* **2009**, *47*, 454–459. [CrossRef]
18. Yang, Z.; Ma, Y.; Bi, W.; Tang, J. Exploring the research landscape of COVID-19-induced olfactory dysfunction: A bibliometric study. *Front. Neurosci.* **2023**, *17*, 1164901. [CrossRef] [PubMed]
19. Lin, L.; Cheng, L. Current and Emerging Treatment Options in Sinus and Nasal Diseases: A Promising Future in the Appropriate Therapies. *J. Clin. Med.* **2022**, *11*, 7398. [CrossRef]
20. Pieniak, M.; Oleszkiewicz, A.; Avaro, V.; Calegari, F.; Hummel, T. Olfactory training—Thirteen years of research reviewed. *Neurosci. Biobehav. Rev.* **2022**, *141*, 104853. [CrossRef]
21. Miwa, T.; Ikeda, K.; Ishibashi, T.; Kobayashi, M.; Kondo, K.; Matsuwaki, Y.; Ogawa, T.; Shiga, H.; Suzuki, M.; Tsuzuki, K.; et al. Clinical practice guidelines for the management of olfactory dysfunction—Secondary publication. *Auris Nasus Larynx* **2019**, *46*, 653–662. [CrossRef] [PubMed]
22. Tabrizi, A.G.; Asadi, M.; Mohammadi, M.; Yekta, A.A.; Sohrabi, M. Efficacy of Platelet-Rich Plasma as an Adjuvant Therapy to Endoscopic Sinus Surgery in Anosmia Patients with Sinonasal Polyposis: A Randomized Controlled Clinical Trial. *Med. J. Islam. Repub. Iran* **2021**, *35*, 156. [CrossRef]
23. Ikumi, A.; Hara, Y.; Yoshioka, T.; Kanamori, A.; Yamazaki, M. Effect of local administration of platelet-rich plasma (PRP) on peripheral nerve regeneration: An experimental study in the rabbit model. *Microsurgery* **2018**, *38*, 300–309. [CrossRef]

24. Sundman, E.A.; Cole, B.J.; Fortier, L.A. Growth factor and catabolic cytokine concentrations are influenced by the cellular composition of platelet-rich plasma. *Am. J. Sports Med.* **2011**, *39*, 2135–2140. [CrossRef] [PubMed]
25. Chellini, F.; Tani, A.; Vallone, L.; Nosi, D.; Pavan, P.; Bambi, F.; Orlandini, S.Z.; Sassoli, C. Platelet-Rich Plasma Prevents In Vitro Transforming Growth Factor-β1-Induced Fibroblast to Myofibroblast Transition: Involvement of Vascular Endothelial Growth Factor (VEGF)-A/VEGF Receptor-1-Mediated Signaling. *Cells* **2018**, *7*, 142. [CrossRef]
26. Mohebbi, A.; Hosseinzadeh, F.; Mohebbi, S.; Dehghani, A. Determining the effect of platelet-rich plasma (PRP) on improving endoscopic sinus surgery: A randomized clinical trial study (RCT). *Med. J. Islam. Repub. Iran* **2019**, *33*, 150. [CrossRef] [PubMed]
27. Nourizadeh, N.; Sharifi, N.S.; Bakhshaee, M.; Ghiasi, S.S.; Rasoulian, B.; Alamdari, D.H. PRP-Fibrin Glue for Pain Reduction and Rapid Healing in Tonsillectomy. *Iran. J. Otorhinolaryngol.* **2022**, *34*, 289. [CrossRef] [PubMed]
28. Albazee, E.; Diab, S.; Awad, A.K.; Aboeldahab, H.; Abdella, W.S.; Abu-Zaid, A. The analgesic and anti-haemorrhagic efficacy of platelet-rich plasma in tonsillectomy: A systematic review and meta-analysis of randomised controlled trials. *Clin. Otolaryngol.* **2023**, *48*, 1–9. [CrossRef]
29. Al-Gerrah, D.A. Use of PRP in Rhinoplasty. *Otolaryngol. Open Access* **2016**, *6*, 1–2. [CrossRef]
30. Yigit, E.; Kirgezen, T.; Ozdemir, O.; Ture, M.; Cagliyan, A.; Yigit, O. The Effect of Platelet-Rich Fibrin on Postoperative Morbidity after Rhinoplasty: A Comparative Analysis with Respect to Edema, Ecchymosis and Pain. *Med. Bull. Haseki/Haseki Tip Bul.* **2022**, *60*, 240–247. [CrossRef]
31. Suresh, A.; Balouch, B.; Martha, V.V.; Sataloff, R.T. Laryngeal Applications of Platelet Rich Plasma and Platelet Poor Plasma: A Systematic Review. *J. Voice* **2024**, *38*, 248.e1–248.e13. [CrossRef] [PubMed]
32. Yasak, A.G.; Yigit, O.; Araz Server, E.; Durna Dastan, S.; Gul, M. The effectiveness of platelet-rich plasma in an anosmia-induced mice model. *Laryngoscope* **2018**, *128*, E157–E162. [CrossRef] [PubMed]
33. Nota, J.; Takahashi, H.; Hakuba, N.; Hato, N.; Gyo, K. Treatment of neural anosmia by topical application of basic fibroblast growth factor-gelatin hydrogel in the nasal cavity: An experimental study in mice. *JAMA Otolaryngol. Head Neck Surg.* **2013**, *139*, 396–400. [CrossRef] [PubMed]
34. Qureshi, M.F.H.; Akhtar, S.; Ghaloo, S.K.; Wasif, M.; Pasha, H.A.; Dhanani, R. Implication of stem cells and platelet rich plasma in otolaryngology, head and neck surgical procedures. *J. Pak. Med. Assoc.* **2023**, *73*, S56–S61. [CrossRef] [PubMed]
35. Schroeder, J.W.; Rastatter, J.C.; Walner, D.L. Effect of vascular endothelial growth factor on laryngeal wound healing in rabbits. *Otolaryngol. Head Neck Surg.* **2007**, *137*, 465–470. [CrossRef]
36. Huang, J.; Shi, Y.; Wu, L.; Lv, C.; Hu, Y.; Shen, Y. Comparative efficacy of platelet-rich plasma applied in myringoplasty: A systematic review and meta-analysis. *PLoS ONE* **2021**, *16*, e0245968. [CrossRef] [PubMed]
37. Sharma, P.; Parida, P.K.; Preetam, C.; Mukherjee, S.; Nayak, A.; Pradhan, P. Outcome of Temporalis Fascia Myringoplasty with and Without use of Platelet Rich Plasma: A Randomized Control Trial. *Indian J. Otolaryngol. Head Neck Surg.* **2022**, *74*, 3832–3840. [CrossRef] [PubMed]
38. Singh Tyagi, B. Treatment of Sensorineural Hearing Loss in Children: Platelet Rich Plasma. *Acta Sci. Otolaryngol.* **2021**, *3*, 7–11. [CrossRef]
39. Khafagy, Y.W.; Abd Elfattah, A.M.; Moneir, W.; Salem, E.H. Leukocyte- and platelet-rich fibrin: A new graft material in endoscopic repair of spontaneous CSF leaks. *Eur. Arch. Otorhinolaryngol.* **2018**, *275*, 2245–2252. [CrossRef]
40. Skarżyńska, M.B.; Kołodziejak, A.; Gos, E.; Sanfis, M.D.; Skarżyński, P.H. Effectiveness of Various Treatments for Sudden Sensorineural Hearing Loss-A Retrospective Study. *Life* **2022**, *12*, 96. [CrossRef]
41. Moffa, A.; Nardelli, D.; Giorgi, L.; Di Giovanni, S.; Carnuccio, L.; Mangino, C.; Baptista, P.; Vacca, M.; Casale, M. Platelet-Rich Plasma for Patients with Olfactory Dysfunction: Myth or Reality? A Systematic Review. *J. Clin. Med.* **2024**, *13*, 782. [CrossRef] [PubMed]
42. Kikuta, S.; Han, B.; Yamasoba, T. Heterogeneous Damage to the Olfactory Epithelium in Patients with Post-Viral Olfactory Dysfunction. *J. Clin. Med.* **2023**, *12*, 5007. [CrossRef] [PubMed]
43. Hu, C.; Gao, Y.; Feng, Y.; Sun, Z.; Yu, Z. Assessment of Factors Influencing the Olfactory Bulb Volume in Patients with Post-Viral Olfactory Dysfunction. *Eur. Arch. Otorhinolaryngol.* **2023**, *280*, 3737–3743. [CrossRef] [PubMed]
44. Wellford, S.A.; Moseman, E.A. Olfactory Immune Response to SARS-CoV-2. *Cell Mol. Immunol.* **2024**, *21*, 134–143. [CrossRef] [PubMed]
45. Park, J.W.; Wang, X.; Xu, R.H. Revealing the Mystery of Persistent Smell Loss in Long COVID Patients. *Int. J. Biol. Sci.* **2022**, *18*, 4795–4808. [CrossRef] [PubMed]
46. Sauve, F.; Nampoothiri, S.; Clarke, S.A.; Fernandois, D.; Ferreira Coêlho, C.F.; Dewisme, J.; Mills, E.G.; Ternier, G.; Cotellessa, L.; Iglesias-Garcia, C.; et al. Long-COVID Cognitive Impairments and Reproductive Hormone Deficits in Men May Stem from GnRH Neuronal Death. *eBioMedicine* **2023**, *96*, 104784. [CrossRef] [PubMed]
47. Saleki, K.; Banazadeh, M.; Saghazadeh, A.; Rezaei, N. The Involvement of the Central Nervous System in Patients with COVID-19. *Rev. Neurosci.* **2020**, *31*, 453–456. [CrossRef] [PubMed]
48. Ho, C.Y.; Salimian, M.; Hegert, J.; O'Brien, J.; Choi, S.G.; Ames, H.; Morris, M.; Papadimitriou, J.C.; Mininni, J.; Niehaus, P.; et al. Postmortem Assessment of Olfactory Tissue Degeneration and Microvasculopathy in Patients with COVID-19. *JAMA Neurol.* **2022**, *79*, 544–553. [CrossRef]
49. Østergaard, L. SARS CoV-2 Related Microvascular Damage and Symptoms during and after COVID-19: Consequences of Capillary Transit-Time Changes, Tissue Hypoxia and Inflammation. *Physiol. Rep.* **2021**, *9*, e14726. [CrossRef]

50. Baldwin, W.M., 3rd; Kuo, H.H.; Morrell, C.N. Platelets: Versatile Modifiers of Innate and Adaptive Immune Responses to Transplants. *Curr. Opin. Organ Transplant.* **2011**, *16*, 41–46. [CrossRef]
51. Ushiro-Lumb, I.; Thorburn, D. Risk of Transmission of Infections to Others after Donor-Derived Infection Transmissions. *Transpl. Infect. Dis.* **2022**, *24*, e13791. [CrossRef] [PubMed]
52. Ince, B.; Yıldırım, M.E.C.; Kilinc, I.; Oltulu, P.; Dadaci, M. Investigation of the Development of Hypersensitivity and Hyperalgesia After Repeated Application of Platelet-Rich Plasma in Rats: An Experimental Study. *Aesthet Surg. J.* **2019**, *39*, 1139–1145. [CrossRef] [PubMed]
53. Perez, A.G.M.; Lana, J.F.S.D.; Rodrigues, A.A.; Luzo, A.C.M.; Belangero, W.D.; Santana, M.H.A. Relevant aspects of centrifugation step in the preparation of platelet-rich plasma. *ISRN Hematol.* **2014**, *2014*, 176060. [CrossRef] [PubMed]
54. Lechien, J.R.; Saussez, S. Injection of Platelet Rich Plasma in the Olfactory Cleft for COVID-19 Patients with Persistent Olfactory Dysfunction: Description of the Technique. *Ear Nose Throat J.* **2022**. [CrossRef] [PubMed]
55. Yan, C.H.; Jang, S.S.; Lin, H.C.; Ma, Y.; Khanwalkar, A.R.; Thai, A.; Patel, Z.M. Use of platelet-rich plasma for COVID-19-related olfactory loss: A randomized controlled trial. *Int. Forum Allergy Rhinol.* **2023**, *13*, 989–997. [CrossRef] [PubMed]
56. Steffens, Y.; Le Bon, S.-D.; Lechien, J.; Prunier, L.; Rodriguez, A.; Saussez, S.; Horoi, M. Effectiveness and safety of PRP on persistent olfactory dysfunction related to COVID-19. *Eur. Arch. Otorhinolaryngol.* **2022**, *279*, 5951–5953. [CrossRef] [PubMed]
57. Abo El Naga, H.A.; El Zaiat, R.S.; Hamdan, A.M. The potential therapeutic effect of platelet-rich plasma in the treatment of post-COVID-19 parosmia. *Egypt. J. Otolaryngol.* **2022**, *38*, 130. [CrossRef]
58. Lechien, J.R.; Le Bon, S.D.; Saussez, S. Platelet-rich plasma injection in the olfactory clefts of COVID-19 patients with long-term olfactory dysfunction. *Eur. Arch. Otorhinolaryngol.* **2023**, *280*, 2351–2358. [CrossRef]
59. Evman, M.D.; Cetin, Z.E. Effectiveness of platelet-rich plasma on post-COVID chronic olfactory dysfunction. *Rev. Assoc. Médica Bras.* **2023**, *69*, e20230666. [CrossRef]
60. Lechien, J.R.; Saussez, S.; Vaira, L.A.; De Riu, G.; Boscolo-Rizzo, P.; Tirelli, G.; Michel, J.; Radulesco, T. Effectiveness of Platelet-Rich Plasma for COVID-19-Related Olfactory Dysfunction: A Controlled Study. *Otolaryngol. Head Neck Surg.* **2024**, *170*, 84–91. [CrossRef]
61. Riccardi, G.; Niccolini, G.F.; Bellizzi, M.G.; Fiore, M.; Minni, A.; Barbato, C. Post-COVID-19 Anosmia and Therapies: Stay Tuned for New Drugs to Sniff Out. *Diseases* **2023**, *11*, 79. [CrossRef] [PubMed]
62. Alrajhi, B.; Alrodiman, O.A.; Alhuzali, A.F.; Alrashed, H.; Alrodiman, Y.A.; Alim, B. Platelet-rich plasma for the treatment of COVID-19 related olfactory dysfunction: A systematic review. *Rhinology* **2023**, *61*, 498–507. [CrossRef]
63. Ohla, K.; Veldhuizen, M.; Green, T.; Hannum, M.; Bakke, A.; Moein, S.; Tognetti, A.; Postma, E.; Pellegrino, R.; Hwang, D.; et al. A follow-up on quantitative and qualitative olfactory dysfunction and other symptoms in patients recovering from COVID-19 smell loss. *Rhinology* **2022**, *60*, 207–217. [CrossRef]
64. Al Aaraj, M.; Boorinie, M.; Salfity, L.; Eweiss, A. The use of Platelet rich Plasma in COVID-19 Induced Olfactory Dysfunction: Systematic Review. *Indian J. Otolaryngol. Head Neck Surg.* **2023**, *75*, 3093–3097. [CrossRef] [PubMed]
65. Yan, C.H.; Mundy, D.C.; Patel, Z.M. The use of platelet-rich plasma in treatment of olfactory dysfunction: A pilot study. *Laryngoscope Investig. Otolaryngol.* **2020**, *5*, 187–193. [CrossRef] [PubMed]
66. Hu, Z.-B.; Chen, H.-C.; Wei, B.; Zhang, Z.-M.; Wu, S.-K.; Sun, J.-C.; Xiang, M. Platelet rich plasma enhanced neuro-regeneration of human dental pulp stem cells in vitro and in rat spinal cord. *Ann. Transl. Med.* **2022**, *10*, 584. [CrossRef] [PubMed]
67. Parrie, L.E.; Crowell, J.A.E.; Telling, G.C.; Bessen, R.A. The cellular prion protein promotes olfactory sensory neuron survival and axon targeting during adult neurogenesis. *Dev. Biol.* **2018**, *438*, 23–32. [CrossRef]
68. Tey, R.V.; Haldankar, P.; Joshi, V.R.; Raj, R.; Maradi, R. Variability in Platelet-Rich Plasma Preparations Used in Regenerative Medicine: A Comparative Analysis. *Stem Cells Int.* **2022**, *2022*, 3852898. [CrossRef]
69. Webster, K.E.; O'Byrne, L.; MacKeith, S.; Philpott, C.; Hopkins, C.; Burton, M.J. Interventions for the prevention of persistent post-COVID-19 olfactory dysfunction. *Cochrane Database Syst. Rev.* **2022**, *2022*, CD013877. [CrossRef]
70. Mavrogeni, P.; Kanakopoulos, A.; Maihoub, S.; Maihoub, S.; Krasznai, M.; Szirmai, A. Anosmia treatment by platelet rich plasma injection. *Int. Tinnitus J.* **2017**, *20*, 102–105. [CrossRef]
71. Shawky, M.A.; Hadeya, A.M. Platelet-rich Plasma in Management of Anosmia (Single Versus Double Injections). *Indian J. Otolaryngol. Head Neck Surg.* **2023**, *75*, 1004–1008. [CrossRef] [PubMed]
72. O'Byrne, L.; Webster, K.E.; MacKeith, S.; Philpott, C.; Hopkins, C.; Burton, M.J. Interventions for the treatment of persistent post-COVID-19 olfactory dysfunction. *Cochrane Database Syst. Rev.* **2022**, *2022*, CD013876. [CrossRef]

Disclaimer/Publisher's Note: The statements, opinions and data contained in all publications are solely those of the individual author(s) and contributor(s) and not of MDPI and/or the editor(s). MDPI and/or the editor(s) disclaim responsibility for any injury to people or property resulting from any ideas, methods, instructions or products referred to in the content.

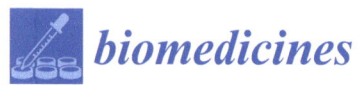 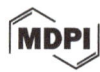

Article

Kidney Function Tests and Continuous eGFR Decrease at Six Months after SARS-CoV-2 Infection in Patients Clinically Diagnosed with Post-COVID Syndrome

Madalina Boruga [1], Susa Septimiu-Radu [2,*], Prashant Sunil Nandarge [3], Ahmed Elagez [4], Gabriela Doros [5], Voichita Elena Lazureanu [6], Emil Robert Stoicescu [2,7], Elena Tanase [2], Roxana Iacob [2,8], Andreea Dumitrescu [9], Adrian Vasile Bota [10], Coralia Cotoraci [10,11] and Melania Lavinia Bratu [2,12,13]

1. Department of Toxicology, Drug Industry, Management and Legislation, Faculty of Pharmacology, "Victor Babes" University of Medicine and Pharmacy Timisoara, 300041 Timisoara, Romania; madalina.boruga@umft.ro
2. Doctoral School, "Victor Babes" University of Medicine and Pharmacy Timisoara, 300041 Timisoara, Romania; stoicescu.emil@umft.ro (E.R.S.); tanase.elena@umft.ro (E.T.); roxana.iacob@umft.ro (R.I.); bratu.lavinia@umft.ro (M.L.B.)
3. Department of General Medicine, D.Y. Patil Medical College Kolhapur, Kolhapur 416005, India; prashantnandarge1997@gmail.com
4. Department of General Medicine, Misr University for Science & Technology, Giza 3236101, Egypt; ahmeddmahmouudd@gmail.com
5. Third Discipline of Pediatrics, "Victor Babes" University of Medicine and Pharmacy Timisoara, 300041 Timisoara, Romania; gdoros@gmail.com
6. Department XIII, Discipline of Infectious Diseases, "Victor Babes" University of Medicine and Pharmacy Timisoara, 300041 Timisoara, Romania; lazureanu.voichita@umft.ro
7. Department of Radiology and Medical Imaging, "Victor Babes" University of Medicine and Pharmacy Timisoara, 300041 Timisoara, Romania
8. Department of Anatomy and Embryology, "Victor Babes" University of Medicine and Pharmacy Timisoara, 300041 Timisoara, Romania
9. Cardioprevent Foundation, 300134 Timisoara, Romania; andreea.dumitrescu@cardioprevent.org
10. Multidisciplinary Doctoral School, "Vasile Goldis" Western University, 310025 Arad, Romania; bota.adrian1@yahoo.com (A.V.B.); rector_vg@uvvg.ro (C.C.)
11. Department of Hematology, Faculty of Medicine, "Vasile Goldis" Western University, 310025 Arad, Romania
12. Center for Neuropsychology and Behavioral Medicine, Discipline of Psychology, Faculty of General Medicine, "Victor Babes" University of Medicine and Pharmacy Timisoara, 300041 Timisoara, Romania
13. Center for Cognitive Research in Neuropsychiatric Pathology, Department of Neurosciences, "Victor Babes" University of Medicine and Pharmacy Timisoara, 300041 Timisoara, Romania
* Correspondence: septimiu.susa@umft.ro

Citation: Boruga, M.; Septimiu-Radu, S.; Nandarge, P.S.; Elagez, A.; Doros, G.; Lazureanu, V.E.; Stoicescu, E.R.; Tanase, E.; Iacob, R.; Dumitrescu, A.; et al. Kidney Function Tests and Continuous eGFR Decrease at Six Months after SARS-CoV-2 Infection in Patients Clinically Diagnosed with Post-COVID Syndrome. *Biomedicines* 2024, 12, 950. https://doi.org/10.3390/biomedicines12050950

Academic Editor: César Fernández De Las Peñas

Received: 6 April 2024
Revised: 18 April 2024
Accepted: 23 April 2024
Published: 24 April 2024

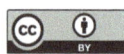

Copyright: © 2024 by the authors. Licensee MDPI, Basel, Switzerland. This article is an open access article distributed under the terms and conditions of the Creative Commons Attribution (CC BY) license (https://creativecommons.org/licenses/by/4.0/).

Abstract: The long-term sequelae of SARS-CoV-2 infection are still under research, since extensive studies showed plenty of systemic effects of the viral infection, extending even after the acute phase of the infection. This study evaluated kidney function tests six months after SARS-CoV-2 infection in patients clinically diagnosed with Post-COVID Syndrome, hypothesizing persistent renal dysfunction evidenced by altered kidney function tests compared to baseline levels. Continuous eGFR decrease <30 at six months post-infection was considered the main study outcome. Conducted at the "Victor Babes" Hospital, this retrospective observational study involved adults with laboratory-confirmed SARS-CoV-2 infection and clinically-diagnosed Post-COVID Syndrome, excluding those with prior chronic kidney disease or significant renal impairment. Kidney function tests, including serum creatinine, blood urea nitrogen (BUN), estimated glomerular filtration rate (eGFR), alongside markers of kidney damage such as proteinuria and hematuria, were analyzed. Among 206 participants, significant differences were observed between the control ($n = 114$) and the Post-COVID group ($n = 92$). The Post-COVID group exhibited higher serum creatinine (109.7 µmol/L vs. 84.5 µmol/L, $p < 0.001$), lower eGFR (65.3 mL/min/1.73 m^2 vs. 91.2 mL/min/1.73 m^2, $p < 0.001$), and elevated BUN levels (23.7 mg/dL vs. 15.2 mg/dL, $p < 0.001$) compared to the control group. Regression analysis highlighted significant predictors of continuous eGFR decrease <30 at six months post-infection. The development of acute kidney injury (AKI) during the initial COVID-19 illness emerged as a strong predictor of reduced eGFR (β = 3.47, $p < 0.001$). Additional factors, including a creatinine increase (23 μmol/L above the normal range) and an elevated Albumin to Creatinine Ratio (ACR) (>11 mg/g above the normal range), were significantly associated with eGFR reduction. Patients with Post-COVID Syndrome demonstrate significant renal impairment six months post-SARS-CoV-2 infection. The study's findings stress the need for ongoing monitoring and intervention strategies for renal health in affected individuals, underscoring the persistent impact of COVID-19 on renal function.

Keywords: COVID-19; SARS-CoV-2; long COVID; Infectious Disease

1. Introduction

As the acute phase of the respiratory syndrome coronavirus 2 (SARS-CoV-2) infection has been extensively studied, attention has increasingly turned to the long-term sequelae of this virus, colloquially known as Post-COVID Syndrome or "Long COVID" [1,2]. This condition encompasses a wide range of persistent symptoms and clinical findings that continue for months beyond the initial infection, affecting multiple organ systems [3]. Among these, renal complications have emerged as a significant concern, given preliminary evidence suggesting that SARS-CoV-2 infection may precipitate or exacerbate kidney dysfunction [4].

Previous viral epidemics, such as those caused by the original SARS-CoV and the Middle East respiratory syndrome coronavirus (MERS-CoV), have been associated with acute kidney injury (AKI) [5–7]. Early data from the current pandemic have similarly highlighted kidney injury as a complication of acute COVID-19, especially in severe cases [8,9]. However, the persistence of renal dysfunction in the aftermath of SARS-CoV-2 infection, particularly in individuals with Post-COVID Syndrome, remains poorly characterized.

The concept of Post-COVID Syndrome encompasses a broad spectrum of symptoms and clinical outcomes, indicating a systemic impact that may involve direct viral injury, immune-mediated damage, or a combination of both [10,11]. While respiratory and cardiovascular sequelae have been the focus of much research, the potential for sustained kidney damage raises concerns about long-term renal health and the risk of chronic kidney disease (CKD) in these patients. Studies have reported that common COVID-19 symptoms such as common cold signs, cough, fever, sore throat, headache, anosmia, and dyspnea were more common in COVID-19 patients without renal disease [12–14]. However, understanding the trajectory of kidney function recovery or decline in the months following SARS-CoV-2 infection is critical for identifying individuals at risk and implementing timely interventions.

Kidney function tests, including serum creatinine, blood urea nitrogen (BUN), and estimated glomerular filtration rate (eGFR), are essential tools for assessing renal health. These biomarkers, alongside urinalysis for proteinuria and hematuria, offer insights into kidney damage and function [15–18]. Despite their importance, there is a paucity of data on the evolution of these parameters in the context of Post-COVID Syndrome, leaving a gap in knowledge that underscores the need for focused studies examining renal outcomes among survivors of SARS-CoV-2 infection.

Therefore, this study aims to evaluate kidney function tests measured at six months after SARS-CoV-2 infection in patients clinically diagnosed with Post-COVID Syndrome. We hypothesize that individuals with Post-COVID Syndrome exhibit persistent renal dysfunction, as evidenced by alterations in kidney function tests, compared to baseline levels. This research seeks to elucidate the extent of renal impairment in this patient population, contributing to a broader understanding of Post-COVID Syndrome's long-term impacts and informing strategies for renal health monitoring and intervention in affected individuals.

2. Materials and Methods

2.1. Study Design and Ethics

This investigation was designed as a retrospective observational study aimed at evaluating kidney function tests in patients clinically diagnosed with Post-COVID Syndrome at approximately six months following SARS-CoV-2 infection. The database search and paper records search extended from January 2023 to December 2023, aligning with the phase where long-term effects of COVID-19 became increasingly recognized across the global medical community. Recruitment and data collection were centered around the "Victor Babes" Hospital affiliated with the "Victor Babes" University of Medicine and Pharmacy from Timisoara, Romania, integrating multidisciplinary expertise to address the complex needs of this patient population. The study received the approval number 2632 from 23 March 2022.

2.2. Patients' Inclusion and Exclusion Criteria

Patients eligible for inclusion in this study were individuals aged 18 years or older who had a laboratory-confirmed SARS-CoV-2 infection, verified either by RT-PCR or rapid antigen tests. Additionally, these individuals must have been diagnosed with Post-COVID Syndrome, characterized by a constellation of symptoms persisting for more than 12 weeks after the acute infection, according to guidelines [19]. These symptoms include, but are not limited to, chronic fatigue, shortness of breath, cognitive disturbances ("brain fog"), joint pain, and ongoing loss of taste or smell, without any alternative diagnosis that could explain these symptoms [20].

Exclusion criteria were established to ensure the safety of participants and the integrity of the study data. Patients were excluded if they had a history of chronic kidney disease or significant renal impairment prior to SARS-CoV-2 infection, as indicated by medical records or baseline kidney function tests showing an eGFR below 60 mL/min/1.73 m^2. Additional exclusion factors included acute renal failure or dialysis within the six months preceding the study, significant cardiovascular disease (e.g., recent myocardial infarction, unstable angina, uncontrolled arrhythmias), severe psychiatric conditions impacting consent or participation ability, and current pregnancy or breastfeeding.

Patients receiving immunosuppressive therapy at the time of SARS-CoV-2 infection or those with a known history of autoimmune diseases affecting kidney function were also excluded. This was to minimize confounding variables that could influence renal function independently of Post-COVID Syndrome. Consent was a prerequisite; thus, individuals who did not agree to participate in the study or who were unable to provide informed consent due to cognitive impairments were excluded.

The study aimed to create a well-defined cohort that accurately represents the spectrum of Post-COVID Syndrome while ensuring that the focus remained on the effects of the condition on kidney function, free from interference by pre-existing renal conditions or other comorbidities that could confound the results. Thus, a control group of patients with COVID-19 who did not develop Post-COVID Syndrome was also included as comparison with the study group, in order to serve as a reference for baseline characteristics of COVID-19 patients.

2.3. Study Variables

The study variables were categorized as follows: (1) Demographic and clinical variables: age, gender, and body mass index (BMI). Additionally, data on the severity of initial SARS-CoV-2 infection, comorbidities, and vaccination status were collected to evaluate their potential impact on Post-COVID Syndrome and kidney function. (2) Laboratory data: key to this study were renal function tests, including serum creatinine, blood urea nitrogen (BUN), and estimated glomerular filtration rate (eGFR), alongside markers of kidney damage such as proteinuria and hematuria assessed through urinalysis. Complementary to these were general health indicators like complete blood count (CBC), electrolytes, C-reactive protein (CRP) for inflammation, and other relevant markers such as ferritin and interleukin-6 (IL-6) to evaluate systemic involvement and inflammation. (4) Symptomatology and Post-COVID Syndrome assessment: a structured assessment of Post-COVID Syndrome symptoms, focusing on duration, severity, and the impact on daily living, was performed. This included documentation of specific symptoms relevant to renal function, such as edema and changes in urination patterns, alongside a comprehensive review of systemic symptoms such as fatigue, cognitive dysfunction, and myalgia. (5) Healthcare utilization and intervention data: information on any interventions, medications related to kidney function or Post-COVID symptoms, and any renal-specific consultations or treatments received during the study period were recorded. This also included data on follow-up visits, hospital readmissions, and any outpatient care specific to renal health or Post-COVID management.

The current study utilized the Chronic Kidney Disease Epidemiology Collaboration (CKD-EPI) Creatinine Equation (2021) for eGFR calculation [21]. This method exclusively uses serum creatinine as the biomarker, adjusted for age, sex, and race, and is widely recognized for its accuracy across varying levels of kidney function.

In our study, COVID-19 severity was characterized according to guidelines [22], based on clinical and laboratory criteria as follows: (1) Mild COVID-19, with the presence of symptoms like fever, cough, sore throat, malaise, headache, muscle pain without shortness of breath, dyspnea, or abnormal chest imaging; (2) Moderate COVID-19 with the evidence of lower respiratory disease during clinical assessment or imaging and a saturation of oxygen (SpO_2) $\geq$94% on room air at sea level; (3) Severe COVID-19, showing a respiratory frequency >30 breaths per minute, blood oxygen saturation $\leq$93% on room air at sea level, ratio of arterial partial pressure of oxygen to fraction of inspired oxygen (PaO_2/FiO_2) <300, or lung infiltrates >50% within 24 to 48 h.

2.4. Statistical Analysis

The statistical processing of data in this study was conducted using the SPSS software, version 26.0. The patient groups were matched by age, gender, and COVID-19 severity. To describe the demographics and clinical characteristics of the participants, descriptive statistics were utilized. This involved summarizing continuous variables by their mean values and standard deviations and representing categorical variables through their counts and percentages. For evaluating differences in categorical data, the Chi-square test and Fisher's exact test were applied as appropriate. Analysis of differences in continuous variables that did not adhere to a normal distribution was carried out using the Mann-Whitney U test. In cases where continuous variables were normally distributed, comparisons were made using the Student's *t*-test for independent samples, reporting mean values and standard deviations. For non-normally distributed data, comparisons of median values and interquartile ranges (IQR) were made with the Mann-Whitney U test. All statistical tests were two-tailed, with a significance level set at a *p*-value of less than 0.05, indicating statistical significance.

3. Results
3.1. Patients' Background

In the current study a detailed demographic analysis was conducted to assess various health and lifestyle variables between the control group (*n* = 114) and the post-COVID group (*n* = 92). The average age of participants in the control group was 55.2 years ($\pm$8.5), while the post-COVID group had an average age of 56.9 years ($\pm$7.6), with the difference not being statistically significant (*p* = 0.136). Gender distribution was also compared, showing a slight difference in proportions with men constituting 51.8% of the control group and 54.3% of the post-COVID group, but this difference was not statistically significant (*p* = 0.710).

There were no significant changes in Body Mass Index (BMI) between the two study groups (*p* = 0.900). The analysis of COVID-19 vaccination status revealed a higher percentage of individuals in the post-COVID group (41.3%) receiving $\geq$2 doses compared to the control group (32.5%), though the difference was not statistically significant (*p* = 0.317).

Antiviral medication requirement showed a higher percentage in the post COVID group (71.7%) compared to the control group (59.6%); [not significant ($p = 0.096$)].

No significant differences were observed in the severity of COVID-19 between the groups ($p = 0.909$) or in personal history variables such as smoking and Charlson Comorbidity Index (CCI) greater than 2 ($p = 0.851$ and $p = 0.904$, respectively). However, notable differences were observed in kidney injury outcomes. The post-COVID group had a significantly higher incidence of acute kidney injury (AKI) during admission (17.4%) compared to the control group (6.1%, $p = 0.014$). Nevertheless, none of the 23 patients who developed AKI required renal replacement therapy during admission. Furthermore, a significant proportion of the post-COVID group experienced a decrease in eGFR below 30 from baseline (27.2%) compared to the control group (9.6%, $p = 0.001$). Additionally, continuous eGFR decrease below 30 at six months was observed exclusively in the post-COVID group (23.9%), as presented in Table 1.

Table 1. Demographic analysis.

Variables	Control Group (n = 114)	Post-COVID Group (n = 92)	p-Value
Age (mean ± SD)	55.2 ± 8.5	56.9 ± 7.6	0.136
Sex			0.710
Men (n,%)	59 (51.8%)	50 (54.3%)	
Women (n,%)	55 (48.2%)	42 (45.7%)	
BMI (n,%)			0.900
Normal weight (18.5–24.9 kg/m^2)	36 (31.6%)	30 (32.6%)	
Overweight (>24.9 kg/m^2)	45 (39.5%)	38 (41.3%)	
Obese (>29.9 kg/m^2)	33 (28.9%)	24 (26.1%)	
COVID-19 vaccination status (n,%)			0.317
1 dose	13 (11.4%)	12 (13.0%)	
≥2 doses	37 (32.5%)	38 (41.3%)	
Unvaccinated	64 (56.1%)	42 (45.7%)	
Antiviral medication requirement (n,%)			0.096
Yes	68 (59.6%)	66 (71.7%)	
No	46 (40.4%)	26 (28.3%)	
Oxygen supplementation (n,%)			0.620
Yes	82 (71.9%)	69 (75.0%)	
No	32 (28.1%)	23 (25.0%)	
COVID-19 severity (n,%)			0.909
Mild	38 (33.3%)	29 (31.5%)	
Moderate	42 (36.8%)	33 (35.9%)	
Severe	34 (29.9%)	30 (32.6%)	
Personal history (n,%)			
Smoking	26 (22.8%)	22 (23.9%)	0.851
CCI > 2	24 (21.1%)	20 (21.7%)	0.904
Kidney injury			
Developed AKI during admission	7 (6.1%)	16 (17.4%)	0.014
eGFR decrease <30 from baseline	11 (9.6%)	25 (27.2%)	0.001
Continuous eGFR decrease <30 at six months	–	22 (23.9%)	–

Data reported as n (%) and calculated using the Chi-square test and Fisher's exact unless specified differently; BMI—Body Mass Index; SD—Standard Deviation; CCI—Charlson Comorbidity Index.

3.2. Laboratory Data

The white blood cell count, a marker of infection and inflammation, was significantly higher in the Post-COVID group (16.6 ± 3.4 1000/mm^3) compared to the control group

(11.8 ± 1.7 1000/mm^3), with a p-value of <0.001, indicating a substantial increase beyond the normal range (4.5–11.0 1000/mm^3). Similarly, levels of C-reactive protein (CRP), an acute-phase reactant indicative of inflammation, were markedly elevated in the Post-COVID group (78.2 ± 24.6 mg/dL) compared to the control group (23.1 ± 2.8 mg/dL), with the difference being statistically significant ($p < 0.001$). Lymphocyte counts, which are critical for the immune response, were significantly lower in the Post-COVID group (1.3 ± 0.6 1000/mm^3) than in the control group (2.7 ± 0.8 1000/mm^3), falling below the normal range (1.0–4.8 1000/mm^3), with a p-value of <0.001.

Significant elevations were also observed in liver enzymes, including aspartate aminotransferase (AST) and alanine aminotransferase (ALT), in the Post-COVID group (47.3 ± 11.8 U/L and 53.7 ± 14.3 U/L, respectively) compared to the control group (21.5 ± 5.2 U/L and 18.6 ± 7.2 U/L, respectively), both with p-values of <0.001. These increases surpass the normal ranges (10–40 U/L for AST and 7–35 U/L for ALT).

Further analysis revealed significant increases in IL-6 (44.6 ± 19.7 pg/mL), procalcitonin (0.48 ± 0.22 ug/L), D-dimers (498.5 ± 198.4 ng/mL), and ferritin (607.5 ± 295.7 ng/mL) levels in the Post-COVID group compared to the control group, all with p-values of <0.001. Hemoglobin levels, vital for oxygen transport, were lower in the Post-COVID group (13.4 ± 1.4 g/dL) compared to the control group (14.7 ± 1.3 g/dL), with the difference being statistically significant ($p < 0.001$) and indicating potential anemia in the Post-COVID group within the context of normal ranges (13.0–17.0 g/dL), as presented in Table 2.

Table 2. Comparative analysis of blood tests between the control group and the Post-COVID group at admission.

Variables	Normal Range	Control Group during Admission (n = 114)	Post-COVID Group During Admission (n = 92)	p-Value
WBC (1000/mm^3)	4.5–11.0	11.8 ± 1.7	16.6 ± 3.4	<0.001
Lymphocytes (1000/mm^3)	1.0–4.8	2.7 ± 0.8	1.3 ± 0.6	<0.001
Hemoglobin (g/dL)	13.0–17.0	14.7 ± 1.3	13.4 ± 1.4	<0.001
AST (U/L)	10–40	21.5 ± 5.2	47.3 ± 11.8	<0.001
ALT (U/L)	7–35	18.6 ± 7.2	53.7 ± 14.3	<0.001
CRP (mg/dL)	0–10	23.1 ± 2.8	78.2 ± 24.6	<0.001
IL-6 (pg/mL)	0.8–6.4	10.3 ± 4.0	44.6 ± 19.7	<0.001
Procalcitonin (ug/L)	0–0.25	0.09 ± 0.06	0.48 ± 0.22	<0.001
D-dimers (ng/mL)	<250	285.2 ± 48.6	498.5 ± 198.4	<0.001
Ferritin (ng/mL)	20–250	292.4 ± 90.8	607.5 ± 295.7	<0.001

WBC—White Blood Cells; AST—Aspartate aminotransferase; ALT—Alanine aminotransferase; CRP—C-reactive protein; IL—Interleukin.

Significant improvements were noted across several blood parameters when comparing values at admission with those six months post-admission. The white blood cell count, initially elevated (16.6 ± 3.4 1000/mm^3) beyond the normal range, decreased significantly to within normal limits (10.9 ± 2.3 1000/mm^3, $p < 0.001$). Similarly, lymphocyte counts showed a notable improvement from a reduced count (1.3 ± 0.6 1000/mm^3) at admission to a healthier level (2.4 ± 0.7 1000/mm^3, $p < 0.001$) within the normal range (1.0–4.8 1000/mm^3), suggesting recovery of immune function. Liver function tests, including aspartate aminotransferase (AST) and alanine aminotransferase (ALT), initially showed marked elevation (47.3 ± 11.8 U/L and 53.7 ± 14.3 U/L, respectively) indicating liver stress or injury. These levels significantly improved to 29.4 ± 7.5 U/L and 24.8 ± 9.1 U/L, respectively, both within the normal ranges (10–40 U/L for AST and 7–35 U/L for ALT), with p-values of <0.001.

Markers of inflammation and infection, such as C-reactive protein, interleukin-6, and procalcitonin, also demonstrated significant reductions. CRP levels decreased from 78.2 ± 24.6 mg/dL to 14.7 ± 9.3 mg/dL, IL-6 from 44.6 ± 19.7 pg/mL to 12.7 ± 4.6 pg/mL, indicating a substantial reduction in systemic inflammation. Additionally, D-dimers and ferritin levels, which were elevated at admission (498.5 ± 198.4 ng/mL and 607.5 ± 295.7 ng/mL, respectively) improved significantly to 295.3 ± 102.7 ng/mL and 248.3 ± 149.2 ng/mL, respectively, with *p*-values of <0.001, although D-dimers remained above the normal range (< 250 ng/mL), as described in Table 3.

Table 3. Intragroup comparison of blood tests between the Post-COVID group at admission and six months after discharge.

Variables	Normal Range	Post-COVID Group during Admission (*n* = 92)	Post-COVID Group Six Months Post-Admission (*n* = 92)	*p*-Value
WBC (1000/mm^3)	4.5–11.0	16.6 ± 3.4	10.9 ± 2.3	<0.001
Lymphocytes (1000/mm^3)	1.0–4.8	1.3 ± 0.6	2.4 ± 0.7	<0.001
Hemoglobin (g/dL)	13.0–17.0	13.4 ± 1.4	14.3 ± 1.2	<0.001
AST (U/L)	10–40	47.3 ± 11.8	29.4 ± 7.5	<0.001
ALT (U/L)	7–35	53.7 ± 14.3	24.8 ± 9.1	<0.001
CRP (mg/dL)	0–10	78.2 ± 24.6	14.7 ± 9.3	<0.001
IL-6 (pg/mL)	0.8–6.4	44.6 ± 19.7	12.7 ± 4.6	<0.001
Procalcitonin (ug/L)	0–0.25	0.48 ± 0.22	0.19 ± 0.08	<0.001
D-dimers (ng/mL)	<250	498.5 ± 198.4	295.3 ± 102.7	<0.001
Ferritin (ng/mL)	20–250	607.5 ± 295.7	248.3 ± 149.2	<0.001

WBC—White Blood Cells; AST—Aspartate aminotransferase; ALT—Alanine aminotransferase; CRP—C-reactive protein; IL—Interleukin.

Creatinine levels were significantly higher in the Post-COVID group (109.7 ± 16.4 µmol/L) compared to the control group (84.5 ± 11.7 µmol/L), with a *p*-value of <0.001, suggesting reduced kidney function in the former. This was further corroborated by the eGFR, which was substantially lower in the Post-COVID group (65.3 ± 12.8 mL/min/1.73 m^2) than in the control group (91.2 ± 7.3 mL/min/1.73 m^2), with a *p*-value of <0.001, indicating significant kidney impairment. BUN levels, another key marker of kidney function, were also significantly higher in the Post-COVID group (23.7 ± 7.2 mg/dL) compared to the control group (15.2 ± 3.6 mg/dL), with a *p*-value of <0.001.

Proteinuria was significantly more pronounced in the Post-COVID group (198.3 ± 91.2 mg/dL) versus the control group (105.1 ± 48.6 mg/dL), with a *p*-value of <0.001. Similarly, albuminuria and the ACR, were markedly higher in the Post-COVID group (52.4 ± 18.9 mg/g and 59.1 ± 23.6 mg/g, respectively) than in the control group (22.7 ± 8.2 mg/g and 24.8 ± 10.1 mg/g, respectively), both with *p*-values of <0.001. Hematuria was significantly more common in the Post-COVID group (3.8 ± 2.1 cells/HPF) compared to the control group (1.5 ± 1.2 cells/HPF), with a *p*-value of <0.001. Urine specific gravity, which measures the concentration of substances in the urine, was lower in the Post-COVID group (1.016 ± 0.008) compared to the control group (1.021 ± 0.004), with a *p*-value of <0.001. Sodium and potassium levels showed no significant differences (Table 4).

Significant improvements were observed in several kidney function parameters over the six-month period. Creatinine levels, which were initially elevated (109.7 ± 16.4 µmol/L) well above the normal range (60–110 µmol/L), indicating impaired kidney function, decreased significantly to 90.4 µmol/L ($p < 0.001$), approaching the upper limit of the normal range and suggesting partial recovery of renal function. The eGFR improved from 65.3 mL/min/1.73 m^2 to 70.6 mL/min/1.73 m^2 ($p = 0.002$). Although this improvement signifies enhanced kidney function, the eGFR values remained below the normal threshold (>90 mL/min/1.73 m^2), indicating and ongoing reduced renal impairment. BUN levels decreased significantly from 23.7 mg/dL to 18.3 mg/dL ($p < 0.001$).

Table 4. Comparative analysis of kidney function tests between the control group and the Post-COVID group at admission.

Variables (Mean ± SD)	Normal Range	Control Group during Admission (n = 114)	Post-COVID Group during Admission (n = 92)	p-Value
Creatinine (μmol/L)	60–110	84.5 ± 11.7	109.7 ± 16.4	<0.001
eGFR (mL/min/1.73 m^2)	>90	91.2 ± 7.3	65.3 ± 12.8	<0.001
BUN (mg/dL)	7–20	15.2 ± 3.6	23.7 ± 7.2	<0.001
Proteinuria (mg/dL)	<150	105.1 ± 48.6	198.3 ± 91.2	<0.001
Hematuria (cells/HPF)	0–3	1.5 ± 1.2	3.8 ± 2.1	<0.001
Albuminuria (mg/g)	<30	22.7 ± 8.2	52.4 ± 18.9	<0.001
ACR (mg/g)	<30	24.8 ± 10.1	59.1 ± 23.6	<0.001
Urine specific gravity	1.005–1.030	1.021 ± 0.004	1.016 ± 0.008	<0.001
Urine osmolality (mOsm/kg)	300–900	600.2 ± 140.3	535.7 ± 195.6	0.006
Sodium (mmol/L)	135–145	139.8 ± 3.9	138.2 ± 4.5	0.138
Potassium (mmol/L)	3.5–5.1	4.3 ± 0.5	4.7 ± 0.6	<0.001

SD—Standard Deviation; ACR—Urine Albumin to Creatinine Ratio; BUN—Blood Urea Nitrogen; eGFR—Estimated Glomerular Filtration Rate.

Markers of renal damage, such as proteinuria, albuminuria, and the ACR, all showed significant decreases, indicating a reduction in kidney damage over time. Improvements were also noted in urine specific gravity and osmolality, both of which returned to within or closer to their normal ranges, indicating better kidney concentrating ability. Furthermore, sodium and potassium levels showed significant normalization, with sodium increasing from 138.2 mmol/L to 140.1 mmol/L ($p < 0.001$) and potassium decreasing from 4.7 mmol/L to 4.5 mmol/L ($p = 0.007$), as presented in Table 5.

Table 5. Intragroup comparison of kidney function tests between the Post-COVID group at admission and six months after discharge.

Variables (Mean ± SD)	Normal Range	Post-COVID Group during Admission (n = 92)	Post-COVID Group Six Months Post-Admission (n = 92)	p-Value
Creatinine (μmol/L)	60–110	109.7 ± 16.4	90.4 ± 13.6	<0.001
eGFR (mL/min/1.73 m^2)	>90	65.3 ± 12.8	70.6 ± 11.1	0.002
BUN (mg/dL)	7–20	23.7 ± 7.2	18.3 ± 5.8	<0.001
Proteinuria (mg/dL)	<150	198.3 ± 91.2	155.9 ± 65.4	0.002
Hematuria (cells/HPF)	0–3	3.8 ± 2.1	2.0 ± 1.7	<0.001
Albuminuria (mg/g)	<30	52.4 ± 18.9	38.8 ± 15.2	<0.001
ACR (mg/g)	<30	59.1 ± 23.6	39.5 ± 16.3	<0.001
Urine specific gravity	1.005–1.030	1.016 ± 0.008	1.022 ± 0.005	<0.001
Urine osmolality (mOsm/kg)	300–900	485.7 ± 195.6	645.8 ± 170.2	<0.001
Sodium (mmol/L)	135–145	138.2 ± 4.5	140.1 ± 3.6	<0.001
Potassium (mmol/L)	3.5–5.1	4.7 ± 0.6	4.5 ± 0.4	0.007

SD—Standard Deviation; ACR—Urine Albumin to Creatinine Ratio; BUN—Blood Urea Nitrogen; eGFR—Estimated Glomerular Filtration Rate.

The findings revealed significant differences between the two groups, indicating ongoing renal impairment in the Post-COVID group six months after discharge. Creatinine levels were significantly higher in the Post-COVID group (90.4 ± 13.6 μmol/L) compared to the control group (84.5 ± 11.7 μmol/L) with a p-value of 0.001, still within the normal range (60–110 μmol/L) but indicative of reduced kidney function. The estimated eGFR was significantly lower in the Post-COVID group (70.6 ± 11.1 mL/min/1.73 m^2) than in the control group (91.2 ± 7.3 mL/min/1.73 m^2), with a p-value of <0.001.

BUN levels were also significantly higher in the Post-COVID group (18.3 ± 5.8 mg/dL) compared to the control group (15.2 ± 3.6 mg/dL), with a p-value of <0.001, indicating a degree of renal stress or impairment. Proteinuria, the presence of excess proteins in the urine, was markedly higher in the Post-COVID group (155.9 ± 65.4 mg/dL) than in the control group (105.1 ± 48.6 mg/dL), with a p-value of <0.001.

Hematuria and proteinuria were significantly more prevalent in the Post-COVID group (2.0 ± 1.7 cells/HPF and 38.8 ± 15.2 mg/g, respectively) compared to the control group (1.5 ± 1.2 cells/HPF and 22.7 ± 8.2 mg/g, respectively), with p-values of 0.014 and <0.001, respectively. The ACR was also significantly elevated in the Post-COVID group (39.5 ± 16.3 mg/g) compared to the control group (24.8 ± 10.1 mg/g), with a p-value of <0.001 (Table 6).

Table 6. Comparison of kidney function tests between the control group at admission and the Post-COVID group at six months post admission.

Variables (Mean ± SD)	Normal Range	Control Group during Admission (n = 114)	Post-COVID Group Six Months Post-Admission (n = 92)	p-Value
Creatinine (µmol/L)	60–110	84.5 ± 11.7	90.4 ± 13.6	0.001
eGFR (mL/min/1.73 m^2)	>90	91.2 ± 7.3	70.6 ± 11.1	<0.001
BUN (mg/dL)	7–20	15.2 ± 3.6	18.3 ± 5.8	<0.001
Proteinuria (mg/dL)	<150	105.1 ± 48.6	155.9 ± 65.4	<0.001
Hematuria (cells/HPF)	0–3	1.5 ± 1.2	2.0 ± 1.7	0.014
Albuminuria (mg/g)	<30	22.7 ± 8.2	38.8 ± 15.2	<0.001
ACR (mg/g)	<30	24.8 ± 10.1	39.5 ± 16.3	<0.001
Urine specific gravity	1.005–1.030	1.021 ± 0.004	1.022 ± 0.005	0.180
Urine osmolality (mOsm/kg)	300–900	600.2 ± 140.3	645.8 ± 170.2	0.036
Sodium (mmol/L)	135–145	139.8 ± 3.9	140.1 ± 3.6	0.289
Potassium (mmol/L)	3.5–5.1	4.3 ± 0.5	4.5 ± 0.4	0.005

SD—Standard Deviation; ACR—Urine Albumin to Creatinine Ratio; BUN—Blood Urea Nitrogen; eGFR—Estimated Glomerular Filtration Rate.

3.3. Risk Assessment

Severe COVID-19 severity showed a significant positive correlation with eGFR decrease, having a β of 2.05 ($p = 0.001$), suggesting that patients who had severe COVID-19 are more likely to experience a notable decline in kidney function, with the CI stretching from 1.89 to 4.21.

AKI was a strong predictor of eGFR decline, with a β of 3.47 ($p < 0.001$) and a CI of 1.97 to 4.97, clearly demonstrating that patients who developed AKI during their initial COVID-19 illness had a significantly higher risk of sustained reduction in kidney function. An increase in creatinine levels of more than 23 µmol/L above the normal range was also a significant predictor of eGFR decline, with a β of 2.21 ($p < 0.001$) and a CI of 1.93 to 3.49, highlighting the impact of kidney injury marked by elevated creatinine on long-term kidney function. Increases in the ACR greater than 11 mg/g above the normal range and BUN increases greater than 8 mg/dL above the normal range were also significantly associated with decreased eGFR, with β coefficients of 1.88 ($p < 0.001$, CI: 1.06 to 4.80) and 1.34 ($p = 0.001$, CI: 1.10 to 5.08), respectively (Table 7, Figure 1).

Table 7. Regression analysis of factors predicting continuous eGFR decrease <30 at six months post SARS-CoV-2 infection.

Independent Variables	Coefficient (β)	Std. Error	p-Value	95% CI
Age	−0.24	0.08	0.004	(−0.40, −0.08)
COVID-19 Severity (Severe = 1)	2.05	0.59	0.001	(1.89, 4.21)
Developed AKI (Yes = 1, No = 0)	3.47	0.76	<0.001	(1.97, 4.97)
Creatinine increase (>23 µmol/L above NR)	2.21	0.65	<0.001	(1.93, 3.49)
ACR increase (>11 mg/g above NR)	1.88	0.47	<0.001	(1.06, 4.80)
BUN increase (>8 mg/dL above NR)	1.34	0.38	0.001	(1.10, 5.08)

CI—Confidence Interval; BUN—Blood Urea Nitrogen; NR—Normal Range; ACR—Urine Albumin to Creatinine Ratio.

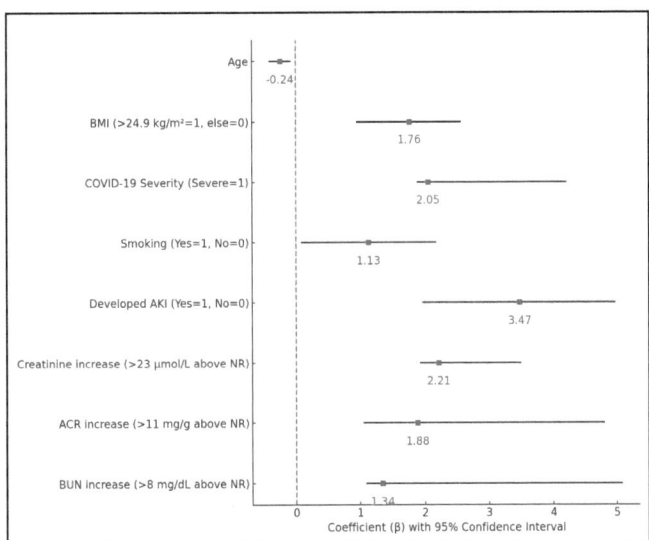

Figure 1. Regression analysis results of factors predicting continuous eGFR decrease <30 at six months post SARS-CoV-2 infection.

4. Discussion

4.1. Literature Findings

The study's findings pointed to significant kidney impairment in Post-COVID patients, especially when noting elevated creatinine levels and reduced eGFR compared to controls. This distinct pattern suggests COVID-19's unique impact on renal health, beyond what's typically observed in acute illness. While some recovery was noted over six months, evidenced by improvements in eGFR and reductions in proteinuria and albuminuria, the continuous abnormalities highlight the risk of developing chronic kidney disease post-COVID. Our analysis revealed significant differences in inflammatory biomarkers between the POST COVID group and the Control group, as detailed in Table 2. This observation aligns with the findings presented in Table 7, where the severity of COVID-19 infection was correlated with a sustained decrease in eGFR to levels below 30 mL/min/1.73 m² at six months post-infection. These results suggest that the inflammatory response elicited by severe COVID-19 may have a prolonged impact on renal function. Despite the partial recovery observed in some kidney function metrics, the persistence of certain abnormalities underlines the potential for long-lasting renal impairment. This raises concerns about the capacity of the kidneys to fully recover after severe COVID-19, pointing to a need for ongoing research into therapeutic strategies that could support renal healing and prevent chronic conditions.

The study findings mirrored those reported by Tannor et al. [23], emphasizing the exacerbated risks and outcomes of COVID-19 on individuals with pre-existing kidney conditions, particularly underlining the severe consequences in low-income settings due to inadequate healthcare infrastructure. Both studies underscored the heightened incidence of acute kidney injury and the progression to chronic kidney disease post-COVID-19 infection, pointing out the global inequities in managing these complications. Similarly, Brogan et al. [24] identified acute kidney injury and potential exacerbation of chronic kidney diseases as critical concerns, noting the unclear role of direct viral infection of kidney cells in these processes. They also highlighted the increased mortality associated with kidney conditions in the context of COVID-19, especially among those with severe disease or on replacement therapy, underscoring the gap in clinical trials for COVID-19 therapies that include patients with severe kidney disease.

Similarly, Žulpaitė et al. [25] reported a significant association between COVID-19 and renal injury, noting that patients with acute kidney injury or chronic kidney disease exacerbated by AKI had higher mortality rates, up to 7.81 times higher for those with AKI and CKD combined compared to those with CKD alone. This study's findings of elevated creatinine levels and reduced eGFR six months post-COVID further underscore the lingering renal impairment, closely echoing Žulpaitė et al.'s [25] observation that COVID-19 patients with renal complications faced longer hospital stays and increased likelihood of death. Mahalingasivam et al. [26] highlighted the global challenge of researching kidney diseases in the COVID-19 context, pointing to variabilities in SARS-CoV-2 testing access and the incidence of infection, complicating the clear classification and management of AKI and CKD. The disparities and methodological hurdles emphasized by Mahalingasivam et al. [26] underline the necessity for a nuanced understanding of COVID-19's impact on renal health, suggesting a convergence in findings across studies that COVID-19 significantly exacerbates risks for patients with kidney diseases, further complicating their prognosis and care.

The study findings, when considered alongside other research provide a comprehensive understanding of COVID-19's impact on renal health, even though the majority of existing studies did not report on the association of CKD with Post-COVID syndrome. Jdiaa et al. [27] highlighted the significantly higher risks of hospitalization and mortality among COVID-19 patients with chronic kidney disease, indicating a hospitalization risk ratio of 1.63 and a mortality hazard ratio of 1.48 for these patients. This correlates with the observed persistent renal impairment in post-COVID patients in the current study, emphasizing the virus's severe effects on individuals with pre-existing renal conditions. Martin de Francisco et al. [28] delved into the categorization of COVID-19 and its long-term manifestations, including persistent symptoms known as long COVID, which has been associated with severe disease phases and pre-existing conditions such as CKD. They also noted a lack of comprehensive renal data in post-COVID syndrome discussions, suggesting a gap in recognizing and addressing renal impairments in these patients.

The findings of the current study, in concert with those presented by Copur et al. [29] and La Porta et al. [30], shed light on the intricate relationship between COVID-19 and renal function. Copur et al., emphasize the significant renal involvement during and post-COVID-19 infection, highlighting a notable decline in renal function up to 12 months following the infection, even in patients who did not exhibit acute kidney injury initially. This observation aligns with the current study's findings, where persistent renal impairment was evident six months post-COVID, suggesting a prolonged impact of the virus on kidney health. La Porta et al., through a retrospective study, identified AKI as a critical factor associated with increased mortality and severity of COVID-19, corroborating the significant role of renal dysfunction in the disease's outcomes as observed in the current study. However, La Porta et al., also noted that baseline kidney function mitigated the role of age in COVID-19 severity and mortality, offering a nuanced view of the interplay between renal function and other risk factors.

Akliu et al.'s research [31] demonstrated a notable decrease in major adverse kidney events (MAKE) among patients with COVID-19-associated AKI, with an adjusted hazard ratio for MAKE of 0.67, indicating a significantly lower risk when compared to AKI from other illnesses. This was further supported by a marked reduction in all-cause mortality, with an adjusted hazard ratio (aHR) of 0.31, and a lower rate of worsened kidney function (aHR, 0.78) in the COVID-AKI group. This suggests that despite the initial severity, patients with COVID-19-associated AKI may have a somewhat more favorable long-term kidney prognosis than those with AKI due to other causes. In contrast, Lin et al. [32] investigated the genetic links between CKD and critical COVID-19, finding a significant association with an odds ratio of 1.28 for the risk of severe COVID-19 in individuals with genetically predicted CKD. However, they did not find a meaningful correlation between severe COVID-19 and CKD when using genome-wide significant SNPs as instrumental variables for critical COVID-19 (OR = 1.03), indicating the complexity of the relationship between

COVID-19 severity and underlying CKD. Together, these studies highlight the nuanced interplay between COVID-19 and renal health, suggesting both a direct impact of the virus on kidney function and a genetic predisposition that may influence disease severity.

To further enhance the understanding of the renal impacts of COVID-19, particularly in severe cases, it is crucial to consider the differential clearance of creatinine and cystatin C. Creatinine, with a molecular weight of 0.11 kDa, and cystatin C, at 13 kDa, provide insights into changes in glomerular filtration barrier properties, potentially indicative of "shrunken pore syndrome" (SPS). SPS, characterized by selective dysfunction in glomerular filtration, may be a critical factor in the renal pathology observed with severe COVID-19. The study by Herget-Rosenthal et al. [33] explored how alterations in the filtration of molecules of different sizes can signal changes in kidney barrier function, relevant in the context of systemic diseases such as COVID-19. However, a 2022 study revealed that in ICU-treated patients, dexamethasone influenced the estimated glomerular filtration rate measured by cystatin C but not by creatinine, suggesting that steroid treatment could impact cystatin C levels and thereby eGFR estimates [34].

Therefore, the current study stands along the existing literature on the COVID-19 long-term outcomes on kidney function, underscoring the necessity of incorporating renal health into the long-term care plan for COVID-19 survivors. With specific risk factors identified, healthcare providers can better target those most at risk of sustained kidney damage, offering a more strategic approach to post-COVID care. The study not only adds to our understanding of COVID-19's extended impact but also calls for a heightened awareness and proactive management of kidney health in recovering patients. As a longer follow-up period can better define long-term consequences of renal function after COVID-19, a larger prospective study will be implemented, and future research on the topic is encouraged to encompass multiple global scenarios.

4.2. Study Limitations

This study, aimed at assessing kidney function in Post-COVID Syndrome patients six months after SARS-CoV-2 infection, inherently faces several limitations. Firstly, its retrospective observational nature limits the ability to establish causality between COVID-19 and observed renal outcomes. The reliance on existing medical records and the potential for incomplete data raise concerns about the comprehensiveness and accuracy of the captured information. Furthermore, the exclusion criteria might have inadvertently omitted individuals with subclinical renal impairment prior to COVID-19, potentially skewing the severity of Post-COVID renal dysfunction observed. Another significant limitation is the study's single-center design, which may limit the generalizability of the findings to broader populations, particularly considering geographical variations in COVID-19 strains and healthcare approaches. The absence of a longitudinal pre-COVID baseline for kidney function in the patients also hinders the ability to definitively attribute observed renal impairments solely to the virus. Additionally, the study's focus on patients who have survived to discharge might introduce survivorship bias, overlooking those with severe COVID-19 who succumbed to the disease or its complications before follow-up kidney function tests could be performed. Another limitation includes the inclusion of participants with eGFR levels between 60–89 mL/min/1.73 m^2, representing mildly decreased renal function, which may influence the purity of our cohort aimed at isolating the renal effects of Post-COVID syndrome. Lastly, the study did not account for variations in the management of acute COVID-19, such as differences in therapeutic interventions that might independently influence kidney function outcomes, nor did it fully explore the impact of COVID-19 vaccination status on renal recovery trajectories.

5. Conclusions

The findings underscore the significant impact of COVID-19 on long-term renal health in patients with Post-COVID Syndrome. The severity of initial infection, AKI development during admission, blood urea nitrogen increase more than 8 units above the threshold, creatinine increase with more than 23 μmol/L during admission, and urine albumin to creatinine ratio increase to more than 11 units above the threshold during COVID-19 admission were identified as key predictors of renal function decline with more than 30 units of eGFR six months post discharge. These results highlight the necessity for ongoing renal health monitoring and tailored intervention strategies to address the chronic renal implications of Post-COVID Syndrome, emphasizing the importance of considering renal outcomes in the holistic management of affected individuals.

Author Contributions: Conceptualization: M.B., M.L.B. and S.S.-R.; methodology: M.B., M.L.B. and S.S.-R.; software: P.S.N. and A.E.; validation: G.D. and V.E.L.; formal analysis: G.D. and V.E.L.; investigation: G.D. and V.E.L.; resources: E.R.S., E.T. and R.I.; data curation: E.R.S., E.T. and R.I.; writing—original draft preparation: M.B., M.L.B. and S.S.-R.; writing—review and editing: P.S.N., A.E., E.R.S., E.T. and R.I.; visualization: A.D., A.V.B. and C.C.; supervision: A.D., A.V.B. and C.C.; project administration: A.D., A.V.B. and C.C. All authors have read and agreed to the published version of the manuscript.

Funding: The APC was funded by "Victor Babes" University of Medicine and Pharmacy, Timisoara, Romania.

Institutional Review Board Statement: The study was conducted according to the guidelines of the Declaration of Helsinki and approved by the Ethics Committee of Victor Babes" Clinical Hospital for Infectious Diseases and Pulmonology in Timisoara (approval number 2632 from 23 March 2022).

Informed Consent Statement: Written informed consent has been obtained from the patients to publish this paper.

Data Availability Statement: Data available on request from the author.

Conflicts of Interest: The authors declare no conflict of interest.

References

1. ReferencesHope, A.A.; Evering, T.H. Postacute Sequelae of Severe Acute Respiratory Syndrome Coronavirus 2 Infection. *Infect. Dis. Clin. N. Am.* **2022**, *36*, 379–395. [CrossRef] [PubMed] [PubMed Central]
2. O'Donnell, J.S.; Chappell, K.J. Chronic SARS-CoV-2, a Cause of Post-acute COVID-19 Sequelae (Long-COVID)? *Front. Microbiol.* **2021**, *12*, 724654. [CrossRef] [PubMed] [PubMed Central]
3. Davis, H.E.; McCorkell, L.; Vogel, J.M.; Topol, E.J. Long COVID: Major findings, mechanisms and recommendations. *Nat. Rev. Microbiol.* **2023**, *21*, 133–146, Erratum in: *Nat. Rev. Microbiol.* **2023**, *21*, 408. [CrossRef] [PubMed] [PubMed Central]
4. Long, J.D.; Strohbehn, I.; Sawtell, R.; Bhattacharyya, R.; Sise, M.E. COVID-19 Survival and its impact on chronic kidney disease. *Transl. Res.* **2022**, *241*, 70–82. [CrossRef] [PubMed] [PubMed Central]
5. Yeung, M.L.; Yao, Y.; Jia, L.; Chan, J.F.; Chan, K.H.; Cheung, K.F.; Chen, H.; Poon, V.K.; Tsang, A.K.; To, K.K.; et al. MERS coronavirus induces apoptosis in kidney and lung by upregulating Smad7 and FGF2. *Nat. Microbiol.* **2016**, *1*, 16004. [CrossRef] [PubMed] [PubMed Central]
6. Menon, T.; Sharma, R.; Kataria, S.; Sardar, S.; Adhikari, R.; Tousif, S.; Khan, H.; Rathore, S.S.; Singh, R.; Ahmed, Z. The Association of Acute Kidney Injury With Disease Severity and Mortality in COVID-19: A Systematic Review and Meta-Analysis. *Cureus* **2021**, *13*, e13894. [CrossRef] [PubMed] [PubMed Central]
7. Chong, W.H.; Saha, B.K. Relationship Between Severe Acute Respiratory Syndrome Coronavirus 2 (SARS-CoV-2) and the Etiology of Acute Kidney Injury (AKI). *Am. J. Med Sci.* **2021**, *361*, 287–296. [CrossRef] [PubMed] [PubMed Central]
8. Chávez-Valencia, V.; Orizaga-de-la-Cruz, C.; Lagunas-Rangel, F.A. Acute Kidney Injury in COVID-19 Patients: Pathogenesis, Clinical Characteristics, Therapy, and Mortality. *Diseases* **2022**, *10*, 53. [CrossRef] [PubMed] [PubMed Central]
9. Sabaghian, T.; Kharazmi, A.B.; Ansari, A.; Omidi, F.; Kazemi, S.N.; Hajikhani, B.; Vaziri-Harami, R.; Tajbakhsh, A.; Omidi, S.; Haddadi, S.; et al. COVID-19 and Acute Kidney Injury: A Systematic Review. *Front. Med.* **2022**, *9*, 705908. [CrossRef] [PubMed] [PubMed Central]
10. Assiri, A.M.; Alamaa, T.; Elenezi, F.; Alsagheir, A.; Alzubaidi, L.; TIeyjeh, I.; Alhomod, A.S.; Gaffas, E.M.; Amer, S.A. Unveiling the Clinical Spectrum of Post-COVID-19 Conditions: Assessment and Recommended Strategies. *Cureus* **2024**, *16*, e52827. [CrossRef] [PubMed] [PubMed Central]
11. Maltezou, H.C.; Pavli, A.; Tsakris, A. Post-COVID Syndrome: An Insight on Its Pathogenesis. *Vaccines* **2021**, *9*, 497. [CrossRef] [PubMed] [PubMed Central]
12. Moeinzadeh, F.; Mortazavi, M.; Shahidi, S.; Mansourian, M.; Yazdani, A.; Zamani, Z.; Seirafian, S. Chronic Kidney Disease and COVID-19 Infection: A Case-Control Study. *Adv. Biomed Res.* **2022**, *11*, 112. [CrossRef] [PubMed] [PubMed Central]
13. Huang, W.; Li, B.; Jiang, N.; Zhang, F.; Shi, W.; Zuo, L.; Liu, S.; Tang, B. Impact of the COVID-19 pandemic on patients with chronic kidney disease: A narrative review. *Medicine* **2022**, *101*, e29362. [CrossRef] [PubMed] [PubMed Central]

14. Pecly, I.M.D.; Azevedo, R.B.; Muxfeldt, E.S.; Botelho, B.G.; Albuquerque, G.G.; Diniz, P.H.P.; Silva, R.; Rodrigues, C.I.S. COVID-19 and chronic kidney disease: A comprehensive review. *Braz. J. Nephrol.* **2021**, *43*, 383–399. [CrossRef] [PubMed] [PubMed Central]
15. Temiz, M.Z.; Hacibey, I.; Yazar, R.O.; Sevdi, M.S.; Kucuk, S.H.; Alkurt, G.; Doganay, L.; Dinler Doganay, G.; Dincer, M.M.; Yuruk, E.; et al. Altered kidney function induced by SARS-CoV-2 infection and acute kidney damage markers predict survival outcomes of COVID-19 patients: A prospective pilot study. *Ren. Fail.* **2022**, *44*, 233–240. [CrossRef] [PubMed] [PubMed Central]
16. Hong, X.W.; Chi, Z.P.; Liu, G.Y.; Huang, H.; Guo, S.Q.; Fan, J.R.; Lin, X.W.; Qu, L.Z.; Chen, R.L.; Wu, L.J.; et al. Characteristics of Renal Function in Patients Diagnosed With COVID-19: An Observational Study. *Front. Med.* **2020**, *7*, 409. [CrossRef] [PubMed] [PubMed Central]
17. Panimathi, R.; Gurusamy, E.; Mahalakshmi, S.; Ramadevi, K.; Kaarthikeyan, G.; Anil, S. Impact of COVID-19 on Renal Function: A Multivariate Analysis of Biochemical and Immunological Markers in Patients. *Cureus* **2022**, *14*, e22076. [CrossRef] [PubMed] [PubMed Central]
18. Al Rumaihi, K.; Khalafalla, K.; Arafa, M.; Nair, A.; Al Bishawi, A.; Fino, A.; Sirtaj, F.; Ella, M.K.; ElBardisi, H.; Khattab, M.A.; et al. COVID-19 and renal involvement: A prospective cohort study assessing the impact of mild SARS-CoV-2 infection on the kidney function of young healthy males. *Int. Urol. Nephrol.* **2023**, *55*, 201–209. [CrossRef] [PubMed] [PubMed Central]
19. Seo, J.W.; Kim, S.E.; Kim, Y.; Kim, E.J.; Kim, T.; Kim, T.; Lee, S.H.; Lee, E.; Lee, J.; Seo, Y.B.; et al. Updated Clinical Practice Guidelines for the Diagnosis and Management of Long COVID. *Infect. Chemother.* **2024**, *56*, 122–157. [CrossRef] [PubMed] [PubMed Central]
20. Srikanth, S.; Boulos, J.R.; Dover, T.; Boccuto, L.; Dean, D. Identification and diagnosis of long COVID-19: A scoping review. *Prog. Biophys. Mol. Biol.* **2023**, *182*, 1–7. [CrossRef] [PubMed] [PubMed Central]
21. Charles, K.; Lewis, M.J.; Montgomery, E.; Reid, M. The 2021 Chronic Kidney Disease Epidemiology Collaboration Race-Free Estimated Glomerular Filtration Rate Equations in Kidney Disease: Leading the Way in Ending Disparities. *Health Equity* **2024**, *8*, 39–45. [CrossRef] [PubMed]
22. Radwan, N.M.; Mahmoud, N.E.; Alfaifi, A.H.; Alabdulkareem, K.I. Comorbidities and severity of coronavirus disease 2019 patients. *Saudi Med. J.* **2020**, *41*, 1165–1174. [CrossRef] [PubMed]
23. Tannor, E.K.; Bajpai, D.; Nlandu, Y.M.; Wijewickrama, E. COVID-19 and Kidney Disease: Progress in Health Inequity From Low-Income Settings. *Semin. Nephrol.* **2022**, *42*, 151318. [CrossRef] [PubMed] [PubMed Central]
24. Brogan, M.; Ross, M.J. COVID-19 and Kidney Disease. *Annu. Rev. Med.* **2023**, *74*, 1–13. [CrossRef] [PubMed]
25. Žulpaitė, G.; Rimševičius, L.; Jančorienė, L.; Zablockienė, B.; Miglinas, M. The Association between COVID-19 Infection and Kidney Damage in a Regional University Hospital. *Medicina* **2023**, *59*, 898. [CrossRef] [PubMed] [PubMed Central]
26. Mahalingasivam, V.; Su, G.; Iwagami, M.; Davids, M.R.; Wetmore, J.B.; Nitsch, D. COVID-19 and kidney disease: Insights from epidemiology to inform clinical practice. *Nat. Rev. Nephrol.* **2022**, *18*, 485–498. [CrossRef] [PubMed] [PubMed Central]
27. Jdiaa, S.S.; Mansour, R.; El Alayli, A.; Gautam, A.; Thomas, P.; Mustafa, R.A. COVID-19 and chronic kidney disease: An updated overview of reviews. *J. Nephrol.* **2022**, *35*, 69–85. [CrossRef] [PubMed] [PubMed Central]
28. de Francisco, Á.M.; Fernández Fresnedo, G. Long COVID-19 renal disease: A present medical need for nephrology. *Nefrologia (Engl. Ed.)* **2023**, *43*, 1–5. [CrossRef] [PubMed] [PubMed Central]
29. Copur, S.; Berkkan, M.; Basile, C.; Tuttle, K.; Kanbay, M. Post-acute COVID-19 syndrome and kidney diseases: What do we know? *J. Nephrol.* **2022**, *35*, 795–805. [CrossRef] [PubMed] [PubMed Central]
30. La Porta, E.; Baiardi, P.; Fassina, L.; Faragli, A.; Perna, S.; Tovagliari, F.; Tallone, I.; Talamo, G.; Secondo, G.; Mazzarello, G.; et al. The role of kidney dysfunction in COVID-19 and the influence of age. *Sci. Rep.* **2022**, *12*, 8650. [CrossRef] [PubMed] [PubMed Central]
31. Aklilu, A.M.; Kumar, S.; Nugent, J.; Yamamoto, Y.; Coronel-Moreno, C.; Kadhim, B.; Faulkner, S.C.; O'Connor, K.D.; Yasmin, F.; Greenberg, J.H.; et al. COVID-19-Associated Acute Kidney Injury and Longitudinal Kidney Outcomes. *JAMA Intern. Med.* **2024**, *184*, 414–423. [CrossRef] [PubMed] [PubMed Central]
32. Lin, H.; Cao, B. Severe COVID-19 and chronic kidney disease: Bidirectional mendelian randomization study. *Virol. J.* **2024**, *21*, 32. [CrossRef] [PubMed] [PubMed Central]
33. Herget-Rosenthal, S.; van Wijk, J.A.; Bröcker-Preuss, M.; Bökenkamp, A. Increased urinary cystatin C reflects structural and functional renal tubular impairment independent of glomerular filtration rate. *Clin. Biochem.* **2007**, *40*, 946–951. [CrossRef] [PubMed]
34. Larsson, A.O.; Hultström, M.; Frithiof, R.; Nyman, U.; Lipcsey, M.; Eriksson, M.B. Differential Bias for Creatinine- and Cystatin C-Derived Estimated Glomerular Filtration Rate in Critical COVID-19. *Biomedicines* **2022**, *10*, 2708. [CrossRef] [PubMed]

Disclaimer/Publisher's Note: The statements, opinions and data contained in all publications are solely those of the individual author(s) and contributor(s) and not of MDPI and/or the editor(s). MDPI and/or the editor(s) disclaim responsibility for any injury to people or property resulting from any ideas, methods, instructions or products referred to in the content.

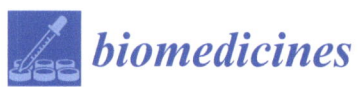 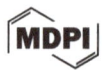

Article

Hemoglobin and Its Relationship with Fatigue in Long-COVID Patients Three to Six Months after SARS-CoV-2 Infection

Somayeh Bazdar [1,2,3], Lizan D. Bloemsma [1,2,3], Nadia Baalbaki [1,2,3], Jelle M. Blankestijn [1,2,3], Merel E. B. Cornelissen [1,2,3], Rosanne J. H. C. G. Beijers [4], Brigitte M. Sondermeijer [5], Yolanda van Wijck [1,2,3], George S. Downward [6,7] and Anke H. Maitland-van der Zee [1,2,3,*,†] on behalf of the P4O2 Consortium

1. Department of Pulmonary Medicine, Amsterdam UMC, University of Amsterdam, 1105 AZ Amsterdam, The Netherlands; s.bazdar@amsterdamumc.nl (S.B.); l.d.bloemsma@amsterdamumc.nl (L.D.B.); j.m.blankestijn@amsterdamumc.nl (J.M.B.); m.e.b.cornelissen@amsterdamumc.nl (M.E.B.C.)
2. Amsterdam Institute for Infection and Immunity, Amsterdam UMC, 1105 AZ Amsterdam, The Netherlands
3. Amsterdam Public Health Research Institute, Amsterdam UMC, 1105 AZ Amsterdam, The Netherlands
4. Department of Respiratory Medicine, Nutrim Institute of Nutrition and Translational Research in Metabolism, Faculty of Health, Medicine and Life Sciences, Maastricht University, 6202 AZ Maastricht, The Netherlands; r.beijers@maastrichtuniversity.nl
5. Department of Pulmonology, Spaarne Gasthuis, 2035 RC Haarlem, The Netherlands; bsondermeijer@spaarnegasthuis.nl
6. Department of Environmental Epidemiology, Institute for Risk Assessment Sciences (IRAS), Utrecht University, 3584 CL Utrecht, The Netherlands; g.s.downward@uu.nl
7. Department of Global Public Health & Bioethics, Julius Center for Health Sciences and Primary Care, University Medical Center Utrecht, 3584 CX Utrecht, The Netherlands
* Correspondence: a.h.maitland@amsterdamumc.nl; Tel.: +31-020-5668137
† Current address: Department of Respiratory Medicine, Amsterdam UMC, 1105 AZ Amsterdam, The Netherlands.

Citation: Bazdar, S.; Bloemsma, L.D.; Baalbaki, N.; Blankestijn, J.M.; Cornelissen, M.E.B.; Beijers, R.J.H.C.G.; Sondermeijer, B.M.; van Wijck, Y.; Downward, G.S.; Maitland-van der Zee, A.H., on behalf of the P4O2 Consortium. Hemoglobin and Its Relationship with Fatigue in Long-COVID Patients Three to Six Months after SARS-CoV-2 Infection. *Biomedicines* **2024**, *12*, 1234. https://doi.org/10.3390/biomedicines12061234

Academic Editors: César Fernández De Las Peñas and Serafino Fazio

Received: 11 February 2024
Revised: 23 May 2024
Accepted: 24 May 2024
Published: 1 June 2024

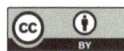

Copyright: © 2024 by the authors. Licensee MDPI, Basel, Switzerland. This article is an open access article distributed under the terms and conditions of the Creative Commons Attribution (CC BY) license (https:// creativecommons.org/licenses/by/ 4.0/).

Abstract: *Background:* While some long-term effects of COVID-19 are respiratory in nature, a non-respiratory effect gaining attention has been a decline in hemoglobin, potentially mediated by inflammatory processes. In this study, we examined the correlations between hemoglobin levels and inflammatory biomarkers and evaluated the association between hemoglobin and fatigue in a cohort of Long-COVID patients. *Methods:* This prospective cohort study in the Netherlands evaluated 95 (mostly hospitalized) patients, aged 40–65 years, 3–6 months post SARS-CoV-2 infection, examining their venous hemoglobin concentration, anemia (hemoglobin < 7.5 mmol/L in women and <8.5 mmol/L in men), inflammatory blood biomarkers, average FSS (Fatigue Severity Score), demographics, and clinical features. Follow-up hemoglobin was compared against hemoglobin during acute infection. Spearman correlation was used for assessing the relationship between hemoglobin concentrations and inflammatory biomarkers, and the association between hemoglobin and fatigue was examined using logistic regression. *Results:* In total, 11 (16.4%) participants were suffering from anemia 3–6 months after SARS-CoV-2 infection. The mean hemoglobin value increased by 0.3 mmol/L 3–6 months after infection compared to the hemoglobin during the acute phase (*p*-value = 0.003). Whilst logistic regression showed that a 1 mmol/L greater increase in hemoglobin is related to a decrease in experiencing fatigue in Long-COVID patients (adjusted OR 0.38 [95%CI 0.13–1.09]), we observed no correlations between hemoglobin and any of the inflammatory biomarkers examined. *Conclusion:* Our results indicate that hemoglobin impairment might play a role in developing Long-COVID fatigue. Further investigation is necessary to identify the precise mechanism causing hemoglobin alteration in these patients.

Keywords: Long-COVID; anemia; hemoglobin; inflammation; fatigue

1. Introduction

Over four years ago, the World Health Organization (WHO) declared COVID-19 a global pandemic. However, infections from SARS-CoV-2 and their long-term consequences remain a global challenge [1,2]. Of particular concern are the many aspects of the long-term outcomes that remain unknown, especially among those who have survived a SARS-CoV-2 infection [3,4]. The term "Long-COVID" refers to the condition in which patients experience a variety of persisting symptoms long after the acute phase of the infection has resolved but often typified by fatigue, dyspnea, brain fog, sleep problems, muscle stiffness, and mental problems [1,5,6]. These symptoms are not restricted to pulmonary manifestations; and just like the acute phase of the disease, organs other than the lungs may be impacted [7,8]. However, many long-term symptoms may not have been present in the acute phase.

Long-COVID is causing widespread disability worldwide, with many potentially developing lifelong disabilities. Nevertheless, current diagnostics and treatments are insufficient, necessitating urgent clinical investigations to address hypothesized underlying biological mechanisms [1]. Whilst the mechanism of long-COVID continues to be unclear due to the wide clinical spectrum and organ involvement, only a thorough understanding of its pathophysiology will allow us to assess and treat the disease's side effects [9]. While persistence of respiratory symptoms, particularly dyspnea and cough, appear to be common in Long-COVID, some of the other persistent symptoms of Long-COVID may be part of a multisystem disease, and interdisciplinary treatment of these chronic sequelae is necessary [10].

A decrease in hemoglobin may be one of the non-respiratory complications of a SARS-CoV-2 infection. In the acute phase of infection, a reduction in hemoglobin is likely mediated via interactions between viral agents and host cells and has previously been found to be a predictive factor for severe respiratory failure in pneumonic COVID-19 patients [11,12]. Based on the results of multivariate regression of a study comprising 1147 COVID-19 patients across five tertiary pediatric hospitals in Asia, higher levels of hemoglobin and platelets were protective against severe/critical COVID-19 infection [11]. A retrospective investigation of 23 COVID-19 hospitalized patients with pneumonia also revealed a significant association between higher levels of hemoglobin and a reduced need for mechanical ventilation administration, with an odds ratio of 0.313 [12]. Various mechanisms for decreased hemoglobin have been proposed, including the conversion of Hb into other forms such as methemoglobin (MetHb) and carboxyhemoglobin (COHb) [13]. While oxidative stress, which is linked to infectious diseases, may contribute [14], medications given during treatment may also be relevant, given that certain medicines such as hydroxychloroquine used to treat COVID-19 have a high potential for oxidation, which can lead to MetHb and COHb [15]. An increase in COHb during SARS-CoV-2 infection may also potentially be related to hemolytic anemia, and an increase in MetHb is a result of hemoglobin oxidation that could also be driven by nitric oxide (NO) [13]. Besides oxidative stress, hyperinflammation may be another reason for developing new-onset anemia during SARS-CoV-2 infection [16]. Investigations of hospitalized patients with COVID-19 disease revealed that increased inflammatory indices such as Interleukin 6 (IL-6) and C-reactive protein (CRP) were increased in those with COVID-19-induced anemia [17].

Anemia is defined as a decrease in hemoglobin (Hb) concentrations and/or red blood cell (RBC) absolute counts leading to an inadequate supply of physiological requirements, and its common diagnostic method is to assess the Hb level [18]. This hematologic disease is typically a multifaceted medical condition, and different factors such as the patient's medical history and the underlying pathological mechanism(s) should be considered while diagnosing and categorizing it [19]. Common manifestations of anemia include a wide range of symptoms such as pale skin, shortness of breath, palpitations, chest pain, dizziness, loss of strength, weakness, and fatigue [20]. According to studies on the prevalence of fatigue and its associated factors, anemia is one of the most frequently found risk factors linked to fatigue in patients with chronic kidney disease (CKD) [21].

Fatigue is the most common symptom in Long-COVID patients [22]. While anemia, psychosocial problems, sleep disorders, and sleep-related respiratory disorders are considered common causes of fatigue in general, cancer, thyroid dysfunction, and other somatic diseases can also be reasons [23]. In a study of 42 men and 33 women, Pasini et.al. reported a mean hemoglobin of 11.5 g/dL (normal range: 14–18 g/dL) among men and 10.9 g/dL (normal range: 12–16 g/dL) among women 60 days following their hospital discharge after COVID-19 [24]. Furthermore, in a 6-month follow-up of 412 ex-COVID-19 patients, it was reported that the average hemoglobin level was significantly lower in patients suffering from fatigue compared to those who were not (13.8 vs. 14.3 g/dL). However, after performing multivariate regression, no statistically significant associations were observed between hemoglobin, other cell blood count measurements (including inflammatory biomarkers), and Long-COVID symptoms [25].

A better understanding of the mechanisms involved in Long-COVID and hemoglobin status/anemia will allow better treatment of those suffering from this condition. While there is some evidence that Long-COVID patients have decreased hemoglobin levels, its link with inflammatory indices as well as its role in developing fatigue symptoms remain unclear. Finding biomarkers that can help to direct optimized care to patients most at risk is crucial, and since hemoglobin is easily assessed by assay and has been associated with Long-COVID, we believe that it is a biomarker worthy of further investigation. The purpose of the current study is therefore to examine the correlations between hemoglobin levels and inflammatory biomarkers and to evaluate the potential role of the inflammatory process in decreasing hemoglobin levels in Long-COVID patients. Furthermore, this study investigates the association between hemoglobin and fatigue in a cohort of Long-COVID patients to evaluate whether hemoglobin levels contribute to developing fatigue in these patients.

2. Methods and Materials

2.1. Study Setting and Participants

The population for the current study consists of participants of the Precision Medicine for More Oxygen (P4O2) COVID-19 cohort. Details on the study design of this cohort have been published elsewhere [26]. In brief, P4O2 COVID-19 is a prospective cohort study that recruited 95 Long-COVID patients, aged 40–65 years, from outpatient Long-COVID clinics in five hospitals in the Netherlands. Two research visits were performed for each patient between months 3–6 and months 12–18 after SARS-CoV-2 infection, during which questionnaires were administered, and physical examinations and biological sampling were performed. There were no specific exclusion criteria for the FU study visit of this cohort, and nine months following the initial study visit, all participants received invitations for a follow-up appointment, but a portion was lost to follow-up. Information about the acute phase of the disease was extracted from patients' medical charts. Participants for whom a hemoglobin measurement was available, either during SARS-CoV-2 infection or their first follow-up (FU) visit 3–6 months after SARS-CoV-2 infection, or both, were eligible for analysis in the current paper. The second study visit was conducted 12–18 months after infection, which included a fairly high number of lost to FU among whom only 11 provided blood samples for hemoglobin.

2.2. Ethical Considerations

The study protocol for the P4O2 COVID-19 cohort was approved by the ethical committee of Amsterdam UMC (reference number NL74701.018.20), and all participants provided written informed consent prior to their enrolment.

2.3. Variables in This Study

Measurements during the acute phase of the SARS-CoV-2 infection (baseline) and FU laboratory measurements of hemoglobin were assessed via venipuncture, performed under aseptic conditions, and analyzed following standard laboratory procedures in each participating hospital. To be eligible for the current study, a hemoglobin level either at baseline or FU (n = 93) was required. A subset of patients (n = 27) did not provide standard venipuncture at the FU visit but most of them did provide a hemoglobin value measured via finger prick test during pulmonary function testing (generally occurring concurrently with the FU visit), which was used instead, and this way all 95 participants were eligible for the current analysis. As this method was expected to provide results somewhat different from those of venipuncture, the hemoglobin values from these participants were only used to examine whether their hemoglobin levels changed by >10% (i.e., clinically significant difference, as described below). Anemia was defined, as per the reference range at the measuring laboratory, as a hemoglobin level less than 7.5 mmol/L in women and less than 8.5 mmol/L in men according to the reference laboratory range. Absolute changes in hemoglobin were calculated as the difference between FU and baseline hemoglobin and were classified into increased, decreased, or unchanged hemoglobin. In addition, "clinically relevant" changes in hemoglobin were determined by an increase or decrease in hemoglobin of 10% or more. As there is no universal definition of a clinically significant change in hemoglobin levels, we utilized the determination of obstetrics and gynecology references which usually recognize a decrease in hemoglobin level if it is more than 10% decrease [27–29].

The Fatigue Severity Scale (FSS) standard questionnaire was used to categorize patients into those with or without fatigue. The total FSS was the sum of the nine questions and the average FSS was calculated by dividing this sum by nine [30]. An average score equal to or more than four was considered as a positive indicator of fatigue, similar to previous research in the P4O2 COVID study [26]. The fatigue severity scale originally utilized a cut-off of 4 or more to indicate severe fatigue. We acknowledge that different cut-offs have been developed, including low (<4), medium/borderline (4–5), and high/severe (>5) [31]. However, for simplicity, and consistency with our other work in this population [26] we have chosen to consistently use 4 as a cut-off point.

Blood samples were also examined for a variety of biomarkers, and markers that indicated the presence of an inflammatory process were included as inflammatory indices in the current study. Identified markers were D-Dimer, Neutrophil/Lymphocyte ratio (NLR), Immature Granulocyte (IG), C-reactive protein (CRP), Creatine phosphokinase (CPK), and Lactate Dehydrogenase (LDH) [32–34]. Normal ranges and analytical approaches were as per the standard operating procedures at participating hospitals.

Additional variables assessed in this paper were: general demographics (i.e., age, sex, and ethnicity), past medical history of underlying diseases (e.g., hypertension, diabetes, cardiovascular disease, kidney diseases, asthma, etc.), history of hospital stay (including length and any ICU admission), dominant SARS-CoV-2 variant during admission, body mass index (BMI), vaccination status, and glomerular filtration rate (GFR—based on serum creatinine).

2.4. Statistical Analysis

Continuous variables were described by mean (SD) for variables with a normal distribution (age, BMI, baseline hemoglobin, FU hemoglobin, hemoglobin change) or median (25th percentile, 75th percentile) for those that were not. Categorical data were described by frequency (percent). Characteristics were also stratified by sex since the reference range for anemia differs between males and females. The Paired-Samples T-test was utilized to compare parametric variables between two timepoints (baseline and first FU visit) and the Independent Samples Test was used to compare parametric variables between two different groups (fatigue patients vs. non-fatigue patients, male vs. female). Chi-square testing was employed while comparing categorical variables between these groups, and for comparing non-parametric variables between them, the Mann–Whitney U test was used. The correlations between hemoglobin levels and inflammatory biomarkers were evaluated via Pearson's correlation test for parametric values and Spearman's correlation for non-parametric ones. A false discovery rate (FDR) was not used as it can be overly conservative especially when validating a smaller number of previously described features or in cases where the effective number of tests is smaller (due to redundancy in similar features measuring the same latent variables) [35,36]. Finally, logistic regression models were developed to assess the relationships between fatigue at 3–6 months after infection and hemoglobin levels (1) in the acute phase, (2) 3–6 months after SARS-CoV-2 infection, and (3) the difference in hemoglobin levels between infection and follow-up. Fatigue was defined as a binary (yes/no) variable based on the pre-defined FSS cutoff of equal or greater than four (yes) or less than four (no). Unadjusted models and models adjusted for age and sex were generated. Covariates for adjustment were identified through the generation of a Directed Acyclic Graph (DAG) (Figure 1) [37]. According to this DAG, age, sex, ethnicity, BMI, underlying diseases, hospital admission, ICU admission, inflammation, and lung function were all identified confounders for the potential pathway of developing fatigue due to hemoglobin alteration. However, considering the sample size and a target of 20 events per covariate, only age and sex, identified as the most important potential confounders, were included in the regression analysis.

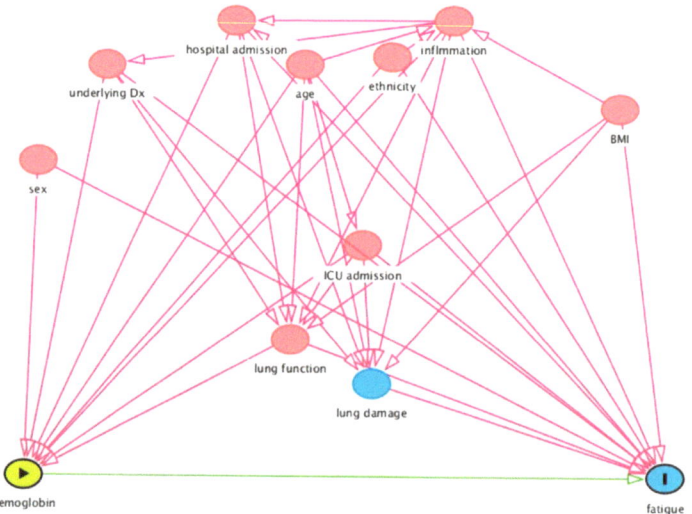

Figure 1. DAG for determining the confounders and effect modifiers in the relationship between hemoglobin levels and fatigue. Figure legend; ⊙ exposure, ⊙ outcome, ● ancestor of outcome, ● ancestor of exposure and outcome, ▬ (potentially) causal path, ▬ biasing path.

Since renal function has the potential to affect both hemoglobin and fatigue, we performed a sensitivity analysis by restricting the regression analysis to those with GFR at follow-up greater than 60 mL/min/1.73 m^2 (n = 56). This cut-off was chosen to differentiate those with normal/mild kidney dysfunction from more severe cases where the prevalence of anemia is higher [38–40]. Furthermore, since a case was detected among the participants with an extreme outlier value for hemoglobin (both baseline and FU), another sensitivity analysis was also performed after excluding this single case. All statistical analyses were performed by SPSS version 28 and a p-value ≤ 0.05 was considered statistically significant for all statistical tests.

3. Results

In total, 1 or more hemoglobin results were available from all 95 participants in the P4O2 COVID cohort, with 59 having data on the Hb level at both the acute phase and at FU (11 participants had missing data during the acute phase and 27 at FU). The mean age of our study population was 54.2 years, and 50.5% of them were men. Most of the participants (89.5%) were suffering from some form of underlying disease, and comorbidities were more common in men than in women (93.8% vs. 85.1%). According to the WHO severity index, most of the infections were categorized as moderate (61.3%)

or severe (28.0%). The characteristics that were significantly different between men and women were fatigue average score during the Long-COVID phase (83.3% in females and 68.9% in males, p-value = 0.026 according to Independent Samples Test), ICU admission (19.1% in women and 38.3% in men, p-value = 0.044 according to Chi-Square test), ICU stay (median 0 (0–0) days in women and median 0 (0–8) days in men, p-value = 0.044 according to Mann–Whitney U test), and BMI (32.2 in women and 28.9 in men, p-value = 0.002 according to Independent Samples Test) (Table 1).

Table 1. Characteristics of the study population.

Population Characteristics		Total (N = 95)	p-Value £	Female (N = 47)	Male (N = 48)
Demographic characteristics					
Age (mean, SD)		54.2 (6.2)	0.765	54.3 (6.1)	54.0 (6.3)
Ethnicity (N, %)	African	8 (9.4%)	0.077	5 (1.6%)	3 (7.0%)
	Asian	3 (3.5%)		2 (4.7%)	1 (2.3%)
	Caucasian	66 (76.7%)		33 (76.7%)	33 (76.7%)
	Latin-American	3 (3.5%)		3 (7.0%)	0 (0.0%)
	Others	6 (7.0%)		0 (0.0%)	6 (14.0%)
Clinical characteristics					
Suffering from any comorbidities (N, %)		85 (89.5%)	0.170	40 (85.1%)	45 (93.8%)
BMI (mean, SD)		30.39 (5.3)	0.002	32.15 (5.4%)	28.85 (4.7)
Dominant SARS-CoV-2 variant at the time of infection (N, %)	Alpha	43 (45.3%)	0.278	23 (48.9%)	20 (41.7%)
	Delta	41 (43.2%)		21 (44.7%)	20 (41.7%)
	Omicron	11 (11.6%)		3 (6.4%)	8 (16.7%)
Hospitalized (N, %)		85 (89.5%)	0.170	40 (85.1%)	45 (93.8%)
Hospital stay (days) (median, percentile 25–75) *		8.00 (4.0–15.2)	0.083	8.00 (3.0–13.0)	10.00 (5.0–21.0)
ICU admission (N, %)		27 (28.7%)	0.40	9 (19.1%)	18 (38.3%)
ICU stay (days) (median, percentile 25–75) *		0.00 (0.0–4.0)	0.044	0.00 (0.0–0.0)	0.00 (0.0–8.0)
One dosage of SARS-CoV-2 vaccination		66 (69.5%)	0.771	32 (68.1%)	34 (70.8%)
Two dosages of SARS-CoV-2 vaccination		41 (43.2%)	0.261	23 (48.9%)	18 (37.5%)
WHO severity index (N, %)	Mild	10 (10.8%)	0.240	7 (15.2%)	3 (6.4%)
	Moderate	57 (61.3%)		30 (65.2%)	27 (57.4%)
	Severe	26 (28.0%)		9 (19.6%)	17 (36.2%)
Average FSS during the 3–6 months visit (median, percentile 25–75) ¥		5.6 (4.1–6.3)	0.026	5.8 (4.7–6.4)	5.3 (3.0–6.3)
Fatigue (Average FSS ≥ 4) during the 3–6 months visit (N, %) ¥			0.116		
Yes		66 (69.5%)		35 (74.5%)	31 (68.9%)
No		21 (22.1%)		7 (14.9%)	14 (29.2%)
Missing		8 (8.4%)		5 (10.6%)	3 (63%)

* The number of days spent in the ICU or hospital for the participants who were not admitted were counted as 0. ¥ Fatigue data were missing for eight (five female and three male) participants. £ p-value for comparing variables between men and women.

3.1. Hemoglobin Levels

The mean hemoglobin level during SARS-CoV-2 infection for our entire study population was 8.6 mmol/L (8.35 mmol/L in women and 8.84 mmol/L in men) (Table 2), which is within the normal laboratory reference range (>7.5 in women and >8.5 in males). During the acute phase, the average hemoglobin concentration was 8.61 mmol/L and

8.70 mmol/L 3–6 months after infection (p-value for difference: 0.003 according to Paired-Samples T-test). Hemoglobin values were significantly different (via Independent Samples Test) between men and women both during the acute phase (8.84 vs. 8.35 mmol/L, respectively, p-value = 0.023) and at follow-up (9.04 vs. 8.36 mmol/L p-value = 0.003,) (Table 2). In patients with hemoglobin levels available at both time points (n = 59), the hemoglobin levels increased on average by 0.3 (from 8.41 mmol/L during the acute phase and 8.71 mmol/L 3–6 months after infection). This was more pronounced in men where the average hemoglobin increased from 8.89 mmol/L to 9.24 mmol/L (mean difference = 0.42 mmol/L). For female participants, the mean hemoglobin value remained the same at baseline and FU (8.35 mmol/L and 8.36 mmol/L, respectively, mean difference = 0.18 mmol/L). However, men and women's differences in hemoglobin change did not reach statistical significance (p-value = 0.222 according to Independent Samples Test). Consistent with this overall increase, hemoglobin levels at FU were higher for 66.1% of our participants (N = 39), with 14 having an increase of greater than 10%. However, 28.8% (N = 17) of the participants had lower hemoglobin levels at FU, with 8 showing a decrease of greater than 10%. Also, in three cases the hemoglobin level during FU remained the same as the baseline value.

Table 2. Hemoglobin level status and the prevalence of anemia in the P4O2 COVID-19 study.

Hb and Anemia Status		Total	Female	Male	p-Value	Experiencing Fatigue 3–6 Months after Infection ¶	No Fatigue 3–6 Months after Infection	p-Value π
Total number of participants		95	47	48	---	66	21	---
Hb ◊ level during the acute phase (mmol/L) (mean, SD) (n = 84)		8.61 (0.99)	8.35 (0.86)	8.84 (1.05)	**0.023**	8.53 (0.99)	8.89 (1.06)	0.171
Hb level during the 3–6 months visit (mmol/L) (mean, SD) (n = 68)		8.70 (0.98)	8.36 (0.87)	9.04 (1.00)	**0.004**	8.54 (0.99)	9.24 (0.99)	**0.046**
Hb level change (mmol/L) (mean, SD) ¥ (n = 59)		0.30 (0.74)	0.18 (0.80)	0.42 (0.67)	0.222	0.19 (0.73)	0.68 (0.69)	0.069
Clinically notable (10%) Hb change (N, %)	Hb decrease ‡	8 (8.4%)	4 (10.50%)	4 (9.50%)	0.881	6 (10.90%)	1 (5.90%)	1.000
	Hb increase Ł	15 (23.7%)	6 (15.80%)	9 (21.40%)	0.519	10 (18.20%)	3 (17.6%)	1.000
Hb level change μ (N, %)	Hb decrease *	17 (28.8%)	10 (34.50%)	7 (23.30%)	0.344	14 (32.20%)	1 (10.00%)	0.249
	Hb increase €	39 (66.1%)	19 (65.50%)	20 (66.70%)	0.926	26 (60.50%)	9 (90.00%)	0.137
Anemia during the acute phase (N, %) £ (n = 84)		19 (22.61%)	5 (12.80%)	14 (31.10%)	**0.046**	13 (23.2%)	4 (20%)	1.000
Anemia during the 3–6 months visit (N, %) £ (n = 68)		11 (16.41%)	5 (13.90%)	6 (18.80%)	0.587	10 (19.2%)	1 (10%)	0.674

Footnotes: ¶ fatigue data were missing for eight cases. π the p-values are related to the comparisons that have been performed for Hb levels/anemia status, between patients experiencing fatigue 3–6 months after infection and those who did not. ◊ normal Hb range is >7.5 in women and >8.5 in males. ¥ follow-up Hb–baseline Hb (difference between baseline and follow-up Hb; there were missing data for 36 (37.90%) cases. ‡ cases with follow-up Hb–baseline Hb < 0.10 × baseline Hb. Ł cases with baseline Hb–follow-up Hb < 0.10 × baseline Hb. * cases with follow-up Hb < baseline Hb. € cases with follow-up Hb > baseline Hb. £ Hb level less than 7.5 mmol/L in women and less than 8.5 mmol/L in men. μ For three cases the baseline Hb was exactly the same as the FH Hb and they had no Hb change. p-values showing statistically significant difference between compared groups have been marked in bold font.

The prevalence of anemia during the acute phase of SARS-CoV-2 infection was 22.6% (19 cases, among whom 7 continued experiencing anemia during follow-up, 8 did not, and data were unavailable for four). This reduced to 16.4% at follow-up (n = 11, 3 were new-onset and 7 were persistent from the acute phase, and data were missing for 1, Table S1). Suffering from anemia was more common in men compared to women during both phases of COVID-19 disease (31.1% versus 12.8% during the acute phase (p-value = 0.046 according to Chi-Square Test) and 18.8% versus 13.9% during the Long-COVID phase (p-value = 0.587 according to Chi-Square Test).

We also examined demographic and clinical characteristics, by dividing the population into notable hemoglobin change (notable decrease versus notable increase or no change). Of note, the group with a notable decrease in hemoglobin had a longer hospital stay than those without (17 days vs. 8 days, Table S2).

When comparing hemoglobin levels between those with and without fatigue 3–6 months after infection, we observed that those experiencing fatigue had lower levels of hemoglobin both at baseline (8.53 vs. 8.89 mmol/L, respectively, p-value = 0.171 according to Independent Samples Test) and at FU (8.54 vs. 9.24 mmol/L, p-value = 0.046 according to Independent Samples Test) than those without fatigue (Table 2). Boxplots displaying the difference in hemoglobin level between those with fatigue versus those without are shown in Figure 2.

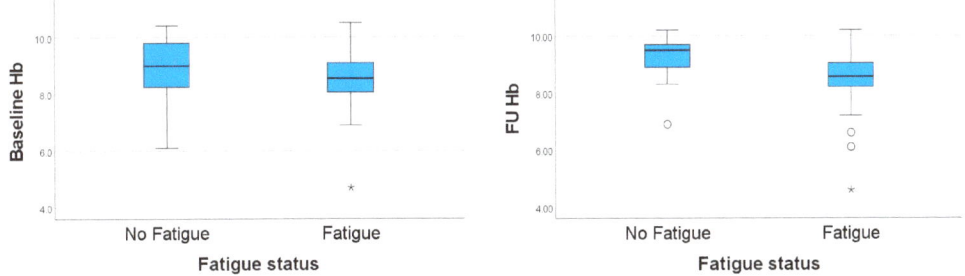

Figure 2. Boxplots for assessing the difference in hemoglobin levels between fatigue and non-fatigue cases. Figure legend: O: mild outlier, *: extreme outlier. *Footnotes:* 1. fatigue status data were missing for 8 cases, and considering the missing data for Hb variables, this graph includes information from 52 cases. 2. The extreme outlier in both baseline and FU figure belongs to the same case.

3.2. Correlations between Hemoglobin and Inflammatory Biomarkers

Results of Spearman correlation tests demonstrated that there were no strong or statistically significant correlations between hemoglobin levels (at baseline, follow-up, and the change in hemoglobin levels) and inflammatory biomarkers (Table 3). Among other variables that were found to be linked with hemoglobin level according to the DAG (Figure 1), the duration of hospital stay, as well as ICU stay had a positive correlation with hemoglobin change (rs = 0.268, and rs = 0.360, respectively) (Table S3).

Table 3. Correlations between hemoglobin measures and inflammatory indices.

Variable	Median (Percentile 25–75)	cc * with Hb Change	N Ɫ	cc with Baseline Hb	N	cc with FU Hb	N
Baseline CRP	91.00 (31.40–152.00)	0.031	59	0.018	84	−0.012	50
FU CRP	2.40 (1.85–6.30)	−0.002	49	NA ‡	50	−0.265	54
Baseline LDH	365.00 (272.00–516.00)	0.082	46	0.012	64	0.089	46
FU LDH	200.00 (170.00–244.75)	0.002	51	NA	51	−0.126	55
Baseline IG	0.03 (0.01–0.08)	0.072	30	0.108	36	0.331	30
FU IG	0.02 (0.01–0.03)	0.075	25	NA	25	−0.006	28
Baseline CPK	102.00 (57.00–298.00)	0.070	34	0.053	52	−0.003	34
FU CPK	72.00 (66.00–100.00)	0.033	31	NA	31	0.084	34
Baseline NLR	5.05 (3.07–7.14)	0.242	46	−0.071	55	0.133	46
FU NLR	1.63 (1.29–2.13)	0.294	36	NA	45	−0.018	49
Baseline D-dimer	0.75 (0.54–2.20)	0.206	55	−0.093	80	−0.030	55

Abbreviations: CRP: C-reactive protein, LDH: Lactate Dehydrogenase, IG: Immature Granulocyte, CPK: creatine phosphokinase, NLR: Neutrophil/Lymphocyte ratio. * Correlation coefficient. Ɫ number of cases in which correlation analysis between them and Hb change has been performed. ‡ NA: not applicable; our research hypothesis did not consider the relationship between FU inflammatory biomarkers and baseline Hb, since the outcome (Hb concentrations) would precede the exposures in this analysis.

3.3. Associations between Hemoglobin Levels and Fatigue

Results of logistic regression analysis indicated that higher venous hemoglobin concentrations were associated with lower odds of fatigue 3–6 months after infection (Table 4). While findings were non-significant, an association between increased Hb, and reduced fatigue was consistently observed. The strongest associations were observed with hemoglobin levels 3–6 months after infection where increased hemoglobin was associated with a reduced likelihood of fatigue. A 1 mmol/L increase in hemoglobin was associated with an adjusted odds ratio of 0.35 for fatigue (95%CI 0.12–1.02). Another strong relationship between fatigue and hemoglobin indices was observed for the change in hemoglobin levels, where a 1 mmol/L positive increase in Hb (i.e., greater in visit 2 than visit 1) resulted in an adjusted OR of 0.38 (95% CI 0.13–1.09). There was also a positive association between fatigue and anemia at both baseline and at follow-up (adjusted OR 1.56 [95% CI 0.42–5.78] and OR 2.25 [95% CI 0.25–20.20], respectively).

Table 4. Associations of hemoglobin levels and anemia with fatigue 3–6 months after SARS-CoV-2 infection (average FSS ≥ 4).

	Unadjusted	Adjusted *
	OR ‡ (95% CI)	OR (95% CI)
Baseline Hb levels	0.676 (0.386–1.184)	0.760 (0.430–1.342)
Follow-up Hb levels	0.370 (0.141–0.969)	0.350 (0.120–1.015)
Hb change	0.380 (0.133–1.081)	0.377 (0.130–1.091)
Baseline anemia	1.209 (0.343–4.259)	1.557 (0.420–5.779)
Follow-up anemia	2.143 (0.243–18.919)	2.246 (0.250–20.203)

* Adjusted for age and sex. ‡ Per 1 mmol/L increase in Hb levels.

Results of the sensitivity analysis where patients with impaired renal function were excluded showed associations that were directionally consistent and comparable to those in the total population. For example, the adjusted ORs of the associations between fatigue and FU hemoglobin and hemoglobin change were, respectively, 0.475 (95% CI 0.159–1.419) per 1 mmol/L increase in hemoglobin, and 0.467 (95% CI 0.150–1.452) per 1 mmol/L increase in hemoglobin (Table S4). In addition, the results of the other sensitivity analysis, which excluded the case with the extreme outlier data for the hemoglobin variable, showed barely any variation from the findings of the regression analysis in the total population (Table S5).

4. Discussion

In the current study, we aimed to assess the role of hemoglobin levels during the acute phase of SARS-CoV-2 infection and 3–6 months after follow-up against inflammatory biomarkers and fatigue in the P4O2 COVID-19 study. Overall, we found that hemoglobin levels increased between the acute and follow-up phases and that the average hemoglobin concentrations in our study population were within the normal range. The proportion of anemic patients also decreased, from 22.6% to 16.4%. However, hemoglobin levels were significantly lower, both at baseline and at follow-up, in patients with fatigue compared to patients without fatigue. No correlations were detected between hemoglobin and inflammatory biomarkers.

Other work examining anemic COVID-19 patients has reported that the SARS-CoV-2 virus is a contributor to both causing and exacerbating anemia [39]. Further, anemia itself has also been shown to play a role in prolonging COVID-19 symptoms [41]. It is therefore possible that anemia, either pre-existing or caused by acute infection, may contribute to some (but not all) of the fatigue symptoms in those who suffer from Long-COVID [42]. In a similar study of 145 former COVID-19 patients, it was reported that while the prevalence of anemia, hyperferritinemia, and systemic thrombo-inflammation all gradually decreased, a sizable portion of the post-COVID population still showed persistent anemia (4.65–11.1%) or iron deficiency (16–35%) at different FU evaluation time points, which may have contributed to their ongoing symptom burden, including fatigue [43].

Fatigue is a multifaceted condition and although its specific etiology can be uncertain, it is usually identified as the main manifestation of anemic patients [44,45] Our regression analysis demonstrated that hemoglobin levels are lower in Long-COVID patients who suffer from fatigue in both the acute phase and 3–6 months afterward. This suggests that hemoglobin may play a role in the fatigue symptoms of Long-COVID patients. Nevertheless, as the current study is observational in nature, further investigation is necessary to establish causation as the link between anemia and fatigue is not always evident. For example, a review of the contributors to persistent fatigue in Myelodysplastic syndrome patients revealed that no clear association has been found between fatigue and anemia. [46]. Therefore, other potential factors including inflammation, sleep-related problems, and oxidative stress may provide alternate explanations.

Another finding in our study suggesting a role of hemoglobin in fatigue is that we also observed a higher percentage of women who reported fatigue (83.3% in women vs. 68.9% in men), while their mean hemoglobin level in the Long-COVID phase was lower than in men (8.36 vs. 9.04). However, BMI was also significantly different between men and women, which can also be associated with fatigue [47,48]. Another characteristic that varied between males and females was hemoglobin change, where men showed a higher rate of increase than women. Previous research has reported that increased erythropoiesis is a secondary outcome of higher testosterone concentrations in men [49], which may explain the difference observed here.

These findings may have potential clinical implications, providing evidence for physicians to consider monitoring the hemoglobin levels in their Long-COVID patients, particularly in those suffering from fatigue as their primary symptom. Whether fatigue can be managed by treating any underlying hemoglobin impairment is outside the scope of the current work; however, it is worth closer evaluation.

We did not observe any correlation between inflammatory markers and hemoglobin concentrations. This stands in contrast to other work such as that of Lanser et al., who examined inflammation-mediated anemia, reporting the impact of *immune* system stimulation and cytokine-mediated alterations on iron homeostasis [16]. The three inflammatory variables that they assessed in their study were ferritin, IL-6, and CRP—of which we only studied CRP. This difference may illustrate that only extremely severe inflammation can affect hemoglobin values, that our sample size was insufficient to identify an effect, or that the inflammatory biomarkers available for use in the current study were not optimal for the evaluation of inflammatory-driven Hb disruption. For example, the erythropoiesis-suppressing effects of specific inflammatory cytokines, such as TNFα, IL-1, and interferon-γ, have been reported in various investigations. Therefore, a broader assessment of inflammatory markers alongside other diagnostic tests for anemia related to inflammation (serum iron, ferritin, and hepcidin), may be a more accurate way to assess the correlation between anemia and inflammation [50]. For example, in an analysis of 214 ex-COVID-19 patients, where all aforementioned variables were included, patients who reported Long-COVID Syndrome months after the acute phase were distinguished by inflammation and abnormal iron homeostasis that lasted longer than two weeks after the onset of symptoms. This led the researchers to conclude that the effects of inflammatory iron dysregulation on erythropoiesis and blood oxygen transportation may be partially responsible for several of the characteristics of Long-COVID [51]. Alternately this might suggest that factors other than inflammation have a more significant role. For example, there is evidence that SARS-CoV-2 infection can produce hemolytic anemia by either generating structural changes in host cells (RBCs) via viral invasion or activating autoantibodies [52]. The fact that we could not validate the same link between inflammation and Hb that was reported by Hanson et al. emphasizes the need to further test the robustness of biomarker analyses [51]. Furthermore, a meta-analysis reviewing the studies evaluating the COVID-19 biomarkers revealed a number of findings, including different results per population, which highlights the significance of validation studies [53]. Especially, since long COVID is a relatively young disease correlations with biomarkers in one population should be validated in other populations. Additional work is therefore needed to further understand the mechanism of hemoglobin decrease in SARS-CoV-2 infection, and how (or if) these factors persist long-term.

An alternative to the proposed hemoglobin and inflammatory biomarkers explored here is the evidence-based association with oxidative stress [54]. Experiments have shown that oxidative stress significantly impacts the structure of hemoporphyrin, which in turn affects hemoglobin function and reduces the efficiency with which hemoglobin binds to oxygen. This process is caused by lipid peroxidation (LPO), which is followed by the formation of LPO's primary and end products [55]. Understanding the potential role of oxidative stress in the development of hemoglobin decrease would be a significant finding that may lead to preventative and therapeutic approaches [56,57].

Among this study's strengths is its well-defined population of Long-COVID patients, who have comprehensive information, including hospital and personal data. Additionally, these patients have an extensive list of fatigue symptoms obtained through standard fatigue questionnaires. However, this study also has some limitations. First, while SARS-CoV-2 infection is the exclusive focus of this investigation, it has been revealed that other viral infections, such as seasonal influenza, may have long-term effects similar to those following SARS-CoV-2 infection [58]. Thus, it is uncertain whether our findings are specific to this particular viral infectious disease, or indicative of post-viral syndromes more broadly. Our limited sample size restricts the overall statistical power, including for regression analysis, and limits the external generalizability of our findings. Further compounding this was missing values for several variables of interest, particularly the baseline variables of inflammatory biomarkers. Such data were only available if they had been ordered during the original presentation and admission in different hospitals. Imputation was considered but ultimately decided against as these were outcome variables. Towards the later part of the pandemic, follow-up visits were more often occurring remotely, meaning that biological sampling at this point was reduced. Furthermore, not having pre-infection hemoglobin data makes evaluating acute changes impossible. In addition, it has been shown that vaccination against SARS-CoV-2 might enhance the likelihood of hematologic problems, such as anemia [59] and on the other hand, that receiving the vaccine prior to SARS-CoV-2 infection might be associated with a lower risk of developing Long-COVID [60]. However, since the vaccination pattern varied greatly (Tables S6 and S7) and our sample size was not large enough, we were unable to analyze the association between anemia and vaccination status in our population. Finally, this cohort was started at a point in time when not much was known about Long-COVID and therefore no specific age group was known to be important at that time, and it seemed that it was mainly affecting individuals of 40 years and older. In addition, because older patients (above 65) are more likely to have more comorbidities that may interfere with the analysis we decided to limit our population to below that age. Thus, the age range of our study population (40 to 65 years) makes us more cautious in generalizing our findings to other age ranges.

5. Conclusions

In our study of Long-COVID patients, we observed that those with fatigue tended to have lower hemoglobin levels than those without. These findings suggest a role of hemoglobin in Long-COVID fatigue. To determine the causes of low hemoglobin levels in Long-COVID patients and in turn, the best course of action for treatment, further studies on the mechanisms influencing hemoglobin levels in Long-COVID are necessary. Furthermore, it is important to perform validation studies to examine whether our findings are reproducible and robust across different cohorts.

Supplementary Materials: The following supporting information can be downloaded at https://www.mdpi.com/article/10.3390/biomedicines12061234/s1, Table S1: Frequency and persistence of anemia in the study population; Table S2: Characteristics of study population according to hemoglobin level change; Table S3: Correlations between hemoglobin levels and demographic and clinical characteristics; Table S4: Results of logistic regression model for Hemoglobin and fatigue (average FSS ≥ 4) for cases with GFR of mild renal dysfunction or better (≥ 60 mL/min/1.73m^2, N = 56); Table S5: Results of logistic regression model for Hemoglobin and fatigue (average FSS ≥ 4) after excluding the case with extreme outlier for hemoglobin; Table S6: Frequency of SARS-CoV-2 vaccination (main dosage) in the study population; Table S7: Type of SARS-CoV-2 vaccination in the study population.

Author Contributions: Conceptualization, S.B., A.H.M.-v.d.Z., G.S.D., L.D.B., Y.v.W. and R.J.H.C.G.B.; methodology, S.B., A.H.M.-v.d.Z., L.D.B., G.S.D. and Y.v.W.; software, S.B., L.D.B. and J.M.B.; validation, S.B., A.H.M.-v.d.Z., G.S.D., L.D.B., Y.v.W., R.J.H.C.G.B., N.B., B.M.S., M.E.B.C. and J.M.B.; formal analysis, S.B. and J.M.B.; investigation, A.H.M.-v.d.Z., Y.v.W., R.J.H.C.G.B., B.M.S., N.B., S.B., M.E.B.C. and L.D.B.; resources, A.H.M.-v.d.Z., Y.v.W., B.M.S., R.J.H.C.G.B., N.B., S.B., M.E.B.C., L.D.B. and J.M.B.; data curation, A.H.M.-v.d.Z., Y.v.W., G.S.D., N.B., S.B., M.E.B.C., L.D.B. and J.M.B.; writing—original draft preparation, S.B.; writing—review and editing, all authors; visualization, S.B.; supervision, A.H.M.-v.d.Z., G.S.D., L.D.B. and Y.v.W.; project administration, A.H.M.-v.d.Z., L.D.B., Y.v.W., N.B. and M.E.B.C.; funding acquisition, A.H.M.-v.d.Z. All authors have read and agreed to the published version of the manuscript.

Funding: Partners in the Precision Medicine for more Oxygen (P4O2) consortium are the Amsterdam UMC, Leiden University Medical Center, Maastricht UMC+, Maastricht University, UMC Groningen, UMC Utrecht, Utrecht University, TNO, Abbvie, Aparito, Boehringer Ingelheim, Breathomix, Clear, Danone Nutricia Research, Fluidda, Ncardia, Olive, Ortec Logiqcare, Philips, Proefdiervrij, Quantib-U, RespiQ, Roche, Smartfish, SODAQ, Thirona, TopMD, Lung Alliance Netherlands (LAN), and the Lung Foundation Netherlands (Longfonds). The consortium is additionally funded by the PPP Allowance made available by Health~Holland, Top Sector Life Sciences & Health (LSHM20104; LSHM20068), to stimulate public-private partnerships and by Novartis. Prof. Dr. Anke-Hilse Maitland-van der Zee is the PI of P4O2.

Institutional Review Board Statement: This study was conducted according to the guidelines of the Declaration of Helsinki, and approved by the ethical committee of Amsterdam UMC (reference number NL74701.018.20), and all participants provided written informed consent prior to their enrolment.

Informed Consent Statement: Informed consent was obtained from all subjects involved in the study.

Data Availability Statement: The data presented in this study are available upon request to the corresponding author. The data are not publicly available due to agreements made by the consortium, that only allow access by each consortium partner to specific data that answer their pre-specified research questions. A request for access to data by organizations outside of the consortium can be submitted to the P4O2 Data Committee (via p4o2@amsterdamumc.nl) and the research will need to be performed in collaboration with one of the P4O2 consortium partners.

Conflicts of Interest: The authors declare no conflicts of interest. The funders had no role in the design of the study; in the collection, analyses, or interpretation of data; in the writing of the manuscript; or in the decision to publish the results.

References

1. Davis, H.E.; McCorkell, L.; Vogel, J.M.; Topol, E.J. Long COVID: Major findings, mechanisms and recommendations. *Nat. Rev. Microbiol.* **2023**, *21*, 133–146. [CrossRef] [PubMed]
2. Saunders, C.; Sperling, S.; Bendstrup, E. A new paradigm is needed to explain long COVID. The Lancet. *Respir. Med.* **2023**, *11*, e12–e13.
3. Wahlgren, C.; Forsberg, G.; Divanoglou, A.; Balkhed Å, Ö.; Niward, K.; Berg, S.; Levi, R. Two-year follow-up of patients with post-COVID-19 condition in Sweden: A prospective cohort study. *Lancet Reg. Health–Eur.* **2023**, *28*, 100595. [CrossRef] [PubMed]
4. COVID, Gemelli Against, and Post-Acute Care Study Group. Post-COVID-19 global health strategies: The need for an interdisciplinary approach. *Aging Clin. Exp. Res.* **2020**, *1*, 1613–1620.
5. NICE. *COVID-19 Rapid Guideline: Managing the Long-Term Effects of COVID-19*; National Institute for Health and Care Excellence (NICE): London, UK, 2020.
6. Crook, H.; Raza, S.; Nowell, J.; Young, M.; Edison, P. Long covid—Mechanisms, risk factors, and management. *BMJ* **2021**, *26*, 374. [CrossRef] [PubMed]
7. Vaes, A.W.; Goërtz, Y.M.; Van Herck, M.; Machado, F.V.; Meys, R.; Delbressine, J.M.; Houben-Wilke, S.; Gaffron, S.; Maier, D.; Burtin, C.; et al. Recovery from COVID-19: A sprint or marathon? 6-month follow-up data from online long COVID-19 support group members. *ERJ Open Res.* **2021**, *7*, 00141-2021. [CrossRef] [PubMed]

8. Ayoubkhani, D.; Khunti, K.; Nafilyan, N.; Maddox, T.; Humberstone, B.; Diamond, S.I.; Banerjee, A. Epidemiology of post-COVID syndrome following hospitalisation with coronavirus: A retrospective cohort study. *MedRxiv* **2021**. [CrossRef]
9. Castanares-Zapatero, D.; Chalon, P.; Kohn, L.; Dauvrin, M.; Detollenaere, J.; de Noordhout, C.M.; Jong, C.P.-D.; Cleemput, I.; Heede, K.V.D. Pathophysiology and mechanism of long COVID: A comprehensive review. *Ann. Med.* **2022**, *54*, 1473–1487. [CrossRef]
10. Montani, D.; Savale, L.; Noel, N.; Meyrignac, O.; Colle, R.; Gasnier, M.; Corruble, E.; Beurnier, A.; Jutant, E.M.; Pham, T.; et al. Post-acute COVID-19 syndrome. *Eur. Respir. Rev.* **2022**, *31*, 163. [CrossRef]
11. Wong, J.J.M.; Abbas, Q.; Liauw, F.; Malisie, R.F.; Gan, C.S.; Abid, M.; Efar, P.; Gloriana, J.; Chuah, S.L.; Sultana, R.; et al. Development and validation of a clinical predictive model for severe and critical pediatric COVID-19 infection. *PLoS ONE* **2022**, *17*, e0275761. [CrossRef]
12. Anai, M.; Akaike, K.; Iwagoe, H.; Akasaka, T.; Higuchi, T.; Miyazaki, A.; Naito, D.; Tajima, Y.; Takahashi, H.; Komatsu, T.; et al. Decrease in hemoglobin level predicts increased risk for severe respiratory failure in COVID-19 patients with pneumonia. *Respir. Investig.* **2021**, *59*, 187–193. [CrossRef]
13. Russo, A.; Tellone, E.; Barreca, D.; Ficarra, S.; Laganà, G. Implication of COVID-19 on Erythrocytes Functionality: Red Blood Cell Biochemical Implications and Morpho-Functional Aspects. *Int. J. Mol. Sci.* **2022**, *23*, 2171. [CrossRef]
14. Lopes, D.V.; Neto, F.L.; Marques, L.C.; Lima, R.B.; Brandão, A.A.G.S. Methemoglobinemia and hemolytic anemia after COVID-19 infection without identifiable eliciting drug: A case-report. *IDCases* **2021**, *23*, e01013. [CrossRef] [PubMed]
15. Scholkmann, F.; Restin, T.; Ferrari, M.; Quaresima, V. The role of methemoglobin and carboxyhemoglobin in COVID-19: A review. *J. Clin. Med.* **2020**, *10*, 50. [CrossRef]
16. Lanser, L.; Burkert, F.R.; Bellmann-Weiler, R.; Schroll, A.; Wildner, S.; Fritsche, G.; Weiss, G. Dynamics in anemia development and dysregulation of iron homeostasis in hospitalized patients with COVID-19. *Metabolites* **2021**, *11*, 653. [CrossRef]
17. Bellmann-Weiler, R.; Lanser, L.; Barket, R.; Rangger, L.; Schapfl, A.; Schaber, M.; Fritsche, G.; Wöll, E.; Weiss, G. Prevalence and predictive value of anemia and dysregulated iron homeostasis in patients with COVID-19 infection. *J. Clin. Med.* **2020**, *9*, 2429. [CrossRef]
18. Chaparro, C.M.; Parminder, S.S. Anemia epidemiology, pathophysiology, and etiology in low-and middle-income countries. *Ann. N. Y. Acad. Sci.* **2019**, *1450*, 15–31. [CrossRef] [PubMed]
19. Cappellini, M.D.; Irene, M. Anemia in Clinical Practice-Definition and Classification: Does Hemoglobin Change with Aging? *Semin. Hematol.* **2015**, *52*, 261–269. [CrossRef] [PubMed]
20. Vieth, J.T.; Lane, D.R. Anemia. *Emerg. Med. Clin.* **2014**, *32*, 613–628. [CrossRef]
21. Gregg, L.P.; Bossola, M.; Ostrosky-Frid, M.; Hedayati, S.S. Fatigue in CKD: Epidemiology, pathophysiology, and treatment. *Clin. J. Am. Soc. Nephrol.* **2021**, *16*, 1445–1455. [CrossRef]
22. Sandler, C.X.; Wyller VB, B.; Moss-Morris, R.; Buchwald, D.; Crawley, E.; Hautvast, J.; Katz, B.Z.; Knoop, H.; Little, P.; Taylor, R.; et al. Long COVID and post-infective fatigue syndrome: A review. In *Open Forum Infectious Diseases*; Oxford University Press: Oxford, UK, 2021; Volume 8.
23. Maisel, P.; Erika, B.; Norbert, D.-B. Fatigue as the Chief Complaint: Epidemiology, Causes, Diagnosis, and Treatment. *Dtsch. Ärzteblatt Int.* **2021**, *118*, 566.
24. Pasini, E.; Corsetti, G.; Romano, C.; Scarabelli, T.M.; Chen-Scarabelli, C.; Saravolatz, L.; Dioguardi, F.S. Serum metabolic profile in patients with long-Covid (PASC) syndrome: Clinical implications. *Front. Med.* **2021**, *1182*, 714426. [CrossRef]
25. Fernández-De-Las-Peñas, C.; Ryan-Murua, P.; Rodríguez-Jiménez, J.; Palacios-Ceña, M.; Arendt-Nielsen, L.; Torres-Macho, J. Serological biomarkers at hospital admission are not related to long-term post-COVID fatigue and dyspnea in COVID-19 survivors. *Respiration* **2022**, *101*, 658–665. [CrossRef] [PubMed]
26. Baalbaki, N.; Blankestijn, J.M.; Abdel-Aziz, M.I.; de Backer, J.; Bazdar, S.; Beekers, I.; Beijers, R.J.H.C.G.; Bergh, J.P.v.D.; Bloemsma, L.D.; Bogaard, H.J.; et al. Precision Medicine for More Oxygen (P4O2)—Study Design and First Results of the Long COVID-19 Extension. *J. Pers. Med.* **2023**, *13*, 1060. [CrossRef] [PubMed]
27. Cardoso, P.; Nielsen, B.B.; Hvidman, L.; Nielsen, J.; Aaby, P. Effect of sublingual misoprostol on severe postpartum haemorrhage in a primary health centre in Guinea-Bissau: Randomised double blind clinical trial. *BMJ* **2005**, *331*, 723.
28. Atukunda, E.C.; Mugyenyi, G.R.; Obua, C.; Atuhumuza, E.B.; Musinguzi, N.; Tornes, Y.F.; Agaba, A.G.; Siedner, M.J. Measuring post-partum haemorrhage in low-resource settings: The diagnostic validity of weighed blood loss versus quantitative changes in hemoglobin. *PLoS ONE* **2016**, *11*, e0152408. [CrossRef] [PubMed]
29. Hamm, R.F.; Wang, E.; Romanos, A.; O'Rourke, K.; Srinivas, S.K. Implementation of quantification of blood loss does not improve prediction of hemoglobin drop in deliveries with average blood loss. *Am. J. Perinatol.* **2018**, *35*, 134–139. [CrossRef]
30. Jerković, A.; Proroković, A.; Matijaca, M.; Katić, A.Ć.; Košta, V.; Mihalj, M.; Dolić, K.; Đogaš, Z.; Vidaković, M.R. Validation of the fatigue severity scale in Croatian population of patients with multiple sclerosis disease: Factor structure, internal consistency, and correlates. *Mult. Scler. Relat. Disord.* **2022**, *58*, 103397. [CrossRef]
31. Lerdal, A. *Fatigue severity scale. Encyclopedia of Quality of Life and Well-Being Research*; Springer International Publishing: Cham, Switzerland, 2021; pp. 1–5.
32. Samprathi, M.; Muralidharan, J. Biomarkers in COVID-19: An up-to-date review. *Front. Pediatr.* **2021**, *8*, 607647. [CrossRef]

33. Budhiraja, S.; Indrayan, A.; Das, P.; Dewan, A.; Singh, O.; Nangia, V.; Singh, Y.P.; Pandey, R.; Gupta, A.K.; Gupta, M.; et al. Relative Importance of Various Inflammatory Markers and Their Critical Thresholds for COVID-19 Mortality. *medRxiv* **2021**. [CrossRef]
34. Alisik, M.; Erdogan, U.G.; Ates, M.; Sert, M.A.; Yis, O.M.; Bugdayci, G. Predictive value of immature granulocyte count and other inflammatory parameters for disease severity in COVID-19 patients. *Int. J. Med. Biochem.* **2021**, *4*, 143–149.
35. Li, J.; Ji, L. Adjusting multiple testing in multilocus analyses using the eigenvalues of a correlation matrix. *Heredity* **2005**, *95*, 221–227. [CrossRef] [PubMed]
36. Wen, S.-H.; Lu, Z.-S. Factors affecting the effective number of tests in genetic association studies: A comparative study of three PCA-based methods. *J. Hum.* **2011**, *56*, 6. [CrossRef]
37. Textor, J.; Van der Zander, B.; Gilthorpe, M.S.; Liśkiewicz, M.; Ellison, G.T. Robust causal inference using directed acyclic graphs: The R package 'dagitty'. *Int. J. Epidemiol.* **2016**, *45*, 1887–1894. [CrossRef] [PubMed]
38. Gluba-Brzózka, A.; Franczyk, B.; Olszewski, R.; Rysz, J. The influence of inflammation on anemia in CKD patients. *Int. J. Mol. Sci.* **2020**, *21*, 725. [CrossRef] [PubMed]
39. Kim, B.; Kim, G.; Kim, E.; Park, J.; Isobe, T.; Sakae, T.; Oh, S. The a body shape index might be a stronger predictor of chronic kidney disease than BMI in a senior population. *Int. J. Environ. Res. Public Health* **2021**, *18*, 12874. [CrossRef] [PubMed]
40. National Kidney Foundation. eGFR Calculator. Available online: https://www.kidney.org/professionals/kdoqi/gfr_calculator (accessed on 27 November 2023).
41. Abu-Ismail, L.; Taha MJ, J.; Abuawwad, M.T.; Al-Bustanji, Y.; Al-Shami, K.; Nashwan, A.; Yassin, M. COVID-19 and anemia: What do we know so far? *Hemoglobin* **2023**, *47*, 122–129. [CrossRef] [PubMed]
42. Lechuga, G.C.; Carlos, M.M.; Salvatore, G.D.-S. Hematological alterations associated with long COVID-19. *Front. Physiol.* **2023**, *14*, 1203472. [CrossRef]
43. Sonnweber, T.; Grubwieser, P.; Sahanic, S.; Böhm, A.K.; Pizzini, A.; Luger, A.; Schwabl, C.; Koppelstätter, S.; Kurz, K.; Puchner, B.; et al. The impact of iron dyshomeostasis and anaemia on long-term pulmonary recovery and persisting symptom burden after COVID-19: A prospective observational cohort study. *Metabolites* **2022**, *12*, 546. [CrossRef]
44. Sobrero, A.; Puglisi, F.; Grossi, F. Fatigue: A main component of anemia symptomatology. In *Seminars in Oncology*; WB Saunders: Philadelphia, PE, USA, 2001; Volume 28.
45. Prochaska, M.T.; Zhang, H.; Alavi, C.; Meltzer, D.O. Fatigability: A new perspective on and patient-centered outcome measure for patients with anemia. *Am. J. Hematol.* **2020**, *95*, E166. [CrossRef]
46. Brownstein, C.G.; Daguenet, E.; Guyotat, D.; Millet, G.Y. Chronic fatigue in myelodysplastic syndromes: Looking beyond anemia. *Crit. Rev. Oncol./Hematol.* **2020**, *154*, 103067. [CrossRef] [PubMed]
47. Lim, W.; Hong, S.; Nelesen, R.; Dimsdale, J.E. The association of obesity, cytokine levels, and depressive symptoms with diverse measures of fatigue in healthy subjects. *Arch. Intern. Med.* **2005**, *165*, 910–915. [CrossRef] [PubMed]
48. Resnick, H.E.; Carter, E.A.; Aloia, M.; Phillips, B. Cross-sectional relationship of reported fatigue to obesity, diet, and physical activity: Results from the third national health and nutrition examination survey. *J. Clin. Sleep Med.* **2006**, *2*, 163–169. [CrossRef] [PubMed]
49. Garcia-Casal, M.N.; Dary, O.; Jefferds, M.E.; Pasricha, S.R. Diagnosing anemia: Challenges selecting methods, addressing underlying causes, and implementing actions at the public health level. *Ann. N. Y. Acad. Sci.* **2023**, *1524*, 37–50. [CrossRef] [PubMed]
50. Nemeth, E.; Tomas, G. Anemia of inflammation. *Hematol./Oncol. Clin. N. Am.* **2014**, *28*, 671–681. [CrossRef] [PubMed]
51. Hanson, A.L.; Mulè, M.P.; Ruffieux, H.; Mescia, F.; Bergamaschi, L.; Pelly, V.S.; Turner, L.; Kotagiri, P.; Göttgens, B.; Hess, C.; et al. Iron dysregulation and inflammatory stress erythropoiesis associates with long-term outcome of COVID-19. *Nat. Immunol.* **2024**, *25*, 471–482. [CrossRef] [PubMed]
52. Al-Kuraishy, H.M.; Al-Gareeb, A.I.; Kaushik, A.; Kujawska, M.; Batiha, G.E.-S. Hemolytic anemia in COVID-19. *Ann. Hematol.* **2022**, *101*, 1887–1895. [CrossRef] [PubMed]
53. Onoja, A.; von Gerichten, J.; Lewis, H.-M.; Bailey, M.J.; Skene, D.J.; Geifman, N.; Spick, M. Meta-Analysis of COVID-19 Metabolomics Identifies Variations in Robustness of Biomarkers. *Int. J. Mol. Sci.* **2023**, *24*, 14371. [CrossRef]
54. Mironova, G.D.; Belosludtseva, N.V.; Ananyan, M.A. Prospects for the use of regulators of oxidative stress in the comprehensive treatment of the novel Coronavirus Disease 2019 (COVID-19) and its complications. *Eur. Rev. Med. Pharmacol. Sci.* **2020**, *24*, 8585–8591.
55. Revin, V.V.; Gromova, N.V.; Revina, E.S.; Samonova, A.Y.; Tychkov, A.Y.; Bochkareva, S.S.; Moskovkin, A.A.; Kuzmenko, T.P. The Influence of Oxidative Stress and Natural Antioxidants on Morphometric Parameters of Red Blood Cells, the Hemoglobin Oxygen Binding Capacity, and the Activity of Antioxidant Enzymes. *BioMed Res. Int.* **2019**, *2019*, 2109269. [CrossRef]
56. Chudow, M.; Beatrice, A. ABC's of vitamin supplementation in critical illness. *J. Pharm. Pract.* **2021**, *34*, 934–942. [CrossRef] [PubMed]
57. Atanasovska, E.; Petrusevska, M.; Zendelovska, D.; Spasovska, K.; Stevanovikj, M.; Kasapinova, K.; Gjorgjievska, K.; Labachevski, N. Vitamin D levels and oxidative stress markers in patients hospitalized with COVID-19. *Redox Rep.* **2021**, *26*, 184–189. [CrossRef] [PubMed]
58. Xie, Y.; Choi, T.; Al-Aly, Z. Long-term outcomes following hospital admission for COVID-19 versus seasonal influenza: A cohort study. *Lancet Infect. Dis.* **2024**, *24*, 239–255. [CrossRef] [PubMed]

59. Choi, H.S.; Kim, M.H.; Choi, M.G.; Park, J.H.; Chun, E.M. Hematologic abnormalities after COVID-19 vaccination: A large Korean population-based cohort study. *medRxiv* **2023**. [CrossRef]
60. Watanabe, A.; Iwagami, M.; Yasuhara, J.; Takagi, H.; Kuno, T. Protective effect of COVID-19 vaccination against long COVID syndrome: A systematic review and meta-analysis. *Vaccine* **2023**, *41*, 1783–1790. [CrossRef] [PubMed]

Disclaimer/Publisher's Note: The statements, opinions and data contained in all publications are solely those of the individual author(s) and contributor(s) and not of MDPI and/or the editor(s). MDPI and/or the editor(s) disclaim responsibility for any injury to people or property resulting from any ideas, methods, instructions or products referred to in the content.

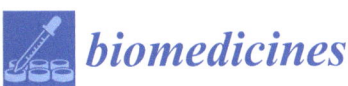

Article

Post-Acute Sequelae of SARS-CoV-2 Infection (PASC) for Patients—3-Year Follow-Up of Patients with Chronic Kidney Disease

Rumen Filev [1,2,*,†], Mila Lyubomirova [1,2], Boris Bogov [1,2], Krassimir Kalinov [3], Julieta Hristova [2,4], Dobrin Svinarov [2,4], Alexander Garev [2,5] and Lionel Rostaing [6,7,†]

1. Department of Nephrology, Internal Disease Clinic, University Hospital "Saint Anna", 1750 Sofia, Bulgaria; mljubomirova@yahoo.com (M.L.); bbogov@yahoo.com (B.B.)
2. Faculty of Medicine, Medical University Sofia, 1504 Sofia, Bulgaria; julieta_sd@yahoo.com (J.H.); dsvinarov@yahoo.com (D.S.); leksgarev@abv.bg (A.G.)
3. Head Biometrics Group, Comac-Medical Ltd., 1404 Sofia, Bulgaria; kkalinov@medistat-bg.com
4. Department of Clinical Laboratory, University Hospital "Alexandrovska", 1431 Sofia, Bulgaria
5. Cardiology Department, University Hospital "Alexandrovska", 1431 Sofia, Bulgaria
6. Nephrology, Hemodialysis, Apheresis and Kidney Transplantation Department, Grenoble University Hospital, 38043 Grenoble, France; lrostaing@chu-grenoble.fr
7. Internal Disease Department, Grenoble Alpes University, 38043 Grenoble, France
* Correspondence: rsfilev@gmail.com
† These authors contributed equally to this work.

Abstract: Post-acute sequelae of SARS-CoV-2 (PASC) is a significant health concern, particularly for patients with chronic kidney disease (CKD). This study investigates the long-term outcomes of individuals with CKD who were infected with COVID-19, focusing on their health status over a three-year period post-infection. Data were collected from both CKD and non-CKD patients who survived SARS-CoV-2 infection and were followed for three years as part of a research study on the impact, prognosis, and consequences of COVID-19 infection in CKD patients. In this prospective cohort study, we analyzed clinical records, laboratory findings, and patient-reported outcomes assessed at intervals during follow-up. The results indicated no permanent changes in renal function in any of the groups analyzed, although patients without CKD exhibited faster recovery over time. Furthermore, we examined the effect of RAAS-blocker therapy over time, finding no influence on PASC symptoms or renal function recovery. Regarding PASC symptoms, most patients recovered within a short period, but some required prolonged follow-up and specialized post-recovery management. Following up with patients in the post-COVID-19 period is crucial, as there is still insufficient information and evidence regarding the long-term effects, particularly in relation to CKD.

Keywords: long COVID; PASC; comorbidity; pain; dyspnea; CKD

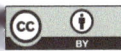

1. Introduction

The COVID-19 pandemic, caused by the novel coronavirus SARS-CoV-2, has forever altered the global health and economic landscape. While significant attention has been focused on the acute phase of the disease, it has become evident that there are long-term health effects in the post-infection period. This phenomenon, characterized by persistent symptoms for months, years, or even longer after the acute infectious phase, continues to challenge healthcare systems.

Long COVID-19 syndrome, also known as post-acute sequelae of SARS-CoV-2 infection (PASC), may have significant implications for individuals with chronic kidney disease (CKD). CKD can be a serious risk factor for complications, as these patients often have compromised immune systems and other underlying health problems. During the acute phase, a common complication is acute kidney injury (AKI). Numerous studies have highlighted that approximately 1 in 10 hospitalized COVID-19 patients experience severe impairment of kidney function [1]. Furthermore, AKI has been identified as a serious risk factor for outcomes, although the incidence and reported outcomes vary widely [1,2]. For example, Hirsch et al. reported a high frequency of AKI (36.6%) in hospitalized COVID-19 patients [2]. Among patients with serious comorbidities, such as cardiovascular disease, hypertension, and diabetes, it is believed that one out of five hospitalized patients will deteriorate to AKI, and around 10% of these patients will require renal replacement therapy (RRT) [3]. This evidence demonstrates that CKD is a significant risk factor for a more severe course of the disease and can worsen the prognosis in some cases. The global prevalence of chronic kidney disease is very high [4].

The COVID-19 pandemic has had a major impact on patients with CKD. AKI is the most common complication of COVID-19 and increases mortality in infected patients, particularly those in intensive care units [5,6]. While most patients who survive COVID-19-associated AKI regain kidney function, up to 30% may remain on dialysis at discharge [7]. The high mortality rate, predisposition to additional complications, and uncertainty about the long-term impact on renal function necessitate serious and thorough follow-up for patients with CKD who have survived COVID-19 infection. A detailed assessment of renal outcomes in the long COVID-19 period is not yet available, and there remains a lack of sufficient information.

PASC is one of the most distressing manifestations reported, characterized by persistent symptoms that can develop within a few weeks after infection and last for months [8]. Despite the severely distressing nature of PASC, long-lasting symptoms can occur in patients who did not experience severe infection or have any comorbidities before the infection [8,9]. Several studies have reported that the most common persistent symptoms after severe COVID-19 infection include fatigue (with or without physical activity), dyspnea, chest pain, cognitive dysfunction, and, in some cases, gastrointestinal problems [8,10,11].

Concerns about PASC syndrome have been raised by reports of increased hospitalizations due to persistent symptoms after surviving COVID-19 infection. In this study, we included patients who were actively followed and who initially participated in a study by our research team to determine early clinical laboratory and prognostic biomarkers for COVID-19 infection outcomes. All participants were successfully cured and were the surviving patients in our cohort at that time. The aim of this study is to determine the risk factors for persistent symptoms of PASC. For all participants, infection was confirmed by a positive PCR test for SARS-CoV-2, following the standardized sample collection protocols [12].

2. Materials and Methods

This single-center study was conducted at Saint Anna Hospital in Sofia, Bulgaria. Patient follow-up occurred between 1 September 2022 and 1 February 2024. All patients tested positive for COVID-19 between 1 February and 31 March 2021. Throughout the follow-up period, patients reported having only one infection. After their recovery, they became more cautious, consistently following infection prevention guidelines and using personal protective equipment, although they chose not to be vaccinated against COVID-19. They did not receive any special treatment that could have influenced the outcomes.

All patients monitored in this study had participated in previous research on biomarkers and COVID-19, having survived the viral infection. They were all hospitalized following a positive PCR test for SARS-CoV-2, with none being outpatients. Only patients older than 18 years without urinary tract infections, as confirmed by microbiology tests and urine sediment, were included. To be classified in the CKD group, patients had to have a known medical history of CKD for at least six months before the COVID-19 infection, documented by kidney ultrasound, serum creatinine levels, and 24 h proteinuria or albumin/creatinine ratio (uACR). Patients without prior CKD diagnosis or documentation were excluded. All participants were unvaccinated against COVID-19 and confirmed their unvaccinated status during follow-up. The cohort consisted exclusively of Caucasian patients. Initially,

160 patients were included: 120 tested positive for COVID-19, and 40 served as controls. Among the controls, 20 had CKD (following the same criteria) but tested negative for COVID-19, while the remaining 20 had no comorbidities and also tested negative for COVID-19. Of the COVID-19 positive group, 70 had CKD (none on hemodialysis), and 50 had no history of kidney disease with normal serum creatinine levels (44–80 μmol/L for women and 62–106 μmol/L for men). The estimated glomerular filtration rate (eGFR) was calculated using the CKD-EPI 2021 formula, and all patients were staged according to KDIGO criteria. Among the hospitalized COVID-19 patients, 23 (21 with CKD) did not survive the infection, resulting in a 14.7% mortality rate. All deceased patients were in the ICU and died of progressive and complicated pneumonia, with no de novo vascular incidents. No patients died during the three-year follow-up period.

During the follow-up phase, each patient had one telephone call and two clinic visits for physical and laboratory examinations. Patients completed a symptom questionnaire (provided in Bulgarian and English in Supplementary Materials) at each of the three follow-up points: the 20th month post-positive test (clinic visit), the 28th month (telephone call), and the 33rd–36th month (clinic visit, with timing extended due to technical reasons). Physical examinations and laboratory tests included blood count, creatinine measurement, eGFR calculation using CKD-EPI 2021, uACR measurement, and kidney ultrasound.

The study adhered to the guidelines of the Declaration of Helsinki and received approval from the KENIMUS Ethics Committee at the Medical University of Sofia, Bulgaria, under protocol No. 12/31.05.2022. All patients provided informed consent and none withdrew from the follow-up program.

This single-center study following CKD patients for three years to examine post-acute sequelae of SARS-CoV-2 infection (PASC) has several strengths and weaknesses. The focus on a specific population allows for a detailed assessment of PASC effects within that group. The single-center nature ensures consistency in data collection and completeness of longitudinal data. Given the paucity of long-term COVID-19 data, following patients for a minimum of three years is crucial. However, single-center studies may have limitations in generalizability and sample size, and the results may be influenced by biases related to the specific population served. Currently, there are no collaborative arrangements with other centers, which could enhance the study's reliability.

Statistical Analysis

Statistical analysis was performed using SAS® version 9.4. The Shapiro–Wilk test was employed to assess the normality of the distribution of creatinine and ACR. The Wilcoxon signed-rank test was used to determine if changes from baseline were significant.

Associations between variables were evaluated using the point biserial correlation coefficient. The odds ratio (OR) was calculated to quantify the association between ACEI/ARB usage and fatigue, cognitive impairment, pain, and sleep problems. A logistic regression model was used to estimate ORs and their significance. A forest plot was used to graphically present the ORs.

Differences between CKD and non-CKD groups, as well as gender differences in follow-up creatinine and ACR, were examined using ANCOVA. The model included follow-up creatinine or ACR as the dependent variable, with the CKD group and gender as factors, and baseline creatinine or ACR and age as covariates.

All comparisons were based on Least Square Means (LSMeans), adjusted for the aforementioned factors and covariates. Differences between LSMeans were graphically presented using a mean–mean scatter plot. A p-value below 0.05 was considered statistically significant.

3. Results

Among the 120 patients confirmed positive for COVID-19, 58.3% (70 patients) had a history of CKD, while the remaining 41.7% (50 patients) did not (Table 1). The overall mortality rate was 14.7% (23 patients), with 19 (82.6%) of the deceased having a history of

CKD. In the surviving group of 97 patients, 51 (52.5%) had CKD, while the remaining 46 (47.5%) did not.

Table 1. Analysis of the cohort at the beginning of the study.

Group	N	Gender	Middle Age Mean (SD)	Race (n%)	Arterial Hypertension	Diabetes	CVD
CKD + COVID-19	70	Female: 21 (42.0%)	56.8 (16.0)	Caucasians 100%	Yes 67 (95.7%)	Yes 40 (57.1%)	Yes 36 (51.4%)
		Male: 29 (58.0%)			No 3 (4.3%)	No 30 (42.9%)	No 34 (47.6%)
Non-CKD + COVID-19	50	Female: 39 (55.7%)	65.9 (12.6)	Caucasians 100%	Yes 12 (24%)	Yes 1 (2%)	Yes 9 (82%)
		Male: 31 (44.3%)			No 38 (76%)	No 49 (98%)	No 41 (18%)
CKD without COVID-19	20	Female: 11 (55%)	66.1 (11.8)	Caucasians 100%	Yes 18 (90%)	Yes 14 (70%)	Yes 9 (45%)
		Male: 9 (45%)			No 2 (10%)	No 6 (30%)	No 11 (55%)
Absolutely healthy	20	Female: 10 (50%)	36.8 (7.8)	Caucasians 100%	None of the patients	None of the patients	None of the patients
		Male: 10 (50%)					
p-values		0.49	<0.0001	NA	<0.0001	<0.0001	<0.0001

Abbreviations: CKD—chronic kidney disease; SD—standard deviation; CVD—cardiovascular diseases.

During the follow-up stage, the median age of CKD patients who tested positive for COVID-19 was 52.6 years, compared to 63.8 years for non-CKD COVID-19 patients ($p = 0.07$). Gender distribution differed between groups, with a total of 43 (44.3%) male patients and 54 (55.6%) female patients ($p = 0.03$). Further analysis revealed that 34 (66.6%) CKD patients were female, while 20 (43.4%) non-CKD patients were female ($p = 0.03$).

During the follow-up, a comparison was conducted between baseline creatinine levels, calculated eGFR, and measured urine albumin/creatinine ratio using the same laboratory tests to evaluate the impact of COVID-19 infection on renal function.

Initially, at baseline, the mean serum creatinine level upon admission was 119.0 μmol/L (range: 50.0–769.0 μmol/L) for the CKD group and 79.0 μmol/L (range: 50.0–295.0 μmol/L) for the non-CKD group (Table 2).

Subsequently, during follow-up, it was observed that patients who survived COVID-19 infection had regained kidney function in terms of serum creatinine levels when comparing the creatinine levels at admission for hospital treatment for COVID-19 infection three years ago to those at the last follow-up. However, no significant differences were noted between the CKD and non-CKD groups regarding renal function recovery (serum creatinine levels), suggesting no substantial distinction in terms of kidney function recovery.

Subsequently, another analysis was conducted comparing all patients at baseline upon admission for hospital treatment with COVID-19 and the follow-up to identify any significant differences regarding creatinine levels. Significant changes were observed in creatinine levels at the last follow-up, with a mean decrease of −4.39 μmol/L (p-value < 0.0001) compared to baseline. However, despite the decrease in creatinine levels, the estimated GFR was found to be lower than at hospital admission for COVID-19 infection three years ago, likely influenced by age as a factor affecting eGFR calculation. Additionally, a statistically significant difference was noted in uACR calculations, with a decrease in measured values by a mean difference of −0.47 g/L (p-value < 0.0001) when comparing overall results at follow-up with those at hospital admission three years ago.

Table 2. Comparison between the groups at the baseline.

Parameter	Statistical Analysis	CKD Patients + COVID-19	Non-CKD Patients + COVID-19	CKD Patients without COVID-19	Healthy Controls	p-Value
Number of patients	n	70	50	20	20	
Creatinine (mcmol/L)	Median (Ranges)	119 (57.0–930.0)	79 (50.0–1295.0)	139.1 (86.0–206.0)	60 (49.0–83.0)	0.0000
eGFR (mL/min)	Mean (SD)	47.9 (23.0)	80.4 (28.9)	62.3 (22.6)	111.1 (13.0)	<0.0001
Urea (mmol/L)	Median (Ranges)	9.2 (2.7–75.2)	5.5 (3.0–82.3)	8.0 (5.0–23.0)	3.0 (2.8–5.0)	0.0000
D-Dimer (mg/L FEU)	Median (Ranges)	0.9 (0.3–10.7)	0.5 (0.3–8.1)	0.7 (0.6–4.7)	0.2 (0.1–0.4)	0.0000
Leucocytes (10^9 cpl)	Mean (SD)	14.8 (11.2)	12.1 (10.5)	8.2 (6.8)	4.5 (2.5)	<0.0001
CRP (mg/L)	Median (Ranges)	50.8 (0.5–320.6)	29.8 (0.1–217.6)	17.0 (1.1–30.0)	1.5 (0.1–5.0)	0.0003

Abbreviation: CKD—chronic kidney disease; eGFR—estimated glomerular filtration rate; CRP—C-reactive protein; SD—standard deviation.

Among the surviving patients, 22 (22.68%) experienced AKI during the COVID-19 infection, classified by KDIGO criteria: Stage I for 13 patients (13.40%), Stage II for 3 patients (3.09%), and Stage III for 6 patients (6.19%). All patients successfully recovered their kidney function, with a median serum creatinine of 113.5 µmol/L (range: 55.00–200.0 µmol/L), and none required renal replacement therapy during or after the COVID-19 infection.

To obtain more precise results, detailed analyses were performed using ANCOVA to analyze the non-CKD and CKD groups. This method was selected as a useful statistical technique for comparing group means while considering the influence of a continuous covariate, allowing for a better understanding of the relationship between groups and dependent variables while controlling for other relevant factors. An analysis was conducted for the follow-up of creatinine and uACR, with the statistical model adjusted for sex and age. Several comparisons were made for creatinine using GLM (Generalized Linear Models) with computation of Least Square Means (LSMEANS) within the context of the GLM results.

When analyzed by this method, similar results were obtained: creatinine significantly improved three years after the infection (p-value < 0.0001). However, differences were observed between the CKD and non-CKD groups, with patients without CKD showing better recovery of renal function than those with any stage of CKD before the COVID-19 infection. Furthermore, females exhibited better recovery of renal function after surviving the COVID-19 infection, while age was found to be non-significant for the results (Table 3 and Figure 1).

Similar analyses were conducted for uACR, yielding comparable results to those for serum creatinine. Significant improvement in uACR was observed three years later, with better improvement noted for non-CKD patients and females exhibiting lower uACR compared to males. Age, again, was found to be non-significant (Tables 4 and 5 and Figure 2).

Table 3. Follow-up results for creatinine divided into groups.

Source	DF	Type III SS	MS	F Value	p-Value
CKD (Yes/No)	1	17,817.1	17,817.1	12.10	0.0008
Gender	1	11,804.1	11,804.1	8.01	0.0057
Age	1	4622.4	4622.4	3.14	0.0798

Abbreviation: CKD—chronic kidney disease; DF—Degrees of Freedom; SS—Sum of Squares; MS—Mean Square; F value—Fisher statistics.

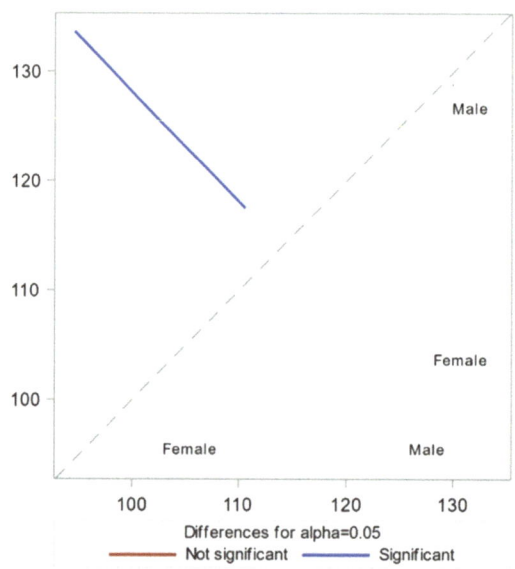

Gender	Follow-Up	p-Values
Female	102.501749	0.0057
Male	125.554974	

Figure 1. Follow-up creatinine (µmol/L) with LSMEAN for gender.

Table 4. Follow-up results for uACR (g/mg).

Source	DF	SS	MS	F Value	p-Value
Model	4	252,699.1	63,174.7	79.72	<0.0001
Error	92	72,904.1	792.4		
Corrected Total	96	325,603.3			

Abbreviation: DF—Degrees of Freedom; SS—Sum of Squares; MS—Mean Square; F value—Fisher statistics.

Table 5. Follow-up results for uACR divided into groups.

Source	DF	Type III SS	MS	F Value	p-Value
CKD (Yes/No)	1	6266.8	6266.8	7.91	0.0060
Gender	1	5358.2	5358.2	6.76	0.0109
Age	1	148.7	148.7	0.19	0.6658

Abbreviation: CKD—chronic kidney disease; DF—Degrees of Freedom; SS—Sum of Squares; MS—Mean Square; F value—Fisher statistics.

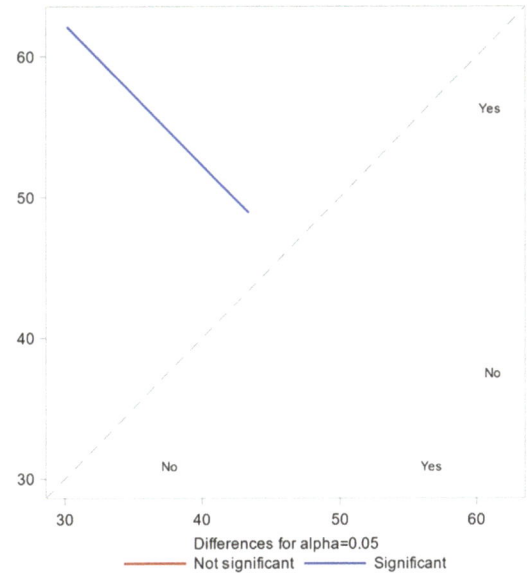

Gender	Follow-Up	*p*-Values
Female	36.7557320	0.0060
Male	55.5077905	

Figure 2. Follow-up uACR with LSMEAN for gender.

The initial follow-up protocols encompassed not only the analysis of laboratory findings but also the comprehensive examination of patients to identify symptoms associated with post-acute sequelae of SARS-CoV-2 (PASC). It is widely acknowledged that symptomatic presentations can vary considerably; however, the symptoms reported by our patients predominantly included fatigue, sleep disturbances, cognitive dysfunction, and notably, a significant proportion of patients reported chest pain or discomfort (Table 6). All symptoms were clearly delineated in the questionnaire, and patients who provided positive responses underwent thorough evaluation. Those requiring further assessment were referred to relevant specialists; for instance, patients reporting chest pain were consulted with a cardiologist and underwent echocardiography ultrasound examinations.

Table 6. Analysis of the PASC symptoms.

Parameter	Medical Examination	Calculations
Fatigue (Up to 12 months)	Yes	57 (58.76%)
	No	40 (41.24%)
Cognitive disfunction (Up to 18 months)	Yes	67 (69.07%)
	No	30 (30.93%)
Chest pain (Up to 6 months)	Yes	35 (36.08%)
	No	62 (63.92%)
Sleep disturbances (Up to 12 months)	Yes	60 (61.86%)
	No	37 (38.14%)

All patients reported that symptoms emerged within a few weeks following the infection, with some enduring for several months (66% of patients), while others persisted for over a year (34% of patients). Subsequent analysis aimed to establish any correlation between the laboratory results and reported post-acute sequelae of SARS-CoV-2 (PASC) symptoms, yet no significant findings or correlations were identified (refer to Table 7). It is noteworthy that no significant differences were observed between the CKD and non-CKD groups, nor between genders, upon comparison. The shortest reported symptom duration was chest pain, lasting up to 6 months, whereas cognitive dysfunction was cited as the most prolonged complaint, enduring for up to 18 months.

Table 7. Correlation between symptoms and follow-up laboratory results.

Laboratory Results and Symptoms	Creatinine (p-Values)	eGFR (p-Values)	ACR (p-Values)
Fatigue	0.4040	0.1506	0.2740
Cognitive disfunction	0.1870	0.0600	0.5398
Chest pain	0.6632	0.1335	0.3814
Sleep disturbances	0.7011	0.2278	0.4360

Abbreviations: eGFR—estimated glomerular filtration rate; ACR—albumin creatinine ratio measured from urine.

Further analysis was conducted concerning reported chest pain, which raised concern for our team due to approximately 35% of patients reporting it in our survey. Patients reporting this symptom underwent additional examinations by pulmonologists and cardiologists. Most patients reported experiencing this symptom for a shorter duration, potentially attributable to reasons such as prolonged coughing or reduced physical activity during COVID-19 recovery, leading to muscle strain or rib discomfort resulting in chest pain. Imaging examinations were conducted to rule out post-COVID inflammation as a cause. In total, 23 patients were assessed by cardiologists, undergoing physical examinations and echocardiography, with five patients further undergoing coronary angiography; however, no additional pathological findings were detected, and no coronary interventions were performed in any cases. With more serious pathological causes for the pain ruled out, patients were incorporated into rehabilitation programs or advised to commence daily physical activity, yielding positive outcomes, particularly for those also reporting fatigue as a symptom.

More than 60% of patients reported experiencing sleeping disturbances and cognitive dysfunction, with many cases involving both symptoms concurrently. Cognitive dysfunction was the longest-lasting symptom, persisting for up to 18 months. Patients described experiencing "brain fog", characterized by difficulties in memory, concentration, and overall mental clarity. The precise etiology of this symptom remained elusive, as even patients with a milder course of COVID-19 exhibited prolonged post-acute sequelae of SARS-CoV-2 (PASC) symptoms. Cognitive rehabilitation involving brain exercises, stress management techniques, and improved sleep hygiene was recommended to these patients. Additionally, some patients reported experiencing depression and anxiety, prompting referrals for specialized follow-up and support from a psychologist. After a year and a half, none of the patients reported such symptoms, including elderly individuals who were closely monitored.

In an earlier phase of the study involving COVID-19 patients, a comprehensive analysis was conducted on the effects of RAAS-blocker therapy. It was concluded that patients receiving ACE inhibitors (ACEi) and angiotensin receptor blockers (ARBs) exhibited a significantly lower mortality rate compared to those receiving other classes of antihypertensive drugs [13]. This analysis was prompted by conflicting information from various trials regarding the use of RAAS blockers at the onset of the pandemic. Subsequently, during follow-up, an investigation was undertaken to assess the impact of ACEi/ARB therapy on laboratory results and to explore any potential correlations with reported PASC symptoms within our patient cohort. Among the surviving patients, 32 individuals (32.9%) were receiving daily RAAS-blocker therapy, which had been initiated prior to COVID-19 infection and continued thereafter. A logistic regression model was employed to examine the effects of RAAS blockers on reported PASC symptoms, including fatigue, cognitive dysfunction, chest pain, and sleep disturbances, using odds ratio analysis. No significant association between symptoms and therapy was identified, leading to the conclusion that RAAS-blocker therapy had no discernible effect during the post-infection period (Figure 3). Similarly, additional analyses conducted on the effects of ACEi/ARBs on kidney function and the albumin/creatinine ratio (ACR) failed to establish any correlation.

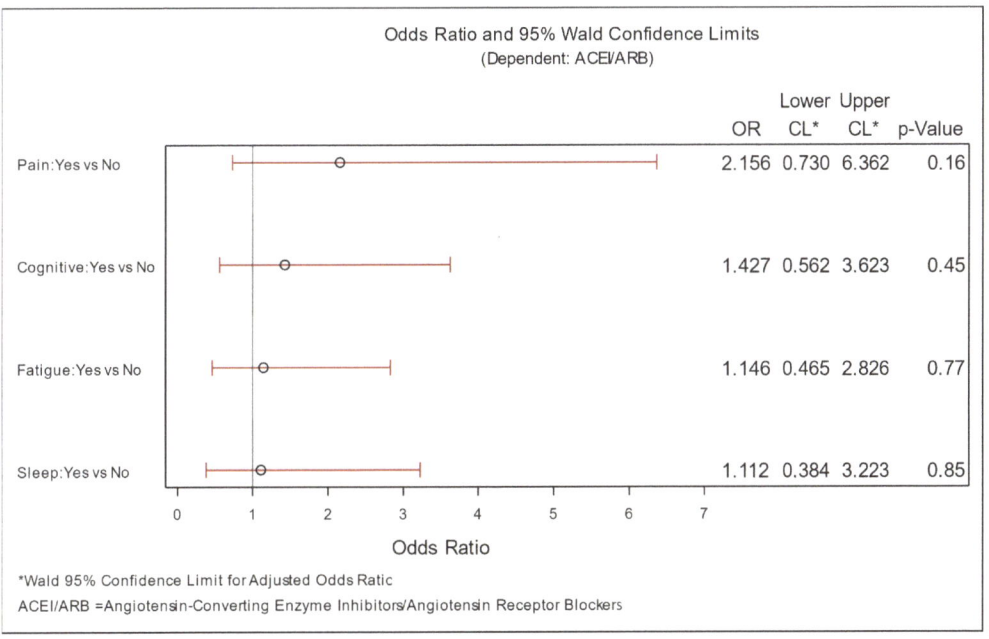

Figure 3. Logistic regression model: odds ratios (dependent: ACEI/ARB).

4. Discussion

The long-term health consequences of COVID-19 remain largely unclear at this point. Studies investigating the long-term health effects of COVID-19 on patients, regardless of hospitalization status, are ongoing. These studies aim to identify the associated risk factors and determine whether they contribute to a more severe course of the disease. While the cohort of surviving COVID-19 patients who were followed up with did not show permanent kidney damage or further progression of chronic kidney disease (CKD), it is strongly recommended that these patients continue to be monitored over time. Additionally, post-acute sequelae of SARS-CoV-2 (PASC) symptoms has been observed to impact individuals' lives, regardless of CKD status or severity of initial COVID-19 symptoms.

Previous reports have indicated that CKD is a predisposing factor for acute kidney injury (AKI), which is a negative prognostic factor for mortality rates [5]. Given the clear and significant data from global analyses, questions have arisen regarding the long-term effects of COVID-19 on kidney function, particularly in CKD patients who may be more vulnerable to complications due to their underlying kidney disease. A study by Benjamin Bowe et al., involving over 1.7 million US veterans, revealed that 30-day survivors of COVID-19 exhibited a higher risk of AKI, a decline in estimated glomerular filtration rate (eGFR), and end-stage kidney disease (ESKD), which subsequently increased the risk of complications for CKD patients [14].

Another important question is whether COVID-19 can induce chronic pathological changes in the kidneys of patients without pre-existing CKD. A retrospective study by Kremec et al. investigated this in 1,008 participants selected from a larger cohort of COVID-19 patients [15]. The study found that surviving patients with mild, moderate, or severe clinical manifestations of COVID-19 did not exhibit an increased risk of kidney outcomes after the acute phase of the disease.

Reports have suggested that COVID-19 patients may experience post-infection complications such as breathing difficulties, heart problems, and pathological changes in kidney structures, potentially indicating lifelong defects in organ structures and functioning. To explore this further, Paidas et al. conducted an in-depth pathohistological investigation using the MHV-1 mouse model of COVID-19 [16]. Their findings indicated long-term recovery in liver and kidney function after infection, but more severe pathological changes in organs such as the brain, lungs, and heart were observed one year post-infection. These findings suggest multi-organ changes with possible implications for long-term prognosis, although the severity of changes in kidney structures may be less pronounced compared to other organs [17,18].

We also found that hospitalized patients with COVID-19 infection exhibit symptoms of post-acute sequelae of SARS-CoV-2 infection (PASC) within the first 2–3 months. Another study reported similar findings among non-hospitalized, PCR-confirmed COVID-19 patients, with one-third of symptomatic participants experiencing persistent symptoms after 4 and 12 weeks [10]. However, there is currently no definitive evidence indicating the duration of PASC symptoms, representing a gap in our knowledge. In our study, all patients reported that their symptoms had completely resolved by the third year. Cross-referencing most publications, it is evident that the most common symptoms persisting for the first 3–6 months post-infection are chest pain, coughing with or without dyspnea, and fatigue [9,19–21]. Patients often describe periods of symptom remission over time [22]. Papers by Nalbandian A et al. and Davis HE et al. noted over 200 symptoms indicating multi-organ involvement [8,23]. In our study, patients reported the previously mentioned common post-infectious symptoms: fatigue, cognitive difficulties, chest pain, and sleep disturbances.

Our results closely align with a study conducted by Alkodaymi et al. [24], although their study assessed PASC symptoms in a much larger population and at different time intervals (≥ 3 to <6, ≥ 6 to <9, ≥ 9 to <12, and ≥ 12 months). The reported results indicate a lower percentage of patients with complaints before the first 6 months, whereas at around the 12-month follow-up, the results became similar to those in our cohort but slightly lower. Tabacof et al. reported cognitive dysfunction in more than half (63%) of the patients analyzed, with one-third experiencing anxiety and depression, similar to our follow-up results [25]. However, it is challenging to draw conclusions about the impact of PASC on anxiety and depression, as the results may be comparable to those in the general population [26]. Notably, the number of patients reporting such psychoneurological symptoms before COVID-19 infection was lower. The pandemic led to a 27.6% increase in cases of major depressive disorders and a 25.6% increase in cases of anxiety disorders globally [27].

A cluster of cardiovascular (CV) abnormalities has been reported in patients in the post-acute phase, including myocardial inflammation, myocardial infarction, right ventricular dysfunction, and arrhythmias. The pathophysiological mechanisms underlying these late cardiac symptoms are not well understood. Numerous reported cases indicate elevated cardiac troponin levels in COVID-19 patients, suggesting myocardial injury and/or ischemia [28], supported by a pathohistological report of microthrombi found in 15 patients [29]. However, the pathological mechanism in the post-COVID phase remains poorly understood. Common to all studies is a slight increase in the percentage of patients with cardiopulmonary symptoms in the first 3 months compared to later stages around 6–9 months [30–34]. Although most PASC cases with cardiopulmonary symptoms do not reveal significant pathological findings requiring intervention, active follow-up, investigation, and diagnostic refinement of these patients are highly recommended. Regarding therapy with RAAS blockers, there are no reported data on the long-term effects on patients post-COVID-19 infection. Current strong evidence supports the benefits of this therapy only during the acute phase of the viral infection, as demonstrated in the early stages of our research on this cohort [13,35].

Additionally, it is important to note that all patients in our cohort were not vaccinated before their COVID-19 infection and did not vaccinate afterward. Some studies have suggested a relationship between long-COVID complications and a full course of vaccination. Watanabe A et al. reported that COVID-19 vaccination before SARS-CoV-2 infection was associated with a lower risk of long COVID after analyzing six observational studies involving 536,291 unvaccinated and 84,603 vaccinated individuals before SARS-CoV-2 infection [36]. Two-dose vaccination was associated with a lower risk of long COVID compared to no vaccination (OR, 0.64; 95% confidence interval [CI], 0.45–0.92) and one-dose vaccination (OR, 0.60; 95% CI, 0.43–0.83). Two-dose vaccination compared to no vaccination was also associated with a lower risk of persistent fatigue (OR, 0.62; 95% CI, 0.41–0.93) and pulmonary disorder (OR, 0.50; 95% CI, 0.47–0.52) [36]. Another study by Gao et al. supported these findings, indicating that COVID-19 vaccines reduce the risk of long COVID. This study highlighted that the protective effect was observed in participants vaccinated with two doses, but not one dose, emphasizing the importance of vaccination before or even after COVID-19 infection, as vaccination was effective against PASC symptoms of long COVID [37]. Notably, during the pandemic, Bulgaria had one of the lowest two-dose vaccination rates and one of the highest mortality rates in the European Union, underscoring the value of vaccination [38].

A significant aspect of PASC symptoms following COVID-19 is the reported differences between hospitalized and non-hospitalized patients. One meta-analysis indicated that the global prevalence of PASC was higher in hospitalized than non-hospitalized patients—54% versus 34% [39]. A meta-analysis by Fernández-de-las-Peñas et al. reported that the most common PASC symptoms among non-hospitalized patients were smell disturbance, taste disturbance, and dyspnea, whereas fatigue was less commonly reported among non-hospitalized patients [40]. Future investigations of PASC should consider patients with varying severity of COVID-19 infection, including those treated in outpatient settings rather than in hospitals. In our cohort, we only included hospitalized patients; thus, further analysis is needed on non-hospitalized patients and the symptoms they reported. However, the data we collected are very similar to that reported for patients who were actively treated in hospitals.

Furthermore, the relationship between PASC and RAAS blockade therapy presents an interesting avenue of research. PASC encompasses a range of persistent symptoms and organ dysfunction following acute COVID-19 infection, and it is intriguing to explore whether there is any relationship between RAAS therapy and the severity of symptoms. Although our research did not find such a relationship, a more in-depth analysis could be considered in the future. The anti-inflammatory effects of RAAS blockers are well known and studied [41], and they could theoretically reduce the chronic inflammation seen in PASC by lowering angiotensin II levels and increasing angiotensin-(1-7). However, the diverse range of PASC symptoms may require more targeted therapies, as neurological symptoms may not respond to RAAS blockers. In the earlier stages of our study, when we analyzed the acute stage of COVID-19, we found a significant effect on the severity of the infection, with patients on ARB/ACEi therapy experiencing fewer transfers to intensive care due to deterioration of their general condition amidst active COVID-19 infection [13]. We believe a thorough analysis should be conducted to determine whether RAAS-blocking therapy has any effect on long-term post-COVID symptoms.

5. Conclusions

Patients with CKD are likely to have long-term sequelae of COVID-19 infection. Although this study did not demonstrate any permanent impairment of renal function or progression of CKD, we strongly recommend that patients with proven renal disease who are survivors of COVID-19 infection be followed up in the future, especially males. We found that even without a direct impact on CKD, PASC can significantly affect the lives of COVID-19 survivors.

Supplementary Materials: The following supporting information can be downloaded at: https://www.mdpi.com/article/10.3390/biomedicines12061259/s1.

Author Contributions: Conceptualization, R.F. and L.R.; methodology, R.F.; software, K.K.; validation, J.H. and D.S.; formal analysis, R.F. and L.R.; investigation, R.F., B.B. and M.L.; resources, R.F.; data curation, R.F.; writing—original draft preparation, R.F.; writing—review and editing, L.R.; visualization, R.F. and A.G.; supervision, L.R.; project administration, R.F.; funding acquisition, L.R. All authors have read and agreed to the published version of the manuscript.

Funding: This research received no external funding.

Institutional Review Board Statement: The study was carried out according to the guidelines of the Declaration of Helsinki and was approved by the KENIMUS Ethics Committee at the Medical University of Sofia, Bulgaria, with protocol No.12/31.05.2022.

Informed Consent Statement: Informed consent was obtained from all subjects involved in the study. Written informed consent has been obtained from the patient(s) to publish this paper.

Data Availability Statement: Data are contained within the article or Supplementary Materials.

Conflicts of Interest: Author Krassimir Kalinov was employed by the company Comac-Medical Ltd. The remaining authors declare that the research was conducted in the absence of any commercial or financial relationships that could be construed as a potential conflict of interest.

Abbreviations

ACEi	Angiotensin-converting enzyme inhibitors
ACOVA	Analysis of covariance AKI—acute kidney injury
ARB	Angiotensin receptor blockers
CKD	Chronic kidney disease
CKD-EPI	Chronic Kidney Disease Epidemiology Collaboration
CV	Cardiovascular
GLM	Generalized Linear Models
eGFR	Estimated glomerular filtration rate
GFR	Glomerular filtration rate
KDIGO	Kidney Disease Improving Global Outcomes
PASC	Post-acute sequelae of SARS-CoV-2 infection
RAAS	Renin–angiotensin–aldosterone blockers
RRT	Renal replacement therapy
uACR	Urine albumin/creatinine ratio

References

1. Bashir, A.M.; Mukhtar, M.S.; Mohamed, Y.G.; Cetinkaya, O.; Fiidow, O.A. Prevalence of Acute Kidney Injury in COVID-19 Patients-Retrospective Single-Center Study. *Infect. Drug Resist.* **2022**, *15*, 1555–1560. [CrossRef] [PubMed]
2. Hirsch, J.S.; Ng, J.H.; Ross, D.W.; Sharma, P.; Shah, H.H.; Barnett, R.L.; Hazzan, A.D.; Fishbane, S.; Jhaveri, K.D.; on behalf of the Northwell COVID-19 Research Consortium and the Northwell Nephrology COVID-19 Research Consortium. Acute kidney injury in patients hospitalized with COVID-19. *Kidney Int.* **2020**, *98*, 209–218. [CrossRef] [PubMed]
3. Schiffrin, E.L.; Flack, J.M.; Ito, S.; Muntner, P.; Webb, R.C. Hypertension and COVID-19. *Am. J. Hypertens.* **2020**, *33*, 373–374. [CrossRef] [PubMed]
4. GBD Chronic Kidney Disease Collaboration. Global, regional, and national burden of chronic kidney disease, 1990-2017: A systematic analysis for the Global Burden of Disease Study 2017. *Lancet* **2020**, *395*, 709–733. [CrossRef] [PubMed] [PubMed Central]
5. Filev, R.; Rostaing, L.; Lyubomirova, M.; Bogov, B.; Kalinov, K.; Svinarov, D. COVID-19 Infection in Chronic Kidney Disease Patients in Bulgaria: Risk Factors for Death and Acute Kidney Injury. *J. Pers. Med.* **2022**, *12*, 1676. [CrossRef]
6. Chang, R.; Elhusseiny, K.M.; Yeh, Y.C.; Sun, W.Z. COVID-19 ICU and mechanical ventilation patient characteristics and outcomes-A systematic review and meta-analysis. *PLoS ONE* **2021**, *16*, e0246318. [CrossRef] [PubMed] [PubMed Central]

7. Chan, L.; Chaudhary, K.; Saha, A.; Chauhan, K.; Vaid, A.; Zhao, S.; Paranjpe, I.; Somani, S.; Richter, F.; Miotto, R.; et al. AKI in Hospitalized Patients with COVID-19. *J. Am. Soc. Nephrol.* **2020**, *32*, 151–160. [CrossRef]
8. Nalbandian, A.; Sehgal, K.; Gupta, A.; Madhavan, M.V.; McGroder, C.; Stevens, J.S.; Cook, J.R.; Nordvig, A.S.; Shalev, D.; Sehrawat, T.S.; et al. Post-acute COVID-19 syndrome. *Nat. Med.* **2021**, *27*, 601–615. [CrossRef] [PubMed] [PubMed Central]
9. Carvalho-Schneider, C.; Laurent, E.; Lemaignen, A.; Beaufils, E.; Bourbao-Tournois, C.; Laribi, S.; Flament, T.; Ferreira-Maldent, N.; Bruyère, F.; Stefic, K.; et al. Follow-up of adults with noncritical COVID-19 two months after symptom onset. *Clin. Microbiol. Infect.* **2020**, *27*, 258–263. [CrossRef] [PubMed] [PubMed Central]
10. Bliddal, S.; Banasik, K.; Pedersen, O.B.; Nissen, J.; Cantwell, L.; Schwinn, M.; Tulstrup, M.; Westergaard, D.; Ullum, H.; Brunak, S.; et al. Acute and persistent symptoms in non-hospitalized PCR-confirmed COVID-19 patients. *Sci. Rep.* **2021**, *11*, 13153. [CrossRef] [PubMed] [PubMed Central]
11. Tenforde, M.W.; Kim, S.S.; Lindsell, C.J.; Billig Rose, E.; Shapiro, N.I.; Files, D.C.; Gibbs, K.W.; Erickson, H.L.; Steingrub, J.S.; Smithline, H.A.; et al. Symptom Duration and Risk Factors for Delayed Return to Usual Health Among Outpatients with COVID-19 in a Multistate Health Care Systems Network—United States, March-June 2020. *MMWR Morb. Mortal. Wkly. Rep.* **2020**, *69*, 993–998. [CrossRef] [PubMed] [PubMed Central]
12. Goodall, B.L.; LeBlanc, J.J.; Hatchette, T.F.; Barrett, L.; Patriquin, G. Investigating the Sensitivity of Nasal or Throat Swabs: Combination of Both Swabs Increases the Sensitivity of SARS-CoV-2 Rapid Antigen Tests. *Microbiol. Spectr.* **2022**, *10*, e0021722. [CrossRef] [PubMed] [PubMed Central]
13. Filev, R.; Rostaing, L.; Lyubomirova, M.; Bogov, B.; Kalinov, K.; Svinarov, D. Renin-angiotensin-aldosterone system blockers in Bulgarian COVID-19 patients with or without chronic kidney disease. *Medicine* **2022**, *101*, e31988. [CrossRef] [PubMed] [PubMed Central]
14. Bowe, B.; Xie, Y.; Xu, E.; Al-Aly, Z. Kidney Outcomes in Long COVID. *J. Am. Soc. Nephrol.* **2021**, *32*, 2851–2862. [CrossRef] [PubMed] [PubMed Central]
15. Kemec, Z.; Akgul, F. Are patients with COVID-19 at risk of long-term chronic kidney disease? *Niger. J. Clin. Pract.* **2023**, *26*, 341–346. [CrossRef] [PubMed]
16. Paidas, M.J.; Cosio, D.S.; Ali, S.; Kenyon, N.S.; Jayakumar, A.R. Long-Term Sequelae of COVID-19 in Experimental Mice. *Mol. Neurobiol.* **2022**, *59*, 5970–5986. [CrossRef] [PubMed] [PubMed Central]
17. Xie, Y.; Xu, E.; Bowe, B.; Al-Aly, Z. Long-term cardiovascular outcomes of COVID-19. *Nat. Med.* **2022**, *28*, 583–590. [CrossRef] [PubMed] [PubMed Central]
18. Teixeira, J.P.; Barone, S.; Zahedi, K.; Soleimani, M. Kidney Injury in COVID-19: Epidemiology, Molecular Mechanisms and Potential Therapeutic Targets. *Int. J. Mol. Sci.* **2022**, *23*, 2242. [CrossRef] [PubMed] [PubMed Central]
19. Cabrera Martimbianco, A.L.; Pacheco, R.L.; Bagattini, Â.M.; Riera, R. Frequency, signs and symptoms, and criteria adopted for long COVID-19: A systematic review. *Int. J. Clin. Pract.* **2021**, *75*, e14357. [CrossRef] [PubMed] [PubMed Central]
20. Davis, H.E.; Assaf, G.S.; McCorkell, L.; Wei, H.; Low, R.J.; Re'em, Y.; Redfield, S.; Austin, J.P.; Akrami, A. Characterizing long COVID in an international cohort: 7 months of symptoms and their impact. *EClinicalMedicine* **2021**, *38*, 101019. [CrossRef] [PubMed] [PubMed Central]
21. Lampl, B.M.J.; Buczovsky, M.; Martin, G.; Schmied, H.; Leitzmann, M.; Salzberger, B. Clinical and epidemiological data of COVID-19 from Regensburg, Germany: A retrospective analysis of 1084 consecutive cases. *Infection* **2021**, *49*, 661–669. [CrossRef] [PubMed] [PubMed Central]
22. Ziauddeen, N.; Gurdasani, D.; O'Hara, M.E.; Hastie, C.; Roderick, P.; Yao, G.; Alwan, N.A. Characteristics and impact of Long Covid: Findings from an online survey. *PLoS ONE* **2022**, *17*, e0264331. [CrossRef] [PubMed] [PubMed Central]
23. Davis, H.E.; McCorkell, L.; Vogel, J.M.; Topol, E.J. Long COVID: Major findings, mechanisms and recommendations. *Nat. Rev. Microbiol.* **2023**, *21*, 133–146; Erratum in *Nat. Rev. Microbiol.* **2023**, *21*, 408. [CrossRef] [PubMed] [PubMed Central]
24. Alkodaymi, M.S.; Omrani, O.A.; Fawzy, N.A.; Shaar, B.A.; Almamlouk, R.; Riaz, M.; Obeidat, M.; Obeidat, Y.; Gerberi, D.; Taha, R.M.; et al. Prevalence of post-acute COVID-19 syndrome symptoms at different follow-up periods: A systematic review and meta-analysis. *Clin. Microbiol. Infect.* **2022**, *28*, 657–666. [CrossRef] [PubMed] [PubMed Central]
25. Tabacof, L.; Tosto-Mancuso, J.; Wood, J.; Cortes, M.; Kontorovich, A.; McCarthy, D.; Rizk, D.; Rozanski, G.; Breyman, E.; Nasr, L.; et al. Post-acute COVID-19 Syndrome Negatively Impacts Physical Function, Cognitive Function, Health-Related Quality of Life, and Participation. *Am. J. Phys. Med. Rehabil.* **2021**, *101*, 48–52. [CrossRef] [PubMed]
26. Pumar, M.I.; Gray, C.R.; Walsh, J.R.; Yang, I.A.; Rolls, T.A.; Ward, D.L. Anxiety and depression-Important psychological comorbidities of COPD. *J. Thorac. Dis.* **2014**, *6*, 1615–1631. [CrossRef] [PubMed] [PubMed Central]
27. COVID-19 Mental Disorders Collaborators. Global prevalence and burden of depressive and anxiety disorders in 204 countries and territories in 2020 due to the COVID-19 pandemic. *Lancet* **2021**, *398*, 1700–1712. [CrossRef] [PubMed] [PubMed Central]
28. Giustino, G.; Croft, L.B.; Stefanini, G.G.; Bragato, R.; Silbiger, J.J.; Vicenzi, M.; Danilov, T.; Kukar, N.; Shaban, N.; Kini, A.; et al. Characterization of Myocardial Injury in Patients With COVID-19. *J. Am. Coll. Cardiol.* **2020**, *76*, 2043–2055. [CrossRef] [PubMed] [PubMed Central]
29. Bois, M.C.; Boire, N.A.; Layman, A.J.; Aubry, M.-C.; Alexander, M.P.; Roden, A.C.; Hagen, C.E.; Quinton, R.A.; Larsen, C.; Erben, Y.; et al. COVID-19-Associated Nonocclusive Fibrin Microthrombi in the Heart. *Circulation* **2021**, *143*, 230–243. [CrossRef] [PubMed] [PubMed Central]

30. Sechi, L.A.; Colussi, G.; Bulfone, L.; Brosolo, G.; Da Porto, A.; Peghin, M.; Patruno, V.; Tascini, C.; Catena, C. Short-term cardiac outcome in survivors of COVID-19: A systematic study after hospital discharge. *Clin. Res. Cardiol.* **2021**, *110*, 1063–1072. [CrossRef] [PubMed] [PubMed Central]
31. Catena, C.; Colussi, G.; Bulfone, L.; Da Porto, A.; Tascini, C.; Sechi, L.A. Echocardiographic Comparison of COVID-19 Patients with or without Prior Biochemical Evidence of Cardiac Injury after Recovery. *J. Am. Soc. Echocardiogr.* **2021**, *34*, 193–195. [CrossRef] [PubMed] [PubMed Central]
32. de Graaf, M.; Antoni, M.; ter Kuile, M.; Arbous, M.; Duinisveld, A.; Feltkamp, M.; Groeneveld, G.; Hinnen, S.; Janssen, V.; Lijfering, W.; et al. Short-term outpatient follow-up of COVID-19 patients: A multidisciplinary approach. *EClinicalMedicine* **2021**, *32*, 100731. [CrossRef] [PubMed] [PubMed Central]
33. Puntmann, V.O.; Carerj, M.L.; Wieters, I.; Fahim, M.; Arendt, C.; Hoffmann, J.; Shchendrygina, A.; Escher, F.; Vasa-Nicotera, M.; Zeiher, A.M.; et al. Outcomes of Cardiovascular Magnetic Resonance Imaging in Patients Recently Recovered From Coronavirus Disease 2019 (COVID-19). *JAMA Cardiol.* **2020**, *5*, 1265–1273; Erratum in *JAMA Cardiol.* **2020**, *5*, 1308. [CrossRef] [PubMed] [PubMed Central]
34. Dennis, A.; Wamil, M.; Alberts, J.; Oben, J.; Cuthbertson, D.J.; Wootton, D.; Crooks, M.; Gabbay, M.; Brady, M.; Hishmeh, L.; et al. Multiorgan impairment in low-risk individuals with post-COVID-19 syndrome: A prospective, community-based study. *BMJ Open* **2021**, *11*, e048391. [CrossRef] [PubMed] [PubMed Central]
35. Zhang, Z.; Wu, S.; Wang, Z.; Wang, Y.; Chen, H.; Wu, C.; Xiong, L. Long-term oral ACEI/ARB therapy is associated with disease severity in elderly COVID-19 omicron BA.2 patients with hypertension. *BMC Infect. Dis.* **2023**, *23*, 882. [CrossRef] [PubMed] [PubMed Central]
36. Watanabe, A.; Iwagami, M.; Yasuhara, J.; Takagi, H.; Kuno, T. Protective effect of COVID-19 vaccination against long COVID syndrome: A systematic review and meta-analysis. *Vaccine* **2023**, *41*, 1783–1790. [CrossRef] [PubMed] [PubMed Central]
37. Gao, P.; Liu, J.; Liu, M. Effect of COVID-19 Vaccines on Reducing the Risk of Long COVID in the Real World: A Systematic Review and Meta-Analysis. *Int. J. Environ. Res. Public Health* **2022**, *19*, 12422. [CrossRef] [PubMed] [PubMed Central]
38. National Statistical Institute of Republic of Bulgaria. COVID 19 Statistical Data. Available online: https://www.nsi.bg/en/content/18120/basic-page/covid-19 (accessed on 10 April 2024).
39. Chen, C.; Haupert, S.R.; Zimmermann, L.; Shi, X.; Fritsche, L.G.; Mukherjee, B. Global Prevalence of Post-Coronavirus Disease 2019 (COVID-19) Condition or Long COVID: A Meta-Analysis and Systematic Review. *J. Infect. Dis.* **2022**, *226*, 1593–1607. [CrossRef] [PubMed] [PubMed Central]
40. Fernández-de-Las-Peñas, C.; Palacios-Ceña, D.; Gómez-Mayordomo, V.; Florencio, L.L.; Cuadrado, M.L.; Plaza-Manzano, G.; Navarro-Santana, M. Prevalence of post-COVID-19 symptoms in hospitalized and non-hospitalized COVID-19 survivors: A systematic review and meta-analysis. *Eur. J. Intern. Med.* **2021**, *92*, 55–70. [CrossRef] [PubMed] [PubMed Central]
41. Martyniak, A.; Tomasik, P.J. A New Perspective on the Renin-Angiotensin System. *Diagnostics* **2022**, *13*, 16. [CrossRef] [PubMed] [PubMed Central]

Disclaimer/Publisher's Note: The statements, opinions and data contained in all publications are solely those of the individual author(s) and contributor(s) and not of MDPI and/or the editor(s). MDPI and/or the editor(s) disclaim responsibility for any injury to people or property resulting from any ideas, methods, instructions or products referred to in the content.

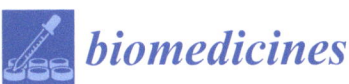

Article

COVID-19 Infection in Autosomal Dominant Polycystic Kidney Disease and Chronic Kidney Disease Patients: Progression of Kidney Disease

Silvia Lai [1,*], Francesca Tinti [1], Adolfo Marco Perrotta [1], Luca Salomone [1], Rosario Cianci [1], Paolo Izzo [2], Sara Izzo [3], Luciano Izzo [2], Claudia De Intinis [2], Chiara Pellicano [4] and Antonietta Gigante [4]

1. Department of Translational and Precision Medicine, UOC Nephrology, Sapienza University of Rome, 00185 Rome, Italy; francesca.tinti@uniroma1.it (F.T.); adolfomarco.perrotta@uniroma1.it (A.M.P.); luca.salomone@uniroma1.it (L.S.); rosario.cianci@uniroma1.it (R.C.)
2. Department of Surgery "Pietro Valdoni", Policlinico Umberto I, Sapienza University of Rome, 00185 Rome, Italy; p_izzo@hotmail.it (P.I.); luciano.izzo@uniroma1.it (L.I.); deintinis.1891513@studenti.uniroma1.it (C.D.I.)
3. Plastic Surgery Unit, Multidisciplinary Department of Medical-Surgical and Dental Specialties, University of Campania "Luigi Vanvitelli", 80138 Naples, Italy; sa_izzo@hotmail.it
4. Department of Translational and Precision Medicine, Sapienza University of Rome, 00185 Rome, Italy; chiara.pellicano@gmail.com (C.P.); antonietta.gigante@uniroma1.it (A.G.)
* Correspondence: silvia.lai@uniroma1.it

Citation: Lai, S.; Tinti, F.; Perrotta, A.M.; Salomone, L.; Cianci, R.; Izzo, P.; Izzo, S.; Izzo, L.; De Intinis, C.; Pellicano, C.; et al. COVID-19 Infection in Autosomal Dominant Polycystic Kidney Disease and Chronic Kidney Disease Patients: Progression of Kidney Disease. *Biomedicines* **2024**, *12*, 1301. https://doi.org/10.3390/biomedicines12061301

Academic Editor: César Fernández De Las Peñas

Received: 22 April 2024
Revised: 5 June 2024
Accepted: 7 June 2024
Published: 12 June 2024

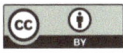

Copyright: © 2024 by the authors. Licensee MDPI, Basel, Switzerland. This article is an open access article distributed under the terms and conditions of the Creative Commons Attribution (CC BY) license (https://creativecommons.org/licenses/by/4.0/).

Abstract: Introduction: the COVID-19 pandemic has brought to light the intricate interplay between viral infections and preexisting health conditions. In the field of kidney diseases, patients with Autosomal Dominant Polycystic Kidney Disease (ADPKD) and Chronic Kidney Disease (CKD) face unique challenges when exposed to the SARS-CoV-2 virus. This study aims to evaluate whether SARS-CoV-2 virus infection impacts renal function differently in patients suffering from ADPKD and CKD when compared to patients suffering only from CKD. Materials and methods: clinical data from 103 patients were collected and retrospectively analyzed. We compared the renal function of ADPKD and CKD patients at two distinct time points: before COVID-19 infection (T0) and 1 year after the infection (T1). We studied also a subpopulation of 37 patients with an estimated glomerular filtration rate (eGFR) < 60 mL/min and affected by ADPKD and CKD. Results: clinical data were obtained from 59 (57.3%) ADPKD patients and 44 (42.7%) CKD patients. At T1, ADPKD patients had significantly higher serum creatinine levels compared to CKD patients, and a significantly lower eGFR was observed only in ADPKD patients with eGFR < 60 mL/min compared to CKD patients ($p < 0.01$, $p < 0.05$; respectively). Following COVID-19 infection, ADPKD–CKD patients exhibited significantly higher variation in both median serum creatinine ($p < 0.001$) and median eGFR ($p < 0.001$) compared to CKD patients. Conclusion: the interplay between COVID-19 and kidney disease is complex. In CKD patients, the relationship between COVID-19 and kidney disease progression is more established, while limited studies exist on the specific impact of COVID-19 on ADPKD patients. Current evidence does not suggest that ADPKD patients are at a higher risk of SARS-CoV-2 infection; however, in our study we showed a significant worsening of the renal function among ADPKD patients, particularly those with an eGFR < 60 mL/min, in comparison to patients with only CKD after a one-year follow-up from COVID-19 infection.

Keywords: autosomal dominant polycystic kidney disease; COVID-19 infection; chronic kidney disease; SARS-CoV-2 virus

1. Introduction

Autosomal Dominant Polycystic Kidney Disease (ADPKD) is one of the most common genetic disorders that affect the kidneys. It is characterized by the development of fluid-filled cysts within the kidneys which can progressively enlarge and impair kidney function over time. Individuals with ADPKD may experience a range of symptoms, including high blood pressure, kidney pain, and, in some cases, kidney failure [1]. The emergence of the COVID-19 pandemic has raised concerns about how this novel coronavirus might impact individuals with preexisting medical conditions, including ADPKD and CKD. COVID-19 is primarily a respiratory illness, but it can have systemic effects on various organs, including the kidneys. Individuals with CKD, such as those with ADPKD, may be at an increased risk of severe complications if they contract the virus [2]. The connection between COVID-19 and ADPKD is not clearly established, although it is known that SARS-CoV-2 virus utilizes Angiotensin-Converting Enzyme 2 (ACE2) receptors on cell membranes to effectively target its host. While it is well-documented that the renin–angiotensin–aldosterone system (RAAS) is more active in ADPKD patients, the extent of hyper-activation or hyper-expression of ACE2 receptors remains unclear. SARS-CoV-2 binding leads to the downregulation of ACE2, potentially disrupting the balance of the RAAS. This can result in increased levels of angiotensin II, which is associated with inflammation, vasoconstriction, and fibrosis. COVID-19 has been linked to acute kidney injury (AKI) and worsening kidney function, particularly in patients with preexisting kidney conditions like ADPKD. The mechanisms include direct viral invasion, cytokine storm, and disruption of the RAAS [3]. Patients with ADPKD are particularly vulnerable due to their already compromised kidney function. The interplay between ADPKD and COVID-19 can lead to a higher risk of AKI and worsening of the renal function. Additionally, the chronic nature of ADPKD means that these patients are at a heightened risk of severe complications from COVID-19, further aggravating their renal condition [4]. Furthermore, the common use of drug treatments involving ACE inhibitors (ACEi) or angiotensin receptor blockers (ARBs) in these patients introduces other clinical implications [1]. Managing COVID-19 in patients with ADPKD requires careful monitoring and treatment adjustments to address both the viral infection and the underlying renal condition.

The aim of the study is to evaluate the progression of renal disease in ADPKD patients as compared to CKD patients after a COVID-19 infection, shedding light on potential differences and implications for clinical management.

2. Materials and Methods

2.1. Study Design and Subjects

In this study, clinical data from 103 consecutive patients were collected and retrospectively analyzed: 59 patients were affected by ADPKD and 44 patients were affected by CKD. The study aimed to compare the renal function of patients with ADPKD and CKD at two distinct time points: before the COVID-19 infection (T0) and 1 year after the infection (T2). The data were obtained from patients at the University Hospital "Policlinico Umberto I" in Rome. The study protocol was approved by the Clinical Research Ethics Committee at the Sapienza University of Rome, Italy, with Ethics Approval acceptance number 298/2020. The study conforms to the principles outlined in the Declaration of Helsinki and we obtained the written consent from each patient enrolled.

2.2. Laboratory Measurements

We performed the following tests with a standard technique: creatinine (mg/dL), serum nitrogen (mg/dL), serum electrolytes (mEq/L), and hemoglobin (g/dL). The eGFR was evaluated according to the Modification of Diet in Renal Disease (MDRD) formula. We evaluated patients with a positive SARS-CoV-2 test using RT-PCR. The negativization of SARS-CoV-2 testing was established following at least two consecutive RT-PCR negative results.

2.3. Blood Pressure Measurements

Blood Pressure (BP) measurements were made in the dominant arm after 10 min of rest in the sitting position using a standard automatic sphygmomanometer. The mean of three measurements was recorded. Hypertension was defined according to international guidelines, as SBP ≥ 140 mmHg or DBP ≥ 90 mmHg on repeated measurements.

2.4. Statistical Analysis

The coefficient of kurtosis was used to evaluate the normal distribution of data. Continuous variables are expressed as median and interquartile range (IQR) and categorical variables are expressed as absolute frequencies and percentages (%). Group comparisons were made through the Mann–Whitney test or the student's t test, as appropriate. The chi-square test or Fisher's exact test, as appropriate, were used to compare categorical variables. A value of $p < 0.05$ was considered to be significant. JASP version 0.17.2.1 software was used for statistical analysis.

3. Results

Clinical data from 103 consecutive patients were collected and retrospectively analyzed in this study. A total of 59 (57.3%) patients were affected by ADPKD and 44 (42.7%) patients were affected by CKD.

3.1. Demographic and Clinical Characteristics of ADPKD and CKD Patients at T0

Demographic and clinical characteristics of ADPKD and CKD patients at T0 are reported in Table 1. The median age of ADPKD patients was 49 years (IQR 34–57) and 31 (52.5%) patients were female. The median systolic blood pressure was 120 mmHg (IQR 112–130), while the median diastolic blood pressure was 80 mmHg (IQR 75–87) and the median heart rate was 65 bpm (IQR 59–75). Median serum creatinine and blood urea nitrogen levels were estimated at 1.06 mg/dL (IQR 0.88–1.5) and 15.4 mg/dL (IQR 12.7–20.3), respectively, whilst the median eGFR was 65.8 mL/min (IQR 46.8–86.9) and 20 (33.9%) ADPKD patients had an eGFR < 60 mL/min. The median serum albumin was 37 g/L (IQR 34–39) and the median urinary protein level was 12.5 mg/dL (IQR 0–30). ADPKD patients with eGFR < 60 mL/min had significantly higher systolic blood pressure [130 mmHg (IQR 120–137.5) vs. 120 mmHg (IQR 110–130), $p < 0.05$] and diastolic blood pressure [85 mmHg (IQR 80–90) vs. 79 mmHg (IQR 70–86), $p < 0.05$] compared to ADPKD patients with eGFR > 60 mL/min. We did not find any other statistically significant difference between ADPKD patients with normal or reduced eGFR at T0.

Table 1. Demographic and clinical characteristics of ADPKD and CKD patients at T0. All data are expressed as median and interquartile range (IQR) or as absolute frequency and percentage (%).

	ADPKD (n = 59)	CKD (n = 44)	p
Age, years	49 (34–57)	65.5 (56.7–76)	<0.001
M/F	28 (47.5)/31 (52.5)	28 (63.6)/16 (36.4)	>0.05
Systolic blood pressure, mmHg	120 (112–130)	140 (126–140)	<0.001
Diastolic blood pressure, mmHg	80 (75–87)	80 (70–80)	>0.05
Heart rate, bpm	65 (59–75)	85.5 (80–97.2)	<0.001
SpO_2, %	98.9 (97.5–99.4)	95 (94–97)	<0.001
Hb, g/dL	12.6 (12–13.8)	13.1 (12–14)	>0.05
Serum creatinine, mg/dL	1.06 (0.88–1.5)	0.9 (0.8–1.35)	>0.05
eGFR, mL/min	65.8 (46.8–86.9)	70 (45–87.2)	>0.05
eGFR < 60 mL/min	20 (33.9)	17 (38.6)	>0.05
Blood urea nitrogen, mg/dL	15.4 (12.7–30.3)	20.5 (12.7–35.2)	<0.001
Na^+, mEq/L	141 (139–144)	135 (132–138)	<0.001
K^+, mEq/L	4.1 (4–4.4)	3.9 (3.6–4.4)	>0.05
Ca^{2+}, mg/dL	9.4 (9–10)	8.5 (8.3–9.2)	>0.05
Serum albumin, g/L	37 (34–39)	38 (33.7–41)	>0.05
Urinary proteins, mg/dL	12.5 (0–30)	15 (0–30)	>0.05

The median age of CKD patients was 65.5 years (IQR 56.7–76) and 16 (36.4%) patients were female. The median systolic blood pressure was 140 mmHg (IQR 126–140), the median diastolic blood pressure was 80 mmHg (IQR 70–80), and the median heart rate was 85 bpm (IQR 80–95). Median serum creatinine and blood urea nitrogen levels were 0.9 mg/dL (IQR 0.8–1.35) and 20.5 mg/dL (IQR 12.7–32.2), respectively, whilst the median eGFR was 70 mL/min (IQR 45–87.2) and 17 (38.6%) CKD patients had an eGFR < 60 mL/min. The median serum albumin was 38 g/L (IQR 33.7–38) and the median urinary protein level was 15 mg/dL (IQR 0–30). CKD patients with eGFR < 60 mL/min were significantly older [76 years (IQR 71–77) vs. 60 years (IQR 54–68), $p < 0.001$] compared to CKD patients with eGFR > 60 mL/min. We did not find any other statistically significant difference between CKD patients with normal or reduced eGFR at T0.

3.2. Demographic and Clinical Characteristics of ADPKD and CKD Patients at T1

Demographic and clinical characteristics of ADPKD and CKD patients at T1 are reported in Table 2. In ADPKD patients, the median serum creatinine level was 1.1 mg/dL (IQR 0.9–1.7), whilst the median eGFR was 59 mL/min (IQR 41–84.5) and 30 (50.8%) ADPKD patients had an eGFR < 60 mL/min. The median serum albumin level was 36 g/L (IQR 33–39.7) and the median urinary protein level was 20 mg/dL (IQR 10–30). We did not find any other statistically significant difference between ADPKD patients with normal or reduced eGFR at T2. In CKD patients, the median serum creatinine level was 0.89 mg/dL (IQR 0.71–1.32), whilst the median eGFR was 81 mL/min (IQR 50.2–94.2) and 12 (27.3%) CKD patients had an eGFR < 60 mL/min. The median serum albumin level was 33.5 g/L (IQR 30–37) and the median urinary protein level was 15 mg/dL (IQR 0.3–30). We did not find any other statistically significant difference between CKD patients with normal or reduced eGFR at T1. At T1, ADPKD patients with an eGFR < 60 mL/min exhibited a significantly lower eGFR compared to CKD patients ($p < 0.05$).

Table 2. Demographic and clinical characteristics of ADPKD and CKD patients at T1. All data are expressed as median and interquartile range (IQR) or as absolute frequency and percentage (%).

	ADPKD ($n = 59$)	CKD ($n = 44$)	p
Serum creatinine, mg/dL	1.1 (0.9–1.74)	0.89 (0.71–1.32)	<0.01
eGFR, mL/min	59 (41–84.5)	81 (50.2–94.2)	>0.05
eGFR < 60 mL/min	28 (47.4)	12 (27.3)	<0.05
Serum albumin, g/L	36 (33–39.7)	33.5 (30–37)	>0.05
Urinary proteins, mg/dL	20 (10–30)	15 (0.3–30)	>0.05

3.3. Comparative Analysis of Renal Function at Each Time Point in ADPKD and CKD Patients

In ADPKD patients, the median serum creatinine was significantly lower at T0 compared to T1 [1.06 mg/dL (IQR 0.88–1.5) vs. 1.1 mg/dL (IQR 0.9–1.7), $p < 0.001$]. In ADPKD patients, the median eGFR was significantly higher at T0 compared to T1 [65.8 mL/min (IQR 46.8–86.9) vs. 59 mL/min (IQR 41–84.5), $p < 0.05$]. There was no statistically significant difference in the variation of eGFR (delta T1_T0) between patients with reduced or normal eGFR at baseline [−6.5 mL/min (IQR −16.2−−1.2) vs. −3.4 mL/min (IQR −15.2–8), $p > 0.05$]. In CKD patients, the median eGFR was significantly lower at T0 compared to T1 [70 mL/min (IQR 45–87.2) vs. 81 mL/min (IQR 50.2–94.2), $p < 0.05$]. There was no statistically significant difference in the variation of eGFR (delta T1_T0) between patients with reduced or normal eGFR at baseline [4 mL/min (IQR 0–19) vs. 9 mL/min (IQR −8.5–16.5), $p > 0.05$]. We observed a significant difference in serum creatinine levels between ADPKD and CKD patients at T1 (and <0.01) (Table 2). Additionally, at T1, ADPKD patients with an eGFR < 60 mL/min exhibited a significantly lower eGFR compared to CKD patients ($p < 0.05$).

3.4. Demographic and Clinical Characteristics of a Subpopulation of ADPKD and CKD Patients with eGFR < 60 mL/min

Clinical data from 37 consecutive patients were collected, 20 (54%) patients were affected by ADPKD and CKD and 17 (46%) patients were affected only by CKD. All patients enrolled had an eGFR < 60 mL/min and were affected by systemic arterial hypertension. ADPKD–CKD patients were significantly younger than CKD patients [46 years (IQR 37.5; 63.5) vs. 76 years (IQR 71;77), $p < 0.001$] and female patients were more frequent among ADPKD–CKD patients compared to CKD patients [10 (50%) vs. 3 (17.6%), $p < 0.05$]. Median systolic [130 mmHg (IQR 120;137) vs. 130 mmHg (IQR 120; 142), $p > 0.05$] and diastolic [85 mmHg (IQR 80; 90) vs. 80 mmHg (IQR 73; 81), $p > 0.05$] blood pressure were similar between ADPKD–CKD patients and CKD patients. CKD patients had a significantly higher median heart rate than ADPKD–CKD patients [92 bpm (IQR 80; 101) vs. 56 bpm (IQR 55; 58), $p < 0.05$]. The median C-Reactive Protein (CRP) level was significantly higher in CKD patients compared to ADPKD–CKD patients [110.4 mg/L (IQR 74.9; 156) vs. 1.8 mg/L (IQR 1.1; 2.3), $p < 0.001$], whilst the median serum D-dimer level [1154 mcg/L (IQR 852; 1663) vs. 774 mcg/L (IQR 513; 1304), $p > 0.05$] and the Neutrophil-to-Lymphocyte Ratio (NLR) [6.25 (IQR 5.33; 11.9) vs. 4.2 (IQR 2.5; 7.3), $p > 0.05$] were similar between the cohorts of patients. The median hemoglobin level was similar between ADPKD–CKD patients and CKD patients [11.8 g/dL (IQR 11.4; 12.7) vs. 12.7 g/dL (IQR 11.9; 13.9), $p > 0.05$], whilst the median ratio of arterial oxygen partial pressure (PaO_2 in mmHg) to fractional inspired oxygen (FiO_2 expressed as a fraction) (P/F ratio) was significantly lower in CKD patients than in ADPKD–CKD patients [321.5 (IQR 241.7; 358.5) vs. 490 (IQR 471; 504.5), $p < 0.05$]. Table 3 shows demographic and clinical characteristics of the enrolled patients.

Table 3. Demographic and clinical characteristics of ADPKD and CKD patients. All data are expressed as median and interquartile range (IQR) or as absolute frequency and percentage (%).

	ADPKD (n = 20)	CKD (n = 17)	p
Age, years, median (IQR)	46 (37.5–63.5)	76 (71–77)	<0.001
M/F, n (%)	10 (50)/10 (50)	3 (17.6)/14 (82.4)	<0.05
SBP, mmHg, median (IQR)	130 (120–137)	130 (120–142)	>0.05
DBP, mmHg, median (IQR)	85 (80–90)	80 (73–81)	>0.05
Heart rate, bpm, median (IQR)	56 (55–58)	92 (80–101)	<0.05
CRP, mg/L, median (IQR)	1.8 (1.1–2.3)	110.4 (74.9–156)	<0.001
D-dimer, mcg/L, median (IQR)	774 (513–1304)	1154 (852–1663)	>0.05
NLR, median (IQR)	4.2 (2.5–7.3)	6.25 (5.33–11.9)	<0.001
Hb, g/dL, median (IQR)	11.8 (11.4–12.7)	12.7 (11.9–13.9)	>0.05
P/F ratio, median (IQR)	490 (471–504.5)	321.5 (241.7–358.5)	<0.05

ADPKD: Autosomal Dominant Polycystic Kidney Disease; CKD: Chronic Kidney Disease; M: male; F: female; SBP: Systolic Blood Pressure; DBP: Diastolic Blood Pressure; CRP: C-Reactive Protein; NLR: Neutrophil-to-Lymphocyte Ratio; Hb: hemoglobin.

At baseline (T0), the median serum creatinine level [1.8 mg/dL (IQR 1.5; 2) vs. 1.7 mg/dL (IQR 1.3; 2.3), $p > 0.05$] and the median eGFR [42.5 mL/min (IQR 39.7; 46.3) vs. 37 mL/min (IQR 27; 54), $p > 0.05$] were similar between ADPKD–CKD patients and CKD patients. Moreover, after SARS-CoV2 infection (T1), the median serum creatinine level [2.2 mg/dL (IQR 1.6; 2.4) vs. 1.5 mg/dL (IQR 1.1; 1.9), $p > 0.05$] and the median eGFR [33.5 mL/min (IQR 26; 44.2) vs. 41 mL/min (IQR 33; 65), $p > 0.05$] were similar between the two cohorts of patients. Table 4 summarizes the comparative analysis of renal function between ADPKD patients and CKD patients. ADPKD–CKD patients had a statistically significant lower median serum creatinine level at T0 than at T1 [1.8 mg/dL (IQR 1.5; 2) vs. 2.2 mg/dL (IQR 1.6; 2.4), $p > 0.05$], with a variation (T1–T0) of 0.29 mg/dL (IQR 0.12; 0.5), and a statistically significant higher eGFR at T0 compared to T1 [42.5 mL/min (IQR 39.7;

46.3) vs. 33.5 mL/min (IQR 26; 44.2), $p < 0.001$], with a variation (T1–T0) of −6.5 mL/min (IQR −16.25; −1.25) (Figure 1A). CKD patients had similar median serum creatinine levels at T0 and at T1 [1.7 mg/dL (IQR 1.3; 2.3) vs. 1.5 mg/dL (IQR 1.1; 1.9), $p > 0.05$], with a variation (T1–T0) of −0.16 mg/dL (IQR −0.3; 0), and a statistically significant lower median eGFR at T0 compared to T1 [37 mL/min (IQR 27; 54) vs. 41 mL/min (IQR 33; 65), $p < 0.01$], with a variation (T1–T0) of 4 mL/min (IQR 0; 19) (Figure 1B).

Table 4. Comparative analysis of renal function between 20 ADPKD patients and 17 CKD patients at baseline T0 and after SARS-CoV2 infection (T1). All results are expressed as median and interquartile range (IQR).

	T0			T1		
	ADPKD	CKD	p	ADPKD	CKD	p
Creatinine, mg/dL	1.8 (1.5; 2)	1.7 (1.3; 2.3)	>0.05	2.2 (1.6; 2.4)	1.5 (1.1; 1.9)	>0.05
eGFR, mL/min	42.5 (39.7; 46.3)	37 (27; 54)	>0.05	33.5 (26; 44.2)	41 (33; 65)	>0.05
	Variation T1–T0					
	ADPKD			CKD		p
Creatinine, mg/dL	0.29 (0.12; 0.5)			−0.16 (−0.3; 0)		<0.001
eGFR, mL/min	−6.5 (−16.25; −1.25)			4 (0; 19)		<0.001

ADPKD: Autosomal Dominant Polycystic Kidney Disease; CKD: Chronic Kidney Disease; eGFR: estimated Glomerular Filtration Rate.

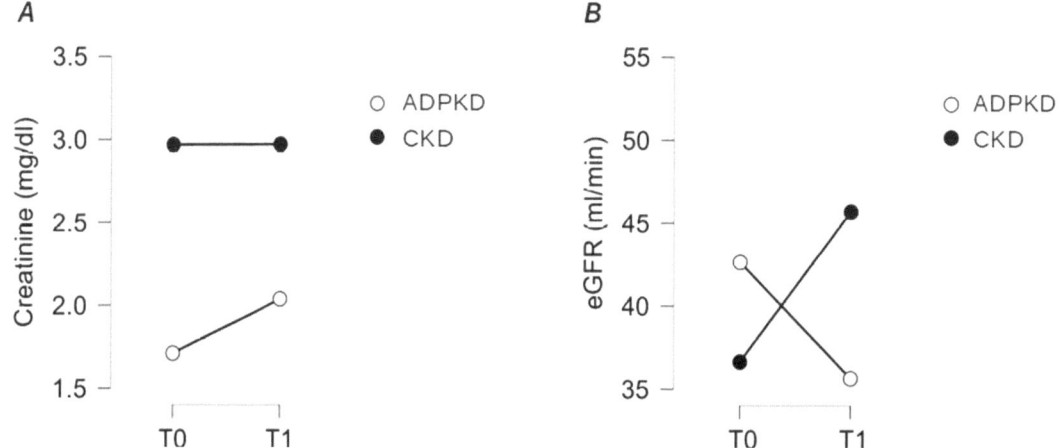

Figure 1. Comparative analysis between 20 ADPKD patients and 17 CKD patients. (**A**) Variation in serum creatinine levels from baseline (T0) to T1 (after SARS-CoV-2 infection); (**B**) variation in serum estimated Glomerular Filtration Rate (eGFR) from baseline (T0) to T1 (after SARS-CoV-2 infection).

ADPKD–CKD patients exhibited a significantly larger variation, compared to CKD patients, in both median serum creatinine levels [0.29 mg/dL (IQR 0.12; 0.5) vs. −0.16 mg/dL (IQR −0.3; 0), $p < 0.001$] and median eGFR [−6.5 mL/min (IQR −16.25; −1.25) vs. 4 mL/min (IQR 0; 19), $p < 0.001$] (Table 2 and Figure 1).

4. Discussion

The interaction between COVID-19 and kidney disease is intricate, potentially yielding distinct implications for patients with ADPKD and CKD. The study's longer follow-up period, in comparison to previous reports, offers an opportunity to better understand the impact of SARS-CoV-2 infection on renal function in individuals with ADPKD and CKD. Schmidt-Lauber et al. conducted a comparative analysis, investigating kidney outcomes in 443 patients following mild-moderate COVID-19 alongside a matched control group of 1328 individuals from the general population without prior COVID-19. Their results, assessed over a median follow-up period of 9 months post non-severe COVID-19, revealed only a slight reduction in the mean eGFR. Importantly, no discernible indications pointed toward an elevated risk of progressive kidney dysfunction [5]. Nevertheless, it is noteworthy that approximately 10% of the study cohort had preexisting CKD, and only a subset of these individuals had a specific underlying etiological diagnosis [6]. Similarly, Bowe et al. [7] reported kidney outcomes following COVID-19 in a population-based study involving US veterans. They identified an elevated risk of AKI, eGFR decline, and ESRD after a median follow-up period of around 6 months [8]. Notably, the mean eGFR in this study exceeded 70 mL/min/1.73 m^2, and the proportion of patients with CKD remained undisclosed [7]. In comparison, our study encompassed patients with different renal diseases, at a higher risk of disease progression. Our cohort exhibited a significantly lower eGFR, and the follow-up period was longer. Consequently, our study could offer an evaluation of whether COVID-19 represents a risk factor for CKD progression in both CKD and ADPKD patients [9]. Indeed, in our cohort, ADPKD patients presented a greater worsening of renal function 1 year after COVID-19 infection; however, this was statistically significant only in patients with eGFR < 60 mL/min. This supports the already known hypothesis that low eGFR can favor the worsening of kidney damage, in our study, in particular, in ADPKD patients. Mirijello et al. [10] showed that patients with reduced eGFR should be considered at high risk of clinical deterioration and death. This further supports the fact that our cohort included patients with a higher risk of CKD progression who may be more prone to worse renal functioning following COVID-19. The impact of SARS-CoV-2 on changes in eGFR has been shown to become more pronounced after a year, suggesting that SARS-CoV-2 infection may have triggered an injury reminiscent of AKI [11]. The association between SARS-CoV-2 infections and AKI is well-established, with proposed mechanisms including virus-related effects as well as those unrelated to the virus (such as sepsis, nephrotoxic agents, cardiovascular instability, etc.) contributing to renal injury. While definitive proof of SARS-CoV-2 renal tropism is lacking, recent data have indicated that SARS-CoV-2-infected pluripotent stem-cell-derived kidney organoids exhibit activation of profibrotic signaling pathways. Hence, SARS-CoV-2 has the capability of directly infecting kidney cells, leading to cellular injury and subsequent fibrosis. These findings offer a potential explanation for both AKI observed in COVID-19 patients and the subsequent development of CKD in individuals experiencing long COVID [11]. Large-scale population studies have sought to evaluate the relationship between CKD and COVID-19 outcomes. A population database study in the United Kingdom, encompassing 17 million patients, revealed a noteworthy association between decreasing eGFR and escalating mortality rates [6]. Individuals with an eGFR ranging from 30 mL/min/1.73 m^2 to 60 mL/min/1.73 m^2 faced a 22% heightened risk of death, whereas those with an eGFR lower than 30 mL/min/1.73 m^2 experienced a 2.5-fold increase in the risk of death. The risk was further elevated in patients on dialysis, the latter experiencing a 3.7-fold increase in the risk of mortality, while those with a solid organ transplant faced a similar 3.5-fold increase in mortality risk [8,9,12]. Specifically focusing on COVID-19 patients with CKD in Mexico, data from 16.000 hospitalized individuals with an eGFR below 60 mL/min/1.73 m^2 have revealed a striking case fatality rate of 39% [13,14]. Additionally, a meta-analysis involving 16 studies and 871 hospitalized kidney transplant patients with COVID-19 reported a pooled case fatality rate of 24% [15]. Consistent findings emerged from similar retrospective studies conducted in Europe, Turkey, and the United States, highlighting an increased risk of mortality due to COVID-19 associated with decreasing renal function, kidney failure, and transplantation [16–18]. While data remain quite limited, there is no evidence to suggest ADPKD increases the likelihood of hospitalization, dialysis, or mortality over and above the risk conferred by the degree of CKD. Other study have not shown an increase in hospitalization, intensive care unit admission, intubation, or mortality following COVID-19 infection in patients with ADPKD compared with patients with other cystic kidney or cystic liver diseases [1,4,5]. While both conditions involve kidney dysfunction, the etiology, progression, and management strategies differ significantly. Limited studies exist on the specific impact of COVID-19 on ADPKD patients. However, it is plausible to speculate that the viral infection may exacerbate the challenges already present in ADPKD. The pro-inflammatory response triggered by COVID-19 could potentially worsen cystic growth, leading to increased pressure within the kidneys and a subsequent decline in renal function. Additionally, the systemic effects of COVID-19, such as hypoxia and coagulopathy, may further compromise kidney health in ADPKD patients [5]. Moreover, it is known that SARS-CoV-2 virus utilizes ACE2 receptors on cell membranes to determine the damage, and it is well-documented that the RAAS is more active in ADPKD patients [1]. The use of ACEIs and ARBs in the context of COVID-19 has been a subject of significant debate and research. ACEIs and ARBs may offer protective effects by mitigating the harmful consequences of elevated angiotensin II levels. By blocking the RAAS pathway, these medications can potentially reduce inflammation and fibrosis, which are exacerbated by COVID-19. There were concerns that ACEIs and ARBs might increase ACE2 expression, potentially facilitating viral entry. However, clinical data have generally not supported this hypothesis. Instead, these medications are thought to stabilize the RAAS, something which might be beneficial in the context of COVID-19. In ADPKD patients, the treatment with ACEi or ARBs is particularly relevant; in fact, these medications are the recommended first-line treatment for hypertension. The HALT-PKD trial has demonstrated that strict blood pressure control with these medications slows the growth of total kidney volume [19]. Early in the pandemic, concerns arose about the use of ACEi and ARBs in COVID-19 patients due to the virus utilizing the ACE2 receptor for cell entry. Competing hypotheses suggest that these medications could either be harmful by increasing the number of ACE2 receptors available for viral binding or beneficial by reducing inflammation and fibrosis leading to lung damage. A systematic review and meta-analysis of 102 observational studies assessed the correlation of ACEi/ARBs use and the likelihood of SARS-CoV-2 infection, mortality, and severe outcomes and showed that prior use of ACEis/ARBs was not associated with an altered risk of SARS-CoV-2 infection or significant change in severe outcomes or mortality after adjustment for confounding factors [20]. The REPLACE COVID trial, a prospective randomized study, was conducted in patients who had previously received a RAAS inhibitor and were admitted to the hospital with COVID-19. A total of 152 participants were enrolled and randomly assigned to either the group continuing or the group discontinuing RAAS inhibitor therapy. The results indicated that participants who continued RAAS inhibition experienced similar lengths of hospital stay, intensive care unit stay, and time on invasive mechanical ventilation compared to those who discontinued RAAS inhibition [21]. Similarly, the BRACE CORONA trial randomized 740 patients with COVID-19 across 29 centers in Brazil to either discontinue or continue ACEi or ARBs. The primary outcome analysis revealed no significant difference in the number of days alive and out of the hospital between the two groups [22]. Studies have shown that continuing ACEIs or ARBs in COVID-19 patients does not increase the risk of severe outcomes and may be associated with improved survival and reduced risk of severe kidney injury. In CKD patients, the relationship between COVID-19 and kidney disease progression is more established. COVID-19 has been associated with AKI, particularly in severe cases [15]. AKI can accelerate the progression of CKD or lead to de novo kidney disease. The virus can directly infect renal cells, causing inflammation and endothelial dysfunction, further contributing to kidney damage. Additionally, the systemic impact of the infection, including cytokine storm and hemodynamic instability, can negatively affect renal function [16]. While both ADPKD and CKD patients face heightened risks following COVID-19 infection, certain nuances differentiate their experiences. ADPKD patients may encounter challenges related to cystic growth and pressure within the kidneys, potentially impacting renal function. In CKD patients, the primary concern lies in the exacerbation of preexisting renal impairment due to COVID-19-induced AKI and systemic effects. Identifying ADPKD patients at higher risk of renal complications following COVID-19 infection can be crucial for early intervention and management. Combining serum and urinary biomarkers of AKI and inflammation and imaging modalities can provide a comprehensive assessment of the risk of renal complications following COVID-19 infection associated with an ADPKD patient. Regular monitoring of serum creatinine, eGFR, and cystatin C can help track kidney function. Urinary biomarkers like NGAL and KIM-1 can provide early warning signs of kidney injury. Imaging studies, particularly MRI or ultrasound, can provide detailed insights into the structural changes in the kidneys [23].

Limitations of the Study

A limitation of our study is the relatively small cohort of CKD and ADPKD patients. Therefore, additional prospective follow-up studies with a larger number of patients are necessary to confirm our results. Moreover, the follow-up period was relatively short.

5. Conclusions

The COVID-19 pandemic has posed challenges for patients with ADPKD and their healthcare providers. Current evidence does not suggest that individuals with ADPKD are at a higher risk of SARS-CoV-2 infection; however, exposure to the virus remains the primary risk factor. For those who contract COVID-19, the risk of hospitalization, intensive care admission, and death is generally increased in individuals with kidney dysfunction, though ADPKD itself does not seem to modify this risk. Despite the lack of increased susceptibility to SARS-CoV-2 infection, our study revealed a significant worsening of renal function among ADPKD patients, particularly those with an eGFR below 60 mL/min, in comparison to patients with CKD after a one-year follow-up from COVID-19 infection. In the nephrological context, it is crucial to stratify patients based on their underlying kidney disease to pinpoint any additional risk or protective factors in the manifestations of COVID-19. This consideration is especially important given the role of the RAAS, a pivotal hormonal system for both kidney function and the evolving pathology of COVID-19. Long-term follow-up is essential to assess the recovery of renal function and mitigate any lasting impacts. Identifying ADPKD patients at higher risk of renal complications following COVID-19 infection involves a multifaceted approach that includes the use of specific biomarkers and imaging modalities. Regular monitoring and early detection are key to managing these risks effectively. Coordination between nephrologists, radiologists, and primary care providers is essential for optimal patient care.

Author Contributions: Conceptualization, S.L. and A.G.; methodology, C.P.; software, L.S.; validation, S.L., A.G., S.I. and A.M.P.; formal analysis, C.D.I. and S.I.; investigation C.P.; resources, L.I.; data curation, P.I.; writing—original draft preparation, S.L.; writing—review and editing, A.G.; visualization, F.T.; supervision, R.C.; project administration, S.L.; funding acquisition, L.S. All authors have read and agreed to the published version of the manuscript.

Funding: This research received no external funding.

Institutional Review Board Statement: The study protocol was approved by the Clinical Research Ethics Committee at the Sapienza University of Rome, Italy, with Ethics Approval acceptance number 298/2020.

Informed Consent Statement: Informed consent was obtained from all subjects involved in the study.

Data Availability Statement: Data are available upon request.

Conflicts of Interest: The authors report no conflicts of interest. The authors alone are responsible for the content and writing of the paper. The manuscript has been seen and approved by all authors. The manuscript is not under consideration for publication elsewhere.

References

1. Kutky, M.; Cross, E.; Treleaven, D.J.; Alam, A.; Lanktree, M.B. The Impact of COVID-19 on Patients With ADPKD. *Can. J. Kidney Health Dis.* **2021**, *8*, 20543581211056479. [CrossRef] [PubMed]
2. Alibrandi, M.T.S.; Vespa, M. Rene, ADPKD e COVID-19: Il doppio ruolo della fragilità renale. *G. Clin. Nefrol. Dial* **2020**, *32*, 99–101. [CrossRef]

3. Banu, N.; Panikar, S.S.; Leal, L.R.; Leal, A.R. Protective role of ACE2 and its downregulation in SARS-CoV-2 infection leading to Macrophage Activation Syndrome: Therapeutic implications. *Rev. Life Sci.* **2020**, *256*, 117905. [CrossRef]
4. Xiang, H.-X.; Fei, J.; Xiang, Y.; Xu, Z.; Zheng, L.; Li, X.-Y.; Fu, L.; Zhao, H. Renal dysfunction and prognosis of COVID-19 patients: A hospital-based retrospective cohort study. *BMC Infect Dis.* **2021**, *21*, 158. [CrossRef]
5. Cui, X.; Gallini, J.W.; Jasien, C.L.; Mrug, M. Autosomal Dominant Polycystic Kidney Disease does not significantly alter major COVID-19 outcomes among veterans. *Kidney360* **2021**, *2*, 983–988. [CrossRef]
6. Ozturk, S.; Turgutalp, K.; Arici, M.; Odabas, A.R.; Altiparmak, M.R.; Aydin, Z.; Cebeci, E.; Basturk, T.; Soypacaci, Z.; Sahin, G.; et al. Mortality analysis of COVID-19 infection in chronic kidney disease, haemodialysis and renal transplant patients compared with patients without kidney disease: A nationwide analysis from Turkey. *Nephrol. Dial. Transplant.* **2020**, *35*, 2083–2095. [CrossRef]
7. Bowe, B.; Xie, Y.; Xu, E.; Al-Aly, Z. Kidney Outcomes in Long COVID. *J. Am. Soc. Nephrol.* **2021**, *32*, 2851–2862. [CrossRef]
8. Williamson, E.J.; Walker, A.J.; Bhaskaran, K.; Bacon, S.; Bates, C.; Morton, C.E.; Curtis, H.J.; Mehrkar, A.; Evans, D.; Inglesby, P.; et al. Factors associated with COVID-19-related death using OpenSAFELY. *Nature* **2020**, *584*, 430–436. [CrossRef]
9. Gansevoort, R.T.; Hilbrands, L.B. CKD is a key risk factor for COVID-19 mortality. *Nat. Rev. Nephrol.* **2020**, *16*, 705–706. [CrossRef]
10. Mirijello, A.; Piscitelli, P.; de Matthaeis, A.; Inglese, M.; D'Errico, M.M.; Massa, V.; Greco, A.; Fontana, A.; Copetti, M.; Florio, L.; et al. Low eGFR Is a Strong Predictor of Worse Outcome in Hospitalized COVID-19 Patients. *J. Clin. Med.* **2021**, *10*, 5224. [CrossRef]
11. Jansen, J.; Reimer, K.C.; Nagai, J.S.; Varghese, F.S.; Overheul, G.J.; de Beer, M.; Puni, R. SARS-CoV-2 infects the human kidney and drives fibrosis in kidney organoids. *Cell Stem Cell.* **2022**, *29*, 217–231.e7. [CrossRef] [PubMed]
12. Parra-Bracamonte, G.M.; Parra-Bracamonte, F.E.; Lopez-Villalobos, N.; Lara-Rivera, A.L. Chronic kidney disease is a very significant comorbidity for high risk of death in patients with COVID-19 in Mexico. *Nephrology* **2021**, *26*, 248–251. [CrossRef] [PubMed]
13. Hilbrands, L.B.; Duivenvoorden, R.; Vart, P.; Franssen, C.F.M.; Hemmelder, M.H.; Jager, K.J.; Kieneker, L.M.; Noordzij, M.; Pena, M.J.; de Vries, H.; et al. COVID-19-related mortality in kidney transplant and dialysis patients: Results of the ERACODA collaboration. *Nephrol. Dial. Transplant.* **2020**, *35*, 1973–1983. [CrossRef]
14. Docherty, A.B.; Harrison, E.M.; Green, C.A.; Hardwick, H.E.; Pius, R.; Norman, L.; Holden, K.A.; Read, J.M.; Dondelinger, F.; Carson, G.; et al. Features of 20 133 UK patients in hospital with COVID-19 using the ISARIC WHO Clinical Characterisation Protocol: Prospective observational cohort study. *BMJ* **2020**, *369*, m1985. [CrossRef] [PubMed]
15. Flythe, J.E.; Assimon, M.M.; Tugman, M.J.; Chang, E.H.; Gupta, S.; Sosa, M.A.; Renaghan, A.D.; Melamed, M.L.; Wilson, F.P.; Neyra, J.A.; et al. Characteristics and outcomes of individuals with pre-existing kidney disease and COVID-19 admitted to intensive care units in the United States. *Am. J. Kidney Dis.* **2021**, *77*, 190–203. [CrossRef] [PubMed]
16. Mikami, T.; Miyashita, H.; Yamada, T.; Harrington, M.; Steinberg, D.; Dunn, A.; Siau, E. Risk factors for mortality in patients with COVID-19 in New York City. *J. Gen. Intern. Med.* **2021**, *36*, 17–26. [CrossRef] [PubMed]
17. Lai, S.; Gigante, A.; Pellicano, C.; Mariani, I.; Iannazzo, F.; Concistrè, A.; Letizia, C.; Muscaritoli, M. Kidney dysfunction is associated with adverse outcomes in internal medicine COVID-19 hospitalized patients. *Eur. Rev. Med. Pharmacol. Sci.* **2023**, *27*, 2706–2714. [PubMed]
18. Perrotta, A.M.; Rotondi, S.; Mazzaferro, S.; Bosi, L.; Letizia, C.; Muscaritoli, M.; Gigante, A.; Salciccia, S.; Pasculli, P.; Ciardi, M.R.; et al. COVID-19 and kidney: Role of SARS-CoV-2 infection in the induction of renal damage. *Eur. Rev. Med. Pharmacol. Sci.* **2023**, *27*, 7861–7867. [PubMed]
19. Chapman, A.B.; Torres, V.E.; Perrone, R.D.; Steinman, T.I.; Bae, K.T.; Miller, J.P.; Schrier, R.W. The HALT Polycystic Kidney Disease Trials: Design and Implementation. *Clin. J. Am. Soc. Nephrol.* **2010**, *5*, 102–109. [CrossRef]
20. Xu, J.; Teng, Y.; Shang, L.; Gu, X.; Fan, G.; Chen, Y.; Tian, R.; Zhang, S.; Cao, B. The effect of prior angiotensin-converting enzyme inhibitor and angiotensin receptor blocker treatment on coronavirus disease 2019 (COVID-19) susceptibility and outcome: A systematic review and meta-analysis. *Clin. Infect Dis.* **2020**, *72*, e901–e913. [CrossRef]
21. Cohen, J.B.; Hanff, T.C.; William, P.; Sweitzer, N.; Rosado-Santander, N.R.; Medina, C.; Chirinos, J.A. Continuation versus discontinuation of renin–angiotensin system inhibitors in patients admitted to hospital with COVID-19: A prospective, randomised, open-label trial. *Lancet Respir. Med.* **2021**, *9*, 275–284. [CrossRef] [PubMed]
22. Lopes, R.D.; Macedo, A.V.; Silva PG DB, E.; Moll-Bernardes, R.J.; Dos Santos, T.M.; Mazza, L. Effect of discontinuing vs. continuing angiotensin-converting enzyme inhibitors and angiotensin II receptor blockers on days alive and out of the hospital in patients admitted with COVID-19: A randomized clinical trial. *JAMA* **2021**, *325*, 254–264. [CrossRef] [PubMed]
23. Shakked, N.P.; de Oliveira, M.H.S.; Cheruiyot, I.; Benoit, J.L.; Plebani, M.; Lippi, G.; Benoit, S.W.; Henry, B.M. Early prediction of COVID-19-associated acute kidney injury: Are serum NGAL and serum Cystatin C levels better than serum creatinine? *Clin. Biochem.* **2022**, *102*, 1–8. [CrossRef] [PubMed]

Disclaimer/Publisher's Note: The statements, opinions and data contained in all publications are solely those of the individual author(s) and contributor(s) and not of MDPI and/or the editor(s). MDPI and/or the editor(s) disclaim responsibility for any injury to people or property resulting from any ideas, methods, instructions or products referred to in the content.

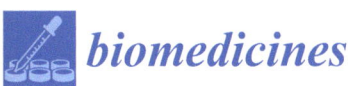

Article

Respiratory SARS-CoV-2 Infection Causes Skeletal Muscle Atrophy and Long-Lasting Energy Metabolism Suppression

Sachiko T. Homma [1,*], Xingyu Wang [2], Justin J. Frere [3], Adam C. Gower [4], Jingsong Zhou [5], Jean K. Lim [3], Benjamin R. tenOever [6] and Lan Zhou [2,*]

1. Department of Neurology, Boston University Chobanian & Avedisian School of Medicine, Boston, MA 02118, USA
2. Department of Neurology, Hospital for Special Surgery, New York, NY 10021, USA
3. Department of Microbiology, Icahn School of Medicine at Mount Sinai, New York, NY 10029, USA
4. Clinical and Translational Science Institute, Boston University Chobanian & Avedisian School of Medicine, Boston, MA 02118, USA
5. College of Nursing and Health Innovation, University of Texas at Arlington, Arlington, TX 76010, USA
6. Department of Microbiology, Grossman School of Medicine, New York University, New York, NY 10016, USA
* Correspondence: shomma@bu.edu (S.T.H.); zhoula@hss.edu (L.Z.); Tel.: +1-617-638-9555 (S.T.H.); +1-212-606-1880 (L.Z.)

Citation: Homma, S.T.; Wang, X.; Frere, J.J.; Gower, A.C.; Zhou, J.; Lim, J.K.; tenOever, B.R.; Zhou, L. Respiratory SARS-CoV-2 Infection Causes Skeletal Muscle Atrophy and Long-Lasting Energy Metabolism Suppression. *Biomedicines* **2024**, *12*, 1443. https://doi.org/10.3390/biomedicines12071443

Academic Editor: César Fernández-de-las-Peñas

Received: 18 May 2024
Revised: 19 June 2024
Accepted: 22 June 2024
Published: 28 June 2024

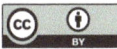

Copyright: © 2024 by the authors. Licensee MDPI, Basel, Switzerland. This article is an open access article distributed under the terms and conditions of the Creative Commons Attribution (CC BY) license (https://creativecommons.org/licenses/by/4.0/).

Abstract: Muscle fatigue represents the most prevalent symptom of long-term COVID, with elusive pathogenic mechanisms. We performed a longitudinal study to characterize histopathological and transcriptional changes in skeletal muscle in a hamster model of respiratory SARS-CoV-2 infection and compared them with influenza A virus (IAV) and mock infections. Histopathological and bulk RNA sequencing analyses of leg muscles derived from infected animals at days 3, 30, and 60 post-infection showed no direct viral invasion but myofiber atrophy in the SARS-CoV-2 group, which was accompanied by persistent downregulation of the genes related to myofibers, ribosomal proteins, fatty acid β-oxidation, tricarboxylic acid cycle, and mitochondrial oxidative phosphorylation complexes. While both SARS-CoV-2 and IAV infections induced acute and transient type I and II interferon responses in muscle, only the SARS-CoV-2 infection upregulated TNF-α/NF-κB but not IL-6 signaling in muscle. Treatment of C2C12 myotubes, a skeletal muscle cell line, with combined IFN-γ and TNF-α but not with IFN-γ or TNF-α alone markedly impaired mitochondrial function. We conclude that a respiratory SARS-CoV-2 infection can cause myofiber atrophy and persistent energy metabolism suppression without direct viral invasion. The effects may be induced by the combined systemic interferon and TNF-α responses at the acute phase and may contribute to post-COVID-19 persistent muscle fatigue.

Keywords: COVID-19; long COVID; influenza; muscle fatigue; muscle atrophy; energy metabolism; mitochondria; interferons; tumor necrosis factor-alpha

1. Introduction

Severe acute respiratory syndrome coronavirus 2 (SARS-CoV-2) has caused a global pandemic of coronavirus disease 2019 (COVID-19) since March 2020. Although the situation has greatly improved, thanks to the development of vaccines, advances in the treatment of acute infections, and the evolution of less virulent strains, many new COVID-19 cases and related morbidity and mortality are encountered every day worldwide. COVID-19 impacts human health beyond acute infection. COVID-19 long-haul symptoms are relatively prevalent across different age groups [1,2], and managing these symptoms has become a challenge. The condition in which the symptoms persist beyond 12 weeks after an acute viral infection with no alternative diagnosis has been defined as post-COVID-19 syndrome [3].

Post-COVID-19 syndrome can manifest many symptoms, the majority of which are neurological and neuropsychiatric, including myalgia, fatigue, brain fog, headaches, insomnia, and anxiety, among others [4,5]. Muscle fatigue represents the most prevalent symptom, as revealed by several large cohort studies, and it can occur regardless of the severity of the initial viral infection [5–9]. Although myalgia and fatigue are common with acute respiratory viral infections such as influenza, the symptoms are often more severe and long-lasting when associated with SARS-CoV-2 [10], implicating prolonged structural and functional abnormalities in skeletal muscle after acute respiratory SARS-CoV-2 infection. There are several published histopathological examinations of the skeletal muscle of patients who suffered from long COVID-19 [11–14]. These studies showed a variety of pathological changes, including muscle atrophy, inflammation, mitochondrial abnormalities, and capillary injury. Recent studies have also shown reduced mitochondrial oxidative capacity in patients with long COVID [12–14].

To better understand the molecular mechanisms underlying the development and persistence of myalgia and fatigue associated with COVID-19, we performed a longitudinal study to characterize the histopathological and transcriptional responses of skeletal muscle to respiratory SARS-CoV-2 infection and benchmarked the findings to influenza A virus (IAV) infection, utilizing the golden hamster as a model system. The hamster model has been proven to largely phenocopy COVID-19 biology, and it displays severe lung morphology and a tropism that matches what is observed in human patients [15–17]. Our study showed no direct viral invasion but myofiber atrophy, which was accompanied by persistent suppression of the genes related to myofibers, ribosomal proteins, and mitochondrial oxidative metabolism in the SARS-CoV-2 group. It downregulated both cytoplasmic and mitochondrial ribosome protein genes, likely impairing protein synthesis. It also downregulated many nuclear genes, but not mitochondrial genes, involved in fatty acid β-oxidation, the tricarboxylic acid (TCA) cycle, and all five oxidative phosphorylation (OXPHOS) complexes. In contrast, no myofiber atrophy or persistent gene expression changes were observed in the IAV-infected hamsters. In addition to the transient type I and type II interferon responses at the acute phase of either infection, only the SARS-CoV-2 infection induced TNF-α but not IL-6 response in skeletal muscle. In vitro co-treatment of differentiated C2C12 cells, a skeletal muscle cell line, with IFN-γ and TNF-α greatly impaired mitochondrial respiration and shifted energy metabolism from mitochondrial oxidative respiration to glycolysis. Our findings suggest that the combined systemic interferon and TNF-α responses during acute respiratory SARS-CoV-2 infection might induce a long-lasting suppression of mitochondrial oxidative energy metabolism and myofiber atrophy, causing acute and persistent muscle symptoms.

2. Materials and Methods

2.1. Golden Hamster Models

Six-week-old male Golden Syrian hamsters (*Mesocricetus auratus*) were obtained from Charles River Laboratories (Wilmington, MA, USA). Hamsters were acclimated to the CDC/USDA-approved Biosafety Level 3 (BSL-3) facility at the Center for Comparative Medicine and Surgery at the Icahn School of Medicine at Mount Sinai (New York, NY, USA). When the hamsters reached 10 weeks of age, they were randomly divided into nine groups for induction of three different kind of infections and for evaluation at three time points post-infection (three hamsters/infection/time point). Three infection groups include (1) mock-infected group: intranasally treated with PBS; (2) SARS-CoV-2-infected group: intranasally infected with 1000 pfu (total volume 100 μL) of SARS-CoV-2 (USA-WA1/2020); and (3) IAV-infected group: intranasally infected with 100,000 pfu (total volume 100 μL) of H1N1 IAV (A/California/04/2009). Intranasal administration was performed under ketamine/xylazine anesthesia. Hamsters were housed for 3-, 30-, and 60 days post-infection (dpi) before being euthanized via sodium pentobarbital and intracardiac perfusion with PBS. After perfusion, quadriceps muscle was exposed and harvested. Half of each sample was placed into a 4% paraformaldehyde (PFA) solution to be fixed for 48 h before being transferred to PBS. The other half was placed into "lysing matrix A" homogenization tubes (MP Biomedicals, Santa Ana, CA, USA) filled with TRIzol (Thermo Fisher Scientific, Waltham, MA, USA) and homogenized before being frozen at −80 °C.

2.2. Hematoxylin and Eosin (H&E) Staining

Paraffin-embedded tissue blocks were cut into 6-μm sections and mounted on charged glass slides (Thermo Fisher Scientific). Sections were deparaffinized by immersion in xylene and rehydrated in decreasing ethanol dilutions. Slides were then stained using the Hematoxylin and Eosin stain kit (Vector Laboratories, Newark, CA, USA) following the manufacturer's instructions. Slides were dehydrated by immersion in increasing concentrations of ethanol, cleared with xylene, and coverslipped. Standard microscope images were acquired using a Nikon E800 microscope with spot camera and software version 5.0 (Diagnostic Instruments Inc., Sterling Heights, MI, USA).

2.3. Immunohistochemistry (IHC)

Paraffin sections were used for immunostaining. Antigen retrieval was performed for 30 min in a pressure cooker with slides immersed in antigen retrieval buffer (Tris/EDTA pH 9.0). Tissue sections were blocked in Tris-Buffered Saline (TBS) with 3% bovine serum albumin and 5% normal goat serum (Vector laboratories) or 5% normal rabbit serum (Vector laboratories) for 2 h at room temperature. For brightfield IHC, the primary antibody of SARS nucleocapsid protein (NP100-56576, Novus Biologicals, Centennial, CO, USA) was added to slides at a 1:250 dilution. Sections were incubated overnight at 4 °C. Slides were washed in TBS with 0.025% Triton X-100 prior to immersion in 0.3% hydrogen peroxide in TBS for 15 min. Slides were washed again, and a horseradish peroxidase-linked secondary antibody system (PK-6100, Vector Laboratories) and diaminobenzidine substrate were used for the detection of immunoreactive signals according to the manufacturer's instructions. Slides were then dehydrated by immersion in increasing concentrations of ethanol, cleared with xylene, and coverslipped. For immunofluorescent microcopy, the sections were incubated overnight at 4 °C with primary antibodies of SARS-CoV-2 N protein (GXT635679, Genetex, Irvine, CA, USA) and SARS-CoV-2 S protein (ZMS1076, Sigma-Aldrich, St. Louis, MO, USA) at a 1:1000 dilution. The sections were then washed and incubated with secondary antibodies conjugated with Alexa Fluor 568 for the N protein and Alexa Fluor 647 for the S protein (A-11011 and A-21235, respectively, Thermo Fisher Scientific) at a 1:1000 dilution for 1 h. The slides were coverslipped after 4′,6-diamidino-2-phenylindole (DAPI) staining of nuclei. Fluorescent microscope images were acquired using a Zeiss Axio Observer microscope and Zen 2.6 (Blue edition) software (Carl Zeiss, White Plains, NY, USA). Autofluorescence was captured by the green fluorescence channel to monitor false-positive cells for SARS-CoV-2 proteins.

2.4. Muscle Fiber Type Composition

After IHC using primary antibodies against slow skeletal myosin heavy chain (ab11083, Abcam, Waltham, MA, USA, 1:200 dilution) and fast skeletal myosin heavy chain (ab51263, Abcam, 1:400 dilution), quantification of the number of each type of myofiber and myofiber cross-sectional area were performed. The fiber type distribution was expressed as a percentage of slow or fast myosin heavy chain expressing fibers in the total fibers on the sections.

2.5. Transmission Electron Microscopy (TEM)

Tissues for TEM were processed and imaged in the Boston University School of Medicine TEM core facility. Tissue blocks of quadriceps were post-fixed with 3% glutaraldehyde solution (Electron Microscopy Sciences, Hatfield, PA, USA) and 3% paraformaldehyde (Electron Microscopy Sciences) in 0.1 M phosphate buffer (PB, pH 7.4) for 24 h at 4 °C. After rinsing in 0.1 M PBS, tissue blocks were fixed with 1% osmium tetroxide (Electron Microscopy Sciences) for 1.5 h, rinsed in water, and then dehydrated in a series of increasing acetone concentrations (50%, 90%, and 100%). The samples were then infiltrated and block-embedded in epoxy resin (Electron Microscopy Sciences). Ultrathin sections (50 nm) were prepared with an ultra-microtome (Leica, Wetzlar, Germany) and collected into copper mesh grids (Ted Pella, Redding, CA, USA). Grids were counterstained with 4% uranyl acetate (Electron Microscopy Sciences) for 5 min at 60 °C, followed by rinses in filtered distilled water and then in 0.4% lead citrate (Ted Pella) for 45 s at room temperature. The sections were imaged and photographed using a JEM1400 electron microscope (JEOL) connected to an AMT NanoSprint-43M-B Mid-Mount CMOS camera (AMT701, Advanced Microscopy Techniques Corp., Woburn, MA, USA). Individual subsarcolemmal (SS) and intermyofibrillar (IMF) mitochondria from three hamsters of each group were manually traced in longitudinal orientation using ImageJ (NIH) and quantified using the morphological and shape descriptors including area (μm^2), perimeter (μm), Feret's diameter (longest distance between any two points within a given mitochondrion, μm), and aspect ratio (major axis divided by minor axis, which is a measure of the length to width ratio).

2.6. Quantitative Reverse-Transcription Polymerase Chain Reaction (qRT-PCR)

Total RNA was isolated from homogenized muscle samples by TRIzol (Thermo Fisher Scientific) and was further cleaned and treated with DNase using Directzol RNA miniprep (Zymo Research, Irvine, CA, USA). One microgram of total RNA from each tissue was reverse-transcribed into cDNA with oligo dT primers using SuperScript IV reverse transcriptase (Thermo Fisher Scientific). Quantitative polymerase chain reaction (qPCR) was performed using primers described in Supplementary Table S1, PowerTrack SYBR Green Master Mix (Applied Biosystems, Waltham, MA, USA), and Quantstudio 12K Flex qPCR system (Applied Biosystems).

2.7. Quantification of Mitochondrial DNA (mtDNA) Content by Real-Time PCR

Total DNA was isolated from paraffin sections of quadriceps using Quick-DNA FFPE MiniPrep (Zymo Research). MtDNA content was gauged by the mtDNA/nuclear DNA (nDNA) ratio measured by qPCR of NADH-ubiquinone oxidoreductase chain 1 gene (*nd1*) and beta-actin gene (*actb*) using primers described in Supplementary Table S1 [18].

2.8. Bulk RNA Sequencing (RNAseq)

One hundred nanograms of total RNA from each sample was enriched for polyadenylated RNA and prepared for next-generation sequencing using NEBNext Ultra II Directional RNA Library Prep Kit (New England Biolabs, Ipswich, MA, USA) and following the manufacturer's instructions. Prepared libraries were sequenced on an Illumina NextSeq 2000 platform. Prepared libraries were sequenced on an Illumina NextSeq 2000 instrument. FASTQ files were aligned to hamster genome build MesAur1.0 using STAR [19] (version 2.7.9a). Ensembl-Gene-level counts were generated using featureCounts (Subread package, version 1.6.2) and Ensembl annotation build 105 (uniquely aligned proper pairs, same strand). FASTQ quality was assessed using FastQC (version 0.11.7) and alignment quality was assessed using RSeQC (version 3.0.0). Differential expression was assessed using Wald test implemented in DESeq2 R package (version 1.32.10). Correction for multiple hypothesis testing was accomplished using Benjamini-Hochberg false discovery rate (FDR). Human homologs of hamster genes were identified using NCBI 'gene orthologs' table (retrieved 28 March 2022). All analyses were performed using R environment for statistical computing (version 4.1.2). Gene Set Enrichment Analysis (GSEA) (version 2.2.1) [20] was used to identify biological terms, pathways, and processes that are coordinately up- or down-regulated within each pairwise comparison. Entrez Gene identifiers of human homologs of all genes in Ensembl Gene annotation were ranked by Wald statistic computed for each pairwise comparison. Ensembl Genes matching multiple hamster Entrez Gene identifiers and hamster genes with multiple human homologs (or vice versa) were excluded prior to ranking, so that the ranked list represents only those human Entrez Gene IDs that match exactly one hamster Ensembl Gene. Each ranked list was then used to perform pre-ranked GSEA analyses (default parameters with random seed 1234) using the Entrez Gene versions of the H (Hallmark), C2 CP (Biocarta, KEGG, PID, Reactome, WikiPathways), C3 (transcription factor and microRNA motif), and C5 (Gene Ontology, GO) gene sets obtained from Molecular Signatures Database (MSigDB), version 7.5.1.

2.9. Cell Culture and Cytokine Treatments

C2C12 mouse myoblasts (CRL-1772) from ATCC (Manassas, VA, USA) were grown in 0.1% gelatin-coated dishes in Dulbecco's modified Eagle's medium (Fisher Scientific) containing 4500 mg/L glucose and supplemented with 10% fetal bovine serum (Thermo Fisher Scientific) and 100 U/mL penicillin/streptomycin (Thermo Fisher Scientific) in a humidified 5% CO_2 incubator at 37 °C. To induce differentiation, proliferating cultures that were near confluence were switched into a low-serum differentiation medium consisting of 2% horse serum (Thermo Fisher Scientific). Cytokine treatments were carried out with differentiating cells that had been in differentiation medium for 3 days after reaching confluence. Differentiating cultures were incubated for 24 and 48 h with mouse TNF-α (410-MT, R&D systems, Minneapolis, MN, USA, 10 ng/mL), universal type I interferon IFN-α (11200, PBL assay science, Piscataway, NJ, USA, 100U), mouse IFN-γ (485-MI, R&D systems, 100U), and mouse IL-6 (406-ML, R&D systems, 10 ng/mL) alone or in combination.

2.10. Immunoblotting

C2C12 myogenic cells were homogenized in RIPA buffer (50 mmol/L Tris-HCl pH 7.4, 150 mmol/L NaCl, 1% NP-40, 0.5% sodium deoxycholic acid, and 0.1% SDS) with protease inhibitors (Thermo Fisher Scientific), sonicated, and then centrifuged at $15,000\times g$ for 15 min. The protein in the supernatant was quantified by a BCA protein assay (Thermo Fisher Scientific). Thirty micrograms of protein were subjected to SDS-PAGE under reducing conditions and transferred to polyvinylidene difluoride (PVDF) membranes (MilliporeSigma, Burlington, MA, USA). Blots were blocked in 3% non-fat skim milk or 3% BSA and washed three times with TBS containing 0.1% Tween. Membranes were incubated with primary antibodies against total OXPHOS cocktail (ab110413, Abcam, 1:250), COX17 (11464-1AP, Proteintech, Rosemont, IL, USA, 1:500), RPS3 (66046-1-lg, Proteintech, 1:500), RPL23 (A305-010A, Bethyl laboratories, Montgomery, TX, USA, 1:1000), or tubulin (2148S, Cell Signaling Technology, Danvers, MA, USA, 1:1000) and then washed. Signals were detected with IRDye 800- or 680-conjugated secondary antibodies (926-68020, 925-68021, LI-COR Biosciences, Lincoln, NE, USA, 1:5000) with appropriate species specificity. Immunoblots were visualized by Image Studio software version 2.1.10 (LI-COR Biosciences) that accompanies the LI-COR Odyssey infrared system (LI-COR Biosciences).

2.11. Bioenergetic Analysis

The oxygen consumption rate (OCR), extracellular acidification rate (ECAR), and ATP production rate of C2C12 cells were determined using an Agilent Seahorse XFe96 Analyzer following the manufacturer's instructions. XF base medium, XFe96 culture plates, and the XF96 Extracellular Flux assay kit were purchased from Agilent Technologies (Santa Clara, CA, USA). C2C12 cells were grown and differentiated on 0.1% gelatin-coated XFe96 culture plates. On the third day in the differentiation medium, cells were treated with cytokine(s) for 24 h, as described above. After the treatment, cells were washed and switched to XF base medium supplemented with 10 mM glucose, 1 mM sodium pyruvate, and 2 mM glutamine and cultured in a CO_2-free incubator at 37 °C for 1 h. OCR and ECAR were measured under basal conditions and after injections of a final concentration of 1 µM oligomycin, 0.5 µM FCCP, and/or 1 µM antimycin A combined with 1 µM rotenone. Following completion of the measurements, cells were washed with PBS and then lysed by adding 25 µL of RIPA lysis buffer to each well. The protein amount of the cell lysate in each well was determined by BCA assay. The OCR and ATP production rates were normalized to the protein amounts.

2.12. Statistics

All non-RNAseq statistical analyses, bar graphs, x-y plots, violin plots, and heat maps were prepared using GraphPad Prism 9 as described in the figure legends. The significance of these analyses was determined utilizing statistical tests, including ANOVA with post-hoc analyses. Specific post-hoc analyses and statistical thresholds are described in the figure legends.

3. Results

3.1. There Is No Evidence of Direct SARS-CoV-2 Viral Invasion of Skeletal Muscle in the Hamster Model

SARS-CoV-2, IAV, or PBS were intranasally delivered to golden hamsters at 10 weeks of age. Inoculation dosages were determined based on the prior studies that achieved comparable kinetics and viral loads in the SARS-CoV-2 and IAV model systems [15–17]. Both respiratory RNA viruses replicated in the lungs of golden hamsters, with the viral levels reaching the highest at 3 dpi and then becoming undetectable by 7 dpi [16,17]. Based on the results, we assessed the SARS-CoV-2 virus at 3 dpi in quadriceps by RNAseq, qRT-PCR, IHC, and TEM. RNAseq analysis detected SARS-CoV-2 transcript of 934.7 ± 503.4 (mean $\pm$ SD) reads per million (RPM) in lungs but only 0.80 ± 0.82 RPM ($p < 0.05$) in muscle at 3 dpi that was most likely from blood contamination, as muscle is rich in blood vessels. The SARS-CoV-2 transcript was not detectable in muscle at 30 or 60 dpi. qRT-PCR detected a high level of SARS-CoV-2 nucleoprotein subgenomic (*sgN*) transcript in the lungs of SARS-CoV-2-infected animals at 3 dpi but not at 30 or 60 dpi or in mock- or IAV-infected animals at any time points (Figure 1A). In quadriceps muscle, no significant expression of *sgN* was detected in any infection groups at any time points (Figure 1B). Immunostaining of SARS-CoV-2 N protein showed robust signals in bronchial epithelial cells (Figure 1C), bronchioles, and alveoli (Supplementary Figure S1B,E) in SARS-CoV-2-infected hamsters at 3 dpi but not 30 dpi (Supplementary Figure S1C,F) or in mock-infected controls at 3 dpi (Supplementary Figure S1A,D). Immunostaining of SARS-CoV-2 S protein showed the same expression pattern (Supplementary Figure S1G–I). No expression of SARS-CoV-2 N protein was detected by immunostaining in quadriceps of SARS-CoV-2-, IAV-, or mock-infected hamsters at 3 dpi (Figure 1D–F), 30 dpi, or 60 dpi. TEM did not show any virus-like particles in the quadriceps. H&E staining showed inflammatory cell infiltrates in bronchioles and alveoli in lungs at 3 dpi (Figure 1G) but not in quadriceps at 3 dpi (Figure 1H–J). Therefore, there is no evidence of direct SARS-CoV-2 invasion of skeletal muscle or persistent viral pneumonia in the COVID-19 hamster model.

3.2. Respiratory SARS-CoV-2 but Not IAV Infection Induces Skeletal Muscle Atrophy

To assess histopathological changes in skeletal muscle post-COVID-19, we stained paraffin sections of quadriceps derived from SARS-CoV-2-, IAV-, or mock-infected hamsters at 3, 30, and 60 dpi with H&E. It showed no myofiber necrosis or regeneration, no endomysial inflammation or fibrosis, and no microthrombi. However, myofiber cross-sectional areas (CSA) were significantly smaller in the SARS-CoV-2 group than in the mock and IAV groups at 60 dpi (Figure 2A and Supplementary Figure S2). Since hamsters and their myofiber size grew during the period of 30–60 dpi (14.3–18.5 weeks of age) [21] (Figure 2A), the respiratory SARS-CoV-2 infection might halt the myofiber growth, causing atrophy.

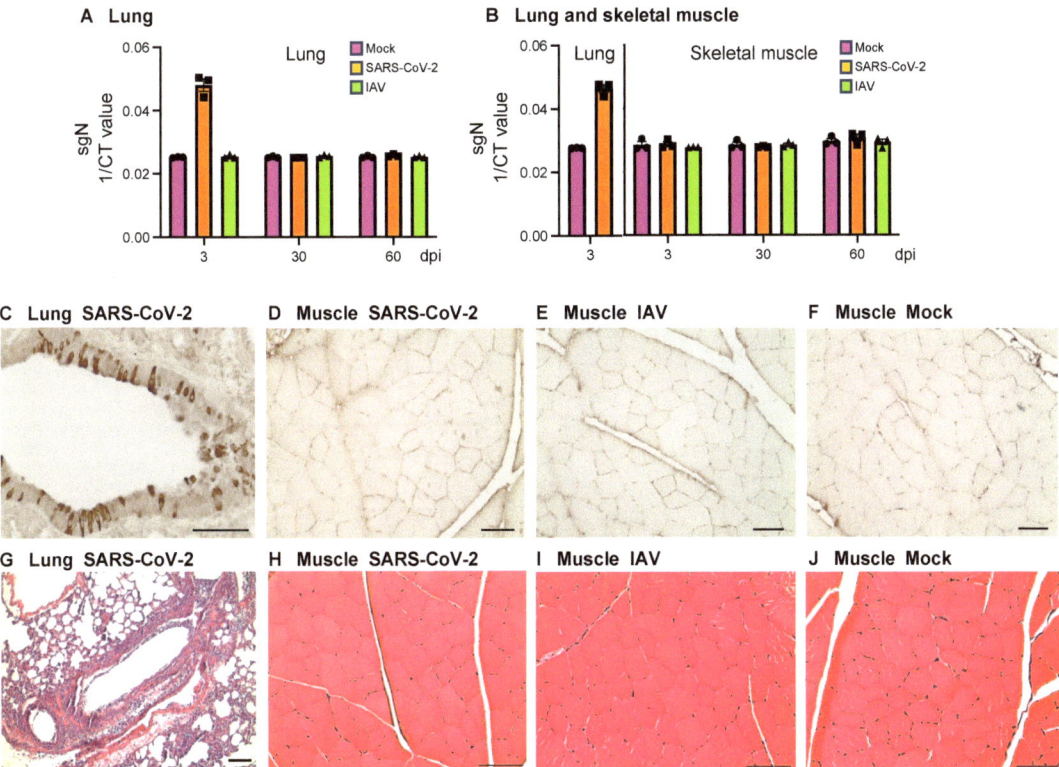

Figure 1. There is no evidence of direct SARS-CoV-2 invasion of skeletal muscle. (**A**,**B**) qRT-PCR of nucleoprotein subgenomic RNA (*sgN*) using RNA samples from lungs (**A**) and quadriceps muscles (**B**) of SARS-CoV-2-, influenza A virus (IAV)-, or mock-infected hamsters at 3-, 30-, and 60-days post-infection (dpi). *n* = 3 hamsters/infection group/time point. Each dot represents mean value of 3 replicates of each sample. Data are expressed as mean ± SEM. CT: cycle threshold. (**C**–**F**) Immunostaining of SARS-CoV-2 N protein using lung tissue from SARS-CoV-2-infected hamsters at 3 dpi (**C**) and quadriceps muscles from SARS-CoV-2- (**D**), IAV- (**E**), and mock- (**F**) infected hamsters at 3 dpi. (**G**–**J**) H&E staining of lung tissue from SARS-CoV-2-infected hamsters at 3 dpi (**G**) and quadriceps muscles from SARS-CoV-2- (**H**), IAV- (**I**), and mock- (**J**)-infected hamsters at 3 dpi. Images are representatives of 3 hamsters/infection group/time point (**C**–**J**). Bar = 50 μm (**C**–**F**). Bar = 100 μm (**G**–**J**).

Skeletal muscle consists of two major fiber types with a differential preference for energy metabolism [22]. To address whether oxidative myofibers (slow twitch fibers) and glycolytic myofibers (fast twitch fibers) were differentially affected by the respiratory SARS-CoV-2 infection, we analyzed the CSA of each myofiber subtype at 60 dpi (Figure 2B–E). CSA of both slow and fast twitch myofiber was significantly smaller ($p < 0.01$) in SARS-CoV-2-infected animals than in mock-infected controls (Figure 2D). In contrast, IAV-infected hamsters retained the size of each type of myofiber. The fiber type distribution was not different among the three groups (Figure 2E).

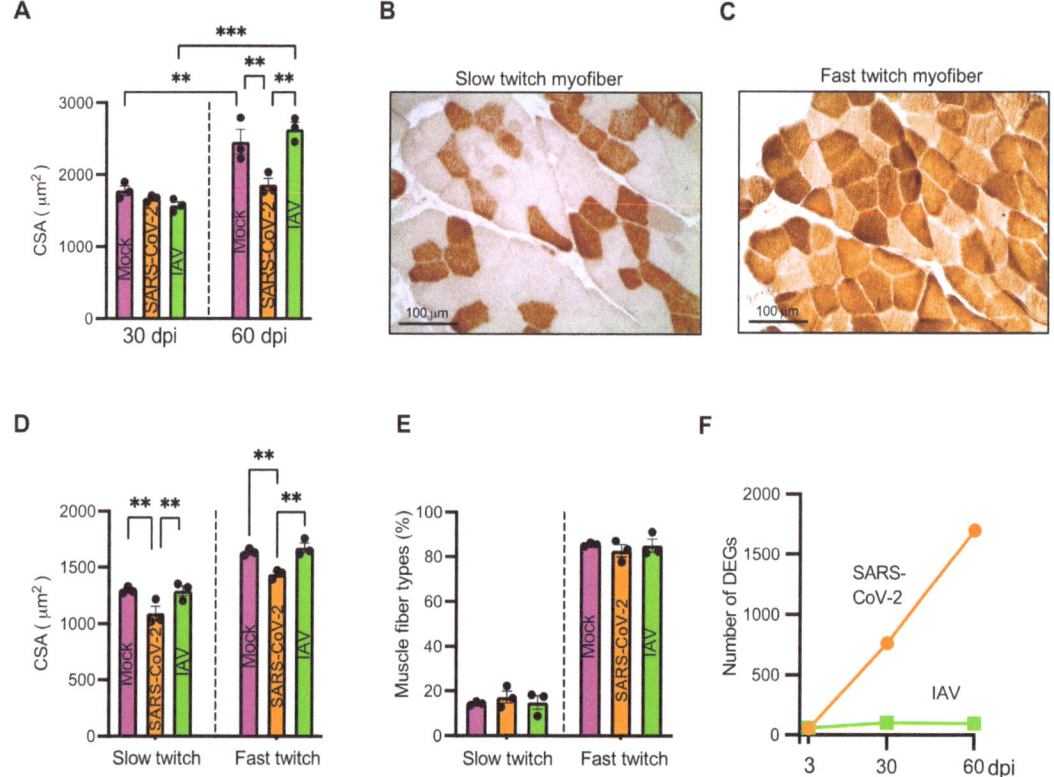

Figure 2. Respiratory infection with SARS-CoV-2 but not influenza A virus (IAV)-induced muscle fiber atrophy. (**A**) Bar graph showing comparison of cross-sectional area (CSA) of myofiber of quadriceps of mock-, SARS-CoV-2-, or IAV-infected hamsters at 30- and 60-days post-infection (dpi). (**B**,**C**) Representative images showing slow twitch myofibers stained intensely by anti-slow skeletal myosin heavy chain antibody (**B**) and fast twitch myofibers stained intensely by anti-fast skeletal myosin heavy chain antibody (**C**). (**D**) Bar graph showing comparison of CSA of slow and fast twitch myofibers of quadriceps from mock-, SARS-CoV-2, or IAV-infected hamsters at 60 dpi. (**E**) Fiber type distribution expressed in relative percent of the total number of myofibers. (**A**,**D**,**E**) Each dot represents mean value of CSA (**A**,**D**) or mean percent of muscle fiber types (**E**) of each hamster. n = 3 hamsters/infection group/time point. Data were analyzed by one-way ANOVA with Tukey's post hoc test and expressed as mean ± SEM. ** $p < 0.01$, *** $p < 0.001$. (**F**) Number of significant differentially expressed genes (DEGs, false discovery rate [FDR] $q < 0.1$) detected by RNAseq of quadriceps muscles derived from SARS-CoV-2 or IAV-infected hamsters at 3, 30, and 60 dpi compared to mock controls. n = 3 hamsters/infection group/time point.

3.3. Respiratory SARS-CoV-2 Infection Induces Long-Lasting Downregulation of Skeletal Muscle Genes, Primarily Affecting Oxidative Myofiber Genes

To assess the transcriptional response, we performed RNAseq using quadriceps obtained from SARS-CoV-2-, IAV-, or mock-infected hamsters at 3, 30, and 60 dpi. We performed Wald tests to compare the SARS-CoV-2 or IAV group with the mock group. While the number of significant (FDR $q < 0.1$) differentially expressed genes (DEGs) remained relatively stable in the IAV-infected hamsters over the 60-day period, the number of significant DEGs increased sharply in the SARS-CoV-2-infected hamsters over the same period (Figure 2F), indicating a much greater and longer skeletal muscle transcriptional response to the respiratory SARS-CoV-2 infection than to the IAV infection.

Since we observed atrophy in both slow and fast twitch myofibers in SARS-CoV-2-infected hamsters, we analyzed the expression of the genes related to each myofiber subtype [23] (Figure 3A,B). In SARS-CoV-2-infected animals, the majority of the genes that are predominantly expressed by slow/intermediate myofibers were consistently downregulated at all three time points, with several genes achieving statistical significance at 30 and 60 dpi; conversely, no genes were significantly downregulated in IAV-infected animals (Figure 3A). In contrast, the fast/type IIb myofiber genes did not show a consistent pattern of regulation at any time point or infection group, with the exception of a trend of upregulation at 60 dpi in the IAV-infected animals (Figure 3B). These findings indicate that the respiratory SARS-CoV-2 infection primarily affected oxidative fibers at the transcriptional level.

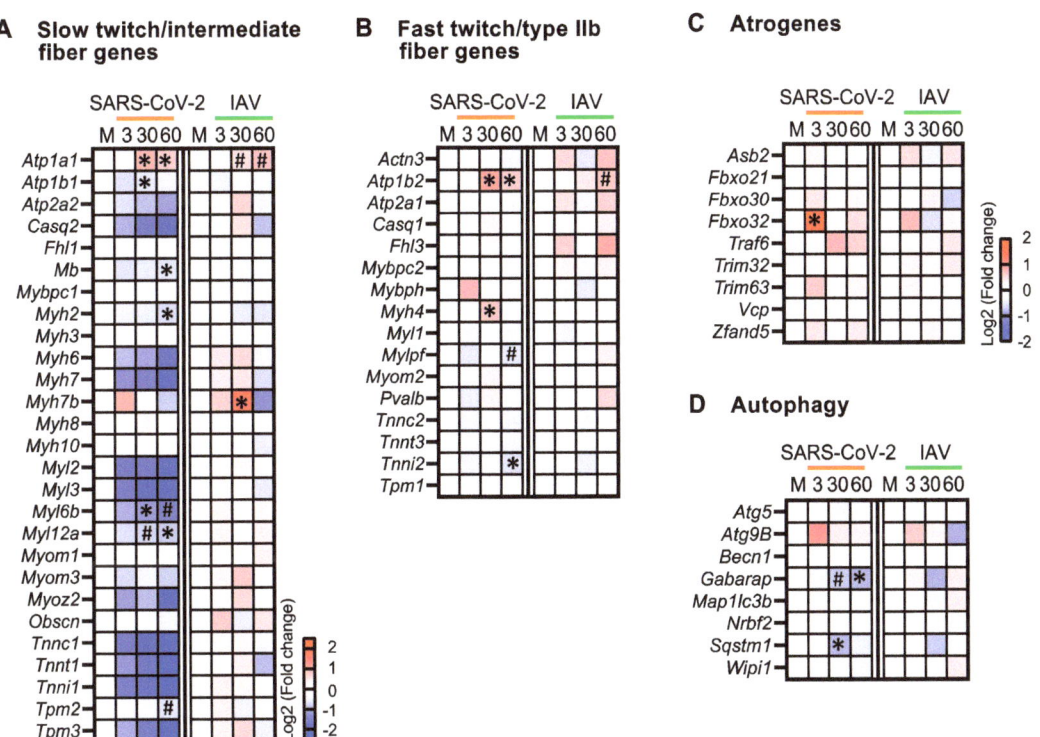

Figure 3. Respiratory SARS-CoV-2 infection induces long-lasting downregulation of oxidative myofiber genes and autophagy genes. (**A–D**) Heatmaps showing changes in the expression of slow twitch/intermediate myofiber genes (**A**), fast twitch/type IIb myofiber genes (**B**), atrogenes (**C**), and autophagy genes (**D**) in quadriceps muscles of SARS-CoV-2- and IAV-infected hamsters at different time points compared to mock controls (M). Blue, white, and red indicate log2 (fold change) values of <-2.5, 0, and >2.5, respectively, for (**A,B**), and log2 values of <-2, 0, and >2, respectively, for (**C,D**). Symbols indicate significant differences compared to mock controls (M) by Wald test (* FDR $q < 0.05$, # FDR $q < 0.1$). $n = 3$ hamsters/infection group/time point.

3.4. Respiratory SARS-CoV-2 Infection Upregulates Atrogenes and Downregulates Autophagy Genes in Skeletal Muscle

Skeletal muscle fiber size is determined by the balance between protein synthesis and degradation. Because the ubiquitin-proteasome system catalyzes the degradation of most proteins in mammalian cells [24], we assessed the expression of atrogenes involved in this system. In the SARS-CoV-2 group, these genes were upregulated at all three time points, with *Fbxo32* significantly upregulated at 3 dpi (Figure 3C). *Fbxo32* encodes skeletal-muscle-specific E3 ubiquitin ligase F-box protein 32 (FBXO32), which is also known as muscle atrophy F-box (MAFbx) and atrogin-1. It is considered one of the master regulators of muscle atrophy [25]. In contrast, there was not a consistent pattern of regulation in the IAV group, with none of the atrogenes significantly upregulated (Figure 3C). The upregulation of atrogenes in SARS-CoV-2-infected animals might therefore contribute to the muscle atrophy detected.

Another proteolytic system that can contribute to muscle atrophy is autophagy. We assessed the expression of the key genes involved in autophagy initiation (*Becn1*, *Wipi1*, *Atg9b*, *Nrbf2*), autophagosome membrane elongation (*Gabarap*, *Map1lc3β*, *Atg5*), and substrate capture (*Sqstm1*) [26]. While the expressions of *Gabarap* and *Sqstm1* were significantly downregulated in the SARS-CoV-2 group at 30 and 60 dpi, none of these genes showed significant changes in the IAV group (Figure 3D). Therefore, the respiratory infection with SARS-CoV-2, but not IAV, might lead to long-lasting impairment of autophagy in skeletal muscle.

3.5. Respiratory SARS-CoV-2 Infection Induces Persistent Downregulation of Genes Involved in Cytoplasmic and Mitochondrial Protein Translation and Mitochondrial Oxidative Phosphorylation (OXPHOS) in Skeletal Muscle

To further characterize the skeletal muscle transcriptional response, we performed GSEA using Wald statistics computed for SARS-CoV-2 and IAV infections at each time point versus mock controls (Supplementary Data S1). There were 415 gene sets with significant coordinate downregulation (normalized enrichment scores [NES] < 0, FDR q < 0.1) in the SARS-CoV-2 group relative to the mock group at both 30 and 60 dpi. These included the Reactome "autophagy" pathway, in accordance with the observed downregulation of autophagy genes (Figure 3D), as well as numerous gene sets related to cytosolic and mitochondrial protein translation, mitochondrial function, and oxidative phosphorylation. We thus assessed the genes involved in these processes.

Muscle atrophy can be caused not only by increased protein degradation but also by reduced protein synthesis. Ribosome biogenesis is a fundamental rate-limiting step for protein synthesis, with each ribosome consisting of large and small RNA-protein complexes. In the SARS-CoV-2 group, 17/39 (44%) of the cytosolic ribosomal protein large subunit (RPL) genes and 16/28 (57%) of the small subunit (RPS) genes were significantly downregulated at 30 dpi, and the number of downregulated genes increased to 37/39 (95%) for RPL and 27/28 (96%) for RPS at 60 dpi (Figure 4A,B). In contrast, none of these genes were significantly changed in the IAV group. Thus, the respiratory SARS-CoV-2 infection may induce a unique, long-lasting suppression of cytoplasmic protein translation machinery in skeletal muscle, contributing to muscle atrophy.

We also analyzed the expression of the genes encoding mitochondrial ribosomal proteins (MRPs). Mitochondrial ribosomes translate mRNAs transcribed from mitochondrial DNA, but the MRPs themselves are encoded by nuclear genes. While both large and small subunit MRP genes were consistently downregulated in the SARS-CoV-2 group, with the majority achieving statistical significance at 60 dpi, none of them were significantly changed in the IAV group (Figure 4C,D). Therefore, mitochondrial protein synthesis may also be suppressed in skeletal muscle by a respiratory SARS-CoV-2 infection.

We next analyzed the mRNA expression of the five mitochondrial OXPHOS complexes that are composed of proteins of structural cores, supernumerary subunits, and assembly factors [27], which are encoded by both mtDNA genes and nDNA genes (Figure 5A–E). While the expression of the 13 mtDNA genes encoding essential proteins of complexes I, III, IV, and V did not change significantly in either the SARS-CoV-2 or the IAV group (Figure 5A,C–E), many nDNA genes encoding proteins of all five complexes were significantly downregulated in the SARS-CoV-2 but not the IAV group, with more significant changes seen at 60 dpi than at 30 dpi (Figure 5A–E). Therefore, the respiratory infection with SARS-CoV-2 induced a global and long-lasting downregulation of nuclear genes involved in skeletal muscle OXPHOS.

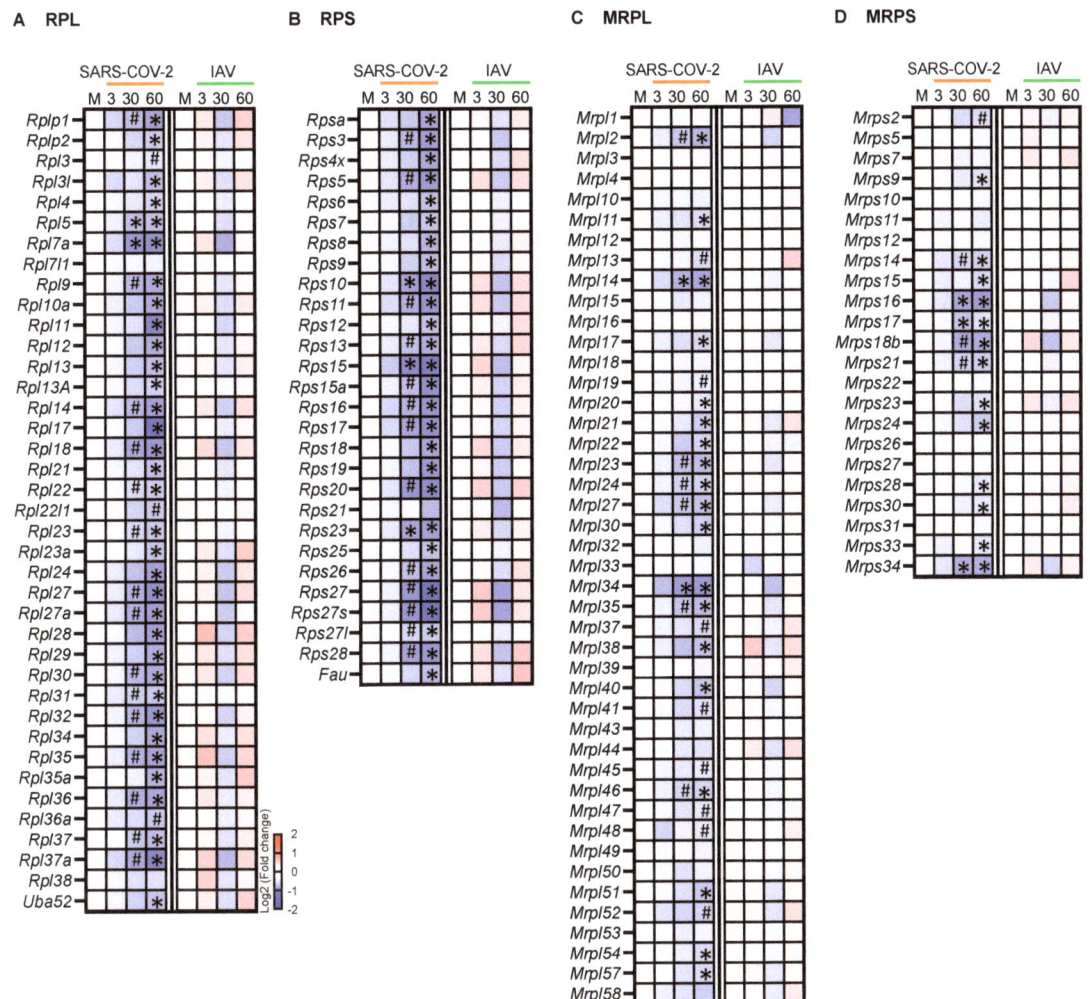

Figure 4. Respiratory infection with SARS-CoV-2 but not influenza A virus (IAV) causes persistent downregulation of many cytosolic and mitochondrial ribosomal protein genes. Heatmaps showing changes in the expression of cytosolic ribosomal protein large subunit (RPL) (**A**), cytosolic ribosomal protein small subunit (RPS) (**B**), mitochondrial ribosomal protein large subunit (MRPL) (**C**), and mitochondrial ribosomal protein small subunit (MRPS) (**D**) genes. Blue, white, and red indicate log2 (fold change) values of <−2, 0, and >2, respectively. Symbols indicate significant differences compared to mock controls (M) by Wald test (* False discovery rate [FDR] $q < 0.05$, # FDR $q < 0.1$). $n = 3$ hamsters/infection group/time point.

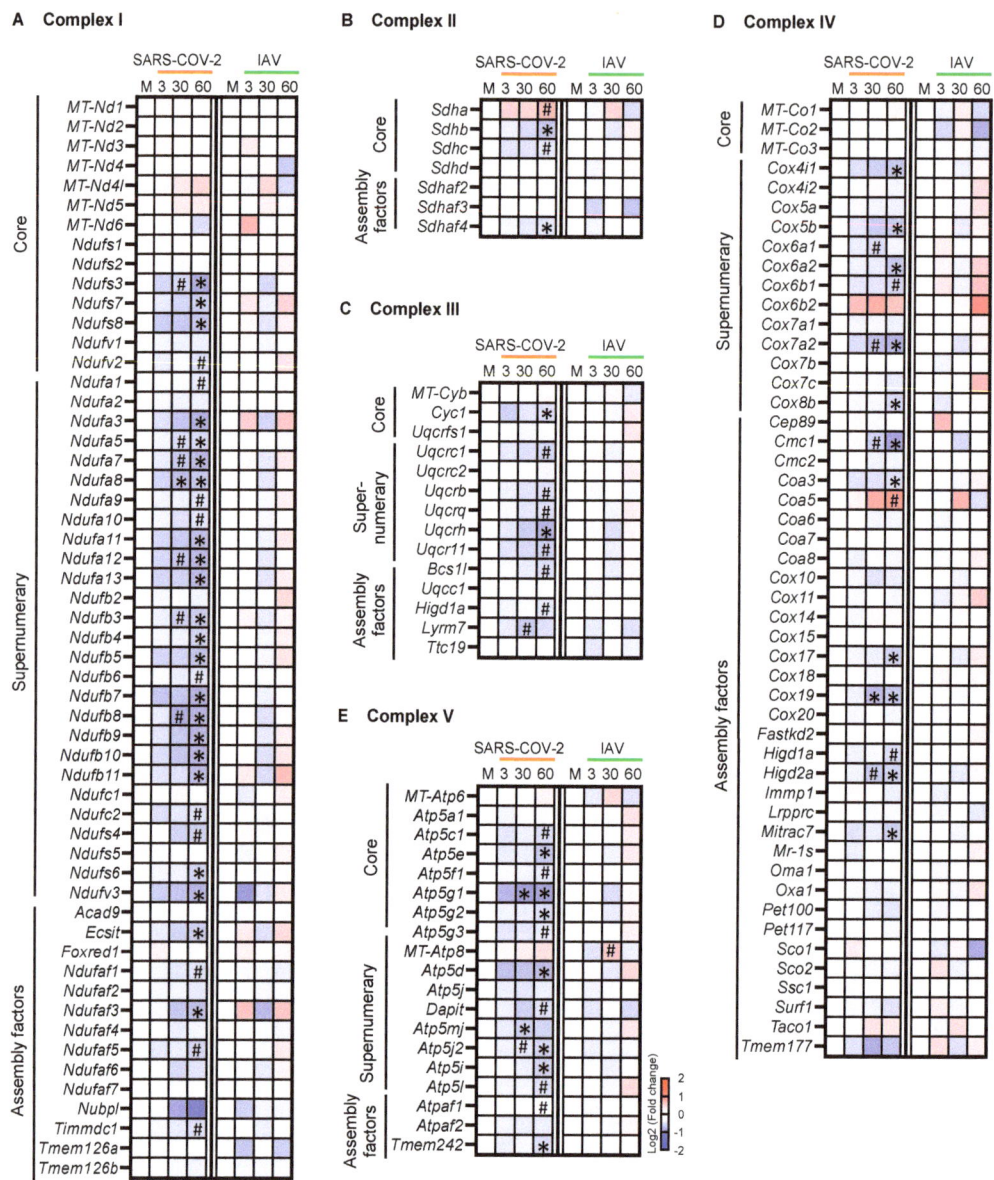

Figure 5. Respiratory infection with SARS-CoV-2 but not influenza A virus (IAV) causes persistent downregulation of nuclear genes encoding core proteins, supernumerary subunit proteins, and assembly factors of all mitochondrial oxidative phosphorylation (OXPHOS) complexes. (**A**–**E**) Heatmaps showing changes in the expression of genes encoding protein components of complex I (**A**), II (**B**), III (**C**), IV (**D**), and V (**E**). Blue, white, and red indicate log2 (fold change) values of <−2, 0, and >2, respectively. Symbols indicate significant differences compared to mock controls (M) by Wald test (* False discovery rate [FDR] $q < 0.05$, # FDR $q < 0.1$). $n = 3$ hamsters/infection group/time point. MT-: mtDNA genes.

Mitochondrial function can be affected by altered mitochondrial biogenesis, dynamics (fusion and fission), and mitophagy. To address whether biogenesis was affected at the transcriptional level, we first estimated the relative amount of cellular mtDNA by the ratio of mtDNA/nDNA. The ratio tended to be lower in the SARS-CoV-2 group than in the IAV and mock groups, but the difference was not significant (Supplementary Figure S3A). We then analyzed the expression of the genes involved in mitochondrial biogenesis [28–30] (Supplementary Figure S3B). There was not a consistent pattern of differential expression, although at 60 dpi in the SARS-CoV-2 group, the estrogen-related receptor α (ESRRA) gene (*Esrra*) was significantly downregulated and the sirtuin-1 gene (*Sirt1*) was significantly upregulated. ESRRA is a downstream target of peroxisome proliferator-activated receptor-γ coactivator-1 α (PGC-1α), which is the master regulator of mitochondrial biogenesis [31,32]. The transcription of the PGC-1α gene (*Ppagc1a*) itself was not differentially regulated with respect to SARS-CoV-2 infection. None of the main genes involved in the regulation of mitochondrial fusion or fission [29,33] showed significant changes (Supplementary Figure S3C). Among mitophagy pathway genes [29,34], although the expression of PTEN-induced kinase 1 gene (*Pink1*) and parkin RBR E3 ubiquitin protein ligase gene (*Prkn*) did not change significantly, the expression of Bcl2 interacting protein 3 gene (*Bnip3*), *Gabarap1*, and *Sqstm1* were significantly downregulated in the SARS-CoV-2 group at 30 and/or 60 dpi (Supplementary Figure S3D). Taken together, the respiratory SARS-CoV-2 infection inhibited mitophagy and, to a lesser degree, mitochondrial biogenesis, but not mitochondrial fusion or fission at the transcriptional level.

3.6. Respiratory SARS-CoV-2 Infection Downregulates Many Enzyme Genes Involved in Fatty Acid β-Oxidation and TCA Cycle

Since the respiratory SARS-CoV-2 infection downregulated OXPHOS genes in skeletal muscle, we next addressed whether the other aspects of the energy metabolism were also affected. To this end, we performed GSEA and analyzed the enzyme genes involved in each catabolic pathway (Figures 6 and 7, and Supplementary Figure S4).

Glycolysis is a cytoplasmic pathway that breaks down glucose into pyruvate. GSEA showed that the genes involved in glycolysis were not coordinately regulated with respect to infection with either SARS-CoV-2 or IAV (Supplementary Figure S4A), although the hexokinase 2 gene (*Hk2*) was significantly upregulated and the lactate dehydrogenase B gene (*Ldhb*) was significantly downregulated in the SARS-CoV-2 group at 30 and 60 dpi (Supplementary Figure S4B,C). In the same manner, the genes participating in amino acid metabolism were not coordinately regulated in response to either infection (Supplementary Figure S4D).

Unlike glycolysis or amino acid metabolism, fatty acid metabolism was coordinately downregulated in the SARS-CoV-2 group at 30 and 60 dpi but not in the IAV group (Figure 6A). While none of the fatty acid synthesis genes showed significant changes (Figure 6B), several genes encoding enzymes involved in the fatty acid β-oxidation showed more significant changes in the SARS-CoV-2 group than in the IAV group at 30 and 60 dpi, among which only the carnitine palmitoyl transferase 1 (CPT1) gene (*Cpt1*) was upregulated at 60 dpi, while the rest were downregulated (Figure 6C,D). β-oxidation is a catabolic process by which fatty acids are broken down to acetyl-CoA. CPT1 is located at the outer mitochondrial membrane to transfer the acyl group from CoA to carnitine, a rate-limiting step in β-oxidation. Within mitochondria, each round of β-oxidation requires the sequential actions of several enzymes, including enoyl-CoA delta isomerase 1 (ECI1), enoyl-CoA hydratase (ECH), hydroxyacyl-CoA dehydrogenase (HADH), and acetyl-Coenzyme A acyltransferase 2 (ACAA2) [35]. The genes encoding these enzymes (*Eci1*, *Echs1*, *Hadh*, and *Acaa2*, respectively) were all significantly downregulated at 60 dpi in the SARS-CoV-2 group but not in the IAV group (Figure 6C,D). Therefore, the respiratory infection with SARS-CoV-2, but not IAV, caused persistent suppression of fatty acid β-oxidation genes.

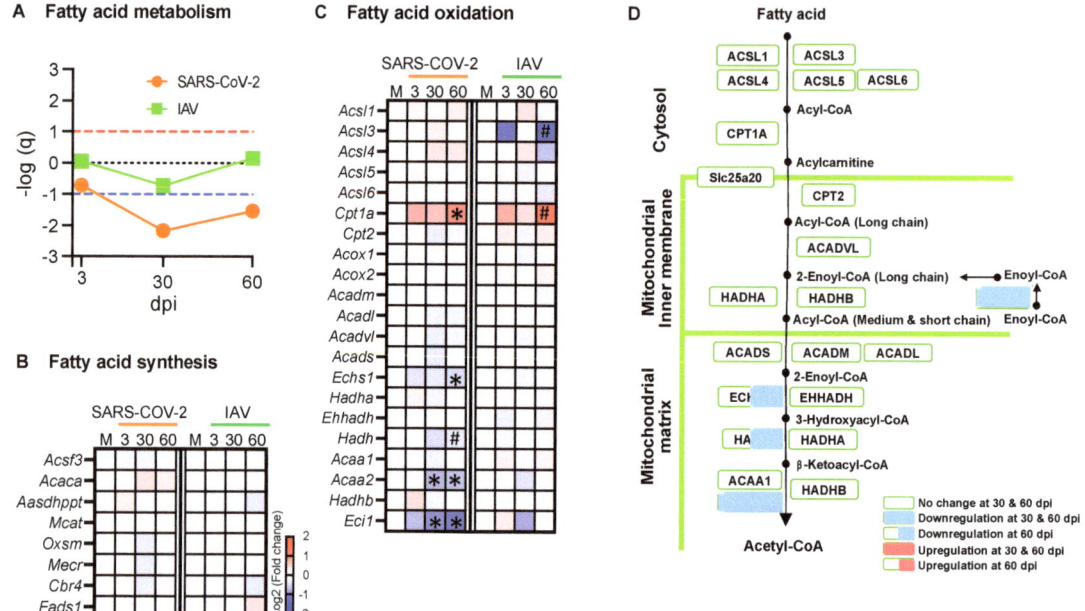

Figure 6. Respiratory SARS-CoV-2 infection downregulates some enzyme genes involved in fatty acid oxidation. (**A**) Summary of Gene Set Enrichment Analysis (GSEA) performed using the Hallmark fatty acid metabolism gene set in SARS-CoV-2 or influenza A virus (IAV)-infected hamsters at 3-, 30-, and 60-days post-infection (dpi) compared to mock controls. Dotted lines indicate false discovery rate (FDR) q value = 0.1 for positive (red) and negative (blue) coordinate regulation. n = 3 hamsters/infection group/time point. (**B**,**C**) Heatmaps showing changes in the expression of enzyme genes involved in fatty acid synthesis (**B**) and fatty acid oxidation (**C**). (**D**) Schematic overview of expression changes in enzyme genes involved in fatty acid oxidation in the SARS-CoV-2 group. Blue, white, and red indicate log2 (fold change) values of <−2, 0, and >2, respectively. Symbols indicate significant differences compared to mock controls (M) by the Wald test (* FDR q < 0.05, # FDR q < 0.1). n = 3 hamsters/infection group/time point.

The TCA cycle is a series of chemical reactions that oxidize acetyl-CoA derived from carbohydrates, lipids, and proteins. GSEA showed significant downregulation of the TCA cycle genes in the SARS-CoV-2 group at 30 and 60 dpi but not in the IAV group (Figure 7A). The isocitrate dehydrogenase gene (*Idh2*), succinate-CoA ligase GDP/ADP-forming subunit alpha gene (*Suclg1*), succinate dehydrogenase genes (*Sdhb* and *Sdhc*), and malate dehydrogenase 1 gene (*Mdh1*) were significantly downregulated by the SARS-CoV-2 infection at 30 and/or 60 dpi (Figure 7B,C). Only *Sdha* was upregulated in the SARS-CoV-2 group at 60 dpi. The findings indicate that the respiratory infection with SARS-CoV-2, but not IAV, induced persistent suppression of the TCA cycle at the transcriptional level.

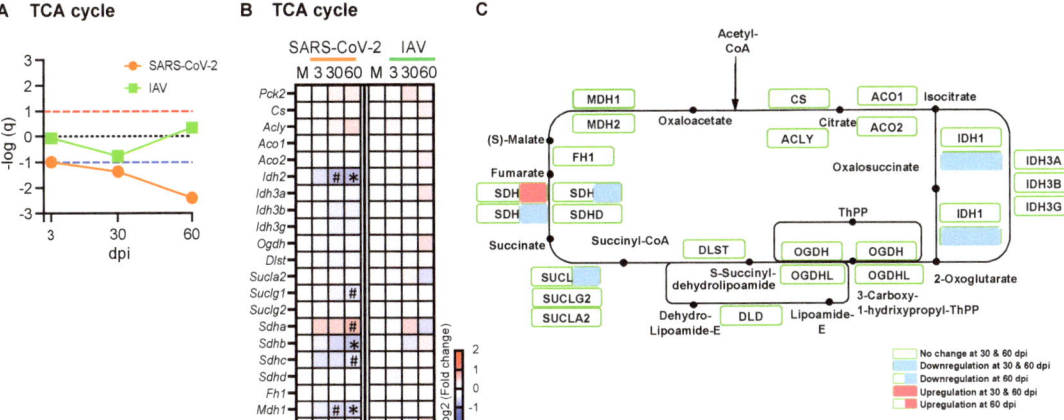

Figure 7. Respiratory SARS-CoV-2 infection downregulates some enzyme genes involved in the TCA cycle. (**A**) Summary of Gene Set Enrichment Analysis (GSEA) performed using the WikiPathways TCA cycle gene set in SARS-CoV-2- or influenza A virus (IAV)-infected hamsters at 3-, 30-, and 60-days post-infection (dpi) compared to mock controls. Dotted lines indicate false discovery rate (FDR) q value = 0.1 for positive (red) and negative (blue) coordinate regulation. n = 3 hamsters/infection group/time point. (**B**) Heatmap showing changes in the expression of enzyme genes involved in TCA cycle. (**C**) Schematic overview of gene expression changes in TCA cycle enzyme genes in the SARS-CoV-2 group. Blue, white, and red indicate log2 (fold change) values of <−2, 0, and >2, respectively. Symbols indicate significant differences compared to mock controls (M) by Wald test (* FDR q < 0.05, # FDR q < 0.1). n = 3 hamsters/infection group/time point.

3.7. Respiratory SARS-CoV-2 or IAV Infection Causes Mild Morphological Changes of Intermyofibrillar Mitochondria

Mitochondria are highly dynamic organelles that remodel their shape, size, and distribution to ensure adaptation to cellular bioenergetic requirements and stress. To address whether there were associated changes in mitochondrial morphology, we performed a TEM study. Scattered subsarcolemmal mitochondrial aggregations were similarly observed in both SARS-CoV-2- and mock-infected hamsters, whereas small intermyofibrillar mitochondrial aggregations were more frequently seen in the SARS-CoV-2 group than in the mock group. In the SARS-CoV-2 group, mitochondrial cristae appeared normal with no inclusions, but focal loss of myofilaments was observed. Enlarged and elongated mitochondria were more frequently seen in SARS-CoV-2 hamsters than in mock-infected controls (Figure 8A,B). We assessed the size and shape of subsarcolemmal (SS) and intermyofibrillar (IMF) mitochondria in quadriceps muscles. IMF mitochondria, but not SS mitochondria (Supplementary Figure S5A–D, Supplementary Table S2), were morphologically different among 3 groups. The IMF mitochondria in the SARS-CoV-2 group were larger in area, perimeter, and Feret's diameter than those in the IAV and mock groups (Figure 8D–F, Supplementary Table S3), indicating that the IMF mitochondria in the SARS-CoV-2 group are more enlarged and elongated, a sign of mitochondria stress [36–38]. Similar changes in mitochondria were seen in a muscle biopsy from a young adult patient who experienced persistent myalgia and fatigue following COVID-19 with no other causes identified (Figure 8C).

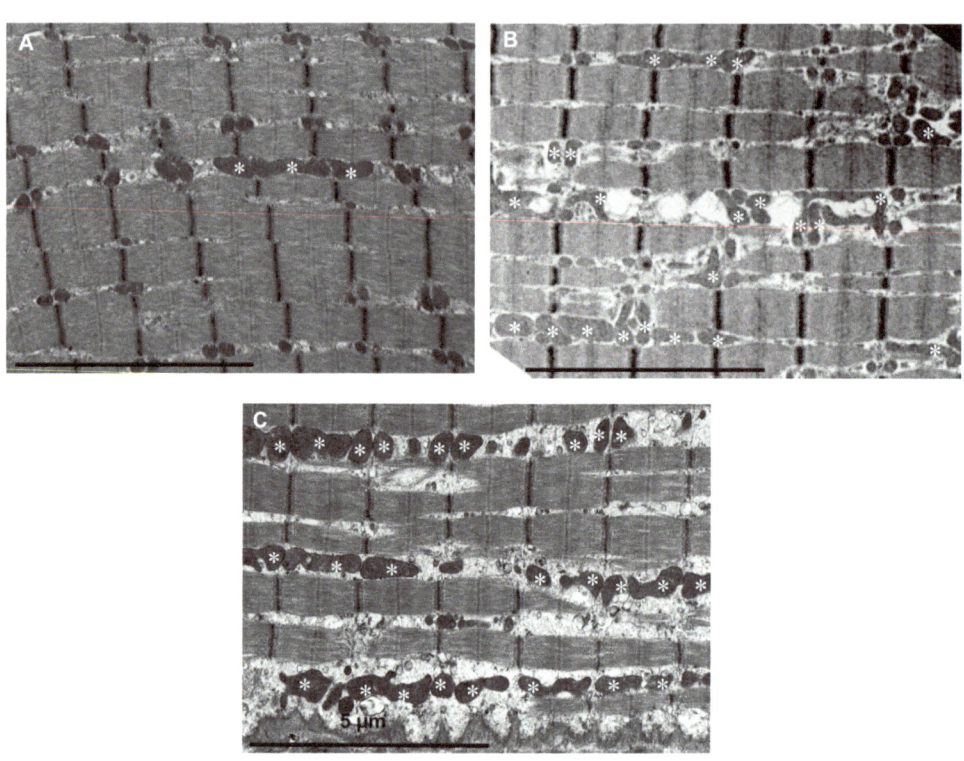

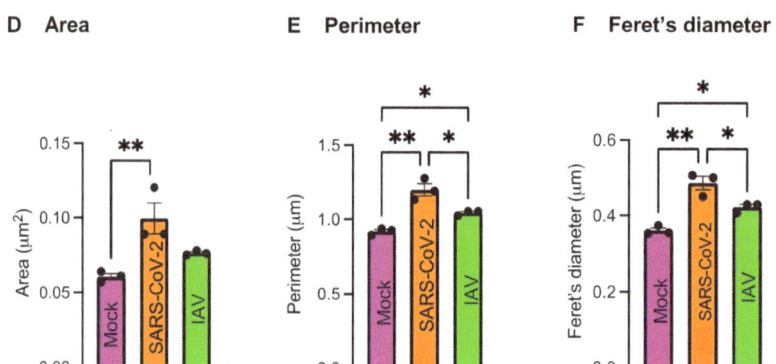

Figure 8. Respiratory SARS-CoV-2 infection causes mitochondrial morphological changes in hamsters and patient. (**A**,**B**) Representative longitudinal electron microscopic images of quadriceps muscle of mock- (**A**) or SARS-CoV-2-infected hamsters (**B**) at day 60 post-infection (dpi) showing an increased number of enlarged and/or elongated mitochondria (white asterisk) in SARS-CoV-2-infected hamsters. (**C**) Longitudinal electron microscopic image of a muscle biopsy from a patient with persistent post-COVID muscle fatigue showing many enlarged and/or elongated mitochondria (white asterisk). (**D**–**F**) Bar graphs showing comparisons of area (**D**), perimeter (**E**), and Feret's diameter (**F**) of intermyofibrillar (IMF) mitochondria of quadriceps muscles of hamsters at 60 dpi. Each dot represents mean value of area (**D**), perimeter (**E**), and Feret's diameter (**F**) of each hamster. $n = 3$ hamsters/infection group. Data were analyzed by one-way ANOVA with Tukey's post hoc test and expressed as mean ± SEM. * $p < 0.05$, ** $p < 0.01$. IAV: Influenza A virus.

3.8. Respiratory SARS-CoV-2 Infection Induces Type I and Type II Interferon (IFN) Responses and Tumor Necrosis Factor-Alpha (TNF-α) Response in Skeletal Muscle

Acute respiratory SARS-CoV-2 infection generates a robust systemic cytokine response in addition to type I and type II interferon responses, and the plasma levels of IFN-α, IFN-γ, IL-1β, IL-6, and TNF-α are significantly increased in human patients with acute COVID-19 [39–43]. Since there is no evidence of direct SARS-CoV-2 viral invasion, we used GSEA to assess whether the transcriptional changes observed in skeletal muscle were triggered by the systemic responses. Both SARS-CoV-2 and IAV respiratory infections induced acute and transient type I and type II interferon responses in skeletal muscle, with strong coordinated upregulation of IFN-α and IFN-γ response genes at 3 dpi but not at 30 or 60 dpi (Figure 9A,B). Likewise, IFN-α and IFN-γ responses were strongly induced at 3 dpi but not at 30 dpi in the lungs (Supplementary Figure S6A,B). TNF-α signaling via NFκB was coordinately upregulated in muscles at 3 and 60 dpi in the SARS-CoV-2 group, but only at 30 dpi in the IAV group (Figure 9C), although the expression of the TNF-α gene (*Tnf*) itself was extremely low in muscles. In the lungs, TNF-α signaling via NFκB was strongly enriched at 3 dpi and then very low at 30 dpi in both SARS-CoV-2 and IAV groups (Supplementary Figure S6C). While IL-6 signaling was strongly induced in the lungs following acute respiratory SARS-CoV-2 infection (Supplementary Figure S6D), it was not coordinately upregulated in skeletal muscle (Figure 9D). These findings suggest an interesting hypothesis that the persistent transcriptional changes in the skeletal muscle of SARS-CoV-2-infected animals might be related to the transient systemic interferon and TNF-α responses during the acute viral infection.

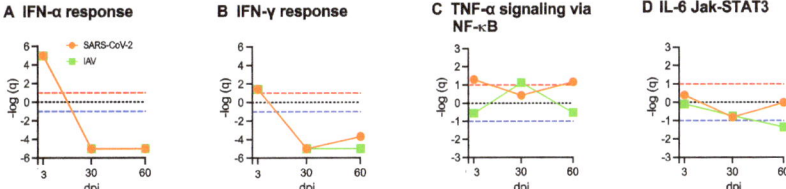

Figure 9. Type I and Type II interferon and TNF-α/NFκB cytokine responses are induced in muscle by respiratory SARS-CoV-2 infection. Summary of Gene Set Enrichment Analysis (GSEA) performed using Hallmark cytokine/inflammation gene sets in SARS-CoV-2- or Influenza A virus (IAV)-infected hamsters at 3-, 30-, and 60-days post infection (dpi) compared to mock controls. Dotted lines indicate false discovery rate (FDR) q value = 0.1 for positive (red) and negative (blue) coordinate regulation. n = 3 hamsters/infection group/time point. Results are shown for IFN-α response (**A**), IFN-γ response (**B**), TNF-α/NF-κB signaling response (**C**), and IL-6/JAK-STAT3 signaling response (**D**).

3.9. Co-Treatment of C2C12 Myotubes with IFN-α, IFN-γ, and TNF-α Markedly Impairs Mitochondrial Respiration and Shifts Energy Metabolism from Oxidative Respiration to Glycolysis

To address whether the combination of interferons and TNF-α could potentially trigger skeletal muscle abnormalities seen in the COVID-19 hamster model, we treated differentiated C2C12 myogenic cells (myotubes) with IFN-α, IFN-γ, and TNF-α individually or in various combinations. Immunoblot analysis showed a significant reduction in NADH dehydrogenase 1 beta subcomplex subunit 8 (NDUFB8, complex I) and succinate dehydrogenase complex iron sulfur subunit B (SDHB, complex II) protein expression after 48 h of treatment with IFN-α/IFN-γ/TNF-α or IFN-γ/TNF-α but not with interferon or TNF-α alone (Figure 10A,B). The expression of selected proteins of complexes III, IV, and V, as well as ribosome small and large units, did not show changes with treatments (Figure 10A and Supplementary Figure S7A,B). To assess mitochondrial oxidative function, we measured the oxygen consumption rate (OCR) using a Seahorse cell metabolic analyzer. Twenty-four hours of treatment with IFN-α/IFN-γ/TNF-α or IFN-γ/TNF-α, but not the others, dramatically reduced basal respiration rate (Figure 10C), but non-mitochondrial respiration did not change by any treatment (Figure 10D). The treatments did not change the total protein amount compared to untreated controls (Supplementary Figure S7C), indicating that the reduction in basal respiration was not caused by cell death. We also measured ATP production rates by mitochondrial oxidation and glycolysis. C2C12 myotubes displayed high oxidative metabolism at baseline; however, IFN-α/IFN-γ/TNF-α and IFN-γ/TNF-α treatments induced a dramatic shift from oxidative respiration towards glycolysis (Figure 10E). The combinations of IL-6 with interferons, including IFN-α/IFN-γ/IL-6 and IFN-γ/IL-6, did not affect OXPHOS protein expression, basal respiration, or oxidative and glycolytic ATP production rates (Figure 10F–I). Therefore, the combination of type II interferon with TNF-α but not IL-6 impaired mitochondrial oxidative functions in skeletal muscle cells in vitro.

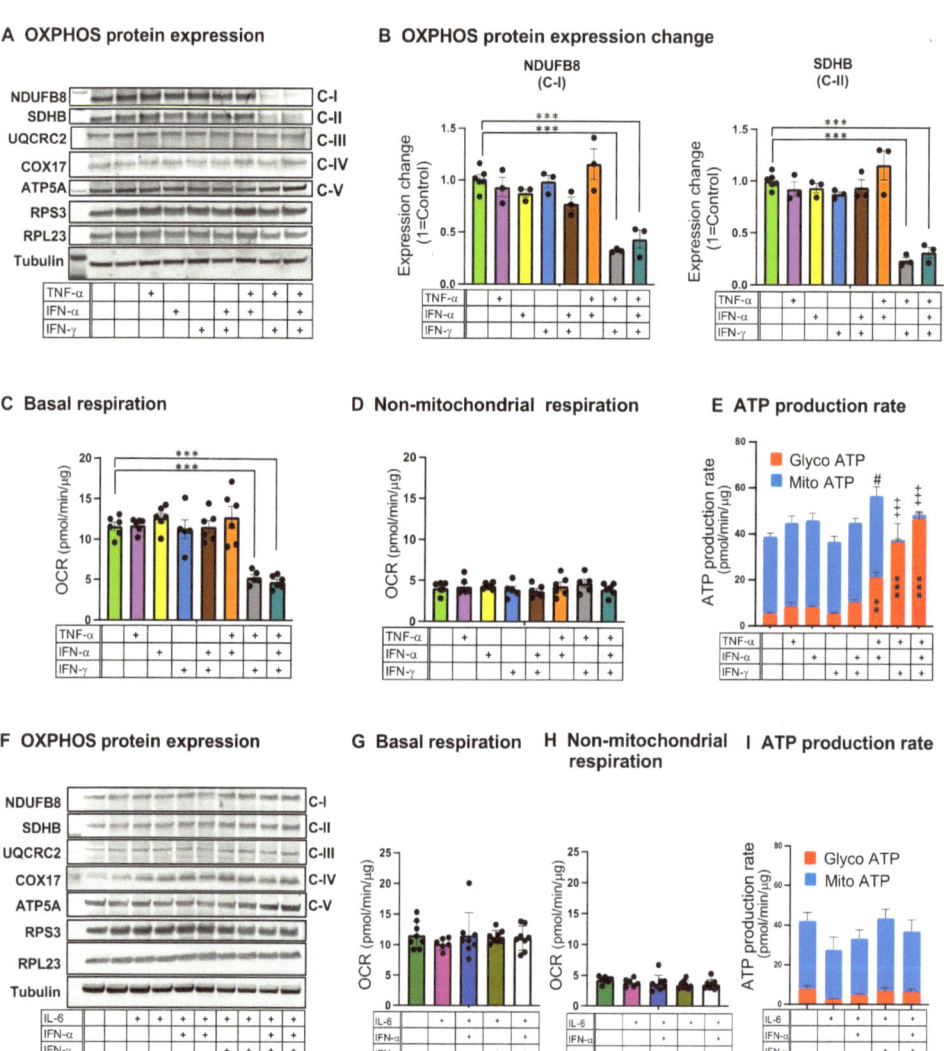

Figure 10. Treatment with a combination of Type II interferon and TNF-α leads to mitochondrial dysfunction in C2C12 myotubes. (**A–E**) Effects of treatments of C2C12 myotubes with IFN-α, IFN-γ, and TNF-α individually or in combinations. (**A**) Immunoblot analysis of OXPHOS protein expression.

(**B**) Quantification of NADH dehydrogenase 1 beta subcomplex subunit 8 (NDUFB8, Complex I; C-I) and succinate dehydrogenase complex iron sulfur subunit B (SDHB, Complex II; C-II) protein expression normalized to tubulin and relative to untreated control. Data were analyzed by one-way ANOVA with Tukey's post hoc test and expressed as mean ± SEM of three independent experiments. (**C**) Oxygen consumption rate under basal conditions (basal respiration). (**D**) Non-mitochondrial respiration. (**E**) Glycolytic (Glyco) ATP production rate (red) and mitochondrial (Mito) ATP production rate (blue). (**F–I**) Effects of treatments of C2C12 myotubes with IFN-α, IFN-γ, and IL-6 individually or in combinations. (**F**) Immunoblot analysis of OXPHOS protein expression. (**G**) basal respiration. (**H**) non-mitochondrial respiration. (**I**) Glycolytic (Glyco) ATP production rate (red) and mitochondrial (Mito) ATP production rate (blue). For (**C–E,G–I**), data were analyzed by one-way ANOVA with Tukey's post hoc test and expressed as mean ± SEM of 3 repetitive experiments with 5 or 6 technical replicates. ** $p < 0.01$, *** $p < 0.001$, # $p < 0.05$, +++ $p < 0.001$. + indicates treatment with IFN-α, IFN-γ, TNF-α, or IL-6.

4. Discussion

Muscle fatigue represents the most common symptom that persists after COVID-19. By characterizing the longitudinal skeletal muscle histopathological and transcriptional changes after acute respiratory SARS-CoV-2 infection in the COVID-19 hamster model, our present study has generated several important findings that shed light on the potential mechanisms underlying muscle symptoms associated with COVID-19 and long COVID.

First, our study supports the notion that SARS-CoV-2 is unlikely to directly invade skeletal muscle after an acute respiratory infection. So far, there has been no convincing evidence that SARS-CoV-2 directly invades skeletal muscle in humans [12,14,44,45]. In the COVID-19 hamster model, our present study shows no evidence of direct SARS-CoV-2 infection of skeletal muscle, as SARS-CoV-2 RNA and protein expression, virus-like particles, and inflammatory cell infiltrates are all absent in skeletal muscle.

Second, despite the absence of direct viral invasion, skeletal muscle in the COVID-19 hamster model undergoes myofiber atrophy and long-lasting transcriptomic changes, which are not observed with acute respiratory IAV infection. Myofiber atrophy has also been reported in muscle biopsies of patients with long COVID [11–13]. Our study further shows that both oxidative and glycolytic myofibers undergo atrophy, which argues against immobilization being the sole cause of the atrophy, as disuse has a primary impact on glycolytic fibers [46]. In parallel with this muscle atrophy, atrogenes are upregulated while many cytoplasmic ribosomal protein genes are downregulated, suggesting that the myofiber atrophy is likely a result of both accelerated protein degradation and impaired protein synthesis.

Another prominent transcriptional response detected in skeletal muscle after respiratory SARS-CoV-2 infection is the long-lasting suppression of genes related to mitochondrial energy metabolism, especially those involved in mitochondrial OXPHOS, fatty acid β-oxidation, and the TCA cycle. Consistent with our findings, reduced expression of OXPHOS proteins, impaired mitochondrial respiration, and altered muscle metabolism with a lower reliance on oxidative metabolism have been observed in patients with exercise intolerance associated with long COVID [13,14]. Our study further shows that the respiratory SARS-CoV-2 infection affects mitochondrial oxidative metabolism at the nuclear gene level, as the 13 protein-encoding mtDNA genes are not affected.

Third, the systemic cytokine response to acute respiratory SARS-CoV-2 infection is likely an important trigger of the persistent histopathological and transcriptional changes observed in skeletal muscle. While respiratory SARS-CoV-2 and IAV infections generate comparable acute and transient type I and II interferon responses in skeletal muscle, the inflammatory cytokine response is different, with the TNF-α/NF-κB signaling pathway being differentially upregulated in the former. SARS-CoV-2 can infect cells and bind to critical host mitochondrial proteins to inhibit mitochondrial function [47,48]. The impaired mitochondrial functions can persist in a variety of non-muscle tissues, even after the virus is cleared [49]. Our present study further shows that the respiratory SARS-CoV-2 infection can persistently suppress mitochondrial oxidative metabolism genes in skeletal muscle without direct infection, which suggests a role of the acute systemic responses in the pathogenesis of muscle abnormalities. There is no evidence of persistent viral pneumonia or a chronic systemic response in our model.

The host interferon response is critical for controlling viral infection, but it can also enhance the inflammatory cytokine response. Exuberant systemic inflammatory cytokine response is a prominent feature of acute respiratory SARS-CoV-2 infection [40]. The plasma levels of type I and type II interferons as well as several inflammatory cytokines, including IFN-α, IFN-γ, IL-6, TNF-α, and IL-1β, are significantly increased in human patients during acute infection [39–43]. While IL-6 signaling is strongly induced in the lungs following acute respiratory SARS-CoV-2 infection [15,40], the genes in this pathway are not coordinately regulated in skeletal muscle, as shown by our transcriptome study. Genes involved in TNF-α/NF-κB signaling, however, are coordinately upregulated in muscle at the acute phase. Given the finding that TNF-α ligand expression is extremely low in skeletal muscle, the circulating TNF-α may act on skeletal muscle to cause muscle abnormalities. The TNF-α/NF-κB signaling pathway is known to induce skeletal muscle atrophy [50–52] by inhibiting muscle protein synthesis and increasing protein breakdown [53]. Activation of TNF-α/NF-κB signaling can also lead to upregulation of *Fbxo32* [54], which is significantly upregulated in skeletal muscle at day 3 post-respiratory SARS-CoV-2 infection. Therefore, the enrichment of this signaling pathway likely contributes to muscle atrophy.

Myalgia and fatigue are common side effects of IFN-α treatment in patients with hepatitis C, which can lead to chronic fatigue. Comparing with healthy controls, one study reported that the patients who developed chronic fatigue after IFN-α treatment showed high serum levels of IL-6 and TNF-α during but not after the treatment [55]. The findings lead us to speculate that although the type I and type II interferon responses are transient in skeletal muscle after the respiratory SARS-CoV-2 infection, the combination of the systemic interferon and TNF-α responses during acute infection might exert a synergistic impact on skeletal muscle and set the stage for chronic muscle fatigue. Importantly, the simultaneous upregulation of IFN-α, IFN-γ, and TNF-α was observed only in SARS-CoV-2-infected hamsters but not in IAV-infected hamsters. This difference might contribute, in part, to the different impact on mitochondrial oxidative function and the persistency of the abnormality. In support of this notion, our in vitro study showed that the treatment of C2C12 myotubes with combined IFN-γ and TNF-α but not IFN-γ or TNF-α alone markedly impaired mitochondrial oxidative function. Although our in vitro study did not demonstrate a significant impact of IFN-α on mitochondrial oxidative function, IFN-α might still play a role in vivo, as this response was also significantly upregulated by the acute SARS-CoV-2 infection. Future studies are needed to further elucidate the mechanisms. Our findings suggest that targeting TNF-α during acute SARS-CoV-2 infection may be beneficial to the prevention or mitigation of persistent muscle fatigue. Drugs, which can boost mitochondrial functions, enhance protein synthesis, and inhibit protein degradation, may also be useful for treating muscle fatigue associated with long COVID.

Our study has several limitations. Our cohort is relatively small and may not have sufficient statistical power to detect all the abnormalities in skeletal muscle. Since no fresh specimens could be withdrawn from the BSL-3 laboratory for serum or tissue protein assays such as ELISA and Western blot, we were unable to assess serum cytokines or muscle proteins to correlate with the transcriptional changes in the hamsters. Many proteins that regulate skeletal muscle atrophy and energy metabolism are activated at the translational and post-translational levels, alterations of which cannot be detected by our transcriptional study. Nevertheless, our study is informative and may help guide future studies and therapy development. The hamster model appears valuable for future studies of muscle abnormalities associated with COVID-19 and long COVID, given the significant histopathological and transcriptional changes detected.

Supplementary Materials: The following supporting information can be downloaded at: https://www.mdpi.com/article/10.3390/biomedicines12071443/s1. Figure S1: Robust expression of SARS-CoV-2 protein in the lung of a SARS-CoV-2 respiratory infected hamster at 3-days post infection (dpi), but no positive expression at 30 dpi; Figure S2: Respiratory infection with SARS-CoV-2 but not IAV-induced skeletal muscle fiber atrophy; Figure S3: Respiratory SARS-CoV-2 infection does not impact the relative amount of mitochondrial DNA, mitochondrial biogenesis genes, or fusion and fission genes, but downregulates some mitophagy genes; Figure S4: Respiratory SARS-CoV-2 infection has mild effects on the expression of genes involved in glycolysis and amino acid metabolism; Figure S5: Limited effects of respiratory SARS-CoV-2 or IAV infection on the morphology of subsarcolemmal mitochondria; Figure S6: Type I and Type II interferon responses, TNF-α/NF-κB and IL6/JAk/STAT3 are induced by SARS-CoV-2 infection at acute phase but not post-recovery phase in lungs; Figure S7: Limited effects of inflammatory cytokine treatments on expressions of some OXPHOS complex and ribosomal proteins in C2C12 myotubes; Table S1: qRT-PCR primer sequences; Table S2: Comparisons of morphometric and shape descriptors of subsarcolemmal mitochondria; Table S3: Comparisons of morphometric and shape descriptors of intermyofibrillar mitochondria; Data S1: Summary of Gene Set Enrichment Analysis (GSEA) results.

Author Contributions: Conceptualization: L.Z., B.R.t. and J.K.L.; methodology: B.R.t., J.K.L. and J.Z.; validation: S.T.H., J.J.F. and X.W.; formal analysis: S.T.H. and J.J.F.; investigation: S.T.H. and J.J.F.; resources: B.R.t., J.K.L., X.W. and L.Z.; data curation: A.C.G.; writing—original draft preparation, S.T.H.; writing—review and editing: L.Z. and A.C.G.; visualization: S.T.H. and A.C.G.; supervision: L.Z., B.R.t. and J.K.L.; project administration: S.T.H., L.Z. and B.R.t.; funding acquisition: S.T.H. and L.Z. All authors have read and agreed to the published version of the manuscript.

Funding: This research was funded by the National Institute of Arthritis and Musculoskeletal and Skin Diseases of the National Institutes of Health under Award Number 5R21AR081655 (L.Z. and S.T.H.) and by Clinical and Translational Science Award UL1TR001430 (A.C.G.).

Institutional Review Board Statement: The animal study protocol was approved by the Institutional Animal Care and Use Committee at Icahn School of Medicine at Mount Sinai (IACUC-2016-0438), and New York University Langone Health (PROTO20210078 and PROTO202000113), and Boston University Institutional Biosafety Committee (#20-2460).

Informed Consent Statement: Patient consent was waived due to muscle biopsy was done for the clinical diagnosis not for research study, EM picture was shown, but no detailed history (age, gender, past medical history, medication list, etc.) was presented.

Data Availability Statement: Raw and processed RNAseq data have been deposited in the Gene Expression Omnibus (GEO) and are accessible through GEO Series accession number GSE231910. This paper does not report the original code. Any additional information required to reanalyze the data reported in this paper is available upon request to the corresponding author (shomma@bu.edu).

Acknowledgments: We would like to thank Yuriy Alekseyev and his team at the Boston University Chobanian & Avedisian School of Medicine Microarray and Sequencing Resource Core Facility for assistance with bulk-RNA sequencing. We thank Maria Medalla, Haiyan Gong, and their team at the Boston University Chobanian & Avedisian School of Medicine TEM Core Facility for their technical assistance with TEM analysis.

Conflicts of Interest: The authors declare no conflicts of interest.

References

1. Bull-Otterson, L.; Baca, S.; Saydah, S. Post–COVID conditions among adult COVID-19 survivors aged 18–64 and $\geq$65 years—United States, March 2020–November 2021. *MMWR Morb. Mortal. Wkly. Rep.* **2022**, *71*, 713–717. [CrossRef]
2. Lopez-Leon, S.; Wegman-Ostrosky, T.; Ayuzo Del Valle, N.C.; Perelman, C.; Sepulveda, R.; Rebolledo, P.A.; Cuapio, A.; Villapol, S. Long-COVID in children and adolescents: A systematic review and meta-analyses. *Sci. Rep.* **2022**, *12*, 9950. [CrossRef] [PubMed]
3. Venkatesan, P. NICE guideline on long COVID. *Lancet Respir. Med.* **2021**, *9*, 129. [CrossRef] [PubMed]
4. Mehandru, S.; Merad, M. Pathological sequelae of long-haul COVID. *Nat. Immunol.* **2022**, *23*, 194–202. [CrossRef]
5. Premraj, L.; Kannapadi, N.V.; Briggs, J.; Seal, S.M.; Battaglini, D.; Fanning, J.; Suen, J.; Robba, C.; Fraser, J.; Cho, S.M. Mid and long-term neurological and neuropsychiatric manifestations of post-COVID-19 syndrome: A meta-analysis. *J. Neurol. Sci.* **2022**, *434*, 120162. [CrossRef]

6. Huang, C.; Huang, L.; Wang, Y.; Li, X.; Ren, L.; Gu, X.; Kang, L.; Guo, L.; Liu, M.; Zhou, X.; et al. 6-Month consequences of COVID-19 in patients discharged from hospital: A cohort study. *Lancet* **2021**, *397*, 220–232. [CrossRef]
7. Huang, L.; Yao, Q.; Gu, X.; Wang, Q.; Ren, L.; Wang, Y.; Hu, P.; Guo, L.; Liu, M.; Xu, J.; et al. 1-Year outcomes in hospital survivors with COVID-19: A longitudinal cohort study. *Lancet* **2021**, *398*, 747–758. [CrossRef]
8. Lopez-Leon, S.; Wegman-Ostrosky, T.; Perelman, C.; Sepulveda, R.; Rebolledo, P.A.; Cuapio, A.; Villapol, S. More than 50 long-term effects of COVID-19: A systematic review and meta-analysis. *Sci. Rep.* **2021**, *11*, 1644. [CrossRef]
9. Rass, V.; Beer, R.; Schiefecker, A.J.; Lindner, A.; Kofler, M.; Ianosi, B.A.; Mahlknecht, P.; Heim, B.; Peball, M.; Carbone, F.; et al. Neurological outcomes 1 year after COVID-19 diagnosis: A prospective longitudinal cohort study. *Eur. J. Neurol.* **2022**, *29*, 1685–1696. [CrossRef]
10. Kucuk, A.; Cumhur Cure, M.; Cure, E. Can COVID-19 cause myalgia with a completely different mechanism? A hypothesis. *Clin. Rheumatol.* **2020**, *39*, 2103–2104. [CrossRef]
11. Soares, M.N.; Eggelbusch, M.; Naddaf, E.; Gerrits, K.H.L.; van der Schaaf, M.; van den Borst, B.; Wiersinga, W.J.; van Vugt, M.; Weijs, P.J.M.; Murray, A.J.; et al. Skeletal muscle alterations in patients with acute Covid-19 and post-acute sequelae of COVID-19. *J. Cachexia Sarcopenia Muscle* **2022**, *13*, 11–22. [CrossRef]
12. Hejbøl, E.K.; Harbo, T.; Agergaard, J.; Madsen, L.B.; Pedersen, T.H.; Østergaard, L.J.; Andersen, H.; Schrøder, H.D.; Tankisi, H. Myopathy as a cause of fatigue in long-term post-COVID-19 symptoms: Evidence of skeletal muscle histopathology. *Eur. J. Neurol.* **2022**, *29*, 2832–2841. [CrossRef]
13. Colosio, M.; Brocca, L.; Gatti, M.F.; Neri, M.; Crea, E.; Cadile, F.; Canepari, M.; Pellegrino, M.A.; Polla, B.; Porcelli, S.; et al. Structural and functional impairments of skeletal muscle in patients with postacute sequelae of SARS-CoV-2 infection. *J. Appl. Physiol.* **2023**, *135*, 902–917. [CrossRef]
14. Appelman, B.; Charlton, B.T.; Goulding, R.P.; Kerkhoff, T.J.; Breedveld, E.A.; Noort, W.; Offringa, C.; Bloemers, F.W.; van Weeghel, M.; Schomakers, B.V.; et al. Muscle abnormalities worsen after post-exertional malaise in long COVID. *Nat. Commun.* **2024**, *15*, 17. [CrossRef]
15. Hoagland, D.A.; Møller, R.; Uhl, S.A.; Oishi, K.; Frere, J.; Golynker, I.; Horiuchi, S.; Panis, M.; Blanco-Melo, D.; Sachs, D.; et al. Leveraging the antiviral type I interferon system as a first line of defense against SARS-CoV-2 pathogenicity. *Immunity* **2021**, *54*, 557–570.e555. [CrossRef]
16. Horiuchi, S.; Oishi, K.; Carrau, L.; Frere, J.; Møller, R.; Panis, M.; tenOever, B.R. Immune memory from SARS-CoV-2 infection in hamsters provides variant-independent protection but still allows virus transmission. *Sci. Immunol.* **2021**, *6*, eabm3131. [CrossRef] [PubMed]
17. Frere, J.J.; Serafini, R.A.; Pryce, K.D.; Zazhytska, M.; Oishi, K.; Golynker, I.; Panis, M.; Zimering, J.; Horiuchi, S.; Hoagland, D.A.; et al. SARS-CoV-2 infection in hamsters and humans results in lasting and unique systemic perturbations after recovery. *Sci. Transl. Med.* **2022**, *14*, eabq3059. [CrossRef] [PubMed]
18. Quiros, P.M.; Goyal, A.; Jha, P.; Auwerx, J. Analysis of mtDNA/nDNA ratio in mice. *Curr. Protoc. Mouse Biol.* **2017**, *7*, 47–54. [CrossRef] [PubMed]
19. Dobin, A.; Davis, C.A.; Schlesinger, F.; Drenkow, J.; Zaleski, C.; Jha, S.; Batut, P.; Chaisson, M.; Gingeras, T.R. STAR: Ultrafast universal RNA-seq aligner. *Bioinformatics* **2013**, *29*, 15–21. [CrossRef]
20. Subramanian, A.; Tamayo, P.; Mootha, V.K.; Mukherjee, S.; Ebert, B.L.; Gillette, M.A.; Paulovich, A.; Pomeroy, S.L.; Golub, T.R.; Lander, E.S.; et al. Gene set enrichment analysis: A knowledge-based approach for interpreting genome-wide expression profiles. *Proc. Natl. Acad. Sci. USA* **2005**, *102*, 15545–15550. [CrossRef]
21. Oklejewicz, M.; Pen, I.; Durieux, G.C.; Daan, S. Maternal and pup genotype contribution to growth in wild-type and tau mutant Syrian hamsters. *Behav. Genet.* **2001**, *31*, 383–391. [CrossRef] [PubMed]
22. Schiaffino, S.; Reggiani, C. Fiber types in mammalian skeletal muscles. *Physiol. Rev.* **2011**, *91*, 1447–1531. [CrossRef]
23. Lynch, C.J.; Xu, Y.; Hajnal, A.; Salzberg, A.C.; Kawasawa, Y.I. RNA sequencing reveals a slow to fast muscle fiber type transition after olanzapine infusion in rats. *PLoS ONE* **2015**, *10*, e0123966. [CrossRef] [PubMed]
24. Zhao, J.; Zhai, B.; Gygi, S.P.; Goldberg, A.L. mTOR inhibition activates overall protein degradation by the ubiquitin proteasome system as well as by autophagy. *Proc. Natl. Acad. Sci. USA* **2015**, *112*, 15790–15797. [CrossRef] [PubMed]
25. Bodine, S.C.; Latres, E.; Baumhueter, S.; Lai, V.K.; Nunez, L.; Clarke, B.A.; Poueymirou, W.T.; Panaro, F.J.; Na, E.; Dharmarajan, K.; et al. Identification of ubiquitin ligases required for skeletal muscle atrophy. *Science* **2001**, *294*, 1704–1708. [CrossRef] [PubMed]
26. Di Malta, C.; Cinque, L.; Settembre, C. Transcriptional regulation of autophagy: Mechanisms and diseases. *Front. Cell Dev. Biol.* **2019**, *7*, 114. [CrossRef] [PubMed]
27. Vercellino, I.; Sazanov, L.A. The assembly, regulation and function of the mitochondrial respiratory chain. *Nat. Rev. Mol. Cell Biol.* **2022**, *23*, 141–161. [CrossRef] [PubMed]
28. Popov, L.D. Mitochondrial biogenesis: An update. *J. Cell. Mol. Med.* **2020**, *24*, 4892–4899. [CrossRef]
29. VanderVeen, B.N.; Fix, D.K.; Carson, J.A. Disrupted skeletal muscle mitochondrial dynamics, mitophagy, and biogenesis during cancer cachexia: A role for inflammation. *Oxid. Med. Cell. Longev.* **2017**, *2017*, 3292087. [CrossRef]
30. Romanello, V.; Sandri, M. Mitochondrial biogenesis and fragmentation as regulators of muscle protein degradation. *Curr. Hypertens. Rep.* **2010**, *12*, 433–439. [CrossRef]

31. Liang, H.; Ward, W.F. PGC-1alpha: A key regulator of energy metabolism. *Adv. Physiol. Educ.* **2006**, *30*, 145–151. [CrossRef] [PubMed]
32. Fernandez-Marcos, P.J.; Auwerx, J. Regulation of PGC-1α, a nodal regulator of mitochondrial biogenesis. *Am. J. Clin. Nutr.* **2011**, *93*, 884S–890S. [CrossRef] [PubMed]
33. Romanello, V.; Guadagnin, E.; Gomes, L.; Roder, I.; Sandri, C.; Petersen, Y.; Milan, G.; Masiero, E.; Del Piccolo, P.; Foretz, M.; et al. Mitochondrial fission and remodelling contributes to muscle atrophy. *EMBO J.* **2010**, *29*, 1774–1785. [CrossRef] [PubMed]
34. Onishi, M.; Yamano, K.; Sato, M.; Matsuda, N.; Okamoto, K. Molecular mechanisms and physiological functions of mitophagy. *EMBO J.* **2021**, *40*, e104705. [CrossRef] [PubMed]
35. Sharpe, A.J.; McKenzie, M. Mitochondrial fatty acid oxidation disorders associated with short-chain enoyl-CoA hydratase (ECHS1) deficiency. *Cells* **2018**, *7*, 46. [CrossRef] [PubMed]
36. Rambold, A.S.; Kostelecky, B.; Elia, N.; Lippincott-Schwartz, J. Tubular network formation protects mitochondria from autophagosomal degradation during nutrient starvation. *Proc. Natl. Acad. Sci. USA* **2011**, *108*, 10190–10195. [CrossRef] [PubMed]
37. Li, J.; Huang, Q.; Long, X.; Guo, X.; Sun, X.; Jin, X.; Li, Z.; Ren, T.; Yuan, P.; Huang, X.; et al. Mitochondrial elongation-mediated glucose metabolism reprogramming is essential for tumour cell survival during energy stress. *Oncogene* **2017**, *36*, 4901–4912. [CrossRef]
38. Tondera, D.; Grandemange, S.; Jourdain, A.; Karbowski, M.; Mattenberger, Y.; Herzig, S.; Da Cruz, S.; Clerc, P.; Raschke, I.; Merkwirth, C.; et al. SLP-2 is required for stress-induced mitochondrial hyperfusion. *EMBO J.* **2009**, *28*, 1589–1600. [CrossRef] [PubMed]
39. Del Valle, D.M.; Kim-Schulze, S.; Huang, H.H.; Beckmann, N.D.; Nirenberg, S.; Wang, B.; Lavin, Y.; Swartz, T.H.; Madduri, D.; Stock, A.; et al. An inflammatory cytokine signature predicts COVID-19 severity and survival. *Nat. Med.* **2020**, *26*, 1636–1643. [CrossRef]
40. Blanco-Melo, D.; Nilsson-Payant, B.E.; Liu, W.C.; Uhl, S.; Hoagland, D.; Møller, R.; Jordan, T.X.; Oishi, K.; Panis, M.; Sachs, D.; et al. Imbalanced host response to SARS-CoV-2 drives development of COVID-19. *Cell* **2020**, *181*, 1036–1045.e1039. [CrossRef]
41. da Silva, R.P.; Goncalves, J.I.B.; Zanin, R.F.; Schuch, F.B.; de Souza, A.P.D. Circulating type I interferon levels and COVID-19 Severity: A systematic review and Meta-analysis. *Front. Immunol.* **2021**, *12*, 657363. [CrossRef]
42. Contoli, M.; Papi, A.; Tomassetti, L.; Rizzo, P.; Vieceli Dalla Sega, F.; Fortini, F.; Torsani, F.; Morandi, L.; Ronzoni, L.; Zucchetti, O.; et al. Blood Interferon-alpha levels and severity, outcomes, and inflammatory profiles in hospitalized COVID-19 patients. *Front. Immunol.* **2021**, *12*, 648004. [CrossRef]
43. Morris, G.; Bortolasci, C.C.; Puri, B.K.; Marx, W.; O'Neil, A.; Athan, E.; Walder, K.; Berk, M.; Olive, L.; Carvalho, A.F.; et al. The cytokine storms of COVID-19, H1N1 influenza, CRS and MAS compared. Can one sized treatment fit all? *Cytokine* **2021**, *144*, 155593. [CrossRef]
44. Manzano, G.S.; Woods, J.K.; Amato, A.A. Covid-19-associated myopathy caused by type I interferonopathy. *N. Engl. J. Med.* **2020**, *383*, 2389–2390. [CrossRef]
45. Stevens, S.; Hendrickx, P.; Snijders, T.; Lambrichts, I.; Stessel, B.; Dubois, J.; van Loon, L.J.C.; Vandenabeele, F.; Agten, A. Skeletal muscles of patients infected with SARS-CoV-2 develop severe myofiber damage upon one week of admission on the intensive care unit. *Appl. Sci.* **2022**, *12*, 7310. [CrossRef]
46. Dubowitz, V.; Sewry, C.A.; Oldfors, A. *Muscle Biopsy: A Practical Approach*, 5th ed.; Elsevier: Amsterdam, The Netherlands, 2020.
47. Gordon, D.E.; Jang, G.M.; Bouhaddou, M.; Xu, J.; Obernier, K.; White, K.M.; O'Meara, M.J.; Rezelj, V.V.; Guo, J.Z.; Swaney, D.L.; et al. A SARS-CoV-2 protein interaction map reveals targets for drug repurposing. *Nature* **2020**, *583*, 459–468. [CrossRef] [PubMed]
48. Stukalov, A.; Girault, V.; Grass, V.; Karayel, O.; Bergant, V.; Urban, C.; Haas, D.A.; Huang, Y.; Oubraham, L.; Wang, A.; et al. Multilevel proteomics reveals host perturbations by SARS-CoV-2 and SARS-CoV. *Nature* **2021**, *594*, 246–252. [CrossRef]
49. Guarnieri, J.W.; Dybas, J.M.; Fazelinia, H.; Kim, M.S.; Frere, J.; Zhang, Y.; Soto Albrecht, Y.; Murdock, D.G.; Angelin, A.; Singh, L.N.; et al. Core mitochondrial genes are down-regulated during SARS-CoV-2 infection of rodent and human hosts. *Sci. Transl. Med.* **2023**, *15*, eabq1533. [CrossRef]
50. Thoma, A.; Lightfoot, A.P. NF-kB and inflammatory cytokine signaling: Role in skeletal muscle atrophy. *Adv. Exp. Med. Biol.* **2018**, *1088*, 267–279. [CrossRef]
51. Sandri, M. Signaling in muscle atrophy and hypertrophy. *Physiology* **2008**, *23*, 160–170. [CrossRef]
52. Sartori, R.; Romanello, V.; Sandri, M. Mechanisms of muscle atrophy and hypertrophy: Implications in health and disease. *Nat. Commun.* **2021**, *12*, 330. [CrossRef]
53. Lang, C.H.; Frost, R.A.; Nairn, A.C.; MacLean, D.A.; Vary, T.C. TNF-alpha impairs heart and skeletal muscle protein synthesis by altering translation initiation. *Am. J. Physiol. Endocrinol. Metab.* **2002**, *282*, E336–E347. [CrossRef] [PubMed]

54. Li, Y.P.; Chen, Y.; John, J.; Moylan, J.; Jin, B.; Mann, D.L.; Reid, M.B. TNF-alpha acts via p38 MAPK to stimulate expression of the ubiquitin ligase atrogin1/MAFbx in skeletal muscle. *FASEB J.* **2005**, *19*, 362–370. [CrossRef] [PubMed]
55. Russell, A.; Hepgul, N.; Nikkheslat, N.; Borsini, A.; Zajkowska, Z.; Moll, N.; Forton, D.; Agarwal, K.; Chalder, T.; Mondelli, V.; et al. Persistent fatigue induced by interferon-alpha: A novel, inflammation-based, proxy model of chronic fatigue syndrome. *Psychoneuroendocrinology* **2019**, *100*, 276–285. [CrossRef] [PubMed]

Disclaimer/Publisher's Note: The statements, opinions and data contained in all publications are solely those of the individual author(s) and contributor(s) and not of MDPI and/or the editor(s). MDPI and/or the editor(s) disclaim responsibility for any injury to people or property resulting from any ideas, methods, instructions or products referred to in the content.

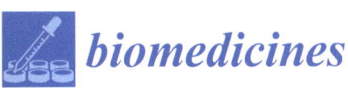

Article

Post-COVID-19 Pain Is Not Associated with DNA Methylation Levels of the *ACE2* Promoter in COVID-19 Survivors Hospitalized Due to SARS-CoV-2 Infection

César Fernández-de-las-Peñas [1,2,*], Gema Díaz-Gil [3], Antonio Gil-Crujera [3], Stella M. Gómez-Sánchez [3], Silvia Ambite-Quesada [1], Anabel Franco-Moreno [4], Pablo Ryan-Murua [4], Juan Torres-Macho [4,5], Oscar J. Pellicer-Valero [6], Lars Arendt-Nielsen [2,7,8] and Rocco Giordano [2,9]

1 Department of Physical Therapy, Occupational Therapy, Rehabilitation and Physical Medicine, Universidad Rey Juan Carlos (URJC), 28922 Alcorcón, Spain; silvia.ambite.quesada@urjc.es
2 Center for Neuroplasticity and Pain (CNAP), Sensory Motor Interaction (SMI), Department of Health Science and Technology, Faculty of Medicine, Aalborg University, DK-9220 Aalborg, Denmark; lan@hst.aau.dk (L.A.-N.); rg@hst.aau.dk (R.G.)
3 Research Group GAMDES, Department of Basic Health Sciences, Universidad Rey Juan Carlos (URJC), 28933 Madrid, Spain; gema.diaz@urjc.es (G.D.-G.); antonio.gil@urjc.es (A.G.-C.); stella.gomez@urjc.es (S.M.G.-S.)
4 Department of Internal Medicine, Hospital Universitario Infanta Leonor-Virgen de la Torre, 28031 Madrid, Spain; anaisabel.franco@salud.madrid.org (A.F.-M.); pablo.ryan@salud.madrid.org (P.R.-M.); juan.torresm@salud.madrid.org (J.T.-M.)
5 Department of Medicine, School of Medicine, Universidad Complutense de Madrid, 28040 Madrid, Spain
6 Image Processing Laboratory (IPL), Universitat de València, Parc Científic, 46980 Paterna, Spain; oscar.pellicer@uv.es
7 Department of Gastroenterology & Hepatology, Mech-Sense, Clinical Institute, Aalborg University Hospital, DK-9000 Aalborg, Denmark
8 Steno Diabetes Center North Denmark, Clinical Institute, Aalborg University Hospital, DK-9000 Aalborg, Denmark
9 Department of Oral and Maxillofacial Surgery, Aalborg University Hospital, DK-9000 Aalborg, Denmark
* Correspondence: cesar.fernandez@urjc.es; Tel.: +34-91-488-88-84

Abstract: One of theories explaining the development of long-lasting symptoms after an acute severe acute respiratory syndrome coronavirus 2 (SARS-CoV-2) infection include changes in the methylation pattern of the host. The current study aimed to investigate whether DNA methylation levels associated with the angiotensin-converting enzyme 2 (*ACE2*) promoter are different when comparing individuals previously hospitalized due to COVID-19 who then developed long-lasting post-COVID pain with those previously hospitalized due to COVID-19 who did not develop post-COVID-19 pain symptoms. Non-stimulated saliva samples were obtained from a cohort of 279 (mean age: 56.3, SD: 13.0 years old, 51.5% male) COVID-19 survivors who needed hospitalization. Clinical data were collected from hospital medical records. Participants were asked to disclose pain symptoms developed during the first three months after hospital admission due to COVID-19 and persisting at the time of the interview. Methylations of five CpG dinucleotides in the *ACE2* promoter were quantified (as percentages). Participants were evaluated up to 17.8 (SD: 5.3) months after hospitalization. Thus, 39.1% of patients exhibited post-COVID-19 pain. Most patients (77.05%) in the cohort developed localized post-COVID-19 pain. Headache and pain in the lower extremity were experienced by 29.4% of the patients. Seven patients received a post-infection diagnosis of fibromyalgia based on the presence of widespread pain characteristics (11.6%) and other associated symptoms. No significant differences in methylation percentages at any CpG location of the *ACE2* promoter were identified when comparing individuals with and without post-COVID-19 pain. The current study did not observe differences in methylation levels of the *ACE2* promoter depending on the presence or absence of long-lasting post-COVID-19 pain symptoms in individuals who needed hospitalization due to COVID-19 during the first wave of the pandemic.

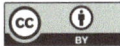

Keywords: methylation; *ACE2*; pain; post-COVID-19; long COVID

1. Introduction

The world has been immersed in the worst worldwide pandemic of the current century due to the rapid spreading of severe acute respiratory syndrome coronavirus 2 (SARS-CoV-2), the agent responsible for causing coronavirus disease 2019 (COVID-19). In addition to millions of deaths and billions of people infected with COVID-19 in the last four years, an important healthcare problem derived from SARS-CoV-2 infection has arisen in the potential development of long-lasting (or persisting) symptoms after an acute SARS-CoV-2 infection. The presence of symptoms once the acute COVID-19 phase has passed has received different names, such as long COVID, post-COVID-19, post-acute COVID-19 syndrome, and chronic post-COVID-19 [1]. A consensus paper proposed that the "post-COVID-19 condition occurs in people with a history of probable or confirmed SARS-CoV-2 infection, usually three months from the onset of infection, with symptoms that last for at least two months and cannot be explained by an alternative medical diagnosis. Common symptoms include, but are not limited to, fatigue, shortness of breath, and cognitive dysfunction, and generally have an impact on everyday functioning" [2].

Different meta-analyses have found that post-COVID-19 symptomatology can be present in up to 25–30% of subjects after recovery from an acute SARS-CoV-2 infection at one [3,4] and even two [5,6] years afterward. Additionally, the presence of post-COVID-19 symptomatology seems to be similar in comparisons between hospitalized and non-hospitalized COVID-19 survivors [3–6]. Although fatigue, dyspnea, or cognitive problems are usually reported as the most prevalent post-COVID-19 symptoms [3–6], pain is also a bothersome post-COVID-19 symptom, one that is experienced by 15–20% of post-COVID-19 survivors in the first six months after the acute infection [7]. A recent meta-analysis found that the prevalence of post-COVID-19 pain ranges between 8% to 17% during the first twelve months after COVID-19, although this prevalence rate depends on the study design, the definition of post-COVID-19 pain, and the outcomes used for collecting data [8]. Of particular relevance is that most published studies included in the two meta-analyses were not specifically focused on post-COVID-19 pain, and the reported prevalence rates are based on an examination of overall post-COVID-19 symptomatology [7,8]. In fact, the prevalence of post-COVID-19 pain has been found to be much higher, reaching up to 60%, when this symptom is specifically investigated [9–12].

Epigenetics has been proposed as one of the potential underlying mechanisms explaining post-COVID-19 pain [13]. Epigenetics include molecular processes that regulate gene expression without inducing changes in the DNA sequence [14]. Several epigenetic processes are described in the literature, methylation being one of the most investigated in COVID-19 research [15]. The potential effect of SARS-CoV-2 on epigenetics has been of interest from the beginning of the COVID-19 pandemic [16]. In fact, studies investigating epigenetics changes induced by SARS-CoV-2 infection are still being conducted [17]. Some studies have previously identified a heterogeneous response in methylation levels in COVID-19 patients at the acute phase of the infection; for instance, some genes such as interferon-related genes exhibited a hypermethylation (higher percentages) pattern, whereas other genes, such as those associated with the inflammatory response, exhibited a hypomethylation (lower percentages) pattern [18,19]. Thus, epigenetic changes in inflammatory-associated genes could explain the development of post-COVID-19 pain symptomatology. Balnis et al. [20] observed that those changes in methylation levels identified at the acute COVID-19 phase persisted at least one year after the infection in a small sample of 15 COVID-19 survivors. These results would suggest the possibility that epigenetics can potentially play a role in the development of post-COVID-19 symptomatology, particularly as to chronic pain. In fact, research work has focused on variations in the dynamics of DNA methylation in chronic pain conditions [21], but no study has specifically investigated DNA methylation changes and the presence of long-lasting post-COVID-19 pain symptomatology.

We have recently investigated the role of the DNA methylation levels of the angiotensin-converting enzyme 2 (*ACE2*) in the development of post-COVID-19 symptoms in individuals who needed hospitalization due to COVID-19 during the first wave of the outbreak [22]. The current paper presents a study, using the same cohort of patients [22], investigating whether DNA methylation levels of the *ACE2* promoter are associated with the development of long-lasting post-COVID-19 pain in individuals who had been hospitalized due to SARS-CoV-2 infection.

2. Methods of the Investigation

2.1. Participants

As described in the earlier paper [22], this study recruited subjects who were previously hospitalized at four urban hospitals in Madrid (Spain) due to COVID-19 during the first wave of the outbreak (March to May 2020). All included participants presented a confirmed positive diagnosis of SARS-CoV-2 infection as well as clinical/radiological findings at hospital admission. The study was approved by the Institutional Ethics Committees of all institutions (URJC0907202015920) and hospitals (HUFA 20/126; HUIL/092-20; HSO25112020; and HCSC20/495E) involved. Participants were informed of the study procedure, read the written informed consent, and signed it if they decided to participate in the study.

2.2. Genome DNA Collection

Evidence shows that using saliva to assess DNA methylation is becoming more common in the literature [23]. In fact, Khare et al. found that salivary DNA is equivalent in quantity and purity to blood DNA [24]. Accordingly, we used a saliva sample rather than a blood sample, because the former is a viable, non-invasive, and stress-free assessment method used to evaluate DNA methylation. In the experiment's scenario, unstimulated whole saliva samples were collected during the morning hours from each patient, using collection tubes and following standardized procedures. Consistent with the manufacturer's instructions, we asked participants to avoid eating, drinking or chewing gum for at least 1 h before saliva sample collection. After collection, samples were centrifuged at 3000 rpm for 15 min to obtain the cell sediment and stored at $-20\ °C$ until the DNA methylation analysis.

A MagMAX™ DNA Multi-Sample Ultra 2.0 Kit (Thermo Fisher Scientific Inc., Hemel Hempstead, UK) and King Fisher Flex purification robot (Thermo Fisher) were used for genomic DNA extraction. Purity and concentration of the resulting DNA were assessed using Quant-iT™ PicoGreen™ dsDNA reagent" (Thermo Fisher).

2.3. Differential Methylation Profiling

We used the same procedures employed in our previous study [22]. Briefly, methylation percentages were calculated in five non-cytosine-phosphate-guanine (CpG) sites of interest within the *ACE2* promoter (CpG1, CpG2, CpG3, CpG4, and CpG5) as previously described [25,26]. The five CpG sites within the *ACE2* promoter were identified with a specific web-based program (http://www.urogene.org/methprimer, last accessed on 10 April 2024). Figure 1 graphs the CpG islands sequence in the promoter region of the *ACE2* receptor.

All methylation analyses procedures were carried out at Fundación Parque Científico de Madrid (FPCM), c/Faraday 7, Madrid, Spain, and have previously been extensively described [22]. For the main analyses, methylation percentage (%) at each position of the *ACE2* promoter (CpG1, CpG2, CpG3, CpG4, and CpG5) was used separately.

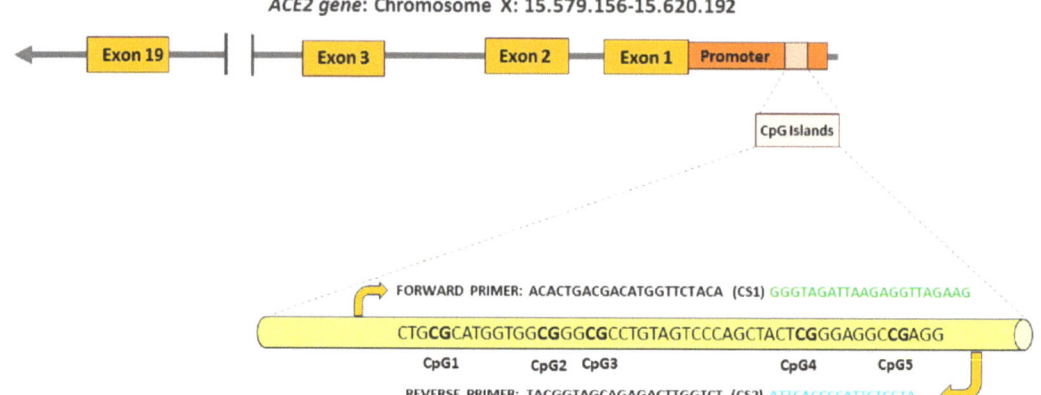

Figure 1. The figure graphs the forward (in green) and reverse (in blue) primers used for DNA methylation sequencing. In addition, each of the five CpG sites analyzed (CG in bold within the sequence) can be visualized in the overall island sequence associated with the *ACE2* promoter region.

2.4. Data Collection

Age, gender, height, weight, pre-existing medical comorbidities, previous chronic pain conditions, days in hospital, COVID-19 onset-associated symptomatology, and need of intensive care unit (ICU) admission were collected from hospital medical records.

Included patients were scheduled for a face-to-face interview conducted by trained healthcare researchers with 15 years of experience in pain management. Thus, participants were asked about the presence of pain symptoms that appeared after their hospital stay due to SARS-CoV-2 infection, over at least the subsequent three months, in absence of any event explaining the developed of pain (e.g., trauma or surgery), and whether the pain persisted at each time of the study (consistent with the definition of a post-COVID-19 condition [2]). They were also asked to describe the location of their pain symptoms (e.g., head, cervical spine, shoulder, elbow–wrist, hip, knee, thorax, lower or upper extremity, or generalized pain). We used the definition of primary chronic musculoskeletal pain proposed by the International Association for the Study of Pain [27].

2.5. Statistical Analysis

The STATA software, version 16.1, was used for data collection, whereas the Python library pandas 0.25.3 was used for data processing. Quantitative data were expressed as means (standard deviations, SD), whereas the categorical data were expressed as numbers of cases (percentages). One-way ANOVA tests were used to determine differences in the methylation percentages (%) between patients with and without post-COVID-19 pain symptoms. The assumption of normality of the data was assessed with the Shapiro–Wilk test. A priori p-values lower than 0.05 were considered statistically significant; the Holm–Bonferroni correction for multiple comparisons was applied.

3. Results

As previously reported [22], a total of 330 individuals who needed hospitalization due to acute SARS-CoV-2 infection during the first wave of the COVID-19 pandemic were invited to participate. Fifty-one (15%) were excluded due to the following reasons: refusal to attend the appointment (n = 15), comorbid diagnosis of fibromyalgia (n = 15), DNA methylation analyses not possible due to contamination of the sample (n = 14), or pregnancy (n = 7). Ultimately, a total of 279 patients (51.3% male, mean age: 56.4 ± 12.8 years old) fulfilled all inclusion criteria.

At the time of the study (mean: 17.8, SD: 5.2 months after hospital discharge), the prevalence of long-lasting post-COVID-19 pain symptomatology was 39.1% (n = 109). Most patients (77.1%) developed localized post-COVID-19 pain symptomatology. Thus, the location of post-COVID-19 pain symptoms is presented in Figure 2. Pain in the head and pain in the lower extremity were the most prevalent locations (29.4%).

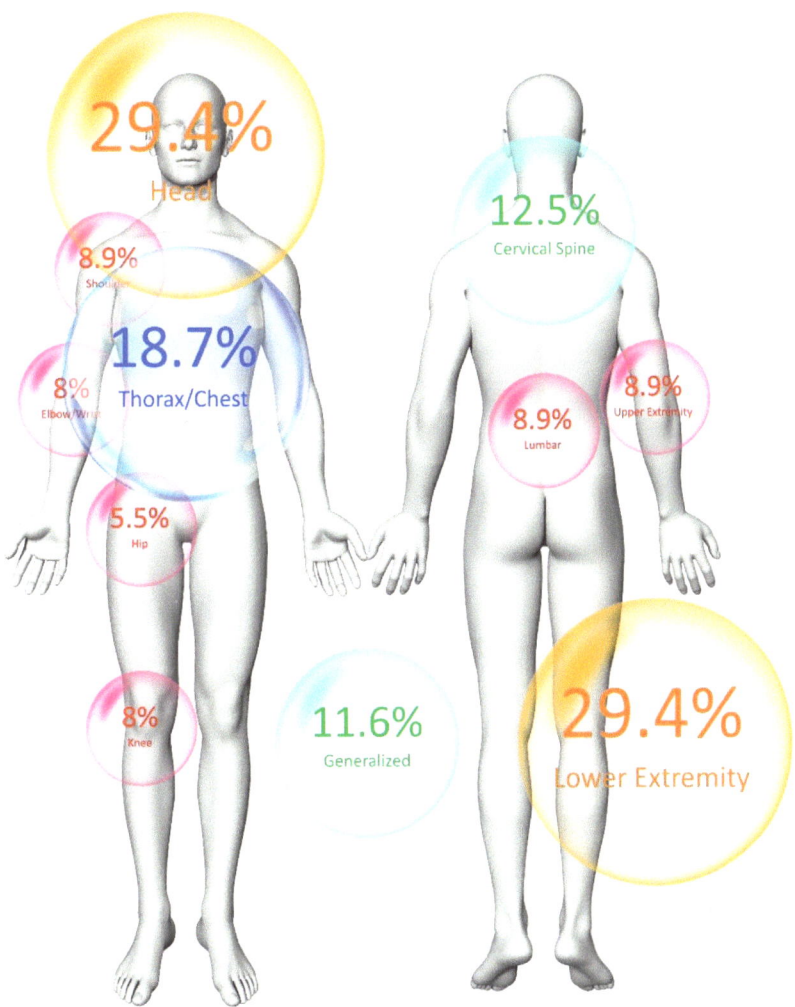

Figure 2. Location of post-COVID-19 pain symptomatology in the cohort analyzed (n = 109).

No significant differences in the presence of previous medical comorbidities were identified between patients who developed post-COVID-19 pain symptomatology and those who did not (Table 1). A significantly higher proportion of females reported post-COVID-19 pain ($p = 0.005$), when compared with males. Further, individuals who developed post-COVID-19 pain exhibited a higher number of COVID-19 onset-associated symptoms at hospitalization ($p = 0.01$), particularly COVID-19 onset-associated headache ($p = 0.008$, Table 1). No significant association was identified between the number of COVID-19 onset-associated symptoms at hospitalization and methylation levels at CpG1 (r = 0.021, $p = 0.829$), CpG2 (r = 0.026, $p = 0.787$), CpG3 (r = 0.061 $p = 0.524$), CpG4 (r = 0.017, $p = 0.861$), or CpG5 (r = 0.091, $p = 0.340$).

Table 1. Demographic, clinical, and methylation percentage of individuals with and without post-COVID-19 pain.

	Post-COVID-19 Pain (n = 109)	No Post-COVID-19 Pain (n = 170)	p Value
Age, mean (SD), years	55.7 (12.2)	57.0 (13.2)	0.443
Sex, male/female (%) *	40 (46.7%)/69 (63.3%)	103 (61.6%)/67 (39.4%)	0.005 *
Weight, mean (SD), kg	80.1 (17.1)	81.6 (16.6)	0.447
Height, mean (SD), cm	167.5 (9.3)	169.0 (9.6)	0.159
Previous medical pathologies (n)	1.25 (1.0)	1.35 (1.0)	0.286
Previous medical pathologies			
Hypertension	36 (33.0%)	59 (34.7%)	0.815
Diabetes	14 (12.8%)	15 (8.8%)	0.309
Cardiovascular Diseases	6 (5.5%)	14 (8.25%)	0.406
Asthma	15 (13.7%)	16 (9.4%)	0.288
Obesity	38 (34.8%)	47 (27.7%)	0.287
Chronic Obstructive Pulmonary Disease	1 (0.9%)	4 (2.35%)	0.382
Number of symptoms associated with COVID-19 at hospital admission, mean (SD) *	3.4 (0.8)	3.1 (1.1)	0.01 *
COVID-19 symptoms at hospitalization			
Fever	36 (70.6%)	125 (73.5%)	0.782
Dyspnea	44 (41.3%)	57 (33.5%)	0.295
Myalgia	42 (38.5%)	74 (43.5%)	0.105
Cough	45 (42.2%)	54 (31.8%)	0.347
Headache *	46 (42.2%)	41 (24.1%)	0.008 *
Diarrhea	19 (17.4%)	35 (20.6%)	0.558
Anosmia	21 (19.3%)	42 (24.7%)	0.351
Ageusia	22 (20.2%)	43 (25.3%)	0.388
Throat Pain	12 (11.0%)	20 (11.7%)	0.855
Vomiting	10 (9.2%)	13 (7.6%)	0.664
Dizziness	6 (5.5%)	10 (5.9%)	0.897
Intensive Care Unit (ICU) admission Yes/No, n (%)	4 (3.7%)/105 (96.3%)	6 (3.5%)/164 (96.5%)	0.905
CpG1 methylation (%)	93.4 (4.3)	93.6 (3.4)	0.608
CpG2 methylation (%)	40.1 (7.2)	40.0 (7.5)	0.881
CpG3 methylation (%)	43.8 (8.5)	43.0 (8.8)	0.445
CpG4 methylation (%)	45.4 (8.0)	45.7 (7.9)	0.784
CpG5 methylation (%)	0.6 (0.3)	0.6 (0.7)	0.971

n: number; SD: standard deviation; * Statistically significant differences between groups ($p < 0.05$).

Overall, no significant differences in methylation percentages in any of the CpG locations of the *ACE2* promoter were identified when comparing COVID-19 survivors who developed post-COVID-19 pain symptoms and those who did not (Table 1). The mean intensity of post-COVID-19 pain was 5.6/10 (SD: 1.7) points. No significant association existed between the intensity of post-COVID-19 pain and methylation levels at CpG1 (r = 0.06, p = 0.959), CpG2 (r = 0.187, p = 0.101), CpG3 (r = 0.078 p = 0.496), CpG4 (r = 0.111, p = 0.325), or CpG5 (r = 0.175, p = 0.184). Similarly, no significant association was observed between the length of pain symptoms and methylation levels at CpG1 (r = 0.11, p = 0.912), CpG2 (r = 0.083, p = 0.381), CpG3 (r = 0.124 p = 0.193), CpG4 (r = 0.011, p = 0.905), or CpG5 (r = 0.115, p = 0.228).

No differences as to the presence of previous chronic pain conditions were identified when comparing the presence or absence of post-COVID-19 pain (Table 2). Seven (6.4%) patients received a diagnosis of fibromyalgia syndrome based on the presence of widespread pain (11.6%) and other associated symptoms. Finally, five (4.6%) and twenty-seven (24.8%) patients received diagnoses of migraine and tension-type headache, respectively (Table 2).

Table 2. Chronic pain condition diagnoses of individuals with and without post-COVID-19 pain.

	Post-COVID-19 Pain (n = 109)	No Post-COVID-19 Pain (n = 170)	p Value
	Pre-COVID-19 Chronic Pain Conditions		
Chronic Pain Symptomatology	60 (55.0%)	70 (41.2%)	0.10
Migraine	10 (9.2%)	7 (4.1%)	0.09
Tension-Type Headache	14 (12.8%)	12 (7.1%)	0.122
Rheumatoid Arthritis	3 (2.75%)	6 (3.5%)	0.724
Osteoarthritis	17 (15.6%)	16 (9.4%)	0.143
	New Post-COVID-19 Chronic Pain Conditions		
Localized Pain	84 (77.05%)	----	----
Migraine	5 (4.6%)	----	----
Tension-Type Headache	27 (24.8%)	----	----
Fibromyalgia Syndrome	7 (6.4%)	----	----
Osteoarthritis	4 (3.7%)	----	----

n: number.

4. Discussion

The present study investigated the potential correlation between methylation levels in the promoter of the *ACE2* gene and the development of long-lasting post-COVID-19 pain symptoms over one-and-a-half years in patients who need hospitalization due to COVID-19 during the first wave of the pandemic. Several studies have highlighted the roles of the surface receptor for S1 of the *ACE2* and the transmembrane protease serine-2 (TMPRSS2) receptor in subjects during the acute COVID-19 phase [28]. It is known that SARS-CoV-2 enters the host cells through the membrane-bound *ACE2* exopeptidase, and hypomethylation of *ACE2* may potentially increase its expression, thereby elevating the risk of infection [29] and accordingly elevating the risk of post-COVID-19 condition. The results obtained in this cohort of COVID-19 survivors did not show a significant correlation between this specific gene investigated and the development of post-COVID-19 pain symptomatology.

4.1. Post-COVID-19 Pain and DNA Methylation Changes

The prevalence of pain symptoms in our cohort of previously hospitalized COVID-19 survivors at a follow-up of 18 months after the infection was 40%. This prevalence rate is higher than those found in published meta-analyses, including studies investigating overall post-COVID-19 symptomatology (including pain) and reporting that 8% to 20% of COVID-19 survivors exhibit post-COVID-19 pain the first year after the infection [7,8], but it is lower in comparison with studies specifically investigating the prevalence of post-COVID-19 pain, where prevalence rates reach to up to 60% of the patients [9–12]. Thus, it is remarkable that most published studies included follow-up periods shorter than one year [7–12]. Since the prevalence of post-COVID-19 pain symptomatology (and also the overall post-COVID-19 condition) tends to decrease with time [30], prevalence data from our sample can be considered representative of this population.

No previous study has investigated DNA methylation changes in individuals with post-COVID-19 pain. It seems that post-COVID-19 pain is associated with the inflammatory response related to COVID-19 [31]. Thus, the fact that individuals who report myalgia as an associated symptom at the acute COVID-19 phase are at a higher risk of developing post-COVID-19 pain [32] supports the finding that muscle pain is specifically sensitive to the cytokine SARS-CoV-2-associated burst. Nevertheless, it has also been reported that long-term post-COVID-19 myalgia is associated with lower levels of inflammatory biomarkers (e.g., interleukins-6) at the acute COVID-19 phase [33].

Interestingly, DNA methylation changes at CpG sites of specific pain genes such as *OPRM1* (opioid receptor Mu 1) and *TRPA1* (Transient Receptor Potential Cation Channel Subfamily A Member 1) have been associated with sensitivity to pain [34]. Therefore, this association could be post-COVID-19-symptom-specific. For instance, Takenaka et al. [35] have observed an association between methylation levels of the *TRPA1* gene promoter region and the presence of neuropathic-like symptoms [35]. Hence, it is possible that the presence of post-COVID-19 pain symptomatology can be associated with DNA methylation changes in genes associated with inflammation, (e.g., *OPRM1* or *TRPA1*) rather than in those genes associated with COVID-19 susceptibility (e.g., *ACE2* promoter) such as those described in our study.

Finally, it is also important to understand that no timeframe can be determined for DNA methylation change identification. In fact, no longitudinal study has investigated those variations of DNA methylation at different timeframes. Thus, it can be hypothesized that COVID-19 could induce different DNA methylation changes at the acute phase of the infection, while these changes reverse afterward. Future studies investigating the longitudinal evolution of DNA methylation changes from the acute COVI-19 phase to the development of post-COVID-19 pain in the context of long-term follow-ups are needed.

4.2. DNA Methylation and Widespread Pain

Among those patients developing post-COVID-19 pain, of particular interest are those developing widespread pain symptomatology, like fibromyalgia syndrome [36,37]. Individuals with widespread pain exhibit nociplastic pain features, which means that these patients need particular medical attention due to the complexity of their clinical presentation [38]. Previous studies have explored DNA methylation changes in patients with chronic widespread pain [39] or fibromyalgia syndrome [40], providing evidence that DNA methylation alterations can be relevant in widespread pain conditions. In the current study, thirteen (11.6%) individuals reported widespread pain symptoms. Among these patients, seven (6.4%) had received a diagnosis of fibromyalgia syndrome one year after the infection. In fact, it has been suggested that SARS-CoV-2 could act as a trigger factor of fibromyalgia syndrome, or as an exacerbator factor, since both conditions share similar mechanisms [41]. Thus, we conducted a secondary analysis looking to see whether COVID-19 survivors with widespread post-COVID-19 pain symptomatology (n = 13) exhibited different DNA methylation percentages than those reporting localized post-COVID-19 pain (n = 96). No significant differences in methylation percentages in any of the CpG sites were seen (Table 3).

Table 3. Methylation percentages in individuals with and without post-COVID-19 widespread pain.

	Widespread Pain (n = 13)	Localized Pain (n = 96)	*p* Value
CpG1 methylation (%)	93.8 (2.8)	93.4 (3.8)	0.703
CpG2 methylation (%)	39.7 (7.0)	40.0 (7.4)	0.860
CpG3 methylation (%)	42.8 (7.5)	43.3 (8.7)	0.841
CpG4 methylation (%)	44.2 (8.4)	45.6 (7.8)	0.527
CpG5 methylation (%)	0.65 (0.3)	0.6 (0.35)	0.739

It is possible that the small sample size of the subgroup of patients with widespread pain symptoms (n = 13) did not permit the detection of significant differences, although this is unlikely. Additionally, it is also possible that DNA methylation changes are gene-specific, since patients with chronic fatigue syndrome and fibromyalgia syndrome are mainly characterized by altered DNA methylation in those genes regulating cellular signaling and immune functioning [42]. Nevertheless, we should recognize that we did not phenotype the type of pain symptomatology and were not able to determine if the symptoms had a nociceptive, neuropathic, or nociplastic pain phenotype.

4.3. Previous Pain Conditions

It has been previously seen that a suffering from musculoskeletal pain before an acute SARS-CoV-2 infection increases the risk (OR1.55, 95%CI 1.27 to 1.89) of post-COVID-19 pain [43]. This finding was confirmed in a large retrospective study determining that the presence of chronic pain conditions before SARS-CoV-2 infection increases the risk of post-COVID-19 pain symptomatology [44]. Although the prevalence of previous chronic pain conditions was higher in COVID-19 survivors who developed post-COVID-19 pain than among those who did not develop pain, the differences were not statistically significant in our study.

4.4. Female Sex

Female sex has been found to be a risk factor associated with overall post-COVID-19 condition [45,46] and also specifically with reference to post-COVID-19 pain [43]. In our cohort, we also saw that the proportion of females reporting post-COVID-19 pain was significantly higher than that of the males. This result could be expected since musculoskeletal pain is more prevalent in females than in males [47,48]. Several biological and sociocultural factors, as well as gender-constructed behaviors, have been proposed as bases for explaining sex differences in COVID-19 and post-COVID-19 responses [49]. An important biological factor associated with the current study is that the expression of the *ACE2* receptor is more pronounced in males than in females, since estrogens can down-regulate its expression [50]. This factor could provide a plausible biological explanation for the reduced severity of COVID-19 in females, but it would not explain the higher prevalence of post-COVID pain in females.

4.5. Limitations

Although this is the first study investigating DNA methylation changes at the *ACE2* promoter and the development of long-lasting post-COVID pain symptomatology, some limitations must also be recognized. First, we included a cohort of patients who need hospitalization when they were infected with a historical SARS-CoV-2 strain; therefore, extrapolation of the current results to other populations should not be attempted. In addition, the sample size could be considered relatively small. Second, the cross-sectional design of our study does not permit the determination of the fluctuating nature of DNA methylation changes. Third, we only analyzed DNA methylation changes at the *ACE2* promoter; hence, we cannot exclude the presence of DNA methylation alterations in pain-associated genes. Finally, we did not collect pain features associated with our sample, so proper characterization of post-COVID pain was not conducted. Therefore, studies including large samples of individuals, hospitalized due to COVID-19 and non-hospitalized, and including whole DNA methylation analyses, might be able to identify epigenetic changes associated with the development of long-lasting post-COVID pain symptomatology.

5. Conclusions

The results from the current study did not find an association between the methylation levels at different CpG sites of *ACE2* promoter and the development of post-COVID pain symptomatology in the one-and-a-half years after suffering from COVID-19 in a cohort of individuals who needed hospitalization due to the infection. Future studies investigating multiple sites where, after infection by SARS-CoV-2, methylation of CpG might more specifically regulate the pain pathways are needed.

Author Contributions: C.F.-d.-l.-P.: conceptualization, visualization, methodology, validation, data curation, writing—original draft, writing—review and editing. G.D.-G.: methodology, validation, data curation, writing—original draft, writing—review and editing. A.G.-C.: methodology, validation, data curation, writing—original draft, writing—review and editing. S.M.G.-S.: validation, data curation, writing—original draft, writing—review and editing. S.A.-Q.: validation, writing—original draft, writing—review and editing. J.T.-M.: validation, writing—original draft writing—review, and editing. P.R.-M.: validation, writing—original draft, writing—review, and editing. A.F.-M.:

validation, writing—original draft, writing—review and editing. O.J.P.-V.: validation, data curation, writing—original draft, writing—review and editing. L.A.-N.: methodology, validation, data curation, writing—original draft, writing—review and editing. R.G.: methodology, validation, supervision, writing—original draft writing—review, and editing. All authors have read and agreed to the published version of the manuscript.

Funding: The project was supported by a grant from the Novo Nordisk Foundation (NNF21OC0067235) (Denmark) and by a grant associated with the Fondo Europeo De Desarrollo Regional—Recursos REACT-UE del Programa Operativo de Madrid 2014–2020, en la línea de actuación de proyectos de I+D+i en materia de respuesta a COVID 19 (LONG-COVID-EXP-CM).

Institutional Review Board Statement: The study design was approved by the Institutional Ethics Committees of all institutions and hospitals involved (URJC0907202015920; H12OCT23/418; HSO 25112020; HUIL/092-20; HCSC20/495E).

Informed Consent Statement: Written informed consent was obtained from all the participants before collecting any data.

Data Availability Statement: The original contributions presented in the study are included in the article, further inquiries can be directed to the corresponding author.

Conflicts of Interest: The authors declare no conflict of interest.

References

1. Akbarialiabad, H.; Taghrir, M.H.; Abdollahi, A.; Ghahramani, N.; Kumar, M.; Paydar, S.; Razani, B.; Mwangi, J.; Asadi-Pooya, A.A.; Malekmakan, L.; et al. Long COVID, a comprehensive systematic scoping review. *Infection* **2021**, *49*, 1163–1186. [CrossRef] [PubMed]
2. Soriano, J.B.; Murthy, S.; Marshall, J.C.; Relan, P.; Diaz, J.V.; WHO Clinical Case Definition Working Group on Post-COVID-19 Condition. A clinical case definition of post-COVID-19 condition by a Delphi consensus. *Lancet Infect Dis.* **2022**, *22*, e102–e107. [CrossRef]
3. Chen, C.; Haupert, S.R.; Zimmermann, L.; Shi, X.; Fritsche, L.G.; Mukherjee, B. Global prevalence of post COVID-19 condition or long COVID: A meta-analysis and systematic review. *J. Infect. Dis.* **2022**, *226*, 1593–1607. [CrossRef] [PubMed]
4. Han, Q.; Zheng, B.; Daines, L.; Sheikh, A. Long-term sequelae of COVID-19: A systematic review and meta-analysis of one-year follow-up studies on post-COVID symptoms. *Pathogens* **2022**, *11*, 269. [CrossRef] [PubMed]
5. Fernández-de-las-Peñas, C.; Notarte, K.I.; Macasaet, R.; Velasco, J.V.; Catahay, J.A.; Therese Ver, A.; Chung, W.; Valera-Calero, J.A.; Navarro-Santana, M. Persistence of post-COVID symptoms in the general population two years after SARS-CoV-2 infection: A systematic review and meta-analysis. *J. Infect.* **2024**, *88*, 77–88. [CrossRef]
6. Rahmati, M.; Udeh, R.; Yon, D.K.; Lee, S.W.; Dolja-Gore, X.; McEVoy, M.; Kenna, T.; Jacob, L.; López Sánchez, G.F.; Koyanagi, A.; et al. A systematic review and meta-analysis of long-term sequelae of COVID-19 2-year after SARS-CoV-2 infection: A call to action for neurological, physical, and psychological sciences. *J. Med. Virol.* **2023**, *95*, e28852. [CrossRef] [PubMed]
7. Fernández-de-las-Peñas, C.; Navarro-Santana, M.; Plaza-Manzano, G.; Palacios-Ceña, D.; Arendt-Nielsen, L. Time course prevalence of post-COVID pain symptoms of musculoskeletal origin in patients who had survived to SARS-CoV-2 infection: A systematic review and meta-analysis. *Pain* **2022**, *163*, 1220–1231. [CrossRef] [PubMed]
8. Kerzhner, O.; Berla, E.; Har-Even, M.; Ratmansky, M.; Goor-Aryeh, I. Consistency of inconsistency in long-COVID-19 pain symptoms persistency: A systematic review and meta-analysis. *Pain Pract.* **2024**, *24*, 120–159. [CrossRef] [PubMed]
9. Bakılan, F.; Gökmen, İ.G.; Ortanca, B.; Uçan, A.; Eker Güvenç, Ş.; Şahin Mutlu, F.; Gökmen, H.M.; Ekim, A. Musculoskeletal symptoms and related factors in postacute COVID-19 patients. *Int. J. Clin. Pract.* **2021**, *75*, e14734. [CrossRef]
10. Karaarslan, F.; Demircioğlu, G.F.; Kardeş, S. Postdischarge rheumatic and musculoskeletal symptoms following hospitalization for COVID-19: Prospective follow-up by phone interviews. *Rheumatol. Int.* **2021**, *41*, 1263–1271. [CrossRef]
11. Soares, F.H.C.; Kubota, G.T.; Fernandes, A.M.; Hojo, B.; Couras, C.; Costa, B.V.; Lapa, J.D.D.S.; Braga, L.M.; Almeida, M.M.; Cunha, P.H.M.D.; et al. "Pain in the Pandemic Initiative Collaborators". Prevalence and characteristics of new-onset pain in COVID-19 survivours, a controlled study. *Eur. J. Pain* **2021**, *25*, 1342–1354. [CrossRef] [PubMed]
12. Bileviciute-Ljungar, I.; Norrefalk, J.R.; Borg, K. Pain burden in post-COVID-19 syndrome following mild COVID-19 infection. *J. Clin. Med.* **2022**, *11*, 771. [CrossRef] [PubMed]
13. Castaldo, M.; Ebbesen, B.D.; Fernández-de-las-Peñas, C.; Arendt-Nielsen, L.; Giordano, R. COVID-19 and musculoskeletal pain: An overview of the current knowledge. *Minerva Anestesiol.* **2023**, *89*, 1134–1142. [CrossRef]
14. Deans, C.; Maggert, K.A. What do you mean, "epigenetic"? *Genetics* **2015**, *199*, 887–896. [CrossRef] [PubMed]
15. Capp, J.P. Interplay between genetic, epigenetic, and gene expression variability: Considering complexity in evolvability. *Evol. Appl.* **2021**, *14*, 893–901. [CrossRef] [PubMed]
16. Mantovani, A.; Netea, M.G. Trained innate immunity, epigenetics, and COVID-19. *N. Engl. J. Med.* **2020**, *383*, 1078–1080. [CrossRef] [PubMed]

17. Behura, A.; Naik, L.; Patel, S.; Das, M.; Kumar, A.; Mishra, A.; Nayak, D.K.; Manna, D.; Mishra, A.; Dhiman, R. Involvement of epigenetics in affecting host immunity during SARS-CoV-2 infection. *Biochim. Biophys. Acta Mol. Basis Dis.* **2023**, *1869*, 166634. [CrossRef] [PubMed]
18. Dey, A.; Vaishak, K.; Deka, D.; Radhakrishnan, A.K.; Paul, S.; Shanmugam, P.; Daniel, A.P.; Pathak, S.; Duttaroy, A.K.; Banerjee, A. Epigenetic perspectives associated with COVID-19 infection and related cytokine storm: An updated review. *Infection* **2023**, *51*, 1603–1618. [CrossRef]
19. Balnis, J.; Madrid, A.; Hogan, K.J.; Drake, L.A.; Chieng, H.C.; Tiwari, A.; Vincent, C.E.; Chopra, A.; Vincent, P.A.; Robek, M.D.; et al. Blood DNA Methylation and COVID-19 outcomes. *Clin. Epigenetics* **2021**, *13*, 118. [CrossRef] [PubMed]
20. Balnis, J.; Madrid, A.; Hogan, K.J.; Drake, L.A.; Adhikari, A.; Vancavage, R.; Singer, H.A.; Alisch, R.S.; Jaitovich, A. Whole-Genome methylation sequencing reveals that COVID-19-induced epigenetic dysregulation remains 1 year after hospital discharge. *Am. J. Respir. Cell Mol. Biol.* **2023**, *68*, 594–597. [CrossRef]
21. Møller Johansen, L.; Gerra, M.C.; Arendt-Nielsen, L. Time course of DNA methylation in pain conditions: From experimental models to humans. *Eur. J. Pain.* **2021**, *25*, 296–312. [CrossRef] [PubMed]
22. Fernández-de-las-Peñas, C.; Díaz-Gil, G.; Gil-Crujera, A.; Gómez-Sánchez, S.M.; Ambite-Quesada, S.; Torres-Macho, J.; Ryan-Murua, P.; Franco-Moreno, A.; Pellicer-Valero, O.J.; Arendt-Nielsen, L.; et al. DNA methylation of the *ACE2* promoter is not associated with post-COVID symptoms in previously hospitalized COVID-19 survivors. *Microorganisms* **2024**, *12*, 1304. [CrossRef]
23. Nishitani, S.; Parets, S.E.; Haas, B.W.; Smith, A.K. DNA methylation analysis from saliva samples for epidemiological studies. *Epigenetics* **2018**, *13*, 352–362. [CrossRef]
24. Khare, P.; Raj, V.; Chandra, S.; Agarwal, S. Quantitative and qualitative assessment of DNA extracted from saliva for its use in forensic identification. *J. Forensic Dent. Sci.* **2014**, *6*, 81–85. [CrossRef] [PubMed]
25. Mikeska, T.; Felsberg, J.; Hewitt, C.A.; Dobrovic, A. Analysing DNA methylation using bisulphite pyrosequencing. *Methods Mol. Biol.* **2011**, *791*, 33–53.
26. Fan, R.; Mao, S.Q.; Gu, T.L.; Zhong, F.D.; Gong, M.L.; Hao, L.M.; Yin, F.Y.; Dong, C.Z.; Zhang, L.N. Preliminary analysis of the association between methylation of the *ACE2* promoter and essential hypertension. *Mol. Med. Rep.* **2017**, *15*, 3905–3911. [CrossRef]
27. Barke, A.; Korwisi, B.; Jakob, R.; Konstanjsek, N.; Rief, W.; Treede, R.D. Classification of chronic pain for the International Classification of Diseases (ICD-11): Results of the 2017 international World Health Organization field testing. *Pain* **2022**, *163*, e310–e318. [CrossRef]
28. Singh, H.O.; Choudhari, R.; Nema, V.; Khan, A.A. *ACE2* and *TMPRSS2* polymorphisms in various diseases with special reference to its impact on COVID-19 disease. *Microb. Pathog.* **2021**, *150*, 104621. [CrossRef]
29. Faramarzi, A.; Safaralizadeh, R.; Dastmalchi, N.; Teimourian, S. Epigenetic-related effects of COVID-19 on human cells. *Infect. Disord. Drug Targets* **2022**, *22*, 21–26. [CrossRef]
30. Fernández-de-las-Peñas, C.; Pellicer-Valero, O.J.; Martín-Guerrero, J.D.; Hernández-Barrera, V.; Arendt-Nielsen, L. Investigating the fluctuating nature of post-COVID pain symptoms in previously hospitalized COVID-19 survivors: The LONG-COVID-EXP multicenter study. *Pain Rep.* **2024**, *9*, e1153. [CrossRef]
31. Cascella, M.; Del Gaudio, A.; Vittori, A.; Bimonte, S.; Del Prete, P.; Forte, C.A.; Cuomo, A.; De Blasio, E. COVID-Pain: Acute and late-onset painful clinical manifestations in COVID-19: Molecular mechanisms and research perspectives. *J. Pain Res.* **2021**, *14*, 2403–2412. [CrossRef] [PubMed]
32. Fernández-de-las-Peñas, C.; Rodríguez-Jiménez, J.; Fuensalida-Novo, S.; Palacios-Ceña, M.; Gómez-Mayordomo, V.; Florencio, L.L.; Hernández-Barrera, V.; Arendt-Nielsen, L. Myalgia as a symptom at hospital admission by severe acute respiratory syndrome coronavirus 2 infection is associated with persistent musculoskeletal pain as long-term post-COVID sequelae: A case-control study. *Pain* **2021**, *162*, 2832–2840. [CrossRef]
33. Sykes, D.L.; Van der Feltz-Cornelis, C.M.; Holdsworth, L.; Hart, S.P.; O'Halloran, J.; Holding, S.; Crooks, M.G. Examining the relationship between inflammatory biomarkers during COVID-19 hospitalization and subsequent long-COVID symptoms: A longitudinal and retrospective study. *Immun. Inflamm. Dis.* **2023**, *11*, e1052. [CrossRef]
34. Bell, J.T.; Loomis, A.K.; Butcher, L.M.; Gao, F.; Zhang, B.; Hyde, C.L.; Sun, J.; Wu, H.; Ward, K.; Harris, J.; et al. Differential methylation of the *TRPA1* promoter in pain sensitivity. *Nat. Commun.* **2014**, *5*, 2978. [CrossRef]
35. Takenaka, S.; Sukenaga, N.; Ohmuraya, M.; Matsuki, Y.; Maeda, L.; Takao, Y.; Hirose, M. Association between neuropathic pain characteristics and DNA methylation of transient receptor potential ankyrin 1 in human peripheral blood. *Medicine* **2020**, *99*, e19325. [CrossRef]
36. Gavrilova, N.; Soprun, L.; Lukashenko, M.; Ryabkova, V.; Fedotkina, T.V.; Churilov, L.P.; Shoenfeld, Y. New clinical phenotype of the Post-COVID syndrome: Fibromyalgia and joint hypermobility condition. *Pathophysiology* **2022**, *29*, 24–29. [CrossRef] [PubMed]
37. Martínez-Lavín, M.; Miguel-Álvarez, A. Hypothetical framework for post-COVID 19 condition based on a fibromyalgia pathogenetic model. *Clin. Rheumatol.* **2023**, *42*, 3167–3171. [CrossRef]
38. Fernández-de-las-Peñas, C.; Nijs, J.; Neblett, R.; Polli, A.; Moens, M.; Goudman, L.; Shekhar Patil, M.; Knaggs, R.D.; Pickering, G.; Arendt-Nielsen, L. Phenotyping post-COVID pain as a nociceptive, neuropathic, or nociplastic pain condition. *Biomedicines* **2022**, *10*, 2562. [CrossRef] [PubMed]

39. Burri, A.; Marinova, Z.; Robinson, M.D.; Kühnel, B.; Waldenberger, M.; Wahl, S.; Kunze, S.; Gieger, C.; Livshits, G.; Williams, F. Are epigenetic factors implicated in chronic widespread pain? *PLoS ONE* **2016**, *11*, e0165548. [CrossRef]
40. Ciampi de Andrade, D.; Maschietto, M.; Galhardoni, R.; Gouveia, G.; Chile, T.; Victorino Krepischi, A.C.; Dale, C.S.; Brunoni, A.R.; Parravano, D.C.; Cueva Moscos, A.S.; et al. Epigenetics insights into chronic pain: DNA hypomethylation in fibromyalgia: A controlled pilot-study. *Pain* **2017**, *158*, 1473–1480. [CrossRef]
41. Fialho, M.F.P.; Brum, E.S.; Oliveira, S.M. Could the fibromyalgia syndrome be triggered or enhanced by COVID-19? *Inflammopharmacology* **2023**, *31*, 633–651. [CrossRef]
42. Fischer, S.; Kleinstäuber, M.; Fiori, L.M.; Turecki, G.; Wagner, J.; von Känel, R. DNA methylation signatures of functional somatic syndromes: Systematic review. *Psychosom. Med.* **2023**, *85*, 672–681. [CrossRef]
43. Fernández-de-las-Peñas, C.; de-la-Llave-Rincón, A.I.; Ortega-Santiago, R.; Ambite-Quesada, S.; Gómez-Mayordomo, V.; Cuadrado, M.L.; Arias-Navalón, J.A.; Hernández-Barrera, V.; Martín-Guerrero, J.D.; Pellicer-Valero, O.J.; et al. Prevalence and risk factors of musculoskeletal pain symptoms as long-term post-COVID sequelae in hospitalized COVID-19 survivors: A multicenter study. *Pain* **2022**, *163*, e989–e996. [CrossRef]
44. Bergmans, R.S.; Clauw, D.J.; Flint, C.; Harris, H.; Lederman, S.; Schrepf, A. Chronic overlapping pain conditions increase the risk of long COVID features, regardless of acute COVID status. *Pain* **2024**, *165*, 1112–1120. [CrossRef]
45. Luo, D.; Mei, B.; Wang, P.; Li, X.; Chen, X.; Wei, G.; Kuang, F.; Li, B.; Su, S. Prevalence and risk factors for persistent symptoms after COVID-19: A systematic review and meta-analysis. *Clin. Microbiol. Infect.* **2024**, *30*, 328–335. [CrossRef]
46. Tsampasian, V.; Elghazaly, H.; Chattopadhyay, R.; Debski, M.; Naing, T.K.P.; Garg, P.; Clark, A.; Ntatsaki, E.; Vassiliou, V.S. Risk factors associated with post-COVID-19 condition: A systematic review and meta-analysis. *JAMA Intern. Med.* **2023**, *183*, 566–580. [CrossRef]
47. Melchior, M.; Poisbeau, P.; Gaumond, I.; Marchand, S. Insights into the mechanisms and the emergence of sex-differences in pain. *Neuroscience* **2016**, *338*, 63–80. [CrossRef]
48. Mills, S.E.E.; Nicolson, K.P.; Smith, B.H. Chronic pain: A review of its epidemiology and associated factors in population-based studies. *Br. J. Anaesth.* **2019**, *123*, e273–e283. [CrossRef]
49. Taslem Mourosi, J.; Anwar, S.; Hosen, M.J. The sex and gender dimensions of COVID-19: A narrative review of the potential underlying factors. *Infect. Genet. Evol.* **2022**, *103*, 105338. [CrossRef]
50. Bwire, G.M. Coronavirus: Why men are more vulnerable to COVID-19 than women? *SN Compr. Clin. Med.* **2020**, *2*, 874–876. [CrossRef]

Disclaimer/Publisher's Note: The statements, opinions and data contained in all publications are solely those of the individual author(s) and contributor(s) and not of MDPI and/or the editor(s). MDPI and/or the editor(s) disclaim responsibility for any injury to people or property resulting from any ideas, methods, instructions or products referred to in the content.

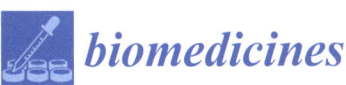

Review

Uncovering the Contrasts and Connections in PASC: Viral Load and Cytokine Signatures in Acute COVID-19 versus Post-Acute Sequelae of SARS-CoV-2 (PASC)

Brandon Compeer [1,2], Tobias R. Neijzen [3], Steven F. L. van Lelyveld [4], Byron E. E. Martina [1], Colin A. Russell [2] and Marco Goeijenbier [2,5,*]

1. Artemis Bioservices B.V., 2629 JD Delft, The Netherlands; b.compeer@artemisbioservices.com (B.C.); b.martina@artemisbioservices.com (B.E.E.M.)
2. Department of Medical Microbiology, University Medical Center Amsterdam (UMC, Amsterdam), 1105 AZ Amsterdam, The Netherlands; c.a.russell@amsterdamumc.nl
3. Department of Intensive Care Medicine, Spaarne Gasthuis, 2035 RC Haarlem, The Netherlands; t.r.neijzen@student.vu.nl
4. Department of Internal Medicine, Spaarne Gasthuis, 2035 RC Haarlem, The Netherlands; s.van.lelyveld@spaarnegasthuis.nl
5. Department of Intensive Care, Erasmus MC University Medical Centre, 3015 GD Rotterdam, The Netherlands
* Correspondence: m.goeijenbier@erasmusmc.nl

Citation: Compeer, B.; Neijzen, T.R.; van Lelyveld, S.F.L.; Martina, B.E.E.; Russell, C.A.; Goeijenbier, M. Uncovering the Contrasts and Connections in PASC: Viral Load and Cytokine Signatures in Acute COVID-19 versus Post-Acute Sequelae of SARS-CoV-2 (PASC). *Biomedicines* **2024**, *12*, 1941. https://doi.org/10.3390/biomedicines12091941

Academic Editor: César Fernández-de-las-Peñas

Received: 9 July 2024
Revised: 13 August 2024
Accepted: 20 August 2024
Published: 23 August 2024

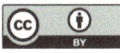

Copyright: © 2024 by the authors. Licensee MDPI, Basel, Switzerland. This article is an open access article distributed under the terms and conditions of the Creative Commons Attribution (CC BY) license (https://creativecommons.org/licenses/by/4.0/).

Abstract: The recent global COVID-19 pandemic has had a profound and enduring impact, resulting in substantial loss of life. The scientific community has responded unprecedentedly by investigating various aspects of the crisis, particularly focusing on the acute phase of COVID-19. The roles of the viral load, cytokines, and chemokines during the acute phase and in the context of patients who experienced enduring symptoms upon infection, so called Post-Acute Sequelae of COVID-19 or PASC, have been studied extensively. Here, in this review, we offer a virologist's perspective on PASC, highlighting the dynamics of SARS-CoV-2 viral loads, cytokines, and chemokines in different organs of patients across the full clinical spectrum of acute-phase disease. We underline that the probability of severe or critical disease progression correlates with increased viral load levels detected in the upper respiratory tract (URT), lower respiratory tract (LRT), and plasma. Acute-phase viremia is a clear, although not unambiguous, predictor of PASC development. Moreover, both the quantity and diversity of functions of cytokines and chemokines increase with acute-phase disease severity. Specific cytokines remain or become elevated in the PASC phase, although the driving factor of ongoing inflammation found in patients with PASC remains to be investigated. The key findings highlighted in this review contribute to a further understanding of PASC and their differences and overlap with acute disease.

Keywords: SARS-CoV-2; COVID-19; PASC; long COVID; cytokines; viral load; upper respiratory tract; lower respiratory tract; plasma

1. Introduction

The COVID-19 pandemic profoundly altered everyday life for an extended duration while claiming the lives of millions [1]. The spectrum of COVID-19 disease ranges from mild subclinical upper respiratory tract (URT) symptoms to acute respiratory distress syndrome (ARDS), with a high mortality. Although most infected individuals undergo a mild acute phase of illness and another large group recovers from more severe disease [2], numerous people have reported persistent symptoms following SARS-CoV-2 infection [3]. Those with Long COVID or Post-Acute Sequelae of COVID-19 (PASC) show pathological damage across diverse organs, including the nervous and immune system, blood vessels, and lungs. This damage manifests in a variety of long-lasting symptoms, most commonly including fatigue, respiratory issues, and neurological problems [3,4]. In an effort to characterize this multisystem disease, recent research has focused on phenotyping according to PASC symptom clustering, which may facilitate linking PASC phenotypes and their underlying mechanisms [5,6]. It should be noted that various terms within COVID-19- and PASC-related research are used, often with varying definitions. Therefore, the key terms used in this review are summarized in an explanatory box (Table 1) providing their definitions as used here. Several studies have investigated the viral load and release of cytokines and chemokines as key factors influencing COVID-19 disease progression and overall outcome. Nasopharyngeal samples of patients with severe disease often display high viral loads [7,8]. Furthermore, the plasma inflammatory markers interleukin (IL-) 6 [9], IL-10, and IL-2 [10] are increased in patients with severe acute phase disease. In the fight against the pandemic, both factors were predominantly studied considering short-term outcomes, including 30-day mortality and Intensive Care Unit (ICU) admission. There remains, however, a scarcity of reviews examining the correlation between viral loads in different organs and the release of cytokines and chemokines among various clinical subsets of COVID-19 disease. Although progress has been made regarding viral and immune dynamics during the acute phase of COVID-19, a clear virological perspective on the link between the cytokine profiles and viral load that dominate acute-phase outcome and subsequent PASC development remains missing. This challenge partly results from the need for long-term studies with extensive follow-up times. Moreover, the diverse symptoms [4] and recently emerging evidence of different PASC phenotypes [11,12] add to the complexity, as the inclusion of a significant number of persons with a diverse range of PASC symptoms is required. In addition, as Greenhalgh et al. [13] have clearly outlined, clinical phenotyping studies have utilized various methods on different samples, therefore leading to different PASC phenotype clusters [4,11–13]. Therefore, here, we review the current body of knowledge on the viral load and cytokine and chemokine release during the acute phase in COVID-19 patients. In addition, we summarize studies that have aimed to establish whether there is a correlation between viral load and increased release of cytokines and chemokines. Determining the existence of such correlations is important, as dysregulated immunity frequently leads to pathophysiological damage. Hence, particularly in hospitalized cases, anticipating heightened cytokine and chemokine release in patients with elevated viral load could be beneficial. Prophylactic medications that inhibit this release may mitigate pathophysiological damage. Finally, this review aims to explore the disparities and associations within cytokine and chemokine profiles among patients during acute disease and those experiencing PASC. This exploration may provide valuable predictive insights into PASC development.

Table 1. Explanatory box with commonly used terms and their corresponding definitions as used here in this review.

Term	Description
PASC or Long COVID	WHO definition of PASC is adopted for this review. This defines PASC as the continuation or development of new symptoms 3 months after the initial SARS-CoV-2 infection, with these symptoms lasting for at least 2 months with no other explanation.
Acute phases spectrum	The phases, asymptomatic, mild, moderate, severe and critical are most often used. However, in this review, the spectrum includes asymptomatic, mild/moderate and severe phase. Rationale for this deviation is that is the review focuses on the differences and progression from non-severe phases (asymptomatic, mild/moderate) to the severe phases.
Asymptomatic	Individuals positive for COVID-19 in absence of infection related symptoms.
Mild/Moderate	Individuals who display mild symptoms including fever, muscle pain and anosmia and moderate symptoms including tachypnea and mild pneumonia without the need for hospitalization.
Severe	Hospitalized patients with clinical signs of pneumonia, severe tachypnea, severe dyspnea and critical symptoms including respiratory and organ failure and coma.

Table 1. *Cont.*

Term	Description
Cytokine storm	State of deregulated immune system, characterized by an excessive production and release of cytokines and chemokines. Release may cause damage to various tissues including lung. Cytokine storm may subsequently trigger acute respiratory stress syndrome leading to organ failure or even death.
Viral load	Commonly quantitatively expressed as concentration in viral copies/mL in plasma. Here, viral load magnitude is defined by the copy number or Ct value determined via (RT-q)PCR. This definition is widely used in the papers cited in this review and is therefore adopted here.
Viremia	Classically defined as the presence of (non-) infectious whole virus or immune neutralized whole virus in serum. Publications referred to here do not use viral culture or staining to determine presence of virus in serum. In turn, the majority uses (RT-q)PCR and adopt the Ct value or quantified copy number as a benchmark for viremia. Therefore, in case the review refers to viremia or viral load, remember that these are Ct values representing RNA copy numbers.
Ct value	Cycle threshold (Ct) value in PCR is the number of cycles needed to indicate that a sample contains the target RNA or DNA. The Ct value negatively correlates with the initial amount of target RNA or DNA, i.e., in this review a low Ct value indicates a high viral load.
Persistent infection	Prolonged presence of SARS-CoV-2 (non-)infectious virus or RNA remnants that is detected for an extended period beyond acute infection. Persistence could be associated with display of symptoms or in absence of symptoms.
URT & LRT	Upper respiratory tract (URT) that includes nasal cavity, pharynx and larynx. Lower respiratory tract (LRT) that includes trachea and lungs.
RNA Load	Copy number of SARS-CoV-2 RNA, detected by (RT-q)PCR on samples from various origin including serum, BAL, nasopharyngeal swabs.
Inoculum	The virus quantity or concentration introduced at the time of host infection.

2. Materials and Methods

We conducted a narrative examination of the current body of literature. The search engines PubMed and Google Scholar were searched for the following keywords, which were additionally combined as ad hoc strings for advanced search: COVID-19; SARS-CoV-2; viral load; disease severity; viremia; cytokines; chemokines; URT; upper respiratory tract; LRT; lower respiratory tract; BAL; serum; plasma; PASC; long COVID. First, relevant research and review articles were selected based on the title and abstract. Next, inclusion for the review was decided based on a thorough analysis of the content.

3. Viral Loads

3.1. Viral Loads during Acute COVID-19

Various studies have shown that the viral loads in the URT are unrelated to clinical presentation [14,15], while others have proposed a correlation [16]. Although distinct factors may explain this contradiction, including timing of sampling (e.g., pre or post symptom onset), differences in population heterogeneity, and outcome assessment, the connection between viral loads in the URT and disease severity is still a subject of debate. On the contrary, high URT viral loads in hospitalized, clinically severe patients were significantly correlated with higher risks of intubation, critical progression, and in-hospital mortality (Figure 1) [14,17–19]. Cytokine storms (Table 1) are more often observed in patients that display critical progression and, in some cases, mortality [20,21]. Given that cytokine storms are characterized by a dysregulation of both the pro- and anti-inflammatory immune response, this dysregulation may lead to loss of control on viral replication. Hence, we hypothesize that, in severe and critical cases, tipping points may be reached where the predisposition or occurrence of a cytokine storm triggers increased viral replication, consequently leading to higher URT viral loads.

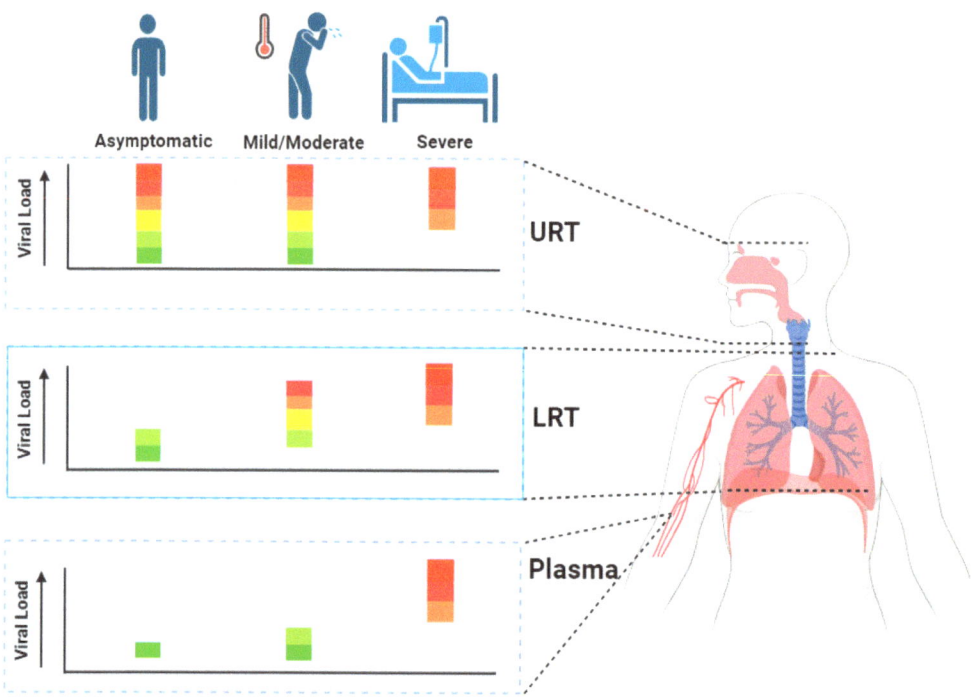

Figure 1. Graphical representation of viral loads observed across clinical classifications of acute-phase COVID-19 disease. Colored bar graphs illustrate viral load levels, ranging from red (high viral load) to green (low viral load). Viral load levels (low-high) are interpretated according to the perspectives of the authors referenced in cited articles. Graphical representation is based on the following references: [14,17–19,22–26]. Figure created using https://www.biorender.com/ (accessed on 12 March 2024).

While mild COVID-19 disease is usually confined to the URT, severe disease often manifests when viral infection reaches the lower respiratory tract (LRT) [27]. Therefore, a correlation between high LRT viral loads and disease progression is anticipated. This has been shown by Ynga-Durand et al., who found that the viral load in bronchoalveolar lavage (BAL) samples obtained from the LRT of severely ill patients admitted to the ICU were linked to fatal outcomes [22]. Furthermore, a retrospective study that analysed sputum obtained from hospital admitted mild-to-moderate ($n = 62$) or severe ($n = 30$) patients found that those with severe disease at baseline displayed higher viral loads in sputum as compared to mild-to-moderate individuals. In addition, the probability of progression to severe disease was positively associated with sputum viral loads at baseline [28]. As noted in the explanatory box (Table 1), the majority of the publications cited here utilized quantitative reverse transcription polymerase chain reaction (RT-qPCR) and adopted the Ct value or quantified copy number as a benchmark for viral load. However, given that RT-qPCR cannot differentiate infectious from non-infectious SARS-CoV-2, no reliable conclusions can be drawn regarding an individual's infectious status.

SARS-CoV-2's main replication sites include ciliated cells of the URT [29] and pneumocytes and macrophages of the LRT [30]. However, leakage of SARS-CoV-2 virus from (damaged) alveolar cells at the LRT to the blood circulation or direct infection of endothelial cells lining the blood circulation are hypothesized to drive SARS-CoV-2 viremia, subsequently leading to systemic spread [31,32]. Given the correlation between LRT viral load and disease severity, it is biologically plausible that a comparable correlation exists in plasma. This relation has been confirmed by studies that have demonstrated the plasma viral load of hospitalized severe patients to correlate with 90-day all-cause mortality [23] or to be linked to an increased likelihood of mortality [24]. It is important to note that most studies cited in this section examined viral loads in patients infected at the time the SARS-CoV-2 wild-type strain (Wuhan-Hu-1) was dominant. Exceptions include studies conducted from March 2020 to April 2021, during which both the Wuhan-Hu-1 and Alpha variants were prevalent [19,22], and one study from March 2020 to January 2022 [24], including various variants. Different variants, such as Omicron, which has reduced LRT replication competence compared to the Wuhan-Hu-1 and Delta strains [33], exhibit distinct viral dynamics. These dynamics may also be influenced by the individual's vaccination status [34,35]. Thus, the provided overview should be interpreted with caution in the context of current variants.

It is interesting to note that viremia is not limited to severe or critically ill patients, as asymptomatic [25] and moderate patients [26] also display viremia, although typically with lower than average loads (Figure 1). We hypothesize that individuals who exhibit viremia but undergo mild illness experience a delayed robust initial immune response, and over time, their immune systems may effectively reduce viral replication and thereby prevent disease progression.

To summarize, hospitalized patients with increased URT, LRT, and plasma viral load show more severe disease and increased mortality [14,17–19,22–26]. It should, however, be noted that most research on SARS-CoV-2 viral loads in the LRT and plasma and, to a lesser extent, the URT, primarily focuses on hospitalized or ICU patients. This group often reflects severe clinical cases. Furthermore, non-hospitalized individuals experiencing mild symptoms during the acute phase are also at risk of developing PASC [3]. Therefore, it is intriguing to map the viral load in the LRT and plasma of asymptomatic and moderate patients, as data from such longitudinal studies could shed light on its potential as an early prognostic indicator for severe COVID-19 and PASC development. The next section will elaborate on research that investigated differences and overlap between the viral loads observed during acute and PASC disease.

3.2. Relation between Acute-Phase Viral Dynamics and PASC Phase

While most SARS-CoV-2 positive individuals typically exhibit a detectable viral load for a brief period, initial case report studies during the pandemic showed persistence of viral RNA and infectious SARS-CoV-2 in patients who experienced prolonged symptoms. For instance, nasopharyngeal swabs from a non-hospitalized person experiencing mild acute infection remained positive, even after 110 days following the initial test. Considering the infection period from June to December 2020, we assume that she was infected with the Wuhan-Hu-1 strain. During this period, she experienced cardiovascular, respiratory, and musculoskeletal PASC-related symptoms [36]. Furthermore, SARS-CoV-2 RNA was detected in the cerebrospinal fluid 114 days after the initial positive nasopharyngeal swabs (first positive test: October 2020) in an individual experiencing prolonged central nervous system (CNS)-related symptoms [37]. Given the initial positive test in October 2020, she most likely contracted the Wuhan-Hu-1 strain, though reinfection with the Alpha variant is possible since it appeared in early 2021 in Czech Republic [38]. A similar trend was revealed in a cohort study, which showed that plasma from a significant portion of vaccinated PASC patients (60%) with ≥ three co-morbidities and who experienced mild/moderate acute COVID-19 remained positive for SARS-CoV-2 RNA over a median follow-up period of 2 years, in contrast to their matched controls (8%) [39]. Moreover, plasma of PASC patients were more frequently found to test positive and displayed higher average viral loads as compared to previously infected persons without PASC [40]. These and other case or cohort studies have addressed the need for longitudinal studies that monitor viral loads over an extended period.

Symptoms of PASC, characterized by memory-related issues, were associated with early SARS-CoV-2 plasma viral load levels in patients with mild-to-critical acute COVID-19 (Table 2) [41]. However, this association was not observed for other PASC subtypes, including anosmia and fatigue. A longitudinal study monitoring hospitalized, severely/critically diseased patients showed that persons with viremia at time of hospital admission were more likely to experience PASC symptoms at 6 months (± 2 months) as compared to hospital-admitted patients without viremia (Table 2) [42]. Similar observations were made by Ram-Mohan et al., who noted that patients who exhibited viremia at baseline were more likely to develop PASC-related symptoms, particularly among those with moderate disease [43]. Furthermore, it was found that a low Ct value in URT swabs, e.g., high viral load (Table 1), was associated with a greater number of PASC-related symptoms (Table 2) [44].

Table 2. Summary of cohort studies on relation between acute-phase viral loads and subsequent PASC development.

Study Population Characteristics	Acute-Phase Viral Load Correlation or Association with PASC Phase	Ref.
Hospitalized (n = 47) Vaccinated Strain variant unknown	Plasma of PASC patients tested positive more frequently (55% vs. 29%) and had higher average viral loads compared to previously infected persons without PASC. In PASC-positive patients, plasma viral load remained unchanged or increased, while in PASC-negative individuals, it decreased or became undetectable over time.	[40]
Mix of mild-to-critical patients. Exact numbers unknown. Unvaccinated * Wuhan-Hu-1 strain	Detectable plasma viral load was associated with memory-related issues, whereas there were no associations with anosmia or fatigue.	[41]
Hospitalized (n = 129) Severe/Critical (≥90% pneumonia)	Viremia at time of hospitalization resulted in a higher chance of PASC symptom development as compared to hospital-admitted patients without viremia.	[42]
Mild/moderate (n = 119) Severe/Critical (n = 8) Unvaccinated * Wuhan-Hu-1 strain **	Patients with detectable plasma viral load at enrollment were more likely to report PASC symptoms one month after confirmed infection as compared to individuals without detectable plasma viral loads (83% vs. 41%).	[43]
Mild/moderate (n = 70) Severe/Critical (n = 6) Vaccination status *** Strain variant unknown	Viral URT loads correlated with an increased number of experienced PASC symptoms.	[44]

* Unvaccinated given that the data of the study were published before the world initiated COVID-19 vaccination campaigns (14 December 2020). ** Given the recruitment period of March 2020–December 2020, we assume that individuals were infected with Wuhan-Hu-1. *** Article did not disclose vaccination status of enrolled individuals. Patient enrollment overlapped with ongoing vaccination campaigns.

What could be the biological rationale behind the increased likelihood of individuals who experienced viremia during the acute phase to develop PASC symptoms? We hypothesize that viremia, potentially leading to systemic dissemination, might result in the infection of multiple organs distant from the initial site of infection, leading to pathophysiological damage and subsequent manifestation of PASC symptoms. However, it is imperative to underscore that the presence of viremia and its subsequent inflammatory response often correlate with severe clinical presentations of acute infection, and the risk of developing PASC is higher among severe cases [45]. Therefore, we also suggest that disease severity may introduce a confounding factor in this context.

Although it was shown that RNA persists in various parts of the bodies of PASC patients [36,37,46], the detection of persistent RNA is generally assessed by PCR (Table 1). Therefore, it remains inconclusive whether the detected persistent RNA originates from RNA remnants or infectious virus. However, considering that RNA is degraded relatively quickly in the human body [47], it is unlikely that the detected RNA concerns remnants of infectious virus originating from the acute phase. Hence, several alternative theories have been proposed to explain RNA persistency, including reverse-transcribed parts of SARS-CoV-2 RNA that are integrated into the host genome, although additional studies are needed to elucidate this theory [40,48]. Moreover, the presence of infectious virus in immune-privileged sites, including the CNS, a mechanism used by other RNA viruses, e.g., Ebola virus and poliovirus [49], may also provide a plausible reason for RNA persistence in PASC patients.

Reports on viral loads in PASC patients primarily focus on plasma samples and, to our best knowledge, limited data are available regarding the relationship between URT and LRT viral loads during acute disease and PASC development. Considering that a notable proportion of PASC patients merely experienced mild acute infection [3], it is interesting to further study viral loads in different body compartments, e.g., LRT and URT, in patients who have experienced mild acute COVID-19. Moreover, not all PASC individuals exhibit sustained viral loads, and thus, viremia is not likely to constitute an unambiguous predictor for PASC development. Yet, the summarized findings indicate that a significant portion of PASC persons remains with detectable viral loads, which could be the direct cause or related to sustained inflammation that is often observed in PASC patients, which will be elaborated on elsewhere in this review. Nevertheless, it remains interesting to speculate about the correlation between viral load and the likelihood of experiencing persistent infection. For instance, it is conceivable that a brief period of high viral load, perhaps just hours, could enable the virus to penetrate various organs and consequently establish persistency. Conversely, it is plausible that persistence merely occurs when an individual maintains a high viral load over an extended period, such as weeks.

4. Cytokines and Chemokines

4.1. Cytokines and Chemokines during Acute COVID-19

Disease severity progression is not solely dictated by viral loads, but is, rather, influenced by the host's response to these viral loads [50]. This complex interplay, referred to as host–pathogen interaction, involves numerous processes, including secretion of cytokines and chemokines initiating a comprehensive immune response, facilitating viral eradication. Given the vast number of cytokines and chemokines that are released during SARS-CoV-2 infection, a particular subset was chosen (Figure 2). This selection was not exclusively because of its frequent mentioning in the literature, but also because the individual cytokines and chemokines play distinct roles in the immune response. For example, IL-17 functions as an inflammation mediator frequently observed in autoimmunity [51], whereas IL-6 is a pleotropic cytokine reported to play a crucial role in viral infections [52]. Furthermore, IL-10 is recognized for its protection from immune-mediated damage [53], whereas TNF-α is involved in initiating tissue necrosis or apoptosis and promoting lung fibrosis [54]. Considering PASC, where lung fibrosis is frequently mentioned [55], highlighting a range of functionally divergent cytokines is important. Lastly, interferon-α and -γ (IFN-α and IFN-γ) were included given their multifunctional role in the frontline defense against viral infections [56].

Reports have shown elevated release of both pro- and anti-inflammatory cytokines in the nasopharynx of patients with varied clinical classifications of COVID-19 disease [57–59]. While there is a scarcity of studies examining asymptomatic patients, Xie et al. concluded that the URT of unvaccinated, asymptomatic patients infected with Wuhan-Hu-1 is characterized by elevated levels of pro-inflammatory IL-2 and IL-6 and decreased levels of anti-inflammatory protein IL-10 [60]. For patients with moderate and severe COVID-19, a higher variety of pro- and anti-inflammatory cytokines and chemokines in the URT was reported to be elevated as compared to their healthy controls (Figure 2). However, this may be biased due to the existence of more reports that have investigated the immune environment of the URT in symptomatic patients as compared to asymptomatic patients. Nevertheless, the overall trend is that increased release of cyto- and chemokines in the URT has been measured in all COVID-19 disease types, and therefore, it appears to be independent of the COVID-19 disease status.

Given that disease severity increases when viral infection extends to the LRT, it is intriguing to investigate whether the cyto- and chemokine profile at this anatomical site is more common in severe COVID-19 cases or independent of the disease status. In patients with moderate COVID-19 disease, only IL-10 levels were found to be increased in the LRT as compared to healthy controls whereas levels of IL-6, IL-1β and TNF-α remained unchanged [59]. In contrast, both the variability in function and the number of upregulated cyto- and chemokines increased with disease severity (Figure 2). This indicates a broader inflammatory state in the LRT of patients with severe disease. Here, results regarding cytokines and chemokines within the LRT of patients with SARS-CoV-2 infection are mainly based on articles that investigated mild/moderate or severe patients predominantly infected with Wuhan-Hu-1 or Alpha variants [59,61–63]. However, as previously mentioned, LRT replication of SARS-CoV-2 seems to vary by variant [33]. Future studies should thus explore whether the cytokine signature in the LRT of patients infected with various variants, including Delta and Omicron, displays similar or distinct patterns.

In the context of viral infections, elevated cyto- and chemokines in plasma indicate severe disease. This has been observed for severe cases of viral respiratory diseases, including MERS, SARS, and highly pathogenic Influenza H7N9 [64–66]. COVID-19 disease does not deviate from this pattern, as elevated plasma cyto- and chemokine levels were more often detected in patients with severe COVID-19 disease (Figure 2). Interestingly, elevated levels of IL-1α, IL-1β, and CCL-2 were observed in the plasma of severe COVID-19 patients [61]. However, in the same patients, BAL analysis revealed that, in addition to the aforementioned cytokines, IL-6 and TNF-α were also significantly higher in severe patients as compared to healthy controls. This illustrates that, in the LRT, an even higher variety of elevated inflammatory mediators is present as compared to plasma. We postulate that this may be attributed to the intricate LRT immune environment, which could lead to a wider array of cytokines and chemokines in response to viral infection compared to those found in plasma, primarily reflecting release from other parts of the body. As enhancers of the early antiviral response, levels of IFN-α and IFN-γ were found to be elevated at both the URT and LRT and in the plasma of patients across various clinical scores (Figure 2). In fact, research has demonstrated the importance of exhibiting a robust early IFN-γ response, as it has been found that low plasma levels of IFN-γ at symptom onset serve as a predictive marker for severe disease, especially when adjusting for factors such as vaccination and comorbidities [67]. Moreover, unvaccinated, fatal COVID-19 cases were characterized by a weak early IFN-γ response in the URT [58]. Thus, in the clinical context, it is of importance to collect samples at the onset of symptoms if IFN-γ is to be used as a biomarker for predicting disease progression and potentially guiding clinical interventions with IFN modulators.

Furthermore, reduced inflammatory levels, including IFN-α and IFN-γ, were found in the plasma of vaccinated as compared with unvaccinated symptomatic individuals [68]. Thus, these results suggest that vaccination may contribute to preventing the excessive inflammatory response often seen in patients with severe disease [20,68].

In conclusion, although the cytokine and chemokine response within the URT appears to be independent of clinical presentation, its release in distant areas from the initial infection site, e.g., LRT and plasma, is associated with disease severity. Determining whether this association aligns with the viral load in these regions may clarify the factors influencing disease progression.

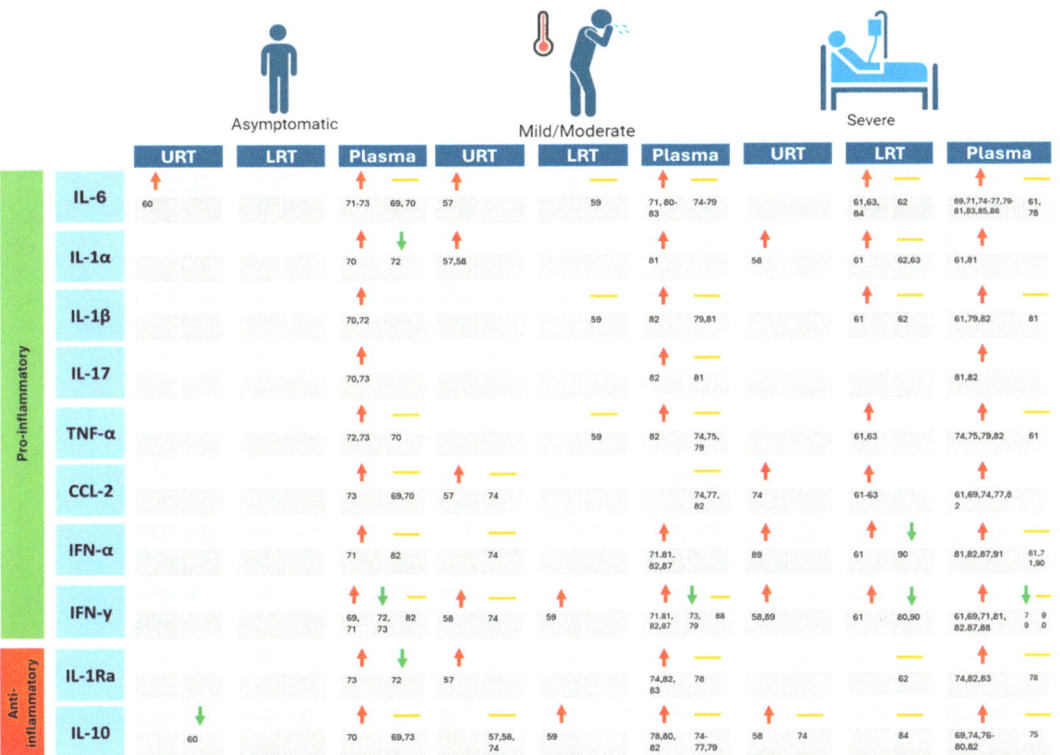

Figure 2. Overview of significant differences in levels of cytokines and chemokines in SARS-CoV-2-positive patients with various clinical acute-phase classifications as compared to healthy, non-infected controls. Red arrow (↑) indicates a significant increase in cytokine or chemokine levels as compared with healthy controls. Orange middle line (—) indicates no significant difference in cytokine or chemokine levels as compared with healthy controls. Green arrow (↓) indicates a significant decrease in cytokine or chemokine levels as compared with healthy controls. Empty tables implicate that no literature regarding this cytokine or chemokine in the context of the clinical classification and sample location could be found. References used include [57–63,69–91], and specific references are found in the corresponding part of the figure.

4.2. Relationship between Viral Load and Cyto- and Chemokine Markers across COVID-19 Disease Subsets

Pathophysiological consequences of viral infections are not solely due to viral replication, but additionally arise from an often dysregulated immune response. Therefore, considering predicting clinical progression, this section elaborates on the question of whether correlations between viral load and release of cyto- and chemokines exist and how these may vary across clinical spectra of acute-phase disease.

Study results on non-vaccinated Wuhan-Hu-1-infected individuals demonstrated a positive correlation between URT viral loads and plasma cytokines IL-6 and IL-10, but not with TNF-α and INF-γ (Table 3) [76]. Furthermore, research showed that in unvaccinated, Wuhan-Hu-1-infected individuals, only plasma CCL-2 levels significantly correlated with URT viral load, whereas such a correlation was absent for a large number of other cytokines and chemokines (Table 3) [77]. In another study investigating a panel of cytokines and chemokines, including IL-6, IL-1α and IL-1β, IL-17, TNF-α, IL-1Ra, IL-10, and CCL-2, only plasma levels of CCL-2 correlated with plasma viral load in unvaccinated, symptomatic patients with confirmed Wuhan-Hu-1 SARS-CoV-2 infection (Table 3) [82]. Nevertheless, it is important to note that these studies did not include stratification based on disease severity.

Table 3. Correlations of SARS-CoV-2 viral loads with markers of inflammation.

Study Population Characteristics *	Viral Load Origin	Cytokine Origin	Correlation with ***	Ref.
Non-stratified ** Mild/Moderate ($n = 26$) Severe/critical ($n = 11$)	URT	Plasma	IL-6, IL-10	[76]
			TNF-α, INF-γ	
Non-stratified ** Asymptomatic ($n = 6$) Mild/Moderate ($n = 17$) Severe/critical ($n = 8$)	URT	Plasma	CCL-2	[77]
			IFN-α, IFN-γ, TNF-α, IL-1β, IL-2, IL-6, IL-7, IL-8, IL-10, IL-12p70, IL-13, IL-17A	
Non-stratified ** Asymptomatic ($n = 4$) Mild/Moderate ($n = 58$) Severe/critical ($n = 8$)	URT	Plasma	CCL-2, VEGF, G-CSF	[82]
			IL-1β, IL-1ra, IL-2, IL-2Rα, IL-6, IL-7, IL-8, IL-9, IL-10, IL-13, IL-15, IL-17, IL-18, IFN-α2, IFN-γ, TNF-α Whole list; see reference	
Hospitalized Severe/critical ($n = 88$)	Plasma	Plasma	IL-6, IL-8, IP10, CCL-2	[32]
			IFN-γ, IL-1RA	
	URT	Plasma	IL-6, IL-8, IP10, CCL-2, IFN-γ	
			IL-1RA	
	LRT	Plasma	IL-6	
			IL-8, IP10, CCL-2, IFN-γ, IL-1RA	
Non-stratified ** Mild/moderate ($n = 15$) Severe/critical ($n = 34$)	Plasma	Plasma	IL-6, CCL-2, CCL-19	[74]
			IFN-α2	
	URT	URT	IFN-γ, IL-33	
			IL-10	

* All patients included in the cited studies were unvaccinated. Given the recruitment period of March 2020–December 2020, we assume that they were infected with the Wuhan-Hu-1 strain. ** Non-stratified = Patients with various clinical classifications (asymptomatic, mild/moderate, severe/critical) were analyzed as a single group. *** Colored table indications: green = positive correlation; orange = no correlation; red = negative correlation.

Research that applied disease stratification has found the plasma, URT, and LRT viral loads of hospitalized, unvaccinated individuals to be correlated with various plasma cytokines, including IL-6, IL-8, and CCL-2 [32]. However, this association was not present for numerous other cytokines and or chemokines including IFN-γ and IL-1RA. Therefore, the authors emphasized that, although viral load could be a direct contributor to the elevated inflammatory markers at several sites in the body, the observed elevated inflammation could be multifactorial. Lastly, Smith et al. showed that, in patients with mild-to-moderate or severe-to-critical disease, the plasma viral load was positively associated with plasma-located TNF-α, IL-6, and anti-inflammatory proteins IL-10 and IL-1RA [74]. On the contrary, URT viral loads were negatively correlated with IFN-γ and IL-33 levels located in the URT (Table 3) [74].

Collectively, there are indications of correlations between viral load and cytokines in the URT, LRT, and plasma of patients with COVID-19. Nevertheless, the lack of stratification based on disease severity impedes the ability to forecast elevations of cytokines and/or chemokines based on viral load. Another limitation is that the data provided herein are based on studies that primarily included patients infected during periods when the Wuhan-Hu-1 strain was predominant.

4.3. Differences and Similarities in Cytokine Profiles in Acute and PASC

Given the diverse range of symptoms associated with PASC, various processes such mitochondrial energy production and latent virus reactivation may play a role in symptom manifestation [4]. Within these processes, cytokines and chemokines are consistently identified as important factors, and thus, investigating the cytokine and chemokine profiles of

PASC patients has become relevant. SchultheiSS et al. demonstrated significant elevations of TNF-α, IL-1β, and IL-6 in PASC patients as compared to previously infected persons without PASC [92]. Within this study, the majority of the individuals were vaccinated (>73%) and primarily experienced mild/moderate COVID-19. However, their results regarding cytokine elevations were not corrected for parameters such as vaccination status or SARS-CoV-2 variants [92]. Likewise, PASC individuals with unreported vaccination statuses demonstrated a 44% elevation in IL-6 levels compared to control subjects without PASC [93]. The majority (84%) of concerned PASC patients who were not hospitalized during acute COVID-19 infection and at least 42% of the included persons displayed at least one comorbidity. Moreover, the highest increase was observed in PASC patients characterized by cardiopulmonary complaints, which demonstrated the degree of IL-6 elevation to vary across PASC disease phenotypes. In another study, IL-6 levels in unvaccinated, Wuhan-Hu-1-infected PASC patients were not statistically different as compared to control subjects without PASC 8 months following initial infection [94]. This contradicting finding is of particular interest as the above studies consisted of PASC patients with comparable clinical conditions, namely, mild-to-moderate acute illness. This emphasizes the heterogeneity of the results regarding the (remained) elevation of specific cytokines in the PASC phase.

Findings from a longitudinal study indicated that PASC patients were characterized by significantly lower IFN responses during their acute period as compared to patients without enduring symptoms [95]. However, this IFN response persisted over time in PASC patients, whereas this was not observed in non-PASC patients. Significantly higher levels of IFN cytokines, specifically IFN-β, were found in PASC patients 8 months post-infection as compared to non-PASC patients [94]. Research conducted by Torres-Ruiz et al. highlighted significantly elevated baseline levels of IL-1α and IP-10, with a trend of higher levels of IL-6, IFN-γ, and IL-1β in patients who later developed PASC as compared to those who recovered from acute infection [96]. On the contrary, no differences were observed for IL-10, IL-13, IL-17, TNF-α, and IL-1RA (Figure 3). This is of particular interest, as we highlighted in the previous section that these cytokines and chemokines were upregulated in the plasma of moderate and severe COVID-19 patients. Therefore, this points out that only several cytokines and chemokines remained or became elevated during the weeks or months after COVID-19 infection in patients who later developed PASC.

Besides pro-inflammatory cytokines, data are available on the levels of anti-inflammatory cytokines in vaccinated PASC patients. For instance, at the metabolite level, patients displayed elevated concentrations of anti-inflammatory metabolites, although anti-inflammatory cytokines and chemokines were not investigated at the protein level during this study [97]. Another study demonstrated that the anti-inflammatory cytokine IL-10 remained elevated in unvaccinated patients suffering from severe PASC as compared to previously infected unvaccinated persons without PASC [98]. Nevertheless, these elevated levels only lasted for 2 months, followed by a smaller difference in IL-10 levels between severe PASC and non-PASC patients, indicating that IL-10 levels return to baseline over time. On the contrary, others reported lower levels of IL-10 and IL-4 in unvaccinated PASC patients as compared to unvaccinated non-PASC individuals, which suggested better control of the inflammatory process [99].

We do realize, however, that the summarized studies show conflicting results regarding the cytokine and chemokine signature in PASC patients. Such discrepancies may be attributed to confounding factors, such as differences in PASC disease phenotype, SARS-CoV-2 variants, vaccination status, comorbidities, and sex. These confounding factors are often not mentioned in all cited articles and are more likely to affect outcomes in studies with relatively small, homogenous populations than in those with larger, more diverse groups. Therefore, additional cohort studies comprising heterogenous study populations that take these confounding factors into account could give more insight into the cytokine and chemokine molecular signatures of persons who later developed PASC. However, the limited number of newly reported COVID-19 and, therefore, PASC cases impedes the set-up of such longitudinal studies. Therefore, retrospective studies using samples taken earlier may offer a solution to study the dynamics involved in PASC development.

Despite conflicting evidence, most current research points out that certain PASC patients show enduring immune activation characterized by sustained levels of pro- and anti-inflammatory cytokines and chemokines. Several cytokines that are elevated at the time of acute COVID-19 remain or become elevated during PASC. These include, but are not limited to, IL-6, IFN-γ, TNF-α, and IL-1β (Figure 3). There have been various hypotheses postulated regarding the underlying biological cause of persistent immune activation. These include viral persistency in reservoir cells, microclot formations, and re-activation of latent (herpes) viruses such as Epstein–Barr virus [100]. These hypotheses are not mutually exclusive and may vary across PASC phenotypes, or they may potentially serve as the underlying cause for the distinct described PASC phenotypes.

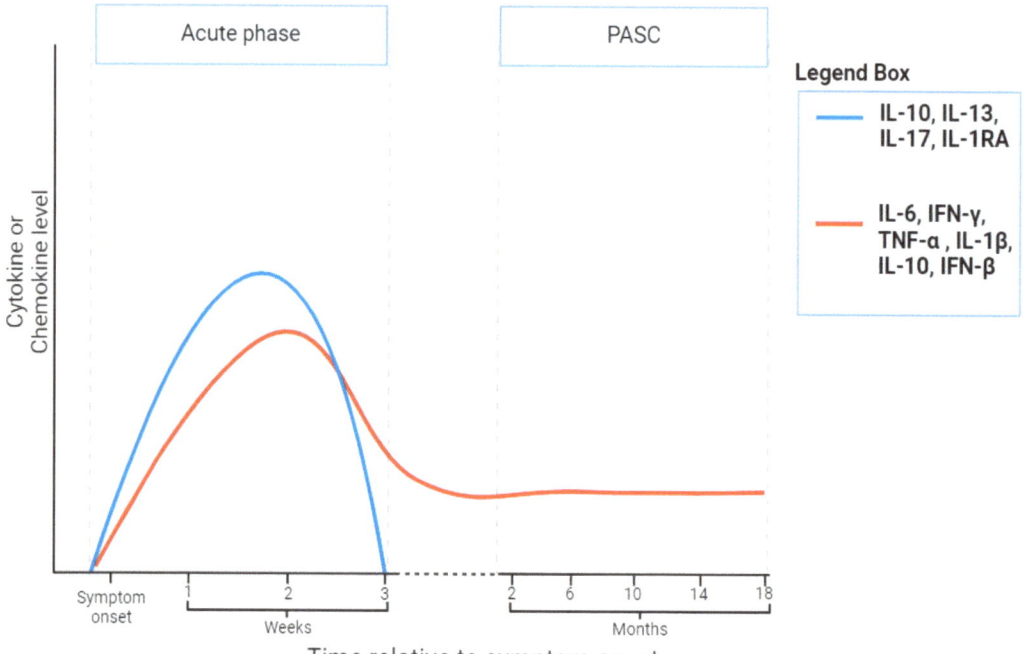

Figure 3. Graphical representation of cytokines and chemokines during acute phase of COVID-19 disease and subsequent PASC phase. Blue line indicates cytokines and chemokines for which literature evidence exists that levels increase during acute phase and diminish during PASC phase. On the contrary, red line indicates cytokines and chemokines that remain elevated during PASC phase. References: blue line: IL-10 [96,99]; IL-13 [96]; IL-17 [96]; IL-1RA [96]. References: red line: IL-6 [92,93,96]; IFN-γ [95,96]; TNF-α [92]; IL-1β [92,96]; IL-10 [98]; IFN-β [94,95]. Note that literature on IL-10 shows conflicting data. Figure created using https://www.biorender.com/ (accessed on 21 March 2024).

5. In Vitro Models and Preclinical Animal Models to Study Acute COVID-19 and PASC

Studying acute COVID-19 and PASC in humans enables researchers to explore the natural progression of infection; nevertheless, drawbacks exist. These include uncontrolled conditions, comorbidities, and resource-intensive procedures. Employing (preclinical) models, from in vitro co-culture systems to animal models, allows researchers to control factors and bypass most described drawbacks. For instance, studies using cultures of human peripheral blood mononuclear cells (PBMCs) from both healthy individuals and severe

COVID-19 patients were conducted to investigate the viral tropism of SARS-CoV-2 [101]. Moreover, in vitro co-culture systems were utilized to examine the initial interaction between immune cells and SARS-CoV-2-infected epithelial cells. This approach allowed researchers to study the underlying factors that might contribute to immune dysregulation in acute COVID-19 [102]. More complex 3D cell culture models, such as organoids and microfluidic devices, have been explored to mimic the viral and immune dynamics of SARS-CoV-2 and serve as a preliminary approach for drug evaluation [103,104]. This approach may have the potential to circumvent the commonly observed, relatively poor translatability of drug efficacy from animal testing to human treatment [105]. Moreover, the number of animal tests for preclinical studies could additionally be reduced by employing 3D cell culture techniques.

Early in the pandemic, several preclinical animal models were quickly mapped to mimic both the acute and PASC phase. Here, we provide a brief overall of the commonly used small animal models (Table 4). This selection is based on the relative ease of utilizing small animal models as compared to non-human primates, which, in addition, presents ethical limitations. Animal models have extensively been described in other review papers [106,107], and therefore, for further information, we recommend consulting those sources. From the overview (Table 4), it can be deducted that several animal models can be employed to answer a range of COVID-19-related questions. For instance, viral replication during asymptomatic infection could be studied using the ferret model [108]. Moreover, both transgenic mice and Syrian hamsters are suitable for studying the efficacy and safety of vaccines and therapeutic drugs. For instance, in Syrian hamsters, both Molnupiravir [109] and Nirmatrelvir [110] showed potent efficacy against various variants, including Omicron. In mice, a combination of Molnupiravir and Nirmatrelvir demonstrated significant inhibition of SARS-CoV-2 replication [111].

Common limitations exist in the currently available in vitro and preclinical models for COVID-19 related research. For instance, the primary health burden of COVID-19 predominantly originates from patients experiencing severe symptoms, often in the presence of comorbidities. Most animal models, however, only display mild disease, with limited reports investigating comorbidities and their effects on acute-phase disease. When it comes to PASC, similar trends apply. Although Syrian hamsters showed PASC-related behavioral changes [112], an animal model that adequately reflects human PASC symptoms remains absent. Moreover, susceptible animal models supporting a long duration of virus replication and competent models to study different hypotheses underlying the molecular mechanisms that drive PASC are still missing. Given that PASC is primarily characterized by behavioral impact, 3D cell culture methods may have limited added value in this area, and thus, animal models remain the preferred choice to study PASC. The various techniques available, from co-culture systems to animal models, should be employed to address the gaps and limitations inherent in each method. In addition, future developments in animal models and 3D cell culture methods may overcome the identified limitations, offering potential benefits for both preclinical studies and therapeutical approaches in the future.

Table 4. Common animal models and their findings in relation to acute COVID-19 and PASC.

Animal	Susceptibility	Severity	Acute Phase	PASC	Ref.
Transgenic Mice	• Upon hACE2 expression • Use of mouse adapted strains	• Mild • Severe	K18-hACE2 mice: • hACE2 overexpression results in systemic virus spread and mortality. • Display lethargy and edema-associated acute lung injury, similar to ARDS. • High titer infection results in upregulation of various cytokines in lung and brain at 7 dpi.	• Mouse-adapted strain induced neuropathological changes in BALB/c mice. May resemble cognitive dysfunction PASC symptom.	[113,114]
Syrian Hamsters	• Natural	• Mild • Severe	• Increases in various cytokines. • High viral loads of 2–8 dpi. Undetectable after ~10 days post infection (dpi). • Inoculum volume impacts severity. • Late and weak immune influx and prolonged weight loss in aged hamsters. • Diet-induced obese hamsters show sustained inflammation and may resemble humans with obese comorbidity.	• Sustained inflammation in olfactory tissue (31dpi); may resemble PASC-like behavior symptoms in humans. • Anosmia caused by olfactory epithelial damage.	[112,115–118]
Ferrets	• Natural	• Asymptomatic • Mild	• Intranasal challenge results in asymptomatic infection with URT virus replication. • Used for transmission studies. • Infection of primarily URT for 8 dpi post-infection with low mortality. • Viral shedding in nasal, saliva, urine, and fecal samples until 8 dpi. • Aged ferrets display higher viral loads, prolonged nasal virus shedding, and severe lung inflammatory cell infiltration. • Used for evaluation of vaccine and antivirals.	• Minimal reported resemblances with human PASC. • Indications for sustained pathological URT abnormalities potentially reflecting long-term impact of infection.	[107,108,118,119]

6. Concluding Remarks and Future Directions

The health, economic, and societal burden of PASC underscores the need to investigate the underlying mechanisms and factors that drive PASC development. Given that PASC is a multifactorial condition with diverse underlying mechanisms, comprehensive understanding and progress in addressing this complex disease necessitate collaborative efforts across various disciplines. Only through translational research integrating insights from clinical, biological, and epidemiological domains can meaningful advancements be made towards unraveling the complexities of PASC. Here, we merely deliver a virologist's perspective in light of available data on the differences in viral loads and cytokine and chemokine responses during the acute and PASC phases. We emphasize that the likelihood of experiencing severe or critical progression increased with viral load levels detected in the URT, LRT, and plasma of hospitalized patients. Acute-phase viremia is a well-characterized, but not unambiguous, predictor of PASC development. Viral RNA, either from infectious virus or remnants, persists in persons that experience PASC. Cytokine and chemokine levels vary significantly across acute-phase clinical conditions. Both the quantity and diversity of functions increase with disease severity. Comparing the acute phase and PASC phase showed that specific cytokines remain or become elevated in the PASC phase. This ongoing inflammation may be the driving factor behind enduring symptoms. The driving factor of ongoing inflammation, whether it be persistent infectious virus hiding in immune-privileged sites, remnants of non-infectious virus, re-activation of latent viruses, or a combination of the potential causes, currently remains unknown.

Author Contributions: Conceptualization, B.C., B.E.E.M. and M.G. Writing and original draft preparation, B.C. with support of T.R.N., M.G. and B.E.E.M. Review and editing, B.E.E.M., S.F.L.v.L., C.A.R. and M.G. Supervision, B.E.E.M., C.A.R. and M.G. All authors have read and agreed to the published version of the manuscript.

Funding: No funding for this manuscript.

Acknowledgments: Figures 1 and 3 were created with www.BioRender.com. The remaining figures and tables were created using Powerpoint.

Conflicts of Interest: Author Brandon Compeer and Byron E. E. Martina were employed by the company "Artemis Bioservices". The remaining authors declare that the re-search was conducted in the absence of any commercial or financial relationships that could be construed as a potential conflict of interest.

References

1. WHO. WHO COVID-19 Dashboard. Available online: https://data.who.int/dashboards/covid19/deaths?n=c (accessed on 5 March 2024).
2. Bulut, C.; Kato, Y. Epidemiology of COVID-19. *Turk. J. Med. Sci.* **2020**, *50*, 563–570. [CrossRef] [PubMed]
3. FAIR Health. *Patients Diagnosed with Post-COVID Conditions an Analysis of Private Healthcare Claims Using the Official ICD-10 Diagnostic Code*; FAIR Health: New York, NY, USA, 2022.
4. Davis, H.E.; McCorkell, L.; Vogel, J.M.; Topol, E.J. Long COVID: Major findings, mechanisms and recommendations. *Nat. Rev. Microbiol.* **2023**, *21*, 133–146. [CrossRef]
5. Liew, F.; Efstathiou, C.; Fontanella, S.; Richardson, M.; Saunders, R.; Swieboda, D.; Sidhu, J.K.; Ascough, S.; Moore, S.C.; Mohamed, N.; et al. Large-scale phenotyping of patients with long COVID post-hospitalization reveals mechanistic subtypes of disease. *Nat. Immunol.* **2024**, *25*, 607–621. [CrossRef] [PubMed]
6. Ozonoff, A.; Jayavelu, N.D.; Liu, S.; Melamed, E.; Milliren, C.E.; Qi, J.; Geng, L.N.; McComsey, G.A.; Cairns, C.B.; Baden, L.R.; et al. Features of acute COVID-19 associated with post-acute sequelae of SARS-CoV-2 phenotypes: Results from the IMPACC study. *Nat. Commun.* **2024**, *15*. [CrossRef] [PubMed]
7. Pujadas, E.; Chaudhry, F.; McBride, R.; Richter, F.; Zhao, S.; Wajnberg, A.; Nadkarni, G.; Glicksberg, B.S.; Houldsworth, J.; Cordon-Cardo, C. SARS-CoV-2 viral load predicts COVID-19 mortality. *Lancet Respir. Med.* **2020**, *8*, e70. [CrossRef]
8. Liu, Y.; Yan, L.-M.; Wan, L.; Xiang, T.-X.; Le, A.; Liu, J.-M.; Peiris, M.; Poon, L.L.M.; Zhang, W. Viral dynamics in mild and severe cases of COVID-19. *Lancet Infect. Dis.* **2020**, *20*, 656–657. [CrossRef]
9. Tjendra, Y.; Al Mana, A.F.; Espejo, A.P.; Akgun, Y.; Millan, N.C.; Gomez-Fernandez, C.; Cray, C. Predicting Disease Severity and Outcome in COVID-19 Patients: A Review of Multiple Biomarkers. *Arch. Pathol. Lab. Med.* **2020**, *144*, 1465–1474. [CrossRef]

10. Huang, C.; Wang, Y.; Li, X.; Ren, L.; Zhao, J.; Hu, Y.; Zhang, L.; Fan, G.; Xu, J.; Gu, X.; et al. Clinical features of patients infected with 2019 novel coronavirus in Wuhan, China. *Lancet* **2020**, *395*, 497–506. [CrossRef]
11. Deer, R.R.; Rock, M.A.; Vasilevsky, N.; Carmody, L.; Rando, H.; Anzalone, A.J.; Basson, M.D.; Bennett, T.D.; Bergquist, T.; Boudreau, E.A.; et al. Characterizing Long COVID: Deep Phenotype of a Complex Condition. *EBioMedicine* **2021**, *74*. [CrossRef]
12. Frontera, J.A.; Thorpe, L.E.; Simon, N.M.; de Havenon, A.; Yaghi, S.; Sabadia, S.B.; Yang, D.; Lewis, A.; Melmed, K.; Balcer, L.J.; et al. Post-acute sequelae of COVID-19 symptom phenotypes and therapeutic strategies: A prospective, observational study. *PLoS ONE* **2022**, *17*, e0275274. [CrossRef]
13. Greenhalgh, T.; Sivan, M.; Perlowski, A.; Nikolich, J. Long COVID: A clinical update. *Lancet* **2024**, *404*, 707–724. [CrossRef] [PubMed]
14. Mitsumura, T.; Okamoto, T.; Tosaka, M.; Yamana, T.; Shimada, S.; Iijima, Y.; Sakakibara, R.; Shibata, S.; Honda, T.; Shirai, T.; et al. Association of SARS-CoV-2 RNA Copy Number with the COVID-19 Mortality Rate and Its Effect on the Predictive Performance of Mortality in Severe Cases. *Jpn. J. Infect. Dis.* **2022**, *75*, 504–510. [CrossRef]
15. Hasanoglu, I.; Korukluoglu, G.; Asilturk, D.; Cosgun, Y.; Kalem, A.K.; Altas, A.B.; Kayaaslan, B.; Eser, F.; Kuzucu, E.A.; Guner, R. Higher viral loads in asymptomatic COVID-19 patients might be the invisible part of the iceberg. *Infection* **2021**, *49*, 117–126. [CrossRef]
16. Puchinger, K.; Castelletti, N.; Rubio-Acero, R.; Geldmacher, C.; Eser, T.M.; Deák, F.; Paunovic, I.; Bakuli, A.; Saathoff, E.; von Meyer, A.; et al. The interplay of viral loads, clinical presentation, and serological responses in SARS-CoV-2—Results from a prospective cohort of outpatient COVID-19 cases. *Virology* **2022**, *569*, 37–43. [CrossRef] [PubMed]
17. Magleby, R.; Westblade, L.F.; Trzebucki, A.; Simon, M.S.; Rajan, M.; Park, J.; Goyal, P.; Safford, M.M.; Satlin, M.J. Impact of Severe Acute Respiratory Syndrome Coronavirus 2 Viral Load on Risk of Intubation and Mortality among Hospitalized Patients with Coronavirus Disease 2019. *Clin. Infect. Dis.* **2021**, *73*, E4197–E4205. [CrossRef] [PubMed]
18. Boyapati, A.; Wipperman, M.F.; Ehmann, P.J.; Hamon, S.; Lederer, D.J.; Waldron, A.; Flanagan, J.J.; Karayusuf, E.; Bhore, R.; Nivens, M.C.; et al. Baseline Severe Acute Respiratory Syndrome Viral Load Is Associated with Coronavirus Disease 2019 Severity and Clinical Outcomes: Post Hoc Analyses of a Phase 2/3 Trial. *J. Infect. Dis.* **2021**, *224*, 1830–1838. [CrossRef]
19. Souverein, D.; van Stralen, K.; van Lelyveld, S.; van Gemeren, C.; Haverkort, M.; Snijders, D.; Soetekouw, R.; Kapteijns, E.; de Jong, E.; Hermanides, G.; et al. Initial Severe Acute Respiratory Syndrome Coronavirus 2 Viral Load Is Associated with Disease Severity: A Retrospective Cohort Study. *Open Forum Infect. Dis.* **2022**, *9*, ofac223. [CrossRef]
20. Liu, Y.; Chen, D.; Hou, J.; Li, H.; Cao, D.; Guo, M.; Ling, Y.; Gao, M.; Zhou, Y.; Wan, Y.; et al. An inter-correlated cytokine network identified at the center of cytokine storm predicted COVID-19 prognosis. *Cytokine* **2021**, *138*, 155365. [CrossRef]
21. Cao, X. COVID-19: Immunopathology and its implications for therapy. *Nat. Rev. Immunol.* **2020**, *20*, 269–270. [CrossRef]
22. Ynga-Durand, M.; Maaß, H.; Milošević, M.; Krstanović, F.; Matešić, M.P.; Jonjić, S.; Protić, A.; Brizić, I.; Šustić, A.; Čičin-Šain, L. SARS-CoV-2 Viral Load in the Pulmonary Compartment of Critically Ill COVID-19 Patients Correlates with Viral Serum Load and Fatal Outcomes. *Viruses* **2022**, *14*, 1292. [CrossRef]
23. Bermejo-Martin, J.F.; García-Mateo, N.; Motos, A.; Resino, S.; Tamayo, L.; Murua, P.R.; Bustamante-Munguira, E.; Curto, E.G.; Úbeda-Iglesias, A.; Torre, M.d.C.d.l.; et al. Effect of viral storm in patients admitted to intensive care units with severe COVID-19 in Spain: A multicentre, prospective, cohort study. *Lancet Microbe* **2023**, *4*, e431–e441. [CrossRef] [PubMed]
24. Giacomelli, A.; Righini, E.; Micheli, V.; Pinoli, P.; Bernasconi, A.; Rizzo, A.; Oreni, L.; Ridolfo, A.L.; Antinori, S.; Ceri, S.; et al. SARS-CoV-2 viremia and COVID-19 mortality: A prospective observational study. *PLoS ONE* **2023**, *18*, e0281052.18. [CrossRef] [PubMed]
25. Karron, R.A.; Hetrich, M.K.; Bin Na, Y.; Knoll, M.D.; Schappell, E.; Meece, J.; Hanson, E.; Tong, S.; Lee, J.S.; Veguilla, V.; et al. Assessment of Clinical and Virological Characteristics of SARS-CoV-2 Infection Among Children Aged 0 to 4 Years and Their Household Members. *JAMA Netw. Open* **2022**, *5*, e2227348. [CrossRef] [PubMed]
26. Jacobs, J.L.; Bain, W.; Naqvi, A.; Staines, B.; Castanha, P.M.S.; Yang, H.; Boltz, V.F.; Barratt-Boyes, S.; Marques, E.T.A.; Mitchell, S.L.; et al. Severe Acute Respiratory Syndrome Coronavirus 2 Viremia Is Associated with Coronavirus Disease 2019 Severity and Predicts Clinical Outcomes. *Clin. Infect. Dis.* **2022**, *74*, 1525–1533. [CrossRef]
27. National Institutes of Health. Coronavirus Disease 2019 (COVID-19) Treatment Guidelines. Available online: https://www.covid19treatmentguidelines.nih.gov/overview/clinical-spectrum/ (accessed on 21 March 2024).
28. Yu, X.; Sun, S.; Shi, Y.; Wang, H.; Zhao, R.; Sheng, J. SARS-CoV-2 viral load in sputum correlates with risk of COVID-19 progression. *Crit. Care* **2020**, *24*, 1–4. [CrossRef]
29. Ahn, J.H.; Kim, J.M.; Hong, S.P.; Choi, S.Y.; Yang, M.J.; Ju, Y.S.; Kim, Y.T.; Kim, H.M.; Rahman, T.; Chung, M.K.; et al. Nasal ciliated cells are primary targets for SARS-CoV-2 replication in the early stage of COVID-19. *J. Clin. Investig.* **2021**, *131*. [CrossRef]
30. V'Kovski, P.; Kratzel, A.; Steiner, S.; Stalder, H.; Thiel, V. Coronavirus biology and replication: Implications for SARS-CoV-2. *Nat. Rev. Microbiol.* **2021**, *19*, 155–170. [CrossRef]
31. McGonagle, D.; Kearney, M.F.; O'Regan, A.; O'Donnell, J.S.; Quartuccio, L.; Watad, A.; Bridgewood, C. Therapeutic implications of ongoing alveolar viral replication in COVID-19. *Lancet Rheumatol.* **2022**, *4*, e135–e144. [CrossRef]
32. Fajnzylber, J.; Regan, J.; Coxen, K.; Corry, H.; Wong, C.; Rosenthal, A.; Worrall, D.; Giguel, F.; Piechocka-Trocha, A.; Atyeo, C.; et al. SARS-CoV-2 viral load is associated with increased disease severity and mortality. *Nat. Commun.* **2020**, *11*, 5493. [CrossRef]
33. Hui, K.P.Y.; Ho, J.C.W.; Cheung, M.-C.; Ng, K.-C.; Ching, R.H.H.; Lai, K.-L.; Kam, T.T.; Gu, H.; Sit, K.-Y.; Hsin, M.K.Y.; et al. SARS-CoV-2 Omicron variant replication in human bronchus and lung ex vivo. *Nature* **2022**, *603*, 715–720. [CrossRef]

34. Puhach, O.; Adea, K.; Hulo, N.; Sattonnet, P.; Genecand, C.; Iten, A.; Jacquérioz, F.; Kaiser, L.; Vetter, P.; Eckerle, I.; et al. Infectious viral load in unvaccinated and vaccinated individuals infected with ancestral, Delta or Omicron SARS-CoV-2. *Nat. Med.* **2022**, *28*, 1491–1500. [CrossRef] [PubMed]
35. Abu-Raddad, L.J.; Chemaitelly, H.; Bertollini, R. Severity of SARS-CoV-2 Reinfections as Compared with Primary Infections. *N. Engl. J. Med.* **2021**, *385*, 2487–2489. [CrossRef] [PubMed]
36. Omololu, A.; Ojelade, B.; Ajayi, O.; Adesomi, T.; Alade, O.; Adebisi, S.; Nwadike, V. "Long COVID": A case report of persistent symptoms in a patient with prolonged SARS-CoV-2 shedding for over 110 days. *SAGE Open Med. Case Rep.* **2021**, *9*, 2050313X211015494. [CrossRef]
37. Viszlayová, D.; Sojka, M.; Dobrodenková, S.; Szabó, S.; Bilec, O.; Turzová, M.; Ďurina, J.; Baloghová, B.; Borbély, Z.; Kršák, M. SARS-CoV-2 RNA in the Cerebrospinal Fluid of a Patient with Long COVID. *Ther. Adv. Infect. Dis.* **2021**, *8*, 204993612110485. [CrossRef]
38. Stadtmüller, M.; Laubner, A.; Rost, F.; Winkler, S.; Patrasová, E.; Šimůnková, L.; Reinhardt, S.; Beil, J.; Dalpke, A.H.; Yi, B. Emergence and spread of a sub-lineage of SARS-CoV-2 Alpha variant B.1.1.7 in Europe, and with further evolution of spike mutation accumulations shared with the Beta and Gamma variants. *Virus Evol.* **2022**, *8*, veac010. [CrossRef] [PubMed]
39. Menezes, S.M.; Jamoulle, M.; Carletto, M.P.; Jamoulle, M.; Carletto, M.P.; Van Holm, B.; Moens, L.; Meyts, I.; Maes, P.; Van Weyenbergh, J. Blood transcriptomics reveal persistent SARS-CoV-2 RNA and candidate biomarkers in Long COVID patients. *medRxiv* **2024**. [CrossRef]
40. Craddock, V.; Mahajan, A.; Krishnamachary, B.; Spikes, L.; Chalise, P.; Dhillon, N.K. Persistent Presence of Spike protein and Viral RNA in the Circulation of Individuals with Post-Acute Sequelae of COVID-19. *medRxiv* **2022**. [CrossRef]
41. Su, Y.; Yuan, D.; Chen, D.G.; Ng, R.H.; Wang, K.; Choi, J.; Li, S.; Hong, S.; Zhang, R.; Xie, J.; et al. Multiple early factors anticipate post-acute COVID-19 sequelae. *Cell* **2022**, *185*, 881–895.e20. [CrossRef]
42. Rombauts, A.; Infante, C.; Lagos, M.d.A.M.d.; Alba, J.; Valiente, A.; Donado-Mazarrón, C.; Carretero-Ledesma, M.; Rodríguez-Álvarez, R.; Omatos, S.; Palacios-Baena, Z.R.; et al. Impact of SARS-CoV-2 RNAemia and other risk factors on long-COVID: A prospective observational multicentre cohort study. *J. Infect.* **2023**, *86*, 154–225. [CrossRef]
43. Ram-Mohan, N.; Kim, D.; Rogers, A.J.; Blish, C.A.; Nadeau, K.C.; Blomkalns, A.L.; Yang, S. Association Between SARS-CoV-2 RNAemia and Postacute Sequelae of COVID-19. *Open Forum Infect. Dis.* **2022**, *9*, ofab646. [CrossRef]
44. Pérez, D.A.G.; Fonseca-Agüero, A.; Toledo-Ibarra, G.A.; Gomez-Valdivia, J.d.J.; Díaz-Resendiz, K.J.G.; Benitez-Trinidad, A.B.; Razura-Carmona, F.F.; Navidad-Murrieta, M.S.; Covantes-Rosales, C.E.; Giron-Pérez, M.I. Post-COVID-19 Syndrome in Outpatients and Its Association with Viral Load. *Int. J. Environ. Res. Public. Health* **2022**, *19*, 15145. [CrossRef]
45. European Centre for Disease Prevention and Control. In *Prevalence of Post COVID-19 Condition Symptoms: A Systematic Review and Meta-Analysis of Cohort Study Data, Stratified by Recruitment Setting Key Facts*; European Centre for Disease Prevention and Control: Solna, Sweeden, 2022.
46. Chen, B.; Julg, B.; Mohandas, S.; Bradfute, S.B.; Force, R.M.P.T.; Hospital, M.G.; Mit; Harvard; Angeles, C.H.L.; States, U. Viral persistence, reactivation, and mechanisms of long COVID. *eLife* **2023**, *12*, e86015. [CrossRef]
47. Proal, A.D.; VanElzakker, M.B. Long COVID or Post-acute Sequelae of COVID-19 (PASC): An Overview of Biological Factors That May Contribute to Persistent Symptoms. *Front. Microbiol.* **2021**, *12*, 698169. [CrossRef]
48. Zhang, L.; Richards, A.; Inmaculada Barrasa, M.; Hughes, S.H.; Young, R.A.; Jaenisch, R. Reverse-transcribed SARS-CoV-2 RNA can integrate into the genome of cultured human cells and can be expressed in patient-derived tissues. *Proc. Nat. Acad. Sci. USA* **2021**, *118*, e2105968118. [CrossRef]
49. Randall, R.E.; Griffin, D.E. Within host RNA virus persistence: Mechanisms and consequences. *Curr. Opin. Virol.* **2017**, *23*, 35–42. [CrossRef] [PubMed]
50. Gao, Y.-D.; Ding, M.; Dong, X.; Zhang, J.-J.; Azkur, A.K.; Azkur, D.; Gan, H.; Sun, Y.-L.; Fu, W.; Li, W.; et al. Risk factors for severe and critically ill COVID-19 patients: A review. *Allergy* **2021**, *76*, 428–455. [CrossRef] [PubMed]
51. Kuwabara, T.; Ishikawa, F.; Kondo, M.; Kakiuchi, T. The Role of IL-17 and Related Cytokines in Inflammatory Autoimmune Diseases. *Mediat. Inflamm.* **2017**, *2017*, 3908061. [CrossRef]
52. Velazquez-Salinas, L.; Verdugo-Rodriguez, A.; Rodriguez, L.L.; Borca, M.V. The Role of Interleukin 6 During Viral Infections. *Front. Microbiol.* **2019**, *10*, 01057. [CrossRef]
53. Carlini, V.; Noonan, D.M.; Abdalalem, E.; Goletti, D.; Sansone, C.; Calabrone, L.; Albini, A. The multifaceted nature of IL-10: Regulation, role in immunological homeostasis and its relevance to cancer, COVID-19 and post-COVID conditions. *Front. Immunol.* **2023**, *14*, 1161067. [CrossRef]
54. Zawawi, Z.M.; Kalyanasundram, J.; Zain, R.M.; Thayan, R.; Basri, D.F.; Yap, W.B. Prospective Roles of Tumor Necrosis Factor-Alpha (TNF-α) in COVID-19: Prognosis, Therapeutic and Management. *Int. J. Mol. Sci.* **2023**, *24*, 6142. [CrossRef]
55. Duong-Quy, S.; Vo-Pham-Minh, T.; Tran-Xuan, Q.; Huynh-Anh, T.; Vo-Van, T.; Vu-Tran-Thien, Q.; Nguyen-Nhu, V. Post-COVID-19 Pulmonary Fibrosis: Facts—Challenges and Futures: A Narrative Review. *Pulm. Ther.* **2023**, *20*, 295–307. [CrossRef] [PubMed]
56. Kim, Y.-M.; Shin, E.-C. Type I and III interferon responses in SARS-CoV-2 infection. *Exp. Mol. Med.* **2021**, *53*, 750–760. [CrossRef]
57. Vu, D.-L.; Martinez-Murillo, P.; Pigny, F.; Vono, M.; Meyer, B.; Eberhardt, C.S.; Lemeille, S.; Von Dach, E.; Blanchard-Rohner, G.; Eckerle, I.; et al. Longitudinal Analysis of Inflammatory Response to SARS-CoV-2 in the Upper Respiratory Tract Reveals an Association with Viral Load, Independent of Symptoms. *J. Clin. Immunol.* **2021**, *41*, 1723–1732. [CrossRef]

58. Sidhu, J.K.; Siggins, M.K.; Liew, F.; Russell, C.D.; Uruchurtu, A.S.S.; Davis, C.; Turtle, L.; Moore, S.C.; E Hardwick, H.; Oosthuyzen, W.; et al. Delayed Mucosal Antiviral Responses Despite Robust Peripheral Inflammation in Fatal COVID-19. *J. Infect. Dis.* **2023**, *230*, e17–e29. [CrossRef]
59. Rolland-Debord, C.; Piéroni, L.; Bejar, F.; Milon, A.; Choinier, P.; Blin, E.; Bravais, J.; Halitim, P.; Letellier, A.; Camuset, J.; et al. Cell and cytokine analyses from bronchoalveolar lavage in non-critical COVID-19 pneumonia. *Intern. Emerg. Med.* **2023**, *18*, 1723–1732. [CrossRef] [PubMed]
60. Xie, C.; Li, Q.; Li, L.; Peng, X.; Ling, Z.; Xiao, B.; Feng, J.; Chen, Z.; Chang, D.; Xie, L.; et al. Association of Early Inflammation with Age and Asymptomatic Disease in COVID-19. *J. Inflamm. Res.* **2021**, *14*, 1207–1216. [CrossRef] [PubMed]
61. Zaid, Y.; Doré, É.; Dubuc, I.; Archambault, A.-S.; Flamand, O.; Laviolette, M.; Flamand, N.; Boilard, É.; Flamand, L. Chemokines and eicosanoids fuel the hyperinflammation within the lungs of patients with severe COVID-19. *J. Allergy Clin. Immunol.* **2021**, *148*, 368–380.e3. [CrossRef]
62. Reynolds, D.; Guillamet, C.V.; Day, A.; Borcherding, N.; Guillamet, R.V.; Choreño-Parra, J.A.; House, S.L.; O'halloran, J.A.; Zúñiga, J.; Ellebedy, A.H.; et al. Comprehensive Immunologic Evaluation of Bronchoalveolar Lavage Samples from Human Patients with Moderate and Severe Seasonal Influenza and Severe COVID-19. *J. Immunol.* **2021**, *207*, 1229–1238. [CrossRef]
63. Grant, R.A.; Poor, T.A.; Sichizya, L.; Diaz, E.; Bailey, J.I.; Soni, S.; Senkow, K.J.; Perez-Leonor, X.G.; Abdala-Valencia, H.; Lu, Z.; et al. Prolonged exposure to lung-derived cytokines is associated with inflammatory activation of microglia in patients with COVID-19. *bioRxiv* **2023**. [CrossRef]
64. Min, C.-K.; Cheon, S.; Ha, N.-Y.; Sohn, K.M.; Kim, Y.; Aigerim, A.; Shin, H.M.; Choi, J.-Y.; Inn, K.-S.; Kim, J.-H.; et al. Comparative and kinetic analysis of viral shedding and immunological responses in MERS patients representing a broad spectrum of disease severity. *Sci. Rep.* **2016**, *6*, 25359. [CrossRef]
65. Wong, C.K.; Lam, C.W.K.; Wu, A.K.L.; Ip, W.K.; Lee, N.L.S.; Chan, I.H.S.; Lit, L.C.W.; Hui, D.S.C.; Chan, M.H.M.; Chung, S.S.C.; et al. Plasma inflammatory cytokines and chemokines in severe acute respiratory syndrome. *Clin. Exp. Immunol.* **2004**, *136*, 95–103. [CrossRef] [PubMed]
66. Wang, Z.; Zhang, A.; Wan, Y.; Liu, X.; Qiu, C.; Xi, X.; Ren, Y.; Wang, J.; Dong, Y.; Bao, M.; et al. Early hypercytokinemia is associated with interferon-induced transmembrane protein-3 dysfunction and predictive of fatal H7N9 infection. *Proc. Natl. Acad. Sci. USA* **2014**, *111*, 769–774. [CrossRef] [PubMed]
67. Cremoni, M.; Allouche, J.; Graça, D.; Zorzi, K.; Fernandez, C.; Teisseyre, M.; Benzaken, S.; Ruetsch-Chelli, C.; Esnault, V.L.M.; Dellamonica, J.; et al. Low baseline IFN-γ response could predict hospitalization in COVID-19 patients. *Front. Immunol.* **2022**, *13*, 953502. [CrossRef] [PubMed]
68. Zhu, X.; Gebo, K.A.; Abraham, A.G.; Habtehyimer, F.; Patel, E.U.; Laeyendecker, O.; Gniadek, T.J.; Fernandez, R.E.; Baker, O.R.; Ram, M.; et al. Dynamics of inflammatory responses after SARS-CoV-2 infection by vaccination status in the USA: A prospective cohort study. *Lancet Microbe* **2023**, *4*, e692–e703. [CrossRef]
69. Martins, M.L.; da Silva-Malta, M.C.F.; Araújo, A.L.; Gonçalves, F.A.; Botelho, M.d.L.; de Oliveira, I.R.; Boy, L.d.S.M.F.; Moreira, H.M.; Barbosa-Stancioli, E.F.; Ribeiro, M.A.; et al. A potent inflammatory response is triggered in asymptomatic blood donors with recent SARS-CoV-2 infection. *Rev. Soc. Bras. Med. Trop.* **2022**, *55*, e0239–2022. [CrossRef]
70. Long, Q.-X.; Tang, X.-J.; Shi, Q.-L.; Li, Q.; Deng, H.-J.; Yuan, J.; Hu, J.-L.; Xu, W.; Zhang, Y.; Lv, F.-J.; et al. Clinical and immunological assessment of asymptomatic SARS-CoV-2 infections. *Nat. Med.* **2020**, *26*, 1200–1204. [CrossRef]
71. Tjan, L.H.; Furukawa, K.; Nagano, T.; Kiriu, T.; Nishimura, M.; Arii, J.; Hino, Y.; Iwata, S.; Nishimura, Y.; Mori, Y. Early Differences in Cytokine Production by Severity of Coronavirus Disease 2019. *J. Infect. Dis.* **2021**, *223*, 1145–1149. [CrossRef]
72. Masood, K.I.; Yameen, M.; Ashraf, J.; Shahid, S.; Mahmood, S.F.; Nasir, A.; Nasir, N.; Jamil, B.; Ghanchi, N.K.; Khanum, I.; et al. Upregulated type I interferon responses in asymptomatic COVID-19 infection are associated with improved clinical outcome. *Sci. Rep.* **2021**, *11*, 22958. [CrossRef]
73. Tripathy, A.S.; Vishwakarma, S.; Trimbake, D.; Gurav, Y.K.; Potdar, V.A.; Mokashi, N.D.; Patsute, S.D.; Kaushal, H.; Choudhary, M.L.; Tilekar, B.N.; et al. Pro-inflammatory CXCL-10, TNF-α, IL-1β, and IL-6: Biomarkers of SARS-CoV-2 infection. *Arch. Virol.* **2021**, *166*, 3301–3310. [CrossRef]
74. Smith, N.; Goncalves, P.; Charbit, B.; Grzelak, L.; Beretta, M.; Planchais, C.; Bruel, T.; Rouilly, V.; Bondet, V.; Hadjadj, J.; et al. Distinct systemic and mucosal immune responses during acute SARS-CoV-2 infection. *Nat. Immunol.* **2021**, *22*, 1428–1439. [CrossRef]
75. Han, H.; Ma, Q.; Li, C.; Liu, R.; Zhao, L.; Wang, W.; Zhang, P.; Liu, X.; Gao, G.; Liu, F.; et al. Profiling serum cytokines in COVID-19 patients reveals IL-6 and IL-10 are disease severity predictors. *Emerg. Microbes Infect.* **2020**, *9*, 1123–1130. [CrossRef] [PubMed]
76. Yin, S.-W.; Zhou, Z.; Wang, J.-L.; Deng, Y.-F.; Jing, H.; Qiu, Y. Viral loads, lymphocyte subsets and cytokines in asymptomatic, mildly and critical symptomatic patients with SARS-CoV-2 infection: A retrospective study. *Virol. J.* **2021**, *18*, 126. [CrossRef] [PubMed]
77. Kwon, J.-S.; Kim, J.Y.; Kim, M.-C.; Park, S.Y.; Kim, B.-N.; Bae, S.; Cha, H.H.; Jung, J.; Lee, M.J.; Choi, S.-H.; et al. Factors of Severity in Patients with COVID-19: Cytokine/Chemokine Concentrations, Viral Load, and Antibody Responses. *Am. J. Trop. Med. Hyg.* **2020**, *103*, 2412–2418. [CrossRef] [PubMed]
78. Ling, L.; Chen, Z.; Lui, G.; Wong, C.K.; Wong, W.T.; Ng, R.W.Y.; Tso, E.Y.K.; Fung, K.S.C.; Chan, V.; Yeung, A.C.M.; et al. Longitudinal Cytokine Profile in Patients with Mild to Critical COVID-19. *Front. Immunol.* **2021**, *12*, 763292. [CrossRef]

79. Huang, W.; Li, M.; Luo, G.; Wu, X.; Su, B.; Zhao, L.; Zhang, S.; Chen, X.; Jia, M.; Zhu, J.; et al. The Inflammatory Factors Associated with Disease Severity to Predict COVID-19 Progression. *J. Immunol.* **2021**, *206*, 1597–1608. [CrossRef]
80. Calabrese, F.; Lunardi, F.; Baldasso, E.; Pezzuto, F.; Kilitci, A.; Olteanu, G.-E.; Del Vecchio, C.; Fortarezza, F.; Boscolo, A.; Schiavon, M.; et al. Comprehensive bronchoalveolar lavage characterization in COVID-19 associated acute respiratory distress syndrome patients: A prospective cohort study. *Respir. Res.* **2023**, *24*, 152. [CrossRef]
81. Lucas, C.; Wong, P.; Klein, J.; Castro, T.B.R.; Silva, J.; Sundaram, M.; Ellingson, M.K.; Mao, T.; Oh, J.E.; Israelow, B.; et al. Longitudinal analyses reveal immunological misfiring in severe COVID-19. *Nature* **2020**, *584*, 463–469. [CrossRef] [PubMed]
82. Chi, Y.; Ge, Y.; Wu, B.; Zhang, W.; Wu, T.; Wen, T.; Liu, J.; Guo, X.; Huang, C.; Jiao, Y.; et al. Serum Cytokine and Chemokine Profile in Relation to the Severity of Coronavirus Disease 2019 in China. *J. Infect. Dis.* **2020**, *222*, 746–754. [CrossRef]
83. Bost, P.; De Sanctis, F.; Canè, S.; Ugel, S.; Donadello, K.; Castellucci, M.; Eyal, D.; Fiore, A.; Anselmi, C.; Barouni, R.M.; et al. Deciphering the state of immune silence in fatal COVID-19 patients. *Nat. Commun.* **2021**, *12*, 1428. [CrossRef]
84. Pandolfi, L.; Fossali, T.; Frangipane, V.; Bozzini, S.; Morosini, M.; D'amato, M.; Lettieri, S.; Urtis, M.; Di Toro, A.; Saracino, L.; et al. Broncho-alveolar inflammation in COVID-19 patients: A correlation with clinical outcome. *BMC Pulm. Med.* **2020**, *20*, 301. [CrossRef]
85. Li, D.; Liu, C.; Liu, J.; Hu, J.; Yang, Y.; Zhou, Y. Analysis of Risk Factors for 24 Patients With COVID-19 Developing from Moderate to Severe Condition. *Front. Cell. Infect. Microbiol.* **2020**, *10*, 548582. [CrossRef] [PubMed]
86. Chen, L.; Wang, G.; Long, X.; Hou, H.; Wei, J.; Cao, Y.; Tan, J.; Liu, W.; Meng, F.; Huang, L.; et al. Dynamics of Blood Viral Load Is Strongly Associated with Clinical Outcomes in Coronavirus Disease 2019 (COVID-19) Patients—A Prospective Cohort Study. *J. Mol. Diagn.* **2021**, *23*, 10–18. [CrossRef]
87. MacCann, R.; Leon, A.A.G.; Gonzalez, G.; Carr, M.J.; Feeney, E.R.; Yousif, O.; Cotter, A.G.; de Barra, E.; Sadlier, C.; Doran, P.; et al. Dysregulated early transcriptional signatures linked to mast cell and interferon responses are implicated in COVID-19 severity. *Front. Immunol.* **2023**, *14*, 1166574. [CrossRef] [PubMed]
88. Laing, A.G.; Lorenc, A.; del Barrio, I.D.M.; Das, A.; Fish, M.; Monin, L.; Muñoz-Ruiz, M.; McKenzie, D.R.; Hayday, T.S.; Francos-Quijorna, I.; et al. A dynamic COVID-19 immune signature includes associations with poor prognosis. *Nat. Med.* **2020**, *26*, 1623–1635. [CrossRef] [PubMed]
89. Santos, J.d.M.B.d.; Soares, C.P.; Monteiro, F.R.; Mello, R.; Amaral, J.B.D.; Aguiar, A.S.; Soledade, M.P.; Sucupira, C.; De Paulis, M.; Andrade, J.B.; et al. In Nasal Mucosal Secretions, Distinct IFN and IgA Responses Are Found in Severe and Mild SARS-CoV-2 Infection. *Front. Immunol.* **2021**, *12*, 595343. [CrossRef] [PubMed]
90. Voiriot, G.; Dorgham, K.; Bachelot, G.; Fajac, A.; Morand-Joubert, L.; Parizot, C.; Gerotziafas, G.; Farabos, D.; Trugnan, G.; Eguether, T.; et al. Identification of bronchoalveolar and blood immune-inflammatory biomarker signature associated with poor 28-day outcome in critically ill COVID-19 patients. *Sci. Rep.* **2022**, *12*, 9502. [CrossRef]
91. Joly, C.; Desjardins, D.; Porcher, R.; Péré, H.; Bruneau, T.; Zhang, Q.; Bastard, P.; Cobat, A.; Resmini, L.; Lenoir, O.; et al. More rapid blood interferon α2 decline in fatal versus surviving COVID-19 patients. *Front. Immunol.* **2023**, *14*, 1250214. [CrossRef]
92. Schultheiß, C.; Willscher, E.; Paschold, L.; Gottschick, C.; Klee, B.; Henkes, S.-S.; Bosurgi, L.; Dutzmann, J.; Sedding, D.; Frese, T.; et al. The IL-1β, IL-6, and TNF cytokine triad is associated with post-acute sequelae of COVID-19. *Cell Rep. Med.* **2022**, *3*, 100663. [CrossRef]
93. Durstenfeld, M.S.; Hsue, P.Y.; Peluso, M.J.; Deeks, S.G. Findings from Mayo Clinic's Post-COVID Clinic: PASC Phenotypes Vary by Sex and Degree of IL-6 Elevation. *Mayo Clin. Proc.* **2022**, *97*, 430–432. [CrossRef]
94. Phetsouphanh, C.; Darley, D.R.; Wilson, D.B.; Howe, A.; Munier, C.M.L.; Patel, S.K.; Juno, J.A.; Burrell, L.M.; Kent, S.J.; Dore, G.J.; et al. Immunological dysfunction persists for 8 months following initial mild-to-moderate SARS-CoV-2 infection. *Nat. Immunol.* **2022**, *23*, 210–216. [CrossRef]
95. Talla, A.; Vasaikar, S.V.; Lemos, M.P.; Moodie, Z.; Lee, P.M.-P.; Henderson, K.E.; Cohen, K.W.; Czartoski, J.L.; Lai, L.; Suthar, M.S.; et al. Longitudinal immune dynamics of mild COVID-19 define signatures of recovery and persistence. *bioRxiv* **2021**. [CrossRef]
96. Torres-Ruiz, J.; Lomelín-Gascón, J.; Luna, J.L.; Castro, A.S.V.; Pérez-Fragoso, A.; Nuñez-Aguirre, M.; Alcalá-Carmona, B.; Absalón-Aguilar, A.; Balderas-Miranda, J.T.; Maravillas-Montero, J.L.; et al. Novel clinical and immunological features associated with persistent post-acute sequelae of COVID-19 after six months of follow-up: A pilot study. *Infect. Dis.* **2023**, *55*, 243–254. [CrossRef] [PubMed]
97. Kovarik, J.J.; Bileck, A.; Hagn, G.; Meier-Menches, S.M.; Frey, T.; Kaempf, A.; Hollenstein, M.; Shoumariyeh, T.; Skos, L.; Reiter, B.; et al. A multi-omics based anti-inflammatory immune signature characterizes long COVID-19 syndrome. *iScience* **2023**, *26*, 105717. [CrossRef]
98. Peluso, M.J.; Lu, S.; Tang, A.F.; Durstenfeld, M.S.; Ho, H.-E.; Goldberg, S.A.; Forman, C.A.; E Munter, S.; Hoh, R.; Tai, V.; et al. Markers of Immune Activation and Inflammation in Individuals with Postacute Sequelae of Severe Acute Respiratory Syndrome Coronavirus 2 Infection. *J. Infect. Dis.* **2021**, *224*, 1839–1848. [CrossRef]
99. Queiroz, M.A.F.; das Neves, P.F.M.; Lima, S.S.; Lopes, J.d.C.; Torres, M.K.d.S.; Vallinoto, I.M.V.C.; de Brito, M.T.F.M.; da Silva, A.L.S.; Leite, M.d.M.; da Costa, F.P.; et al. Cytokine Profiles Associated with Acute COVID-19 and Long COVID-19 Syndrome. *Front. Cell. Infect. Microbiol.* **2022**, *12*, 922422. [CrossRef]
100. Pretorius, E.; Vlok, M.; Venter, C.; Bezuidenhout, J.A.; Laubscher, G.J.; Steenkamp, J.; Kell, D.B. Persistent clotting protein pathology in Long COVID/Post-Acute Sequelae of COVID-19 (PASC) is accompanied by increased levels of antiplasmin. *Cardiovasc. Diabetol.* **2021**, *20*, 172. [CrossRef] [PubMed]

101. Pontelli, M.C.; Castro, Í.A.; Martins, R.B.; La Serra, L.; Veras, F.P.; Nascimento, D.C.; Silva, C.M.; Cardoso, R.S.; Rosales, R.; Gomes, R.; et al. SARS-CoV-2 productively infects primary human immune system cells in vitro and in COVID-19 patients. *J. Mol. Cell Biol.* **2022**, *14*. [CrossRef] [PubMed]
102. Leon, J.; Michelson, D.A.; Olejnik, J.; Chowdhary, K.; Oh, H.S.; Hume, A.J.; Galvan-Pena, S.; Zhu, Y.; Chen, F.; Vijaykumar, B.; et al. A virus-specific monocyte inflammatory phenotype is induced by SARS-CoV-2 at the immune-epithelial interface. *Proc. Natl. Acad. Sci. USA* **2022**, *119*, e2116853118. [CrossRef]
103. de Dios-Figueroa, G.T.; Aguilera-Marquez, J.d.R.; Camacho-Villegas, T.A.; Lugo-Fabres, P.H. 3D Cell Culture Models in COVID-19 Times: A Review of 3D Technologies to Understand and Accelerate Therapeutic Drug Discovery. *Biomedicines* **2021**, *9*, 602. [CrossRef]
104. Clevers, H. COVID-19: Organoids go viral. *Nat. Rev. Mol. Cell Biol.* **2020**, *21*, 355–356. [CrossRef]
105. Marshall, L.J.; Bailey, J.; Cassotta, M.; Herrmann, K.; Pistollato, F. Poor Translatability of Biomedical Research Using Animals—A Narrative Review. *Altern. Lab. Anim.* **2023**, *51*, 102–135. [CrossRef]
106. Chu, H.; Chan, J.F.-W.; Yuen, K.-Y. Animal models in SARS-CoV-2 research. *Nat. Methods* **2022**, *19*, 392–394. [CrossRef] [PubMed]
107. Fan, C.; Wu, Y.; Rui, X.; Yang, Y.; Ling, C.; Liu, S.; Liu, S.; Wang, Y. Animal models for COVID-19: Advances, gaps and perspectives. *Signal Transduct. Target. Ther.* **2022**, *7*, 220. [CrossRef] [PubMed]
108. Jansen, E.B.; Orvold, S.N.; Swan, C.L.; Yourkowski, A.; Thivierge, B.M.; Francis, M.E.; Ge, A.; Rioux, M.; Darbellay, J.; Howland, J.G.; et al. After the virus has cleared—Can preclinical models be employed for Long COVID research? *PLoS Pathog.* **2022**, *18*. [CrossRef] [PubMed]
109. Rosenke, K.; Okumura, A.; Lewis, M.C.; Feldmann, F.; Meade-White, K.; Bohler, W.F.; Griffin, A.J.; Rosenke, R.; Shaia, C.; Jarvis, M.A.; et al. Molnupiravir inhibits SARS-CoV-2 variants including Omicron in the hamster model. *J. Clin. Investig.* **2022**, *7*, e160108. [CrossRef]
110. Abdelnabi, R.; Foo, C.S.; Jochmans, D.; Vangeel, L.; De Jonghe, S.; Augustijns, P.; Mols, R.; Weynand, B.; Wattanakul, T.; Hoglund, R.M.; et al. The oral protease inhibitor (PF-07321332) protects Syrian hamsters against infection with SARS-CoV-2 variants of concern. *Nat. Commun.* **2022**, *13*, 719. [CrossRef]
111. Jeong, J.H.; Chokkakula, S.; Min, S.C.; Kim, B.K.; Choi, W.-S.; Oh, S.; Yun, Y.S.; Kang, D.H.; Lee, O.-J.; Kim, E.-G.; et al. Combination therapy with nirmatrelvir and molnupiravir improves the survival of SARS-CoV-2 infected mice. *Antivir. Res.* **2022**, *208*, 105430. [CrossRef]
112. Frere, J.J.; Serafini, R.A.; Pryce, K.D.; Zazhytska, M.; Oishi, K.; Golynker, I.; Panis, M.; Zimering, J.; Horiuchi, S.; Hoagland, D.A.; et al. SARS-CoV-2 Infection in Hamsters and Humans Results in Lasting and Unique Systemic Perturbations after Recovery. *Sci. Translational Med.* **2022**, *14*, eabq3059. [CrossRef]
113. Yinda, C.K.; Port, J.R.; Bushmaker, T.; Offei Owusu, I.; Purushotham, J.N.; Avanzato, V.A.; Fischer, R.J.; Schulz, J.E.; Holbrook, M.G.; Hebner, M.J.; et al. K18-hACE2 mice develop respiratory disease resembling severe COVID-19. *PLoS Pathog.* **2021**, *17*, e1009195. [CrossRef]
114. Gressett, T.E.; Leist, S.R.; Ismael, S.; Talkington, G.; Dinnon, K.H.; Baric, R.S.; Bix, G. Mouse Adapted SARS-CoV-2 Model Induces "Long-COVID" Neuropathology in BALB/c Mice. *bioRxiv* **2023**. [CrossRef]
115. Handley, A.; Ryan, K.A.; Davies, E.R.; Bewley, K.R.; Carnell, O.T.; Challis, A.; Coombes, N.S.; Fotheringham, S.A.; Gooch, K.E.; Charlton, M.; et al. SARS-CoV-2 Disease Severity in the Golden Syrian Hamster Model of Infection Is Related to the Volume of Intranasal Inoculum. *Viruses* **2023**, *15*, 748. [CrossRef] [PubMed]
116. Reyna, R.A.; Kishimoto-Urata, M.; Urata, S.; Makishima, T.; Paessler, S.; Maruyama, J. Recovery of anosmia in hamsters infected with SARS-CoV-2 is correlated with repair of the olfactory epithelium. *Sci. Rep.* **2022**, *12*, 628. [CrossRef] [PubMed]
117. Osterrieder, N.; Bertzbach, L.D.; Dietert, K.; Abdelgawad, A.; Vladimirova, D.; Kunec, D.; Hoffmann, D.; Beer, M.; Gruber, A.D.; Trimpert, J. Age-Dependent Progression of SARS-CoV-2 Infection in Syrian Hamsters. *Viruses* **2020**, *12*, 779. [CrossRef] [PubMed]
118. Briand, F.; Sencio, V.; Robil, C.; Heumel, S.; Deruyter, L.; Machelart, A.; Barthelemy, J.; Bogard, G.; Hoffmann, E.; Infanti, F.; et al. Diet-Induced Obesity and NASH Impair Disease Recovery in SARS-CoV-2-Infected Golden Hamsters. *Viruses* **2022**, *14*, 2067. [CrossRef]
119. van de Ven, K.; van Dijken, H.; Wijsman, L.; Gomersbach, A.; Schouten, T.; Kool, J.; Lenz, S.; Roholl, P.; Meijer, A.; van Kasteren, P.B.; et al. Pathology and Immunity After SARS-CoV-2 Infection in Male Ferrets Is Affected by Age and Inoculation Route. *Front. Immunol.* **2021**, *12*, 750229. [CrossRef]

Disclaimer/Publisher's Note: The statements, opinions and data contained in all publications are solely those of the individual author(s) and contributor(s) and not of MDPI and/or the editor(s). MDPI and/or the editor(s) disclaim responsibility for any injury to people or property resulting from any ideas, methods, instructions or products referred to in the content.

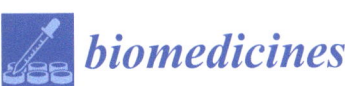

Systematic Review

New Onset of Acute and Chronic Hepatic Diseases Post-COVID-19 Infection: A Systematic Review

Ahamed Lebbe [1,†], Ali Aboulwafa [1,†], Nuran Bayraktar [1], Beshr Mushannen [1], Sama Ayoub [1], Shaunak Sarker [1], Marwan Nour Abdalla [1], Ibrahim Mohammed [2], Malik Mushannen [3], Lina Yagan [4] and Dalia Zakaria [5,*]

1. Medical Department, Weill Cornell Medicine-Qatar, Doha 24144, Qatar; aaa4010@qatar-med.cornell.edu (A.L.); aaa4001@qatar-med.cornell.edu (A.A.); nub4001@qatar-med.cornell.edu (N.B.); sna4001@qatar-med.cornell.edu (S.A.); shs4020@qatar-med.cornell.edu (S.S.); msn4002@qatar-med.cornell.edu (M.N.A.)
2. Department of Medicine, Albany Medical College, New York, NY 12208, USA; mohammi3@amc.edu
3. Department of Medicine, New York-Presbyterian Brooklyn Methodist Hospital, New York, NY 12208, USA
4. Department of Medicine, University of Pennsylvania, Philadelphia, PA 19104, USA
5. Premedical Department, Weill Cornell Medicine-Qatar, Doha 24144, Qatar
* Correspondence: dez2003@qatar-med.cornell.edu
† These authors contributed equally to this work.

Abstract: The SARS-CoV-2 virus caused a pandemic in the 2020s, which affected almost every aspect of life. As the world is recovering from the effect of the coronavirus, the concept of post-COVID-19 syndrome has emerged. Multiple organ systems have been implicated, including the liver. We aim to identify and analyze the reported cases of severe and long-term parenchymal liver injury post-COVID-19 infection. Several databases were used to conduct a comprehensive literature search to target studies reporting cases of severe and long-term parenchymal liver injury post-COVID-19 infection. Screening, data extraction, and cross checking were performed by two independent reviewers. Only 22 studies met our inclusion criteria. Our results revealed that liver steatosis, non-alcoholic fatty liver disease (NAFLD), and cirrhosis were the most reported liver associated complications post-COVID-19 infection. Moreover, complications like acute liver failure, hepatitis, and liver hemorrhage were also reported. The mechanism of liver injury post-COVID-19 infection is not fully understood. The leading proposed mechanisms include the involvement of the angiotensin-converting enzyme-2 (ACE-2) receptor expressed in the liver and the overall inflammatory state caused by COVID-19 infection. Future studies should incorporate longer follow-up periods, spanning several years, for better insight into the progression and management of such diseases.

Keywords: COVID-19; SARS-CoV-2; post-COVID-19 sequelae; long-COVID; liver injury; hepatic injury; parenchymal liver disease

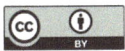

1. Introduction

A new coronavirus emerged in 2019, causing a debilitating pandemic in 2020. The coronavirus was called severe acute respiratory syndrome coronavirus 2 (SARS-CoV-2), and the disease caused was called coronavirus disease 2019 (COVID-19). The infection ranged from asymptomatic and mild to severe, with infection of lung parenchyma and multiorgan dysfunction, often affecting those with comorbidities and underlying immunodeficiency [1].

As the world recovered from the pandemic, the concept of "long COVID" or post-acute sequelae of SARS-CoV-2 infection (PASC) and "post-COVID syndrome" came about as patients who recovered from the illness experienced a wide variety of symptoms. Some of the complications were short term. Symptoms occurring between 4 and 12 weeks after infection are referred to as post-COVID-19 condition, as per the Centers for Disease Control and Prevention (CDC), whereas long COVID typically refers to issues persisting after the 12-week period [2].

The SARS-CoV-2 virus affects many organs throughout the body, and the liver and biliary system have been implicated in long COVID manifestations [3]. SARS-CoV-2 is among many viruses that are associated with liver disease. Hepatitis associated with viral hemorrhagic fevers brought on by the likes of Dengue fever, as well as fulminant liver necrosis induced by the likes of adenoviruses, are just some examples of this [4]. Herpes viruses, in their unique manner, can remain dormant and reactivate at later stages of life, causing catastrophic disease ranging from fulminant hepatitis to lymphocyte proliferation and transformation into lymphoma [4]. Similar to SARS-CoV-2, respiratory viruses such as influenza viruses often display milder symptoms that more closely represent that of SARS-CoV-2. Many patients have abnormal liver chemistries post-COVID-19 infection; however, the clinical implications and long-term manifestations of liver injury inflicted by COVID-19 are not well defined in the literature. The liver injury observed is usually classified by deriving an R-factor suggestive of a hepatocellular or cholestatic pattern of injury. Parenchymal liver injury comprises a variety of lesions that include inflammatory infiltration, hepatocellular degenerative changes, and liver cell death via necrosis or apoptosis. Inflammatory infiltration is a common characteristic in cases of hepatitis and can sometimes go unnoticed through lab studies; hence, it is confirmed via imaging. Steatosis, bile stasis, ballooning, and Mallory–Denk bodies are just some features of hepatocellular degenerative changes observed in fatty liver diseases, such as NAFLD. A clear distinction between steatosis and steatohepatitis is important to observe in these cases, given the latter's greater potential to progress to fibrosis and cirrhosis. These two characteristics can often be seen in conjunction, along with sclerosis as a long-term outcome. These characteristics often have a temporal relationship in parenchymal liver injury. Inflammation transitions to hepatocellular changes in response to the acute injury that may then progress gradually into cell death and its associated changes (fibrosis, sclerosis, etc.). Hepatocellular injury is specific to liver parenchyma, while cholestatic injury is reflective of injury that is biliary in origin. The degree of liver injury correlates to the severity of COVID-19 infection. Conversely, patients with pre-existing liver disease were noted to have an increased risk for severe COVID-19 infection and intensive care unit (ICU) admission [5]. Interestingly, non-alcoholic fatty liver disease (NAFLD) has been associated with a longer viral shedding time [5].

The objective of this systematic review is to look at the patterns and manifestations of parenchymal liver injury reported in individuals either after recovering from COVID-19 infection or those that occurred during the active infection and lasted and/or required treatment for 12 weeks or longer.

2. Materials and Methods

The preferred reporting items for systematic reviews and meta-analysis (PRISMA) statement was used to develop the protocol of this systematic review [6].

2.1. Information Sources and Search Strategy

This study is part of a large project that investigates the long-term and severe complications of COVID-19. A comprehensive search was conducted by an information professional who prioritized sensitivity to retrieve all relevant studies. The following databases were searched in October 2023: PubMed, Medline (Ovid, 1946–Current), Embase (Ovid, 1974–2021), Scopus, Web of Science, Science Direct, and Cochrane Library. The search was designed around keywords and controlled vocabulary that focused on "Long COVID" and variants (see Supplementary Materials S1 for full search details). No language or date restrictions were used. All database search results were imported into EndNote (version 19) and exported to Covidence, where duplicates were removed prior to initial screening (Supplementary Materials S1).

2.2. Eligibility Criteria

No restrictions were made based on gender, age, or country. Duplicates were removed and any articles that were not in English or did not have primary data, such as review articles, were excluded from the study. All conference abstracts were excluded, and only full articles were included. During the full-text screening, any studies that reported parenchymal liver injury were included if a clear diagnosis was reported. Any studies reporting only liver function test (LFT) derangement were excluded. We only included severe and/or long-term parenchymal liver complications. The inclusion criteria related to this point included any patients who developed a parenchymal liver injury after recovering from COVID-19. If the injury was diagnosed after at least a month post-COVID-19 diagnosis or if the study reported that anti-SARS-CoV-2 IgG but not IgM antibodies were detected, the study was included. The studies that reported parenchymal liver injury diagnosis during the active COVID-19 infection were included only if the patient did not recover from the liver injury within 12 weeks or required treatment for 12 weeks or more. The study was also included if the patient died within 12 weeks, which indicates severity. Any cases with parenchymal liver injury that were diagnosed during the active infection of COVID-19 and fully recovered within less than 12 weeks were excluded.

2.3. Study Selection and Data Collection

Title, abstract screening, and full-text screening were conducted by two independent reviewers for each study using Covidence. Disagreements were resolved by consensus. Data were extracted and cross checked by two independent reviewers.

2.4. Data Items

Demographic and clinical data, including age, sex, comorbidities, treatments, and outcomes, were collected. Continuous variables were expressed as mean ± standard deviation or range of results. Categorical variables were expressed as percentages.

2.5. Risk of Bias and Quality Assessment

The quality assessment was conducted using different methods depending on the type of study. The Newcastle–Ottawa Quality Assessment Scale (NOS) was used to assess the cohort studies [7]. The scale developed by Murad et al. was used to assess the case reports and case series [8]. Quality assessment was conducted and cross checked by two independent reviewers.

2.6. Data Analysis

The parenchymal liver disorders reported by the included studies were classified under the following categories: steatosis and NAFLD; liver fibrosis, sclerosis, and cirrhosis; hepatitis; acute liver failure; liver inflammation by imaging; hepatomegaly; and any other parenchymal liver disorders that do not fall under the above categories.

3. Results

Figure 1 shows the flow diagram of our protocol. After removing the duplicates, the titles and abstracts of 38148 studies were screened, of which 273 were selected for full-text screening. Only 22 studies met our inclusion criteria. Of the two hundred fifty-one excluded studies, one hundred thirty-four were irrelevant, eighteen had no primary data, forty-one were conference abstracts, forty-three did not have enough data, fourteen were not in English, and one was duplicate. Supplementary Table S1 summarizes the demographic and clinical data of the included subjects as well as the quality assessment score for each study [9–30].

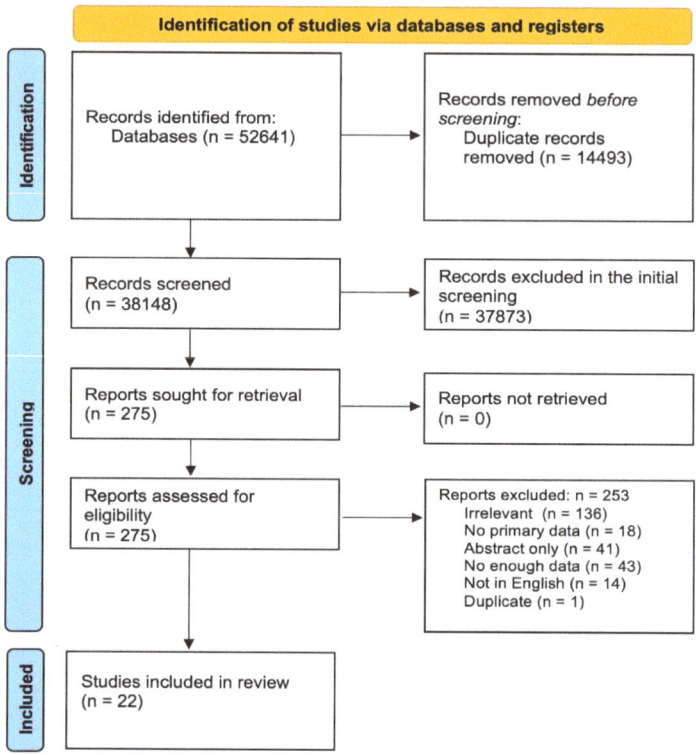

Figure 1. Protocol of database search, screening, and study selection.

3.1. Types of Studies and Demographic Data

Of the twenty-two included studies, nine were case reports, ten were cohort studies, one was a case series and one was a cross-sectional study. Among the twenty-two included studies, two were from the USA, three from India, four from the UK, two from Indonesia, two from Latvia, two from Romania, and one from Brazil, Israel, Taiwan, UAE, China, Hungary, and Italy each.

The total number of patients reported by 22 studies (case series and case reports) was 161,594. Of these patients, 500 sustained post-COVID-19 parenchymal liver disease. Approximately 48% of patients were males. Furthermore, the age of the included patients ranged from 3 months to 88 years (Supplementary Table S1).

3.2. Clinical Data

The reported disorders related to the liver parenchyma post-COVID-19 were categorized into: steatosis and NAFLD, liver fibrosis, sclerosis, cirrhosis, acute liver failure, liver inflammation by imaging, hepatomegaly, hepatitis, and other post-COVID-19 parenchymal liver diseases that do not fall under the previous groups. An overlap exists, as certain studies reported various mechanisms of parenchymal liver injury. Therefore, some studies were included under multiple categories and some patients were counted under different categories (Supplementary Table S1). Figure 2 summarizes the types of reported parenchymal injury post-COVID-19 infection and the reported outcomes.

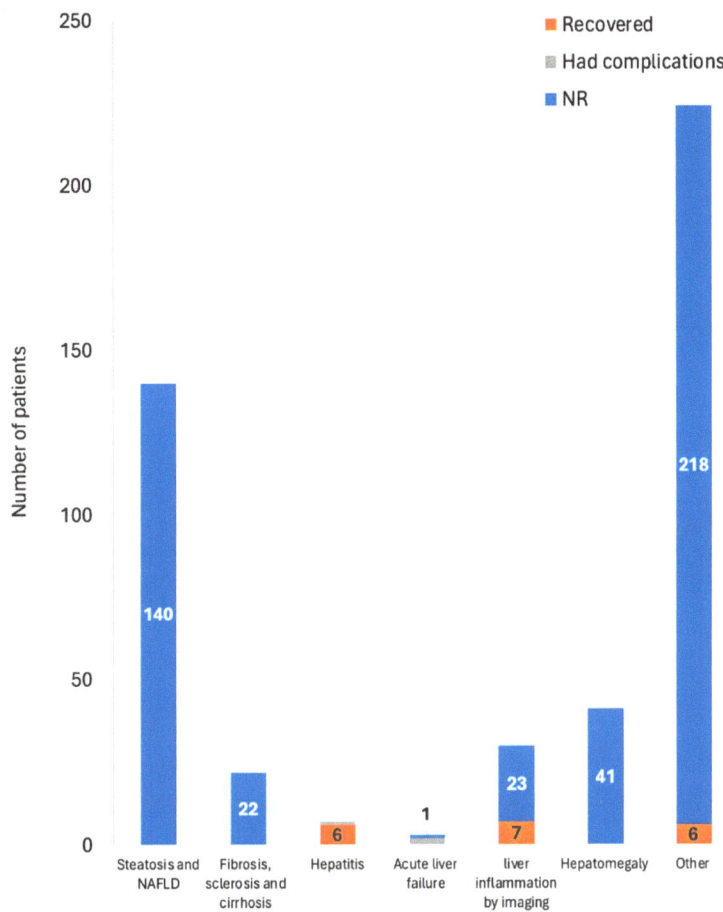

Figure 2. Types of the reported parenchymal liver injury post-COVID-19 infection and the reported outcomes. Only 1 death was reported by the 22 included studies. NAFLD: non-alcoholic fatty liver disease, NR: not reported.

3.2.1. Steatosis and NAFLD

Steatosis and NAFLD were reported by 7 studies on 140 patients whose age ranged from 52 to 74 years. This was excluding Ma et al., who reported that the hazard ratio (HR) of developing NAFLD was 1.33 (1.15 to 1.55 with $p < 0.001$) in patients who recovered from COVID-19 as compared to healthy controls.

Of the included 140 patients, 35 were reported to have steatosis, and 105 had NAFLD. The prevalence of steatosis among COVID-19 patients was 26% according to Roman et al. at the 6 month follow-up. Out of the 140 patients, 24 had severe COVID-19, but no deaths were reported (Table 1). Figure 3a summarizes the reported types of post-COVID-19 steatosis/NAFLD.

Table 1. Post-COVID-19 steatosis and NAFLD.

Study	Study Type/County	N (Total)/Gender (%M)	n/N (%)/Type of LPD	* Age (Years)	Previous Liver Disease	COVID-19 Severity	Follow-Up Time/Outcome
[11]	Prospective longitudinal study/UK	Baseline 536/(27%M)	NR Liver steatosis	NR	NR	13% hospitalized	196 (182–209) days
		Follow-up (over 1 year) 331/(27%M)	NR	NR	NR	NR	NA
[19] ^	Large-scale prospective population cohort study/UK	COVID-19 group 112,311/(45.2%M)	NR NAFLD	NR	NR	Non-hospitalized Hospitalized Severe	254 (IQR 184–366) days
		Contemporary control group 359,671/(44.6%M)	NR NAFLD	NR	NR	NR	254 (184–366) days
		Historical control group 370,979/(55%M)	NAFLD	56.94	NR	NR	254 (IQR 184–367) days
[22]	Observational cohort study/Latvia	Post-COVID-19 56/(50%M)	NR Steatosis	NR	NR	Moderate: 10/30 (33%) Severe: 7/30 (23%)	NR
		Control 34/(38%M)	NR Steatosis Fibrosis	NR	NR	NR	NR
[23] ^	Observational cohort study/Hungary	150/(54%M)	99/(66%) Steatosis (n = 147): F3: 15 F2: 29 F1: 49 F0: 54	NR	NR	83 ICU	NR
[25] ^	Prospective cohort study/Romania	78/(56%M)	58 (74%) Hepatic steatosis: 20/(26%)	NR	NR	NR 60 non-severe 18 severe	6 months
[26]	Retrospective cohort study/Italy	235/(68.9%M)	105/(77%) NAFLD	61 (52–72.5)	None	Patients with IV/NIV: 45	NR
		105/(63.8%M) No NAFLD at follow-up	NR Median reported PACS symptoms: 3	63 (52–74)	None	Patients with IV/NIV: 21 ($p = 0.9$)	As above
		130/(73.1%M) NAFLD at follow-up	NR ** NAFLD	60 (52–70)	None	patients with IV/NIV: 24	As above
[27]	Prospective cohort study/Romania	Pulmonary injury group 53/(43.4%M)	NR Steatosis	NR	None	NR	NR
		Non-pulmonary injury group 44/(31.8%M)	NR	NR	None	NR	NR

ICU: intensive care unit, IV: invasive ventilation, LPD: liver parenchymal disease, M: male, NIV: noninvasive ventilation, NAFLD: non-alcoholic fatty liver disease, NR: not reported. * Mean ± SE/Median (IQR), ** Criteria: Presence of liver steatosis (score > 36 on hepatic steatosis index) + body mass index (BMI) > 25 or type 2 diabetes militis (T2DM). Median reported PACS system: 2. ^ Includes patients with multiple types of parenchymal liver injury.

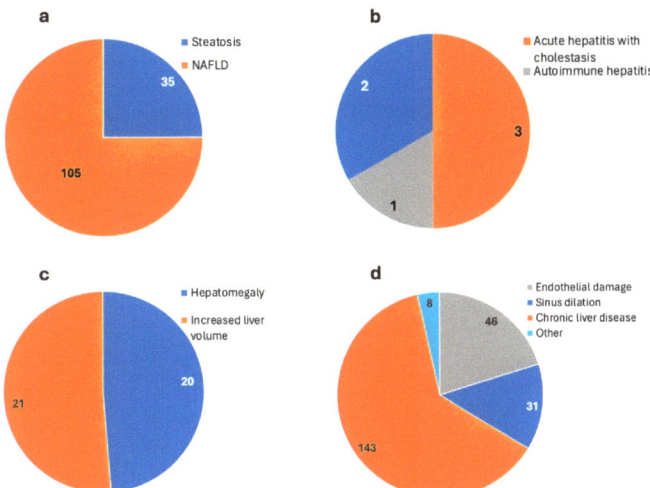

Figure 3. Types of post-COVID-19 parenchymal liver injury as reported by 22 included studies. The numbers in the figures show the reported number of patients. (**a**) Post-COVID-19 steatosis and NAFLD as reported by 7 included studies. (**b**) Post-COVID-19 acute hepatitis with cholestasis and autoimmune hepatitis as reported by 4 included studies. (**c**) Post-COVID-19 hepatomegaly and increased liver volume as reported by 2 included studies. (**d**) Post-COVID-19 endothelial damage, sinus dilation, chronic liver disease, or other disorders as reported by 11 included studies. The other disorders were reported only in 8 patients, such as autoimmune hemolytic anemia, acute liver injury with calcified liver nodule, portal venous thrombosis, liver abscesses, hemophagocytic lymphohistiocytosis, deranged LFTs with ascites, and congestive hepatopathy. Liver stiffness was also reported but the number of patients was not reported (NR). Liver fibrosis was reported in 7 patients while sclerosis and cirrhosis post-COVID-19 were reported without reporting the number of patients (4 studies). Acute liver failure was reported by 3 case reports and liver inflammation (by imaging) was reported in 29 patients by 2 studies. The last 3 categories were not presented as pie charts due to the lack of number of patients or because there were no different types to show on the pie chart. NAFLD: non-alcoholic fatty liver disease, NR: not reported.

3.2.2. Liver Fibrosis, Sclerosis, and Cirrhosis

Post-COVID-19 liver fibrosis, sclerosis, and cirrhosis were reported by four studies on 22 patients (Table 2).

Table 2. Post-COVID-19 liver fibrosis, sclerosis, and cirrhosis.

Study	Study Type/County	N (Total)/Gender (%M)	n/N (%)/Type of LPD	* Age (Years)	Previous Liver Disease	COVID-19 Severity	Follow-Up Time/Outcome
[17]	Cross-sectional, single-center study/Latvia	Acute COVID-19 group 66/(50%M)	NR Liver fibrosis	NR	NR	NR	No follow-up
		Post-COVID-19 group 58/(53%M)	NR Liver fibrosis	NR	NR	NR	No follow-up
		Control group 17/(53%M)	NR	NR	NR	NR	No follow-up

Table 2. Cont.

Study	Study Type/County	N (Total)/Gender (%M)	n/N (%)/Type of LPD	* Age (Years)	Previous Liver Disease	COVID-19 Severity	Follow-Up Time/Outcome
[19] ^	Large-scale prospective population-based cohort study/UK	COVID-19 group 112,311/(45.2%M)	NR Hepatic sclerosis or cirrhosis	NR	NR	Non-hospitalized Hospitalized Severe	254 (IQR 184–366) days
		Contemporary control group 359,671/(44.6%M)	NR Hepatic sclerosis or cirrhosis	NR	NR	NR	254 (184–366) days
		Historical control group 370,979/(55%M)	Hepatic sclerosis or cirrhosis	56.94	NR	NR	254 (IQR 184–367) days
[22]	Observational cohort study/Latvia	Post- COVID-19 56/(50%M)	NR Fibrosis	NR	NR	Moderate: 10/30 (33%) Severe: 7/30 (23%)	NR
		Control 34/(38%M)	NR Fibrosis	NR	NR	NR	NR
[23]	Observational cohort study/Hungary	150/(54%M)	99 (66%) Cirrhosis F4 fibrosis: 7 F3 fibrosis: 3 F1/2 fibrosis: 68 No fibrosis/F0: 72	NR	NR	83 cases ICU	NR

ICU: intensive care unit, LPD: liver parenchymal disease, M: male, NR: not reported. * Mean ± SE/Median (IQR). ^ Includes patients with multiple types of parenchymal liver injury.

3.2.3. Hepatitis

Post-COVID-19 hepatitis was reported by four studies on six patients whose age ranged from 8 months to 25 years. Of the six patients, none of them were reported to have severe COVID-19, all six of them recovered from liver injury, and no deaths were reported (Table 3). Figure 3b summarizes the reported types of post-COVID-19 hepatitis.

Table 3. Post-COVID-19 hepatitis.

Study	Study Type/County	N (Total)/Gender (%M)	n/N (%)/Type of LPD	* Age (Years)	Previous Liver Disease	COVID-19 Severity	Follow-Up Time/Outcome
[13]	Case report/Romania	1 M	1/(100%) Immune hepatitis	21	None	Mild COVID-19	ALT normalization 20 days after peak on follow-up
[14]	Retrospective case series/Israel	5/(100%M)					
			Patient 3: Acute hepatitis with cholestasis	8	None	Mild	4 months
			Patient 4: Acute hepatitis with cholestasis	8	NAFLD	Mild	4 months

Table 3. Cont.

Study	Study Type/County	N (Total)/Gender (%M)	n/N (%)/Type of LPD	* Age (Years)	Previous Liver Disease	COVID-19 Severity	Follow-Up Time/Outcome
			Patient 5: Acute hepatitis with cholestasis	13	None	Mild	45 days
[27]	Case report/UAE	1/(100%M)	1/(100%) Autoimmune hepatitis	33	None	Mild	7 months after hospitalization (asymptomatic)
[30]	Case report/India	1 F	1/(100%) Acute hepatitis	25	NR	Mild	5 months after presentation

ALT: alanine transaminase, F: female, LPD: liver parenchymal disease, M: male, NR: not reported. * Mean ± SE/Median (IQR).

3.2.4. Acute Liver Failure

Acute liver failure was reported by three studies on three patients whose age ranged from 3 months to 65 years. Of the three patients, none of them were reported to have severe COVID-19, and two of them had remarkable complications of NAFLD and Hemophagocytic lymphohistiocytosis following the liver insult, but no deaths were reported (Table 4).

Table 4. Post-COVID-19 acute liver failure.

Study	Study Type/County	N (Total)/Gender (%M)	n/N (%)/Type of LPD	* Age (Years)	Previous Liver Disease	COVID-19 Severity	Follow-Up Time/Outcome
[14]	Retrospective case series/Israel	5/(100%M)	5/(100%) Patient 1: Acute liver failure	Patient 1: 3-month-old	None	Mild	NR
			Patient 2: Acute liver failure	Patient 2: 5-month-old	None	NR	NR
[19] ˆ	Large-scale prospective population-based cohort study/UK	COVID-19 group 112,311/(45.2%M)	NR Liver failure	NR	NR	Non-hospitalized Hospitalized Severe	254 (IQR 184–366) days
		Contemporary control group 359,671/(44.6%M)	NR Liver failure	NR	NR	NR	254 (184–366) days
		Historical control group 370,979/(55%M)	Liver failure	56.94	NR	NR	254 (IQR 184–367) days
[20]	Case report/USA	1 F	1 (100%) Acute liver failure	68		NR	NR

F: female, LPD: liver parenchymal disease, M: male, NR: not reported. * Mean ± SE/Median (IQR). ˆ Includes patients with multiple types of parenchymal liver injury.

3.2.5. Liver Inflammation by Imaging

Liver inflammation was reported by two studies on 29 patients whose age ranged from 56 to 88 years. Of the twenty-nine patients, seven of them were reported to have severe COVID-19 but no deaths were reported (Table 5).

Table 5. Post-COVID-19 liver inflammation by imaging.

Study	Study Type/County	N (Total)/Gender (%M)	n/N (%)/Type of LPD	* Age (Years)	Previous Liver Disease	COVID-19 Severity	Follow-Up Time/Outcome
[10] ˆ	Prospective study/China	COVID-19 cohort 7/(42%M)	7/(100%) ** Liver inflammation by imaging	66 (56–88)	HLD: 0/7 (0%)	Severe	16.1 days after discharge (on average)
[12] ˆ	Prospective observational cohort study/UK	Experimental cohort (post-COVID-19 syndrome patients) 201/(29.4%M)	56/(28%) Increased liver inflammation (≥784 ms cT1) 11.5%	NR	NR	NR 19% hospitalized	NR
		Control cohort (healthy individuals) 36/(88.6%M)	NR Increased Liver inflammation (≥784 ms cT1) 0%	NR	NR	NR	NR

HLD: Hyperlipidemia, M: male, NR: not reported. * Mean ± SE/Median (IQR). ** SUVavg, SUVmax in liver—significantly higher ($p < 0.05$) vs. controls. No significant difference b/w CTmax and CTavg vs. controls. LPD: liver parenchymal disease. ˆ Includes patients with multiple types of parenchymal liver injury.

3.2.6. Hepatomegaly

Hepatomegaly was reported by two studies on 41 patients. Of the 41, 20 were reported to have hepatomegaly and 21 had increased liver volume by imaging. No deaths were reported (Table 6). Figure 3c summarizes the reported types of post-COVID-19 hepatomegaly.

Table 6. Post-COVID-19 hepatomegaly.

Study	Study Type/County	N (Total)/Gender (%M)	n/N (%)/Type of LPD	* Age (Years)	Previous Liver Disease	COVID-19 Severity	Follow-Up Time/Outcome
[11] ˆ	Prospective longitudinal study/UK	Baseline 536/(27%M)	NR	NR	NR	13% hospitalized due to COVID-19	196 (182–209) days
		Follow-up (over 1 year) 331/(27%M)	20/(14%) Hepatomegaly	NR	NR		NR
[12] ˆ	Prospective observational cohort study/UK	Experimental cohort (post-COVID-19 syndrome patients) 201/(29.4%M)	56/(28%) Increased liver volume (≥1935 mL) 10.4%	NR	NR	NR 19% of patients hospitalized	NR
		Control cohort (healthy individuals) 36/(88.6%M)	NR Increased liver volume (≥1935 mL) 2.9%	NR	NR	NR	NR

LPD: liver parenchymal disease, M: male, NR: not reported. * Mean ± SE/Median (IQR). ˆ Includes patients with multiple types of parenchymal liver injury.

3.2.7. Other Parenchymal Liver Diseases

There were 11 further studies describing various other liver diseases experienced after COVID-19 in 225 patients (Table 7). Ayoubkhani et al. described 140 patients having unspecified chronic liver disease and reported that chronic liver disease was diagnosed in 0.3% of patients after discharge due to COVID-19 infection [9]. Daid et al. reported a case of intraparenchymal liver hemorrhage in a 43-year-old, and Liemarto et al. reported a case of liver hemorrhage with abscess and necrosis in a 49-year-old patient, who passed away on the 20th day of admission (Table 6 and Figure 3d) [18,24].

Table 7. Other parenchymal liver post-COVID-19 complications.

Study	Study Type/County	N (Total)/Gender (%M)	n/N (%)/Type of HPD	* Age (Years)	Previous Liver Disease	COVID-19 Severity	Follow-Up Time/Outcome
[9]	Retrospective cohort study/UK	Experimental group (COVID-19 group) 47,780/(54.9%M)	143/(0.3%) Chronic liver disease NR	NR	NR	10% of patients needed ICU	Mean follow-up 140 ± 50 days Maximum 253 days
		Matched control group (individuals who did not test positive for COVID-19) 47,780/(54.9%M)	NR	NR	NR	NR	Mean follow-up 153 ± 33 days Maximum 253 days
[15]	Case study/India	1/(100%M)	Congestive hepatopathy	17	None	Mild COVID-19	3 months Discharged
[16]	Single-center prospective observational study/India	78/(34.6%M)	NR Deranged LFTs: 40/78 Ascites: 1/78	NR	NR	NR	No follow-up
[18]	Case study/USA	1 F	100% Intraparenchymal liver hemorrhage	43	NR	Severe COVID-19 infection	Until discharge only
[21]	Case report/Brazil	1 M	1/(100%) hemophagocytic lymph histiocytosis	57	None	Mild COVID-19 infection	NR
[23]^	Observational cohort study/Hungary	150/(54%M)	99/(66%) Endothelial damage (n = 119): F3: 46 F2: 52 F1: 21 F0: 0 Sinus dilatation (n = 119): F3: 31 F2: 52 F1: 36 F0: 0	NR	NR	83 cases requiring ICU	NR
[24]	Case report/Indonesia	1 M	1/(100%) Liver abscesses with hemorrhage and parenchymal necrosis	49	None	Severe COVID-19 pneumonia admitted to ICU	Died on day 20
[25]^	Prospective cohort study/Romania	78/(56%M)	58/(74%) Portal venous system thrombosis: 2 (2.5%)	NR	NR	NR 60 non-severe 18 severe	6 months
[27]^	Prospective cohort study/Romania	Pulmonary injury group 53/(43.4%M)	NR Liver stiffness	NR	None	NR	NR
		Non-pulmonary injury group 44/(31.8%M)	NR Liver stiffness	NR	None	NR	NR

Table 7. Cont.

Study	Study Type/County	N (Total)/Gender (%M)	n/N (%)/Type of HPD	* Age (Years)	Previous Liver Disease	COVID-19 Severity	Follow-Up Time/Outcome
[29]	Case report/Taiwan	1 F	1/(100%) Acute liver injury + calcified liver nodule	60	None	Mild	Over 3 months, LFTs trended down until returning to normal by the last follow-up visit
[30]	Case report/India	1 F	1/(100%) Autoimmune hemolytic anemia	25	NR	Mild	5 months after presentation

F: female, ICU: intensive care unit, LFTs: liver function tests, M: male, NR: not reported. * Mean ± SE/Median (IQR). ^ Includes patients with multiple types of parenchymal liver injury.

4. Discussion

Numerous studies have explored the hepatic manifestations associated with COVID-19 infection. This systematic review compiles data reporting parenchymal liver injury following COVID-19 infection to elucidate the underlying mechanisms, prevalence, and clinical implications of hepatic involvement as one of the severe and long-term complications of COVID-19.

This systematic review involves 22 studies from 13 different countries reporting 500 patients who had post-COVID-19 parenchymal liver injury. The most common manifestation was steatosis and NAFLD in addition to acute liver failure, hepatitis, fibrosis, and sclerosis.

4.1. Post-COVID-19 Steatosis and NAFLD

Non-alcoholic fatty liver disease (NAFLD), now referred to as metabolic dysfunction-associated steatotic liver disease (MASLD), encompasses a spectrum of liver conditions characterized by excessive fat accumulation in the liver without significant alcohol consumption or other secondary causes. NAFL is defined by hepatic steatosis without evidence of hepatocellular injury, such as ballooning degeneration of hepatocytes, while Nonalcoholic steatohepatitis (NASH) involves hepatic steatosis accompanied by inflammation and hepatocellular injury, which can progress to fibrosis, cirrhosis, and liver-related morbidity and mortality (Han S. et al.) [31]. The term MASLD was suggested to more accurately reflect the pathogenesis of the disease, with the diagnosis being made in the presence of hepatic steatosis and one of the following criteria: overweight/obesity, type 2 diabetes mellitus, and evidence of metabolic dysregulation [30]. The development of NAFLD is also influenced by genetic factors, with many studies having identified genetic drivers of NAFLD, beyond the established factors of metabolic syndrome and insulin resistance. Notably, the phospholipase domain-containing protein 3 (PNPLA3) and transmembrane 6 superfamily member 2 (TM6SF2) nucleotide polymorphisms were found to affect the development and progression of the disease [30]. Genes involved in carbohydrate and lipid metabolism, insulin signaling pathways, inflammatory pathways, oxidative stress, and fibrogenesis have also been linked with NAFLD/NASH development and progression [30]. Mitochondrial dysfunction is the key mediator triggering oxidative stress and is brought on by an imbalance of oxidants and antioxidants. Most notably, the uncoupling between β-oxidation, the tricarboxylic acid (TCA) cycle, and the electron transport chain (ETC) frequently results in inefficient lipid metabolism and reactive oxygen species (ROS) overproduction in the liver [32]. The capacity of antioxidant defense is further suppressed by ROS overproduction, leading to further oxidative damage [32].

Steatosis and NAFLD were among the most reported post-COVID-19 liver manifestations as reported by seven studies on 140 patients, of which 24 had severe COVID-19. Pesti et al. found that 15 of the 147 autopsies had steatosis [23]. However, a correlation between the severity of infection and the development of steatosis was not established by

Pestii et al. [23]. However, Dennies et al. reported a more frequent incidence of steatosis in symptomatic groups [11]. Roman et al. reported that 26% of the patients had steatosis at the 6 month follow-up [25]. Furthermore, they reported that patients with severe COVID-19 were more likely to have persistent alanine transaminase (ALT) elevation at 6 months compared to those with non-severe COVID-19. Bende et al. investigated the outcomes of COVID-19 patients with and without pulmonary injury, delineating that pulmonary injury correlates with a severe disease course [27]. They found that patients with pulmonary injury were more likely to have steatosis. Ma et al. reported that the hazard ratio (HR) of developing post-COVID-19 NAFLD was 1.33 (CI 95%, 1.15 to 1.55 with $p < 0.001$) as compared to healthy controls [19]. Radzina et al. used attenuation imaging (ATI) to detect steatosis and found that post-COVID-19 individuals had significantly increased steatosis compared to healthy controls [22]. Milic et al. reported that 55% of patients had NAFLD on follow-up, while only 37% were calculated to have NAFLD during the initial admission [26]. This finding correlated to the weight changes during and after COVID-19 (−6 kg during, +5 kg after), leading the authors to suggest that the loss of muscle during the acute phase and a buildup of fat in the liver during the chronic/post-acute phase is what leads to NAFLD in individuals who recovered from COVID-19 infection.

A prominent theory regarding the mechanism of liver injury is that the angiotensin-converting enzyme-2 (ACE-2) receptor serves as a gateway for the virus. The spike protein on the virus surface binds to the ACE-2 receptor, facilitating this process. The ACE-2 receptor is reported to be expressed in hepatocytes and more frequently in cholangiocytes. Although there is not much evidence that the biliary tree is affected more than hepatocytes, interestingly, it is highly expressed in the endothelial layer of small blood vessels but is absent in the sinusoidal epithelium [33]. SARS-CoV-2 competes with Ang II for binding to ACE2, and when the virus binds, it inhibits ACE2 activity and decreases its expression on the cell membrane [34]. This can potentially disrupt the balance of the renin–angiotensin–aldosterone system (RAAS), leading to angiotensin-2 mediated vasoconstriction and a decrease in angiotensin (1-7)-mediated vasodilation that may contribute to inflammation [35]. Additionally, the kallikrein–kinin system (KKS), often considered an antagonist to the RAAS, mitigates inflammatory effects by reducing the generation of reactive oxygen species and lowering blood pressure [36]. The internalization of ACE-2 due to viral binding can further disrupt this balance by increasing bradykinin levels, which can activate the bradykinin (B) 2 receptor and enhance inflammation, particularly through the cytokine storm [37].

4.2. Post-COVID-19 Liver Fibrosis, Sclerosis, and Cirrhosis

Liver fibrosis occurs due to the excessive accumulation of extracellular matrix proteins, including collagen, in the liver, as a result of chronic liver injury or persistent inflammation [38]. Cirrhosis is the most advanced stage of liver fibrosis, where extensive scarring has disrupted the normal architecture of the liver, leading to the formation of nodules and impaired liver function. It is characterized by the presence of regenerative nodules surrounded by fibrous bands [39]. Our results revealed that three studies reported fibrosis and two studies reported cirrhosis as post-COVID-19 complications. Kolesova et al. reported that 65% of patients with acute COVID-19 exhibited an abnormal Fibrosis-4 Index (FIB-4), possibly serving as a derivative for systemic inflammation, hepatocellular damage, and infection severity [17]. FIB-4 scores may have been falsely elevated in the acute setting in the setting of inflammation, and a decrease in the index was observed post-recovery. In the post-COVID-19 group, 5% had increased levels of FIB-4. A history of liver disease did not influence FIB-4 in the post-COVID-19 group, suggesting that COVID-19 infection is the cause of liver fibrosis. Therefore, it is essential to monitor liver chemistries post-COVID-19 to facilitate early diagnosis and prevent liver damage [17]. Similarly, Pesti et al. reported fibrosis post-COVID-19 in seven patients out of one hundred fifty in an autopsy study [23]. Moreover, significantly increased fibrosis, viscosity, and steatosis were reported by Radzina et al. in post-COVID-19 patients compared to controls [22]. Finally, they reported a significantly positive relationship between ALT, gamma-glutamyl transferase (GGT), and body mass index (BMI) with liver fibrosis seen on shear wave dispersion (SWD).

Conversely, Pesti et al. suggested that fibrosis is likely due to pre-existing comorbidities or treatments rather than COVID-19 infections, as they found no association with the severity of COVID-19 and fibrosis or cirrhosis [23]. They observed signs of apoptosis in histopathology slides of the liver without detectable COVID-19 protein/RNA. This suggests that liver damage may occur indirectly due to other factors such as hypoxia caused by COVID-19 rather than through direct cytopathic mechanisms.

4.3. Post-COVID-19 Hepatitis

Hepatitis is inflammation of the liver, which can be caused by various factors such as viruses, heavy alcohol use, certain medications, and autoimmune disorders. This inflammation can lead to swelling and damage to the liver, affecting its function [40]. A total of six patients were reported to have hepatitis across four studies. Most patients were asymptomatic. Daga et al. described a patient with abdominal pain and nausea, who was later diagnosed with acute cholecystitis in addition to hepatitis [30]. Shorbagi et al. also reported a patient with abdominal pain and diarrhea who was found to have ulcerative colitis, potentially confounding the clinical picture [28]. However, it was later found that the patient had ulcerative colitis-like syndrome, which may have caused the symptoms. The patient was diagnosed with autoimmune hepatitis, identified by an elevated antinuclear antibody (ANA) and anti-smooth muscle antibody titers. Three patients were reported with cholestasis along with hepatitis by Cooper et al. and Dragenescu reported a case of isolated hepatitis in a 21-year-old [13,14]. All patients had mild COVID-19, which was supportively managed.

4.4. Post-COVID-19 Acute Liver Failure

Acute liver failure is characterized by the rapid deterioration of liver function, leading to the development of hepatic encephalopathy and impaired synthetic function. This often results in coagulopathy and altered mental status in individuals without preexisting liver disease [41]. Acute liver failure was reported by three studies on three patients, excluding Ma et al., who did not report data on liver failure [19]. Cooper et al. reported that two patients, one 3 months old and one 5 months old, required liver transplant [14]. The first case had a mild infection, but both cases presented with encephalopathy and deteriorated over the hospital course, requiring liver transplantation at the end. The case reported by Anguiano-Albarran et al. also presented with encephalopathy and renal failure [20]. The patient was treated with supportive measures for liver failure with fluid resuscitation and intravenous albumin. The patient recovered and was ultimately followed-up as a case of NAFLD.

It was proposed that the cytokine storm seen in critically ill COVID-19 patients is marked by an overactive immune response leading to biliary sclerotic alterations and liver dysfunction, which in turn contributes to multiorgan failure [20].

4.5. Post-COVID-19 Liver Inflammation by Imaging

Liver inflammation is a condition characterized by the swelling and damage of liver tissue. This inflammation is the body's natural response to injury or infection [42]. Two studies reported 29 patients with liver inflammation on imaging via positron emission tomography (PET) scan: Bai et al., with magnetic resonance imaging (MRI), and Dennis et al. [10,11]. The imaging, conducted 16 days on average after discharge, showed that post-COVID-19 patients had significantly higher standardized uptake values (SUV)max and (SUV)avg compared to controls ($p < 0.05$) (Bai et al.). All patients had severe COVID-19, in addition to evidence of inflammation in various other organs. No follow-up data were reported by this study. On the other hand, Dennis et al. followed the patients over 4 months and showed that liver inflammation was detected to a greater extent in post-COVID-19 patients than controls. Furthermore, they reported that liver inflammation and fibrosis (referred to as fibro inflammation together) were associated with cognitive dysfunction.

4.6. Post-COVID-19 Hepatomegaly

Hepatomegaly is a physical finding that may suggest intrinsic liver dysfunction and is a non-specific finding in many liver-related conditions [43]. Hepatomegaly was reported by two studies on 41 patients. Dennis et al. reported increased liver volume in 10.4% of the patients who were followed after COVID-19 infection, which was significantly higher than the control group ($p < 0.0001$) [11]. Furthermore, Dennis et al. reported hepatomegaly in 20 of the patients in the follow-up cohort, and it was associated with a poor quality of life [12]. However, no specifics were mentioned regarding other symptoms or impairments. The study also mentioned that liver impairment was more common in obese individuals and women.

4.7. Other Post-COVID-19 Parenchymal Liver Disorders

Congestive hepatopathy is a liver disorder that occurs due to prolonged passive venous congestion of the liver, commonly because of right-sided heart failure [44]. Congestive hepatopathy was reported in one patient by Ahmed et al.; the patient was described to have dilated cardiomyopathy 2 weeks after his COVID-19 infection diagnosis with deranged liver chemistries, which resolved after diuresis [15]. This was attributed to either COVID-19 or drug-induced liver injury (DILI) from herbal medicine, which the patient took prior to admission. Deranged LFTs are very common following viral infections and are non-specific. Lai et al. reported a case of deranged LFTs with a calcified liver nodule seen on imaging, while Sai et al. reported a case of deranged LFTs and ascites [16,29]. However, the clinical significance and outcome were not clearly defined.

Two cases reported liver hemorrhage post-COVID-19 infection. Daid et al. described a patient who developed right upper quadrant (RUQ) pain and abnormal liver chemistries around 2 weeks after her admission for COVID-19 infection, which was treated with N-acetylcysteine [18]. The mechanism of injury was believed to involve endothelial cell damage caused by widespread vascular thrombosis accompanied by microangiopathy, as demonstrated in earlier studies [45,46]. The study suggests that physicians should consider intraparenchymal hepatic hemorrhage when encountering a patient who recovered from COVID-19 and is presenting with RUQ pain and elevated transaminase levels.

Hepatomegaly was reported by Liemarto et al. in a 49-year-old patient who presented, a month after his COVID-19 infection recovery, with abdominal pain and hepatomegaly [24]. It was found that the patient had two abscesses with hemorrhage, which were drained via an exploratory laparotomy (ex-lap). The study suggests many etiologies for liver damage after COVID-19 infection, including direct damage from SARS-CoV-2 proliferation in the liver, systemic changes due to inflammation, hypoxia, and microvascular damage [47]. It was also suggested to be drug-induced, as the patient received tocilizumab, which has been reported to cause liver injury through the IL-6 signaling relating to liver recovery [48].

Soldera et al. described a case of Hemophagocytic Lymphohistiocytosis (HLH) after COVID-19 infection [21]. HLH is a rare but severe systemic inflammatory syndrome characterized by excessive immune activation and an uncontrolled proliferation of activated lymphocytes and macrophages. This condition leads to widespread inflammation and tissue damage, affecting multiple organs [49]. The patient presented with high-grade fever, upper abdominal pain, and transaminitis. Bone marrow biopsy confirmed HLH, and it was successfully treated with etoposide, dexamethasone, and cyclosporine. Soldera et al. emphasized that severe cases of COVID-19 can result in liver injury, potentially leading to the development of HLH [21]. It is recommended to assess patients with post-COVID-19 liver injury for HLH, particularly if they exhibit a high-grade fever and have a history of rheumatic diseases. Prompt diagnosis and treatment of HLH following a COVID-19 infection are essential to avoid adverse outcomes [21].

A case of cold autoimmune hemolytic anemia was reported by Daga et al. a month after the resolution of the patient's COVID-19 infection [30]. Of note, the patient also had acute icteric hepatitis. The hypothesized mechanism involves post-infectious impact of COVID-19 causing a viral reactivation, as the patient later tested positive for Epstein–Barr virus (EBV) IgG and cytomegalovirus (CMV) IgG titers. The presence of these antibodies, along with the autoimmune hemolytic anemia and the absence of other hepatic insults, suggests a possible relationship between the post-COVID inflammatory phase and latent viral pathogens.

An association between pulmonary injury and liver stiffness was reported by Bende et al. [27]; it was revealed that patients who had pulmonary injury had significantly higher liver stiffness measured via liver elastography after 3 to 11 weeks following the subsidization of symptoms from COVID-19 infection. Therefore, it was concluded that it may be beneficial to routinely investigate patients within 12 weeks following COVID-19 infection to detect early signs of fibrosis and prevent progression.

Interestingly, Ayoubkhani et al. looked at rates of chronic liver disease after COVID-19 infection and found that chronic liver disease was diagnosed in 0.3% of patients after discharge, and this was 2.8 times more frequently diagnosed than controls [9]. However, the types of liver disease were not reported.

4.8. Study Limitations

The limitations of this study included the possible overlap between the categories of the parenchymal liver disorders and between the hepatobiliary and parenchymal injury. Patients with multiple types of injury were reported by some studies. These patients were clustered without describing the individual cases. Therefore, some patients were counted multiple times under different categories due to the inability to specify which patient had which combination of disorders. The small number of the included studies is another limitation, which is attributed to excluding conference abstracts. Only full article journal publications were selected to maintain the quality of the included studies and to avoid duplication when the work is published in both conferences and journals. Furthermore, another limitation was the small number of cohort studies as most of the included studies were either case series or case reports. This did not provide enough data to calculate the rate of incidence of parenchymal liver injury post-COVID-19 infection. However, the case reports provided enough details about the individual cases, which gave a better insight into the included cases with more details about prognosis and management.

5. Conclusions

This systematic review looked at the acute and chronic parenchymal liver complications of COVID-19. Common chronic complications that were found in patients' weeks after their COVID-19 infection included liver steatosis, fibrosis, NAFLD, and chronic liver disease. Complications like hepatitis, acute liver failure, and hemorrhage were observed shortly after recovery. Most of the patients were described as recovered or recovering from liver injury. However, two patients with acute liver failure had to undergo liver transplants, and one patient with liver abscess and hemorrhage died. The mechanism of SARS-CoV-2's direct viral attack affecting the liver centers around the expression of the ACE-2 receptor by the hepatocytes. The indirect mechanisms include the overall inflammatory state of COVID19 infection, drug side effects, and previous comorbidities. The acute complications are usually severe and should be monitored for patients who recently recovered from COVID-19. Chronic complications, like steatosis, fibrosis, and cirrhosis are typically not as symptomatic; thus, it is important for clinicians to monitor patients for these complications. The association between vaccination status and long COVID-19 liver injury is unclear, mostly due to underreporting of vaccination status in the studies. The connection between the severity of COVID-19 and the risk of long COVID-19-related liver injury is not well documented in most studies. Milic et al. found that 18% of patients who developed NAFLD required invasive ventilation, compared to 20% of those who did not develop NAFLD.

Further research is necessary to determine whether the severity of COVID-19 influences the likelihood of long-term liver complications. Further studies should focus on how comorbidities and factors surrounding the COVID-19 infection influence the development of liver complications following infection. To gain a more comprehensive understanding of liver injury in post-COVID-19 patients, future studies should incorporate longer follow-up periods, spanning several years after recovering from COVID-19.

Supplementary Materials: The following supporting information can be downloaded at https://www.mdpi.com/article/10.3390/biomedicines12092065/s1, Table S1: Demographic and clinical data for patients reported with parenchymal liver injury reported post-COVID-19 infection.; Supplementary S1: Database search strategy.

Author Contributions: Conceptualization, A.L., A.A., D.Z., M.M., L.Y. and I.M.; methodology, D.Z.; software, D.Z.; validation, D.Z.; formal analysis A.L. and D.Z; investigation D.Z.; resources, D.Z.; data curation, A.L. and D.Z.; writing—original draft preparation, A.L, A.A, N.B., B.M., S.A., S.S. and M.N.A.; writing—review and editing, A.L., L.Y., M.M. and D.Z.; visualization, D.Z.; supervision, D.Z.; project administration, D.Z.; cross-checking, M.M., L.Y., I.M., A.A. and A.L.; screening, A.L, A.A, N.B., B.M., S.A., S.S. and M.N.A.; data extraction, A.L, A.A, N.B., B.M., S.A., S.S. and M.N.A. All authors have read and agreed to the published version of the manuscript.

Funding: The publication of this article was funded by the Weill Cornell Medicine–Qatar Health Sciences Library.

Data Availability Statement: All extracted data for this systematic review are submitted as Supplementary Materials.

Acknowledgments: We would like to thank Sa'ad Laws for his help during the early phases of this project, including developing the search strategy and importing papers. We would like also to thank Weill Cornell Medicine-Qatar for the continuous support.

Conflicts of Interest: The authors declare no conflicts of interest.

References

1. Fung, M.; Babik, J.M. COVID-19 in Immunocompromised Hosts: What We Know So Far. *Clin. Infect. Dis.* **2021**, *72*, 340–350. [CrossRef] [PubMed]
2. Gottlieb, M.; Wang, R.C.; Yu, H.; Spatz, E.S.; Montoy, J.C.C.; Rodriguez, R.M.; Chang, A.M.; Elmore, J.G.; Hannikainen, P.A.; Hill, M.; et al. Severe Fatigue and Persistent Symptoms at 3 Months Following Severe Acute Respiratory Syndrome Coronavirus 2 Infections During the Pre-Delta, Delta, and Omicron Time Periods: A Multicenter Prospective Cohort Study. *Clin. Infect. Dis.* **2023**, *76*, 1930–1941. [CrossRef] [PubMed]
3. Desai, A.D.; Lavelle, M.; Boursiquot, B.C.; Wan, E.Y. Long-Term Complications of COVID-19. *Am. J. Physiol. Cell Physiol.* **2022**, *322*, C1–C11. [CrossRef]
4. Buonomano, P.; Di Stasio, G.D.; Sinisi, A.A.; Rambaldi, P.F.; Mansi, L. Gamma Emitters in the Primary or Secondary Pathologies of the Adrenal Cortex. In *Nuclear Medicine and Molecular Imaging: Volume 1–4*; Elsevier: Amsterdam, The Netherlands, 2022; Volume 2, pp. 224–238.
5. Zhao, X.; Lei, Z.; Gao, F.; Xie, Q.; Jang, K.; Gong, J. The Impact of Coronavirus Disease 2019 (COVID-19) on Liver Injury in China: A Systematic Review and Meta-Analysis. *Medicine* **2021**, *100*, e24369. [CrossRef]
6. Moher, D.; Liberati, A.; Tetzlaff, J.; Altman, D.G. Preferred Reporting Items for Systematic Reviews and Meta-Analyses: The PRISMA Statement. *Int. J. Surg.* **2010**, *8*, 336–341. [CrossRef]
7. Wells, G.A.; Shea, B.; O'Connell, D.; Peterson, J.; Welch, V.; Losos, M.; Tugwell, P. The Newcastle-Ottawa Scale (NOS) for Assessing the Quality of Nonrandomised Studies in Meta-Analyses 2021. Available online: https://www.ohri.ca/programs/clinical_epidemiology/oxford.asp (accessed on 12 August 2024).
8. Murad, M.H.; Sultan, S.; Haffar, S.; Bazerbachi, F. Methodological Quality and Synthesis of Case Series and Case Reports. *BMJ Evid. Based Med.* **2018**, *23*, 60–63. [CrossRef] [PubMed]
9. Ayoubkhani, D.; Khunti, K.; Nafilyan, V.; Maddox, T.; Humberstone, B.; Diamond, I.; Banerjee, A. Post-COVID Syndrome in Individuals Admitted to Hospital with COVID-19: Retrospective Cohort Study. *BMJ* **2021**, *372*, n693. [CrossRef] [PubMed]
10. Bai, Y.; Xu, J.; Chen, L.; Fu, C.; Kang, Y.; Zhang, W.; Fakhri, G.E.; Gu, J.; Shao, F.; Wang, M. Inflammatory Response in Lungs and Extrapulmonary Sites Detected by [18F] Fluorodeoxyglucose PET/CT in Convalescing COVID-19 Patients Tested Negative for Coronavirus. *Eur. J. Nucl. Med. Mol. Imaging* **2021**, *48*, 2531–2542. [CrossRef]

11. Dennis, A.; Cuthbertson, D.J.; Wootton, D.; Crooks, M.; Gabbay, M.; Eichert, N.; Mouchti, S.; Pansini, M.; Roca-Fernandez, A.; Thomaides-Brears, H.; et al. Multi-Organ Impairment and Long COVID: A 1-Year Prospective, Longitudinal Cohort Study. *J. R. Soc. Med.* **2023**, *116*, 97–112. [CrossRef]
12. Dennis, A.; Wamil, M.; Alberts, J.; Oben, J.; Cuthbertson, D.J.; Wootton, D.; Crooks, M.; Gabbay, M.; Brady, M.; Hishmeh, L.; et al. Multiorgan Impairment in Low-Risk Individuals with Post-COVID-19 Syndrome: A Prospective, Community-Based Study. *BMJ Open* **2021**, *11*, e048391. [CrossRef]
13. Drăgănescu, A.C.; Săndulescu, O.; Bilașco, A.; Kouris, C.; Streinu-Cercel, A.; Luminos, M.; Streinu-Cercel, A. Transient Immune Hepatitis as Post-Coronavirus Disease Complication: A Case Report. *World J. Clin. Cases* **2021**, *9*, 4032–4039. [CrossRef]
14. Cooper, S.; Tobar, A.; Konen, O.; Orenstein, N.; Kropach Gilad, N.; Landau, Y.E.; Mozer-Glassberg, Y.; Bar-Lev, M.R.; Shaoul, R.; Shamir, R.; et al. Long COVID-19 Liver Manifestation in Children. *J. Pediatr. Gastroenterol. Nutr.* **2022**, *75*, 244–251. [CrossRef] [PubMed]
15. Ahmed, M.; Green, S.R.; Sundar, D. Dilated Cardiomyopathy with Congestive Hepatopathy in Post COVID-19 PatientA Case Report. *J. Clin. Diagn. Res.* **2022**, *16*, 4. [CrossRef]
16. Sai, B.V.K.; Kumar, H.; Arun Babu, T.; Chaitra, R.; Satapathy, D.; Kalidoss, V.K. Clinical Profile and Outcome of Multisystem Inflammatory Syndrome in Children (MIS-C) Associated with COVID-19 Infection: A Single-Center Observational Study from South India. *Egypt. Pediatr. Assoc. Gaz.* **2023**, *71*, 4. [CrossRef]
17. Kolesova, O.; Vanaga, I.; Laivacuma, S.; Derovs, A.; Kolesovs, A.; Radzina, M.; Platkajis, A.; Eglite, J.; Hagina, E.; Arutjunana, S.; et al. Intriguing Findings of Liver Fibrosis Following COVID-19. *BMC Gastroenterol.* **2021**, *21*, 370. [CrossRef]
18. Daid, S.S.; Toribio, A.D.; Lakshmanan, S.; Sadda, A.; Epstein, A. Spontaneous Intraparenchymal Hepatic Hemorrhage as a Sequela of COVID-19. *Cureus* **2020**, *12*, e10447. [CrossRef] [PubMed]
19. Ma, Y.; Zhang, L.; Wei, R.; Dai, W.; Zeng, R.; Luo, D.; Jiang, R.; Wu, H.; Zhuo, Z.; Yang, Q.; et al. Risks of Digestive Diseases in Long COVID: Evidence from a Large-Scale Cohort Study. *MedRxiv* **2023**. [CrossRef]
20. Anguiano-Albarran, R.; Cain, D.; Ashfaq, M.; Modi, A.; Gautam, S. Multiorgan Failure and Omicron: A Suspected Case of Post-COVID-19 Cholangiopathy. *Cureus* **2023**, *15*, e35010. [CrossRef]
21. Soldera, J.; Bosi, G.R. Haemophagocytic Lymphohistiocytosis Following a COVID-19 Infection: Case Report. *J. Infect. Dev. Ctries.* **2023**, *17*, 302–303. [CrossRef]
22. Radzina, M.; Putrins, D.S.; Micena, A.; Vanaga, I.; Kolesova, O.; Platkajis, A.; Viksna, L. Post-COVID-19 Liver Injury: Comprehensive Imaging with Multiparametric Ultrasound. *J. Ultrasound Med.* **2022**, *41*, 935–949. [CrossRef]
23. Pesti, A.; Danics, K.; Glasz, T.; Várkonyi, T.; Barbai, T.; Reszegi, A.; Kovalszky, I.; Vályi-Nagy, I.; Dobi, D.; Lotz, G.; et al. Liver Alterations and Detection of SARS-CoV-2 RNA and Proteins in COVID-19 Autopsies. *GeroScience* **2023**, *45*, 1015–1031. [CrossRef]
24. Liemarto, A.K.; Budiono, B.P.; Chionardes, M.A.; Oliviera, I.; Rahmasiwi, A. Liver Abscess with Necrosis in Post COVID-19: A Case Report. *Ann. Med. Surg.* **2021**, *72*, 103107. [CrossRef] [PubMed]
25. Roman, A.; Moldovan, S.; Stoian, M.; Tilea, B.; Dobru, D. SARS-CoV-2 Associated Liver Injury: A Six-Month Follow-up Analysis of Liver Function Recovery. *Med. Pharm. Rep.* **2022**, *95*, 393–399. [CrossRef]
26. Milic, J.; Barbieri, S.; Gozzi, L.; Brigo, A.; Beghé, B.; Verduri, A.; Bacca, E.; Iadisernia, V.; Cuomo, G.; Dolci, G.; et al. Metabolic-Associated Fatty Liver Disease Is Highly Prevalent in the Postacute COVID Syndrome. *Open Forum Infect. Dis.* **2022**, *9*, ofac003. [CrossRef] [PubMed]
27. Bende, F.; Tudoran, C.; Sporea, I.; Fofiu, R.; Bâldea, V.; Cotrău, R.; Popescu, A.; Sirli, R.; Ungureanu, B.S.; Tudoran, M. A Multidisciplinary Approach to Evaluate the Presence of Hepatic and Cardiac Abnormalities in Patients with Post-Acute COVID-19 Syndrome—A Pilot Study. *J. Clin. Med.* **2021**, *10*, 2507. [CrossRef]
28. Shorbagi, A.I.; Obaideen, A.; Jundi, M. Post-COVID-19 Polyautoimmunity—Fact or Coincidence: A Case Report. *Front. Med.* **2023**, *10*, 1013125. [CrossRef]
29. Lai, P.-H.; Ding, D.-C. Acute Liver Injury in a COVID-19 Infected Woman with Mild Symptoms: A Case Report. *World J. Clin. Cases* **2023**, *11*, 472–478. [CrossRef] [PubMed]
30. Daga, M.; Mawari, G.; Singh, S.; Hussain, M.; Srivastava, S.; Sonika, U.; Sakhuja, P. A Case of Hepatitis: Post—Acute Sequelae of Asymptomatic COVID-19 Infection. *J. Int. Med. Sci. Acad.* **2021**, *34*, 322–325.
31. Han, S.K.; Baik, S.K.; Kim, M.Y. Non-Alcoholic Fatty Liver Disease: Definition and Subtypes. *Clin. Mol. Hepatol.* **2023**, *29*, S5–S16. [CrossRef]
32. Hong, T.; Chen, Y.; Li, X.; Lu, Y. The Role and Mechanism of Oxidative Stress and Nuclear Receptors in the Development of NAFLD. *Oxidative Med. Cell. Longev.* **2021**, *2021*, 6889533. [CrossRef]
33. Jothimani, D.; Venugopal, R.; Abedin, M.F.; Kaliamoorthy, I.; Rela, M. COVID-19 and the Liver. *J. Hepatol.* **2020**, *73*, 1231–1240. [CrossRef]
34. Glowacka, I.; Bertram, S.; Herzog, P.; Pfefferle, S.; Steffen, I.; Muench, M.O.; Simmons, G.; Hofmann, H.; Kuri, T.; Weber, F.; et al. Differential Downregulation of ACE2 by the Spike Proteins of Severe Acute Respiratory Syndrome Coronavirus and Human Coronavirus NL63. *J. Virol.* **2010**, *84*, 1198–1205. [CrossRef] [PubMed]
35. Murray, E.; Tomaszewski, M.; Guzik, T.J. Binding of SARS-CoV-2 and Angiotensin-Converting Enzyme 2: Clinical Implications. *Cardiovasc. Res.* **2020**, *116*, e87–e89. [CrossRef]
36. Madeddu, P.; Emanueli, C.; El-Dahr, S. Mechanisms of Disease: The Tissue Kallikrein–Kinin System in Hypertension and Vascular Remodeling. *Nat. Rev. Nephrol.* **2007**, *3*, 208–221. [CrossRef] [PubMed]

37. Karmouty-Quintana, H.; Thandavarayan, R.A.; Keller, S.P.; Sahay, S.; Pandit, L.M.; Akkanti, B. Emerging Mechanisms of Pulmonary Vasoconstriction in SARS-CoV-2-Induced Acute Respiratory Distress Syndrome (ARDS) and Potential Therapeutic Targets. *Int. J. Mol. Sci.* **2020**, *21*, 8081. [CrossRef] [PubMed]
38. Dawood, R.M.; El-Meguid, M.A.; Salum, G.M.; El Awady, M.K. Key Players of Hepatic Fibrosis. *J. Interferon Cytokine Res.* **2020**, *40*, 472–489. [CrossRef]
39. Ginès, P.; Krag, A.; Abraldes, J.G.; Solà, E.; Fabrellas, N.; Kamath, P.S. Liver Cirrhosis. *Lancet* **2021**, *398*, 1359–1376. [CrossRef]
40. Gregorio, G.V.; Mieli-Vergani, G.; Mowat, A.P. Viral Hepatitis. *Arch. Dis. Child.* **1994**, *70*, 343–348. [CrossRef]
41. Vasques, F.; Cavazza, A.; Bernal, W. Acute Liver Failure. *Curr. Opin. Crit. Care* **2022**, *28*, 198–207. [CrossRef]
42. Koyama, Y.; Brenner, D.A. Liver Inflammation and Fibrosis. *J. Clin. Investig.* **2017**, *127*, 55–64. [CrossRef]
43. Walker, W.A.; Mathis, R.K. Hepatomegaly. An Approach to Differential Diagnosis. *Pediatr. Clin. N. Am.* **1975**, *22*, 929–942. [CrossRef]
44. Fortea, J.I.; Puente, Á.; Cuadrado, A.; Huelin, P.; Pellón, R.; González Sánchez, F.J.; Mayorga, M.; Cagigal, M.L.; García Carrera, I.; Cobreros, M.; et al. Congestive Hepatopathy. *Int. J. Mol. Sci.* **2020**, *21*, 9420. [CrossRef]
45. Varga, Z.; Flammer, A.J.; Steiger, P.; Haberecker, M.; Andermatt, R.; Zinkernagel, A.S.; Mehra, M.R.; Schuepbach, R.A.; Ruschitzka, F.; Moch, H. Endothelial Cell Infection and Endotheliitis in COVID-19. *Lancet* **2020**, *395*, 1417–1418. [CrossRef] [PubMed]
46. Ackermann, M.; Verleden, S.E.; Kuehnel, M.; Haverich, A.; Welte, T.; Laenger, F.; Vanstapel, A.; Werlein, C.; Stark, H.; Tzankov, A.; et al. Pulmonary Vascular Endothelialitis, Thrombosis, and Angiogenesis in COVID-19. *N. Engl. J. Med.* **2020**, *383*, 120–128. [CrossRef] [PubMed]
47. Nardo, A.D.; Schneeweiss-Gleixner, M.; Bakail, M.; Dixon, E.D.; Lax, S.F.; Trauner, M. Pathophysiological Mechanisms of Liver Injury in COVID-19. *Liver Int.* **2021**, *41*, 20–32. [CrossRef]
48. Muhović, D.; Bojović, J.; Bulatović, A.; Vukčević, B.; Ratković, M.; Lazović, R.; Smolović, B. First Case of Drug-induced Liver Injury Associated with the Use of Tocilizumab in a Patient with COVID-19. *Liver Int.* **2020**, *40*, 1901–1905. [CrossRef]
49. Zoref-Lorenz, A.; Ellis, M.; Jordan, M.B. Inpatient Recognition and Management of HLH. *Hematology* **2023**, *2023*, 259–266. [CrossRef]

Disclaimer/Publisher's Note: The statements, opinions and data contained in all publications are solely those of the individual author(s) and contributor(s) and not of MDPI and/or the editor(s). MDPI and/or the editor(s) disclaim responsibility for any injury to people or property resulting from any ideas, methods, instructions or products referred to in the content.

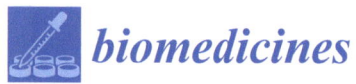 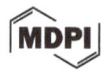

Article

Mortality Risk and Urinary Proteome Changes in Acute COVID-19 Survivors in the Multinational CRIT-COV-U Study

Justyna Siwy [1], Felix Keller [2], Mirosław Banasik [3], Björn Peters [4,5], Emmanuel Dudoignon [6], Alexandre Mebazaa [6], Dilara Gülmez [7], Goce Spasovski [8], Mercedes Salgueira Lazo [9], Marek W. Rajzer [10], Łukasz Fuławka [11,12], Magdalena Dzitkowska-Zabielska [13,14], Harald Mischak [1], Manfred Hecking [7], Joachim Beige [15,16,17], Ralph Wendt [17,*] and UriCoV Working Group [†]

1. Mosaiques Diagnostics GmbH, 30659 Hannover, Germany; siwy@mosaiques-diagnostics.com (J.S.)
2. Department of Internal Medicine IV (Nephrology and Hypertension), Medical University of Innsbruck, 6020 Innsbruck, Austria
3. Department of Nephrology and Transplantation Medicine, Wrocław Medical University, 50-556 Wrocław, Poland
4. Department of Molecular and Clinical Medicine, Institute of Medicine, The Sahlgrenska Academy at University of Gothenburg, 413 45 Gothenburg, Sweden
5. Department of Nephrology, Skaraborg Hospital, 541 85 Skövde, Sweden
6. Department of Anaesthesiology and Critical Care, Saint Louis-Hôpital Lariboisière, AP-HP, 75010 Paris, France
7. Department of Epidemiology, Medical University of Vienna, 1090 Vienna, Austria
8. Department of Nephrology, University Sts. Cyril and Methodius, 1000 Skopje, North Macedonia
9. Virgen Macarena Hospital, University of Seville, 41009 Seville, Spain
10. First Department of Cardiology, Interventional Electrocardiology and Arterial Hypertension, Jagiellonian University Medical College, 30-688 Kraków, Poland
11. Department of Clinical and Experimental Pathology, Wrocław Medical University, 50-556 Wrocław, Poland
12. Molecular Pathology Centre Cellgen, 50-353 Wrocław, Poland
13. Faculty of Physical Education, Gdańsk University of Physical Education and Sport, 80-336 Gdańsk, Poland
14. Centre of Translational Medicine, Medical University of Gdańsk, 80-210 Gdańsk, Poland
15. Kuratorium for Dialysis and Transplantation (KfH) Leipzig, 04129 Leipzig, Germany
16. Department of Internal Medicine II, Martin-Luther-University Halle-Wittenberg, 06120 Halle, Germany
17. Department of Nephrology, St. Georg Hospital Leipzig, 04129 Leipzig, Germany
* Correspondence: ralph.wendt@sanktgeorg.de
† Membership of the UriCoV Working Group is provided in the Acknowledgments.

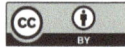

Abstract: Background/Objectives: Survival prospects following SARS-CoV-2 infection may extend beyond the acute phase, influenced by various factors including age, health conditions, and infection severity; however, this topic has not been studied in detail. Therefore, within this study, the mortality risk post-acute COVID-19 in the CRIT-COV-U cohort was investigated. Methods: Survival data from 651 patients that survived an acute phase of COVID-19 were retrieved and the association between urinary peptides and future death was assessed. Data spanning until December 2023 were collected from six countries, comparing mortality trends with age- and sex-matched COVID-19-negative controls. A death prediction classifier was developed and validated using pre-existing urinary peptidomic datasets. Results: Notably, 13.98% of post-COVID-19 patients succumbed during the follow-up, with mortality rates significantly higher than COVID-19-negative controls, particularly evident in younger individuals (<65 years). These data for the first time demonstrate that SARS-CoV-2 infection highly significantly increases the risk of mortality not only during the acute phase of the disease but also beyond for a period of about one year. In our study, we were further able to identify 201 urinary peptides linked to mortality. These peptides are fragments of albumin, alpha-2-HS-glycoprotein, apolipoprotein A-I, beta-2-microglobulin, CD99 antigen, various collagens, fibrinogen alpha, polymeric immunoglobulin receptor, sodium/potassium-transporting ATPase, and uromodulin and were integrated these into a predictive classifier (DP201). Higher DP201 scores, alongside age and BMI, significantly predicted death. Conclusions: The peptide-based classifier demonstrated significant predictive value for mortality in post-acute COVID-19 patients, highlighting the utility of urinary peptides in prognosticating post-acute COVID-19 mortality, offering insights for targeted interventions. By utilizing these defined biomarkers in the clinic, risk stratification, monitoring, and personalized interventions can be significantly improved. Our data also suggest that mortality should be considered as one possible symptom or a consequence of post-acute sequelae of SARS-CoV-2 infection, a fact that is currently overlooked.

Keywords: long COVID; PASC; biomarker; mortality; peptides; urine

1. Introduction

The life expectancy of SARS-CoV-2 survivors remains a subject of critical inquiry, affected by various factors such as age, pre-existing health conditions, and the severity of the initial infection [1]. While much attention has been directed toward understanding the acute phase of COVID-19, there is a growing recognition of the long-term health implications for those who have recovered. It has become increasingly evident that the impact of SARS-CoV-2 extends beyond the immediate symptoms experienced during the acute phase of the disease. The COVID-19 pandemic has markedly elevated global mortality [2], with a significant proportion of COVID-19 survivors facing lingering health challenges and increased morbidity in the months and years following recovery from acute infection.

Among those at risk for severe outcomes, older individuals with pre-existing health conditions such as cardiovascular disease, diabetes, and respiratory disorders are particularly vulnerable [3,4]. Studies have shown that male sex and ethnicity—specifically Black or South Asian backgrounds—as well as the severity of the initial infection correlate with higher rates of COVID-19-related death [5]. These factors contribute to a complex interplay of risks that affect the long-term prognosis of COVID-19 survivors. Some patients experience persisting or new developing disease burdens after the acute SARS-CoV-2 infection that cannot be attributed to any alternative diagnosis. This phenomenon is also documented after other acute respiratory infections but to a lesser extent [6]. Common symptoms include fatigue, shortness of breath, cognitive dysfunction, and reduced ability to perform daily activities of life, and new symptoms are also being observed [7]. The overlapping conditions and the variable onset of symptoms were recently reviewed in detail [8]. In October 2021, the World Health Organisation established the first clinical case definition for long COVID (LC), which was recently redefined [9–12]. Given the estimate that 10% of persons with SARS-CoV-2 acquire LC, there are at least 65 million individuals around the world affected [8]. Vaccination has been shown to reduce the incidence of LC [13,14]. Because of the absence of any biomarkers for LC, the diagnosis is almost entirely reliant on reported symptoms and questionnaires [15]. Investigations in large cohorts show a large variety of new or persisting symptoms in up to 45% of COVID-19 survivors [16]; however, correcting for individual pre-existing symptoms and comparing with symptom dynamics in COVID-19-negative populations during the pandemic leads to a much lower prevalence of LC [17]. The average duration of LC symptom clusters is estimated to be 9.0 months for hospitalized individuals and 4.0 months for non-hospitalized individuals, with 15.1% who continue to experience symptoms at 12 months [12]. Women are clearly more affected [12].

The pathophysiology of LC remains insufficiently understood. Persistent SARS-CoV-2 in the body has been considered a potential factor [18,19]. Patients with persisting infection showed more than 50% higher odds of self-reporting LC [20]. The COVID-19 duration was also associated with cognitive deficits after recovery [21]. Additionally, reduced serotonin levels may contribute to the neurocognitive symptoms associated with viral persistence in LC [22]. Persisting immunological dysfunction in LC patients might also play an important role [23]. Further analyses revealed significant heterogeneity and large biological diversity in LC with clusters and subsets with distinct signatures, reaching from persistent inflammation to non-inflammatory LC [23,24]. Multidimensional immune phenotyping identified discriminating biological features associated with LC [25]. Despite the growing body of research on acute COVID-19 and LC, the long-term mortality among COVID-19 survivors is poorly understood, with specific underlying mechanisms remaining elusive. It is hypothesized that the prolonged effects and ongoing physiological stress and organ damage caused by persistent COVID-19 symptoms could contribute to an increased risk of mortality, especially among those with pre-existing conditions or those who experienced severe acute infection [26]. This study seeks to address this knowledge gap by examining mortality rates among patients who have survived the acute phase of the illness and by identifying specific urinary peptides that may be associated with future death. Urinary peptides are short sequences of amino acids that can reflect pathological processes in the body, and their identification could potentially serve as biomarkers for predicting long-term health outcomes in COVID-19 survivors.

Staessen et al. in the study *"Prospective Validation of a Proteomic Urine Test for Early and Accurate Prognosis of Critical Course Complications in Patients with SARS-CoV-2 Infection"* (CRIT-COV-U) investigated urinary peptides in 1012 adults with PCR-confirmed COVID-19 [27]. The research focused on the acute phase of the disease with a median follow-up of 10 days. The authors demonstrated that it is possible to predict adverse COVID-19 outcomes within the acute phase of the illness using specific urinary peptides, and this prediction can be made within 4 days of a positive PCR test [27]. Within this study, mortality rates among patients who have survived the acute phase of COVID-19 are investigated to identify potential predictors of long-term post-acute COVID-19 mortality (PACM), including demographic factors, clinical characteristics, and laboratory parameters. Additionally, the role of urinary peptides as biomarkers of future death is examined, leveraging recent advances in proteomic technology to explore their predictive value. Detection of urinary peptides associated with future mortality could have significant implications for risk stratification and personalized care among COVID-19 survivors.

Incorporating these biomarkers into clinical practice could allow healthcare providers to better identify individuals at high risk of adverse outcomes and tailor interventions accordingly. This would ultimately improve long-term outcomes and quality of life for survivors of COVID-19, contributing to more effective management of the pandemic. By integrating advanced biomarker detection with traditional clinical assessments, the ability to predict, monitor, and manage the long-term health impacts of COVID-19 can be enhanced, ensuring that survivors receive the comprehensive care they need to mitigate future health risks.

2. Materials and Methods

2.1. Study Population

Post-acute survival data of 651 unvaccinated patients were gathered from the *"Prospective Validation of a Proteomic Urine Test for Early and Accurate Prognosis of Critical Course Complications in Patients with SARS-CoV-2 Infection"* (CRIT-COV-U) study, spanning until December 2023 across six countries and nine centers (Table S1) [27]. These patients were enrolled during the initial and subsequent waves of the pandemic in 2020–2021, predominantly infected with the wild-type virus, and had survived the acute phase of COVID-19. Urine peptide data of first urine samples collected within 3 days of a positive PCR were used. The cohort was stratified into discovery (n = 324) and validation (n = 327) sets through random partitioning. This project complied with the Helsinki Declaration. The Ethics Committee of the German–Saxonian Board of Physicians (Dresden, Germany; number EK-BR-70/23-1) and the Institutional Review Boards of the recruiting sites provided ethical approval. To assess the impact of age on mortality within this cohort, comparisons were made against age- and sex-matched data from individuals not infected with SARS-CoV-2 (n = 5192), sourced from the Human Urinary Database [28].

2.2. Urinary Peptidomics

Data were extracted from the Human Urinary Proteome Database, which contains datasets acquired using capillary electrophoresis coupled with mass spectrometry (for details on the CE-MS analysis, please see [29]) as described previously [28]. Data were evaluated using MosaFinder software (version 1.4) and normalized based on the abundance of 29 collagen peptides [30]. Of the 5071 sequenced peptides identified to date, only those present in at least 50% of the entire discovery cohort of 324 individuals (923 peptides) were retained for further analyses.

2.3. Statistical Analysis

As descriptive statistics for the samples, the median and interquartile range (IQR) were used for continuous variables and absolute (N) and relative frequencies (%) for categorical variables. Hypotheses of no differences in scale or distribution of patient characteristics between the death and non-death groups were tested with Wilcoxon–Mann–Whitney test for continuous variables and with χ^2 homogeneity tests for categorical variables. Adjustment for multiple testing was implemented according to Benjamini [31,32]. Visualized are kernel density estimates of the distribution of the scores split by mortality groups. Mortality per person–time stratified by age and DP201 groups, is estimated as the ratio of the number of the deceased to the sum of all patients' observation times within each group scaled to 100 person-years. The corresponding mortality probabilities and their 95% confidence intervals (CI) for each group represent estimates from a logistic regression including all 651 patients.

2.4. Classifier Development

A classifier combining multiple features (peptides) into a single variable was developed using support vector machine modeling as described in [33]. All peptides demonstrating a significant difference (adjusted for the false-discovery rate set at 0.05) between cases and controls were included in the classifier. Classification was performed by determining the Euclidian distance (classification score) of the vector to a separating hyperplane. The optimal parameters for C (cost of misclassification) and gamma (flexibility of the separating hyperplane) were determined via leave-one-out cross-validation error estimation, as described in more detail in [34].

3. Results

3.1. Assessment of Mortality in Acute COVID-19 Survivors

Of the 893 patients from the CRIT-COV-U study surviving acute COVID-19, follow-up data from 651 patients could be obtained (Table 1). At the time of inclusion in the CRIT-COV-U study (and urine sampling), the median age of the 651 patients was 63 years (IQR: 48–76)), with a male predominance of 53.5%. The median body mass index (BMI) recorded was 27.0 (IQR: 24.4–30.3) kg/m^2, and the estimated glomerular filtration rate (eGFR) was 90.0 (IQR: 70–111) mL/min/1.73 m^2. The majority of patients, 56.4%, had no recorded comorbidities. The entry WHO scores were 1–3 in 311 (48%) participants, 4–5 in 317 (49%) participants, and 6 in 23 (4%) participants. Throughout the follow-up period, spanning a median of 2.92 years (IQR: 2.67–3.09), pertinent data were collected to assess mortality outcomes in survivors of the acute phase of COVID-19.

Among the 651 patients who survived the acute phase of COVID-19 and could be followed up on, 91 individuals (13.98%) succumbed during the follow-up duration, with 55 (8.45%) of these fatalities occurring within the first year post-infection. In stark contrast, among the age- and sex-matched controls totaling 5192 individuals, a markedly lower proportion of 92 (1.77%) deaths were recorded within the same time frame. Notably, mortality displayed an age-dependent pattern across both cohorts, with significantly elevated rates observed among those who had survived COVID-19 compared to their COVID-19-negative counterparts (Figure 1A–E). Specifically, within the first year post-infection, mortality rates surged up to 4.7 times higher in patients younger than 65 years compared to the COVID-19-negative controls.

Table 1. Baseline cohort characteristics. Median and IQR are shown for continuous variables and absolute (N) and relative frequencies (%) for categorical variables.

	No Death (n = 560)	Death (n = 91)	*p*-Value
Age	60 (45–73)	78 (70–83)	<0.0001
BMI [kg/m^2]	27.1 (24.5–30.3)	26.5 (23.7–29.9)	0.1929
Number of comorbidities	0.0 (0.0–1.0)	1 (0.3–2.0)	<0.0001
eGFR [mL/min/1.73 m^2]	92.47 (76.00–112.17)	69 (52.00–90.00)	<0.0001
Heart rate [beats per min]	80.0 (72.0–80.0)	80.0 (70.0–86.5)	0.1827
Diastolic blood pressure [mm Hg]	78.0 (70.0–82.0)	73.0 (64.3–80.0)	0.0494
Systolic blood pressure [mm Hg]	128 (115.0–140.0)	128 (110.0–140.0.)	0.5809
sex, men (%)	289 (51.6)	58 (63.7)	0.0416
WHO score admission	3 (2–4)	4 (3–4)	<0.0001

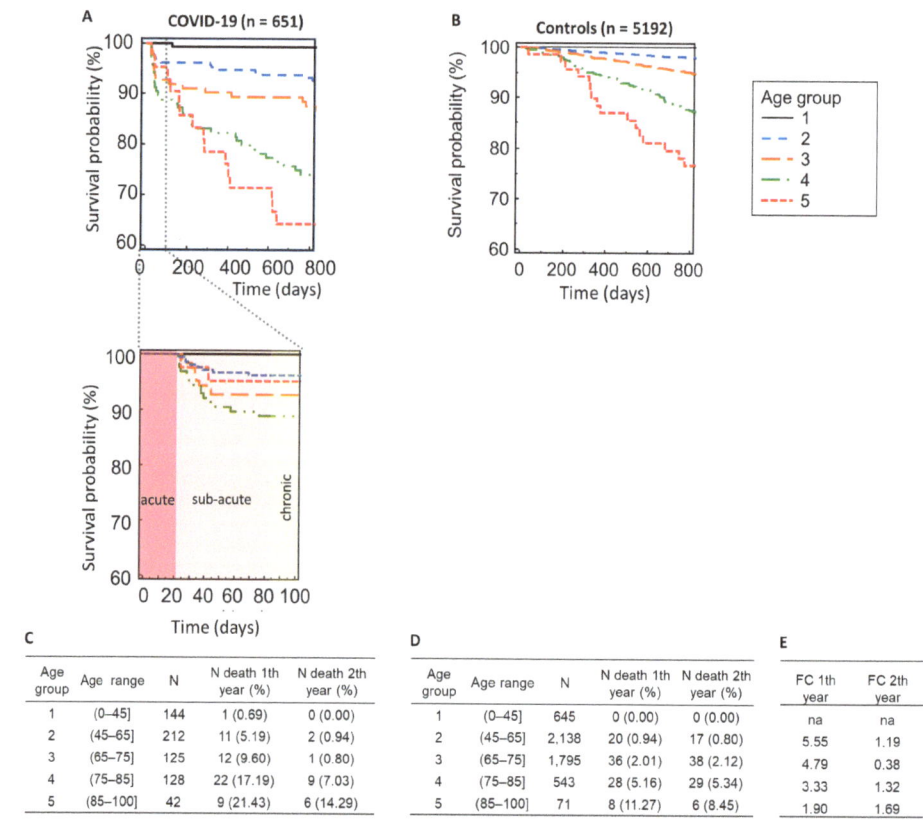

Figure 1. Age-dependent mortality in the post-acute COVID-19 cohort and healthy controls. Kaplan–Meier survival curves are shown for the cohort who survived acute-phase COVID-19 (**A**), including zoomed-in view of the acute (without detected deaths) and sub-acute phases, which highlight that only those who survived the acute phase were followed up, and age- and sex-matched COVID-19-negative healthy controls (**B**). The number of deaths per age group in the post-acute COVID-19 cohort (**C**) and controls (**D**) as well as the calculated fold change (FC) between the COVID-19 and controls (**E**) is given.

3.2. Identification of Biomarkers Associated with Post-Acute COVID-19 Mortality

For the identification of biomarkers potentially associated with mortality after surviving the initial acute phase of COVID-19, the previously acquired urinary peptidomics datasets from baseline samples of COVID-19-diagnosed patients within the CRIT-COV-U study were utilized. These datasets were stratified into discovery (n = 324) and validation cohort (n = 327) sets through random partitioning. Urinary peptides potentially associated with PACM were defined by applying the Mann–Whitney test to compare 44 deceased and 280 surviving patients within the discovery set. Subsequently, adjustments for multiple testing were implemented to ensure statistical robustness.

The analysis of urinary peptidome datasets within the discovery set enabled the identification of 201 peptides (listed in Table S2) as significantly associated with PACM when comparing deceased and surviving patients. These peptides encompassed upregulated fragments of albumin, alpha-2-HS-glycoprotein, apolipoprotein A-I, and beta-2-microglobulin, alongside downregulated fragments of CD99 antigen, various collagens, fibrinogen alpha, polymeric immunoglobulin receptor, sodium/potassium-transporting ATPase, and uromodulin. Among these peptides, 14 overlapped with the previously established Cov50 classifier designed for prognosticating unfavorable COVID-19 outcomes during the acute phase [35].

3.3. Establishment and Validating a Classifier Predicting Post-Acute COVID-19 Mortality

The 201 peptides significantly associated with PACM were combined to form a support-vector machine-based classifier (DP201). This classifier enabled separating the discovery set with 80% sensitivity and 83% specificity upon complete leave-one-out cross-validation (area under the curve (AUC) = 0.86, Figure 2A). Subsequently, this classifier was applied to the independent validation cohort, consisting of 47 deceased and 280 surviving patients, which resulted in significant separation of the groups with an AUC of 0.78, as shown in Figure 2B.

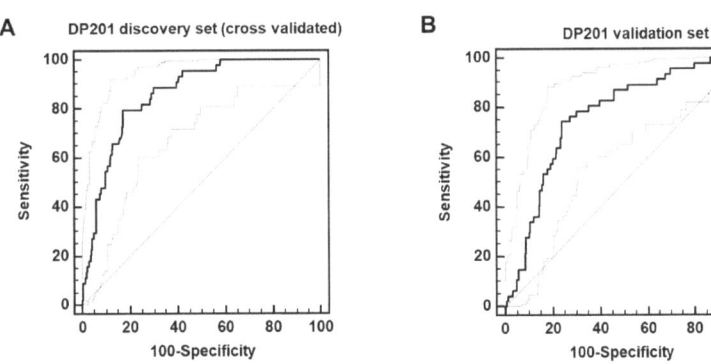

Figure 2. ROC curves (displayed as solid lines) for the classification of the deceased and surviving patients in the complete leave-one-out cross-validated discovery cohort (**A**) and independent validation cohort (**B**). Dotted lines display 95% confidence bounds.

The resultant outcomes in relation to follow-up time are depicted in Figure 3A,B, illustrating a clear correlation between higher classification scores and heightened mortality risk. Further Cox regression analysis revealed that age, BMI, and DP201 were significantly associated with PACM, while sex, number of comorbidities, eGFR, and COVID-19 WHO score did not exhibit statistical significance. Integration of these three parameters into Cox's model yielded a hazard ratio of 6.28 (95%CI: 3.54–11.44) compared to age and DP201 alone (Figure 3C,D).

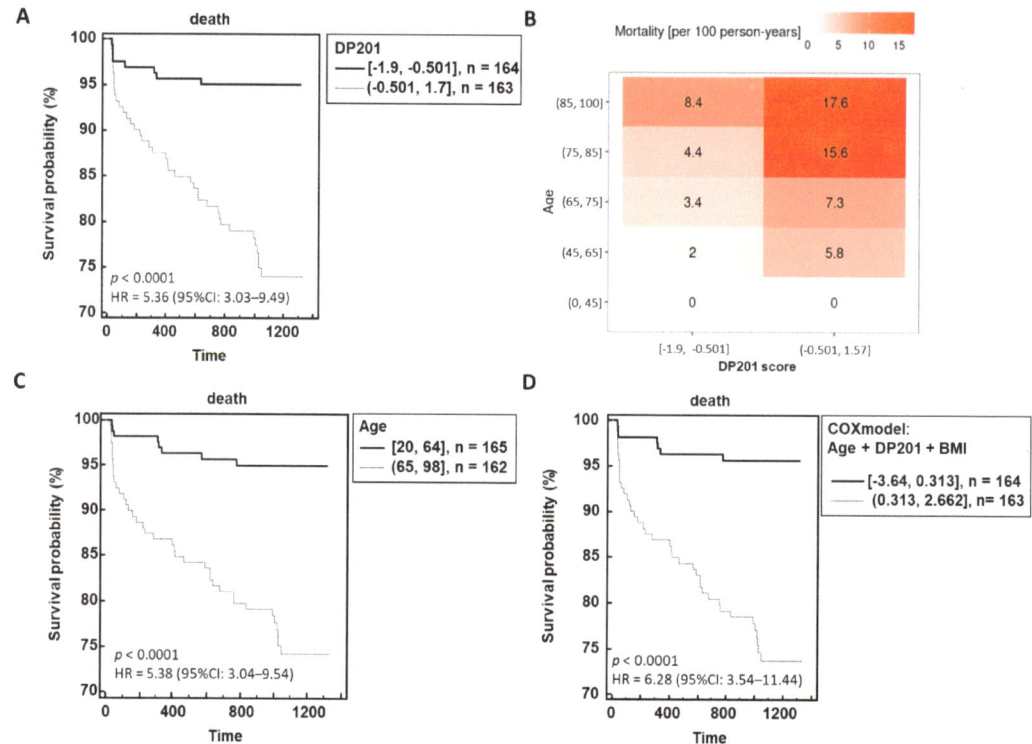

Figure 3. Performance of the urinary peptide-based death prediction classifier in the independent validation data. The risk of death is significant dependent on the DP201 score (**A**) although the age dependency can still be observed (**B**). The hazard ratio for survival probability DP201 classifier (**A**) and age (**C**) could be increased using a model including DP201, age, and BMI (**D**).

4. Discussion

Our findings first and foremost demonstrate that COVID-19 is associated with a highly significantly increased risk of mortality even after the acute phase of the disease. To date, this issue was apparently not well-covered by the studies, which either investigated the immediate outcome of the acute infection or the long-term effect in the context of the post-acute sequelae of SARS-CoV-2 infection (PASC). However, PASC was typically only assessed in patients still alive. Our data indicate that a significant number of patients may have died as a result of the consequences associated with the previous SARS-CoV-2 infection. The mortality in post-acute COVID-19 patients was significantly higher than in age- and sex-matched controls and the deaths could be potentially labeled as PASC-related deaths.

A retrospective analysis of 13,638 patients with COVID-19 hospitalization documented a significantly increased risk for future mortality; increased 12-month mortality was observed in patients with severe COVID-19 compared to COVID-19-negative patients, which was concluded to be an under-investigated sequela of COVID-19 [36].

Another large retrospective analysis of long-term outcomes of 22,571 adult patients hospitalized due to COVID-19 in Austria in the year 2020 found an increased mortality compared to 217,295 propensity score matched controls [37]. Similar to our results, the difference between patients and controls remained significant in the younger age groups (41–64 years and 65–74 years, $p < 0.001$) but not in the oldest age group ($p = 0.078$) [37].

An investigation was conducted on the long-term risks in over 800,000 COVID-19 patients compared the risk of post-discharge death with 56,409 Influenza patients as a historical control; patients who were discharged alive from a COVID-19-related hospitalization admission had nearly twice the risk of post-discharge death compared to historical controls admitted to hospital with influenza [38].

Data from a large study with 47,780 English patients discharged alive after COVID-19 hospitalization showed an increased risk of readmission and mortality during a follow-up of 140 days. The post-discharge mortality risk was eight times greater than in matched controls and with the largest differences in the age group < 70 years [26].

A report from the US investigated the mortality after recovery from the initial episode of COVID-19 and reported a significantly higher 24-month-adjusted all-cause mortality risk for patients with severe COVID-19 compared to COVID-19-negative comparators (HR 2.01). The risk of excess death was highest during days 0 to 90 after infection (aHR 6.36) and still elevated during days 91 to 180 (aHR 1.18). Beyond 180 days after infection there was no excess mortality during the next 1.5 years [39]. A recent large US cohort of 135,161 people with SARS-CoV-2 infection and 5,206,835 controls were followed for 3 years to estimate risks of death and PASC. Among non-hospitalized individuals, the increased risk of death was no longer present after the first year of infection, while among hospitalized individuals, risk of death was high in the first year (incidence rate ratio: 3.17) and declined but remained significantly elevated even in the third year after infection (IRR 1.29) [40].

SARS-CoV-2 infection obviously poses a persistent threat to individuals even beyond the acute phase. Importantly, among those who successfully navigate the acute phase of COVID-19, the risk of mortality escalates significantly during the subsequent follow-up period. Particularly noteworthy is the observation that within the first year following infection, mortality rates surge dramatically among individuals who have survived the acute phase of the illness when compared to a COVID-19-negative control cohort. What is striking is that this increase in mortality risk is most pronounced among younger individuals, highlighting a concerning trend that defies conventional assumptions regarding age-related vulnerability to severe outcomes. The most abundant significantly changed peptides in patients experiencing death during follow-up are derived from β2-microglobulin (B2M). Higher B2M serum concentrations are associated with higher mortality in the general population, non-dialyzed chronic kidney disease patients, and patients receiving hemodialysis (HD) [41].

The data also show a consistently higher level of uromodulin peptides in patients without event. This is in very good agreement with a recent study presented by Vasquez-Rios and colleagues, where increased levels of uromodulin were found associated with a lower risk of cardiovascular death [42]

Thymosin beta4 (TB4) is an abundant actin-sequestering protein that has been described in the context of multiple (patho)physiological processes, among others, including wound healing, angiogenesis, and migration, to name just a few. It has also been described as increased in kidney disease, with the highest levels detected in patients with end-stage kidney disease [43]. Drum and colleagues found TB4 to be significantly increased in women with heart failure with preserved ejection fraction and associated with mortality. The strict association with female sex may be the result of TB4 being an X-linked gene product, which consequently is also found higher in women [44].

The Sodium/potassium-transporting ATPase subunit gamma (FYXD2) is found to be highly expressed in the kidney distal tubulus. In previous studies, a reduced abundance of peptides derived from FYXD2 has been observed as associated with the progression of CKD, specifically of IgA nephropathy [45].

Reduced levels of a peptide derived from S100A9 consequently reduced degradation of this protein and likely results in increased levels of calprotectin, which was described as associated with an increased risk of mortality [46].

Reduced abundance of peptides from the polymeric immunoglobulin (PIGR) receptor was previously found associated with acute COVID-19 mortality [35]. Similarly, increased complement activation, which result in an increase in complement-derived urine peptides, was also described as associated with increased COVID-19 mortality [47].

The most pronounced effect is on collagen fragments, with both an increase and decrease in specific collagen-derived peptides being observed. A change in collagen peptides has been described for multiple diseases and was also found to be associated with mortality, including mortality in the context of COVID-19 [27,48]. As observed here, both the up- and downregulation of collagen fragments were observed. This was interpreted as disruption of collagen degradation, leading to increased fibrosis. Two urinary peptide-based classifiers, CKD273 [49] and FPP_BH29 [50]—both based on multiple specific collagen peptides—were presented as highly significantly associated with fibrosis. To investigate if the changes observed in this study are associated with increased fibrosis, we applied these two classifiers onto the data and compared the scoring in the survivors vs. patients experiencing death in follow-up. As shown in Figure 4, we observe a highly significant increase in both scores, indicating increased fibrosis in the case group.

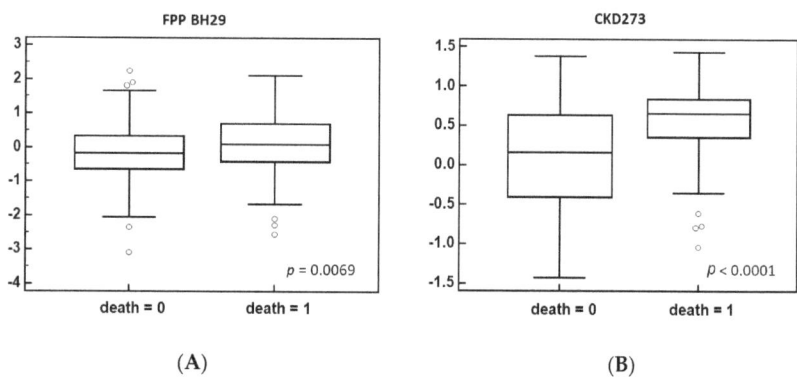

Figure 4. Distribution of the classification scores between the deceased and surviving patients for the fibrosis-related classifier FPP BH29 (**A**) and CKD273 classifier (**B**).

Also, a consistent reduction in CD99 was observed in severe cases of COVID-19, where a significant reduction in CD99 also was found on the surface of peripheral blood lymphocytes [51]. Based on the data, the authors hypothesized that reduction in CD99 may have a negative impact on the endothelial barrier integrity, a well-known phenomenon in severe COVID-19.

The increase in urinary albumin, fetuin, and apolipoprotein A1 may all be consequences of a similar underlying mechanism: endothelial dysfunction resulting in a loss of functionality of the glomerular filtration barrier. In fact, an increase in albuminuria is well-known and associated with an increased risk of mortality.

The increase in alpha 1 antitrypsin, a major plasma inflammatory protein, was found associated with increased mortality in the Nagahama study based on 9682 subjects [52]. This is in line with the observed increase associated with PACM in our study, which may be further exacerbated by the proteinuria, as mentioned above.

Furthermore, the identification of specific urinary peptides capable of predicting heightened mortality risk at the outset of SARS-CoV-2 infection underscores the intricate interplay between molecular biomarkers and clinical outcomes. These peptides serve as early indicators of the likelihood of mortality, providing valuable insights into the underlying pathophysiological mechanisms driving adverse outcomes in COVID-19 patients. By leveraging these predictive biomarkers, healthcare professionals can proactively identify individuals at elevated risk of mortality and implement targeted interventions aimed at mitigating this risk, thereby potentially altering the trajectory of the disease course, like already shown for chronic kidney and heart diseases [53].

A shortcoming of this study may be that the patients investigated were not immunized against SARS-CoV-2 as at the time of the initial study, the vaccine was generally not available. While mortality due to acute COVID-19 has been reduced dramatically as a result of immunization, it is not certain that immunity protects from PACM equally well, and this needs to be investigated in a subsequent study.

5. Conclusions

Our findings underscore the multifaceted nature of SARS-CoV-2 infection, extending far beyond the acute phase and exerting a lasting impact on mortality outcomes. The acute phase of COVID-19 appears to initiate a complex disease trajectory in many survivors. Apparently, recovery from the acute phase does not necessarily equate to a return to pre-infection health. Instead, many survivors experience ongoing health challenges, often referred to "long COVID" or PASC, which includes persistent fatigue, cardiovascular complications, cognitive impairments, and other chronic conditions. Our study adds mortality risk in COVID-19 survivors to the list of symptoms. This risk is driven by the interplay between demographic factors (such as age), pre-existing health conditions (like cardiovascular disease, diabetes mellitus, and respiratory disorders), and molecular changes, detectable in the urinary peptidome. Understanding these interactions may help in identifying individuals who are at higher risk of adverse outcomes, enabling more precise and effective healthcare interventions.

The identified predictive biomarkers represent a significant advancement in our ability to foresee and manage long-term health risks in COVID-19 survivors. These biomarkers offer a window into the biological processes that continue to affect patients long after the initial infection has resolved. The approach applied here not only enhances our understanding of the disease but also holds the promise of improving monitoring and treatment of COVID-19 survivors. By integrating predictive biomarkers into clinical practice, a more effective risk stratification and personalized interventions can be achieved. Personalized interventions, informed by a patient's unique biomarker profile [53], can improve management strategies and optimize treatment plans, ultimately leading to better health outcomes.

This research lays the groundwork for improved clinical management and patient outcomes by providing a robust framework for predicting and mitigating long-term risks associated with SARS-CoV-2 infection, consequently offering a path toward more proactive and patient-centered care. By focusing on the long-term health of COVID-19 survivors, their quality of life can be enhanced and mortality rates could be reduced.

Supplementary Materials: The following supporting information can be downloaded at: https://www.mdpi.com/article/10.3390/biomedicines12092090/s1, Table S1: Distribution of patients across participating enters; Table S2: Urinary peptides significantly associated with PACM.

Author Contributions: Conceptualization, J.S., R.W. and the UriCoV working group; methodology, J.S., R.W., F.K. and J.B.; software, H.M.; validation, J.S. and R.W.; formal analysis, F.K.; investigation and resources, J.S., R.W., F.K., M.B., B.P., E.D., A.M., D.G., G.S., M.S.L., M.W.R., Ł.F., M.D.-Z., M.H. and the UriCoV working group; resources and data curation, J.S., F.K. and the UriCoV working group; writing—original draft preparation, J.S., R.W. and J.B.; writing—review and editing, J.S., R.W., F.K., B.P., H.M. and J.B.; visualization, F.K. and J.S.; funding acquisition, J.S., R.W., M.B., A.M., B.P., H.M., M.H. and J.B. All authors have read and agreed to the published version of the manuscript.

Funding: This project was supported by the Federal Ministry of Health (BMG) via grant number 2523FSB114; by the German Ministry for Education and Science (BMBF) via grant 01KU2309; by the Sweden's innovation agency (Vinnova) via grant 2022-00542; by the National Centre for Research and Development (Narodowe Centrum Badań i Rozwoju) via grant number: PerMed/V/80/UriCov/2023; by the Austrian Science Fund (FWF) via Project number I 6464, Grant-DOI 10.55776/I6464; by the French National Research Agency—Agence Nationale de la Recherche (ANR)—under the grant ANR-22-PERM-0014; and in part by the Austrian Science Fund (FWF) via Project number I 6471, Grant-DOI 10.55776/I6471 under the frame of ERA PerMed.

Institutional Review Board Statement: This study was conducted in accordance with the Declaration of Helsinki and approved by the Institutional Review Board (or Ethics Committee) of the German–Saxonian Board of Physicians (Dresden, Germany; number EK-BR-70/23-1) and the Institutional Review Boards of the recruiting sites.

Informed Consent Statement: Informed consent was obtained from all subjects involved in this study.

Data Availability Statement: The data that support the findings of this study are available on request from the corresponding author.

Acknowledgments: UriCoV Working Group: Justyna Siwy, Mosaiques Diagnostics GmbH, Hannover, Germany; Ralph Wendt, Department of Nephrology, St. Georg Hospital, Leipzig, Germany; Joachim Beige, Division of Nephrology, St. Georg Hospital, Leipzig, Department of Internal Medicine II, Martin-Luther-University Halle-Wittenberg, Halle, Germany, and Kuratorium for Dialysis and Transplantation (KfH) Leipzig, Leipzig, Germany; Miroslaw Banasik, Department of Nephrology and Transplantation Medicine, Wrocław Medical University, Wroclaw, Poland; Björn Peters, Department of Molecular and Clinical Medicine, Institute of Medicine, the Sahlgrenska Academy at University of Gothenburg, Gothenburg, Sweden, and Department of Nephrology, Skaraborg Hospital, Region Västra Götaland, Skövde, Sweden; Emmanuel Dudoignon, Hospital Saint Louis-Lariboisière, Paris, France; Dilara Gülmez, Lenka Grula, Amelie Kurnikowski, and Manfred Hecking, all from the Department of Epidemiology, Medical University of Vienna, Vienna, Austria; Magdalena Krajewska, Justyna Zachciał, Dorota Bartoszek, Patryk Wawrzonkowski, and Krzysztof Wiśnicki from the Department of Nephrology and Transplantation Medicine, Wrocław Medical University, Wroclaw, Poland; Emelie Sarenmalm, Department of Infectious Diseases, Skaraborg Hospital, Region Västra Götaland, Skövde, Sweden; Åsa Nilsson, Research, Education, Development, and Innovation Department, Skaraborg Hospital, Skövde, Sweden; Goce Spasovski, University Sts. Cyril and Methodius, Skopje, Republic of North Macedonia; Mercedes Salgueira Lazo, Virgen Macarena Hospital and University of Seville, Sevill, Spain; Maria Isabel García Sánchez, Biobank Node at Virgen Macarena Hospital, Seville, integrated in the Spanish National Biobanks Network (PT23/00134); Marek W Rajzer from the First Department of Cardiology, Interventional Electrocardiology and Arterial Hypertension, Jagiellonian University Medical College, Kraków, Poland; Beata Czerwieńska, from the Department of Nephrology, Endocrinology, and Metabolic Diseases, Medical University of Silesia, Katowice, Poland; Magdalena Dzitkowska—Zabielska from the Faculty of Physical Education, Gdańsk University of Physical Education and Sport and Centre of Translational Medicine, Medical University of Gdańsk, Gdańsk, Poland; Łukasz Fuławka from Molecular Pathology Centre Cellgen, Wrocław, Poland; Elena Nowacki, University of Patients–Sorbonne University, Paris, France; Catherine Tourette-Turgis, University of Patients, research chair "Compétences & vulnérabilités" Sorbonne University, France; Morgane Michel, Université Paris Cité, ECEVE, UMR 1123, Inserm, Paris, France; Assistance Publique-Hôpitaux de Paris, Hôpital Robert Debré, Unité d'épidémiologie clinique, Paris, France.

Conflicts of Interest: H.M. is the co-founder and co-owner of Mosaiques Diagnostics. J.S. is employed by Mosaiques Diagnostics GmbH. All other authors declare no conflicts of interest. Authors must identify and declare any personal circumstances or interests that may be perceived as inappropriately influencing the representation or interpretation of reported research results. The funders had no role in the design of the study; in the collection, analyses, or interpretation of data; in the writing of the manuscript; or in the decision to publish the results.

References

1. Zhang, X.; Wang, F.; Shen, Y.; Zhang, X.; Cen, Y.; Wang, B.; Zhao, S.; Zhou, Y.; Hu, B.; Wang, M.; et al. Symptoms and Health Outcomes Among Survivors of COVID-19 Infection 1 Year After Discharge From Hospitals in Wuhan, China. *JAMA Netw. Open* **2021**, *4*, e2127403. [CrossRef] [PubMed]
2. GBD 2021 Demographics Collaborators. Global age-sex-specific mortality, life expectancy, and population estimates in 204 countries and territories and 811 subnational locations, 1950–2021, and the impact of the COVID-19 pandemic: A comprehensive demographic analysis for the Global Burden of Disease Study 2021. *Lancet* **2024**, *403*, 1989–2056.
3. Williamson, E.J.; Walker, A.J.; Bhaskaran, K.; Bacon, S.; Bates, C.; Morton, C.E.; Curtis, H.J.; Mehrkar, A.; Evans, D.; Inglesby, P.; et al. Factors associated with COVID-19-related death using OpenSAFELY. *Nature* **2020**, *584*, 430–436. [CrossRef]
4. Docherty, A.B.; Harrison, E.M.; Green, C.A.; Hardwick, H.E.; Pius, R.; Norman, L.; Holden, K.A.; Read, J.M.; Dondelinger, F.; Carson, G.; et al. Features of 20,133 UK patients in hospital with covid-19 using the ISARIC WHO Clinical Characterisation Protocol: Prospective observational cohort study. *BMJ* **2020**, *369*, m1985. [CrossRef]

5. Apea, V.J.; Wan, Y.I.; Dhairyawan, R.; Puthucheary, Z.A.; Pearse, R.M.; Orkin, C.M.; Prowle, J.R. Ethnicity and outcomes in patients hospitalised with COVID-19 infection in East London: An observational cohort study. *BMJ Open* **2021**, *11*, e042140. [CrossRef]
6. Vivaldi, G.; Pfeffer, P.E.; Talaei, M.; Basera, T.J.; Shaheen, S.O.; Martineau, A.R. Long-term symptom profiles after COVID-19 vs. other acute respiratory infections: An analysis of data from the COVIDENCE UK study. *EClinicalMedicine* **2023**, *65*, 102251. [CrossRef] [PubMed]
7. Morin, L.; Savale, L.; Pham, T.; Colle, R.; Figueiredo, S.; Harrois, A.; Gasnier, M.; Lecoq, A.L.; Meyrignac, O.; Noel, N.; et al. Four-Month Clinical Status of a Cohort of Patients After Hospitalization for COVID-19. *JAMA* **2021**, *325*, 1525–1534.
8. Davis, H.E.; McCorkell, L.; Vogel, J.M.; Topol, E.J. Long COVID: Major findings, mechanisms and recommendations. *Nat. Rev. Microbiol.* **2023**, *21*, 133–146. [CrossRef]
9. Ely, E.W.; Brown, L.M.; Fineberg, H.V. Long Covid Defined. *N. Engl. J. Med.* **2024**. [CrossRef]
10. Thaweethai, T.; Jolley, S.E.; Karlson, E.W.; Levitan, E.B.; Levy, B.; McComsey, G.A.; McCorkell, L.; Nadkarni, G.N.; Parthasarathy, S.; Singh, U.; et al. Development of a Definition of Postacute Sequelae of SARS-CoV-2 Infection. *JAMA* **2023**, *329*, 1934–1946. [CrossRef]
11. Chou, R.; Herman, E.; Ahmed, A.; Anderson, J.; Selph, S.; Dana, T.; Williams, L.; Ivlev, I. Long COVID Definitions and Models of Care: A Scoping Review. *Ann. Intern. Med.* **2024**, *177*, 929–940. [CrossRef] [PubMed]
12. Wulf, H.S.; Abbafati, C.; Aerts, J.G.; Al-Aly, Z.; Ashbaugh, C.; Ballouz, T.; Blyuss, O.; Bobkova, P.; Bonsel, G.; Borzakova, S.; et al. Estimated Global Proportions of Individuals With Persistent Fatigue, Cognitive, and Respiratory Symptom Clusters Following Symptomatic COVID-19 in 2020 and 2021. *JAMA* **2022**, *328*, 1604–1615.
13. Ayoubkhani, D.; Bosworth, M.L.; King, S.; Pouwels, K.B.; Glickman, M.; Nafilyan, V.; Zaccardi, F.; Khunti, K.; Alwan, N.A.; Walker, A.S. Risk of Long COVID in People Infected With Severe Acute Respiratory Syndrome Coronavirus 2 after 2 Doses of a Coronavirus Disease 2019 Vaccine: Community-Based, Matched Cohort Study. *Open Forum Infect. Dis.* **2022**, *9*, ofac464. [CrossRef] [PubMed]
14. Xie, Y.; Choi, T.; Al-Aly, Z. Postacute Sequelae of SARS-CoV-2 Infection in the Pre-Delta, Delta, and Omicron Eras. *N. Engl. J. Med.* **2024**, *391*, 515–525. [CrossRef] [PubMed]
15. Klok, F.A.; Boon, G.J.A.M.; Barco, S.; Endres, M.; Geelhoed, J.J.M.; Knauss, S.; Rezek, S.A.; Spruit, M.A.; Vehreschild, J.; Siegerink, B. The Post-COVID-19 Functional Status scale: A tool to measure functional status over time after COVID-19. *Eur. Respir. J.* **2020**, *56*, 2001494. [CrossRef]
16. O'Mahoney, L.L.; Routen, A.; Gillies, C.; Ekezie, W.; Welford, A.; Zhang, A.; Karamchandani, U.; Simms-Williams, N.; Cassambai, S.; Ardavani, A.; et al. The prevalence and long-term health effects of Long Covid among hospitalised and non-hospitalised populations: A systematic review and meta-analysis. *EClinicalMedicine* **2023**, *55*, 101762. [CrossRef]
17. Ballering, A.V.; van Zon, S.K.R.; Olde Hartman, T.C.; Rosmalen, J.G.M. Persistence of somatic symptoms after COVID-19 in the Netherlands: An observational cohort study. *Lancet* **2022**, *400*, 452–461. [CrossRef]
18. Tejerina, F.; Catalan, P.; Rodriguez-Grande, C.; Adan, J.; Rodriguez-Gonzalez, C.; Munoz, P.; Aldamiz, T.; Diez, C.; Perez, L.; Fanciulli, C.; et al. Post-COVID-19 syndrome. SARS-CoV-2 RNA detection in plasma, stool, and urine in patients with persistent symptoms after COVID-19. *BMC Infect. Dis.* **2022**, *22*, 211. [CrossRef]
19. Stein, S.R.; Ramelli, S.C.; Grazioli, A.; Chung, J.Y.; Singh, M.; Yinda, C.K.; Winkler, C.W.; Sun, J.; Dickey, J.M.; Ylaya, K.; et al. SARS-CoV-2 infection and persistence in the human body and brain at autopsy. *Nature* **2022**, *612*, 758–763. [CrossRef]
20. Ghafari, M.; Hall, M.; Golubchik, T.; Ayoubkhani, D.; House, T.; MacIntyre-Cockett, G.; Fryer, H.R.; Thomson, L.; Nurtay, A.; Kemp, S.A.; et al. Prevalence of persistent SARS-CoV-2 in a large community surveillance study. *Nature* **2024**, *626*, 1094–1101. [CrossRef]
21. Hampshire, A.; Azor, A.; Atchison, C.; Trender, W.; Hellyer, P.J.; Giunchiglia, V.; Husain, M.; Cooke, G.S.; Cooper, E.; Lound, A.; et al. Cognition and Memory after Covid-19 in a Large Community Sample. *N. Engl. J. Med.* **2024**, *390*, 806–818. [CrossRef] [PubMed]
22. Wong, A.C.; Devason, A.S.; Umana, I.C.; Cox, T.O.; Dohnalova, L.; Litichevskiy, L.; Perla, J.; Lundgren, P.; Etwebi, Z.; Izzo, L.T.; et al. Serotonin reduction in post-acute sequelae of viral infection. *Cell* **2023**, *186*, 4851–4867. [CrossRef] [PubMed]
23. Phetsouphanh, C.; Darley, D.R.; Wilson, D.B.; Howe, A.; Munier, C.M.L.; Patel, S.K.; Juno, J.A.; Burrell, L.M.; Kent, S.J.; Dore, G.J.; et al. Immunological dysfunction persists for 8 months following initial mild-to-moderate SARS-CoV-2 infection. *Nat. Immunol.* **2022**, *23*, 210–216. [CrossRef] [PubMed]
24. Talla, A.; Vasaikar, S.V.; Szeto, G.L.; Lemos, M.P.; Czartoski, J.L.; MacMillan, H.; Moodie, Z.; Cohen, K.W.; Fleming, L.B.; Thomson, Z.; et al. Persistent serum protein signatures define an inflammatory subcategory of long COVID. *Nat. Commun.* **2023**, *14*, 3417. [CrossRef]
25. Klein, J.; Wood, J.; Jaycox, J.R.; Dhodapkar, R.M.; Lu, P.; Gehlhausen, J.R.; Tabachnikova, A.; Greene, K.; Tabacof, L.; Malik, A.A.; et al. Distinguishing features of long COVID identified through immune profiling. *Nature* **2023**, *623*, 139–148. [CrossRef]
26. Ayoubkhani, D.; Khunti, K.; Nafilyan, V.; Maddox, T.; Humberstone, B.; Diamond, I.; Banerjee, A. Post-covid syndrome in individuals admitted to hospital with covid-19, retrospective cohort study. *BMJ* **2021**, *372*, n693. [CrossRef]
27. Staessen, J.A.; Wendt, R.; Yu, Y.L.; Kalbitz, S.; Thijs, L.; Siwy, J.; Raad, J.; Metzger, J.; Neuhaus, B.; Papkalla, A.; et al. Predictive performance and clinical application of COV50, a urinary proteomic biomarker in early COVID-19 infection: A prospective multicentre cohort study. *Lancet Digit. Health* **2022**, *10*, e727–e737. [CrossRef]

28. Latosinska, A.; Siwy, J.; Mischak, H.; Frantzi, M. Peptidomics and proteomics based on CE-MS as a robust tool in clinical application: The past, the present, and the future. *Electrophoresis* **2019**, *40*, 2294–2308. [CrossRef]
29. Mavrogeorgis, E.; Mischak, H.; Latosinska, A.; Siwy, J.; Jankowski, V.; Jankowski, J. Reproducibility Evaluation of Urinary Peptide Detection Using CE-MS. *Molecules* **2021**, *26*, 7260. [CrossRef]
30. Jantos-Siwy, J.; Schiffer, E.; Brand, K.; Schumann, G.; Rossing, K.; Delles, C.; Mischak, H.; Metzger, J. Quantitative Urinary Proteome Analysis for Biomarker Evaluation in Chronic Kidney Disease. *J. Proteome Res.* **2009**, *8*, 268–281. [CrossRef]
31. Benjamini, Y.; Hochberg, Y. Controlling the false discovery rate: A practical and powerful approach to multiple testing. *J. R. Stat. Soc. B (Methodol.)* **1995**, *57*, 125–133. [CrossRef]
32. Benjamini, Y.; Yekutieli, D. The control of the false discovery rate under dependency. *Ann. Stat.* **2001**, *29*, 1165–1188. [CrossRef]
33. Good, D.M.; Zürbig, P.; Argiles, A.; Bauer, H.W.; Behrens, G.; Coon, J.J.; Dakna, M.; Decramer, S.; Delles, C.; Dominiczak, A.F.; et al. Naturally occurring human urinary peptides for use in diagnosis of chronic kidney disease. *Mol. Cell Proteom.* **2010**, *9*, 2424–2437. [CrossRef]
34. Farmakis, D.; Koeck, T.; Mullen, W.; Parissis, J.; Gogas, B.D.; Nikolaou, M.; Lekakis, J.; Mischak, H.; Filippatos, G. Urine proteome analysis in heart failure with reduced ejection fraction complicated by chronic kidney disease: Feasibility, and clinical and pathogenetic correlates. *Eur. J. Heart Fail.* **2016**, *18*, 822–829. [CrossRef]
35. Wendt, R.; Thijs, L.; Kalbitz, S.; Mischak, H.; Siwy, J.; Raad, J.; Metzger, J.; Neuhaus, B.; Leyen, H.V.; Dudoignon, E.; et al. A urinary peptidomic profile predicts outcome in SARS-CoV-2-infected patients. *EClinicalMedicine* **2021**, *36*, 100883. [CrossRef] [PubMed]
36. Mainous, A.G., III; Rooks, B.J.; Wu, V.; Orlando, F.A. COVID-19 Post-acute Sequelae Among Adults: 12 Month Mortality Risk. *Front. Med.* **2021**, *8*, 778434. [CrossRef] [PubMed]
37. Graf, A.C.; Reichardt, D.; Wagenlechner, C.; Krotka, P.; Traxler-Weidenauer, D.; Mildner, M.; Mascherbauer, J.; Aigner, C.; Auer, J.; Wendt, R. Baseline Drug Treatments and Long-Term Outcomes in COVID-19-Hospitalized Patients: Results of the 2020 AUTCOV Study. *medRxiv* **2024**. [CrossRef]
38. Oseran, A.S.; Song, Y.; Xu, J.; Dahabreh, I.J.; Wadhera, R.K.; de Lemos, J.A.; Das, S.R.; Sun, T.; Yeh, R.W.; Kazi, D.S. Long term risk of death and readmission after hospital admission with covid-19 among older adults: Retrospective cohort study. *BMJ* **2023**, *382*, e076222. [CrossRef]
39. Iwashyna, T.J.; Seelye, S.; Berkowitz, T.S.; Pura, J.; Bohnert, A.S.B.; Bowling, C.B.; Boyko, E.J.; Hynes, D.M.; Ioannou, G.N.; Maciejewski, M.L.; et al. Late Mortality After COVID-19 Infection Among US Veterans vs Risk-Matched Comparators: A 2-Year Cohort Analysis. *JAMA Intern. Med.* **2023**, *183*, 1111–1119. [CrossRef]
40. Cai, M.; Xie, Y.; Topol, E.J.; Al-Aly, Z. Three-year outcomes of post-acute sequelae of COVID-19. *Nat. Med.* **2024**, *30*, 1564–1573. [CrossRef]
41. Maruyama, Y.; Nakayama, M.; Abe, M.; Yokoo, T.; Minakuchi, J.; Nitta, K. Association between serum beta2-microglobulin and mortality in Japanese peritoneal dialysis patients: A cohort study. *PLoS ONE* **2022**, *17*, e0266882. [CrossRef] [PubMed]
42. Vasquez-Rios, G.; Katz, R.; Levitan, E.B.; Cushman, M.; Parikh, C.R.; Kimmel, P.L.; Bonventre, J.V.; Waikar, S.S.; Schrauben, S.J.; Greenberg, J.H.; et al. Urinary Biomarkers of Kidney Tubule Health and Mortality in Persons with CKD and Diabetes Mellitus. *Kidney360* **2023**, *4*, e1257–e1264. [CrossRef] [PubMed]
43. Mina, I.K.; Mavrogeorgis, E.; Siwy, J.; Stojanov, R.; Mischak, H.; Latosinska, A.; Jankowski, V. Multiple urinary peptides display distinct sex-specific distribution. *Proteomics* **2023**, *24*, e2300227. [CrossRef]
44. Drum, C.L.; Tan, W.K.Y.; Chan, S.P.; Pakkiri, L.S.; Chong, J.P.C.; Liew, O.W.; Ng, T.P.; Ling, L.H.; Sim, D.; Leong, K.G.; et al. Thymosin Beta-4 Is Elevated in Women With Heart Failure With Preserved Ejection Fraction. *J. Am. Heart Assoc.* **2017**, *6*, e005586. [CrossRef]
45. Rudnicki, M.; Siwy, J.; Wendt, R.; Lipphardt, M.; Koziolek, M.J.; Maixnerova, D.; Peters, B.; Kerschbaum, J.; Leierer, J.; Neprasova, M.; et al. Urine proteomics for prediction of disease progression in patients with IgA nephropathy. *Nephrol. Dial. Transpl.* **2020**, *37*, 42–52. [CrossRef]
46. Didriksson, I.; Lengquist, M.; Spangfors, M.; Leffler, M.; Sievert, T.; Lilja, G.; Frigyesi, A.; Friberg, H.; Schiopu, A. Increasing plasma calprotectin (S100A8/A9) is associated with 12-month mortality and unfavourable functional outcome in critically ill COVID-19 patients. *J. Intensive Care* **2024**, *12*, 26. [CrossRef] [PubMed]
47. Barratt-Due, A.; Pettersen, K.; Borresdatter-Dahl, T.; Holter, J.C.; Gronli, R.H.; Dyrhol-Riise, A.M.; Lerum, T.V.; Holten, A.R.; Tonby, K.; Troseid, M.; et al. Escalated complement activation during hospitalization is associated with higher risk of 60-day mortality in SARS-CoV-2-infected patients. *J. Intern. Med.* **2024**, *296*, 80–92. [CrossRef]
48. Keller, F.; Beige, J.; Siwy, J.; Mebazaa, A.; An, D.; Mischak, H.; Schanstra, J.P.; Mokou, M.; Perco, P.; Staessen, J.A.; et al. Urinary peptides provide information about the risk of mortality across a spectrum of diseases and scenarios. *J. Transl. Med.* **2023**, *21*, 663. [CrossRef]
49. Magalhães, P.; Pejchinovski, M.; Markoska, K.; Banasik, M.; Klinger, M.; Svec-Billa, D.; Rychlik, I.; Rroji, M.; Restivo, A.; Capasso, G.; et al. Association of kidney fibrosis with urinary peptides: A path towards non-invasive liquid biopsies? *Sci. Rep.* **2017**, *7*, 16915. [CrossRef]
50. Catanese, L.; Siwy, J.; Mavrogeorgis, E.; Amann, K.; Mischak, H.; Beige, J.; Rupprecht, H. A Novel Urinary Proteomics Classifier for Non-Invasive Evaluation of Interstitial Fibrosis and Tubular Atrophy in Chronic Kidney Disease. *Proteomes* **2021**, *9*, 32. [CrossRef]

51. Siwy, J.; Wendt, R.; Albalat, A.; He, T.; Mischak, H.; Mullen, W.; Latosinska, A.; Lubbert, C.; Kalbitz, S.; Mebazaa, A.; et al. CD99 and polymeric immunoglobulin receptor peptides deregulation in critical COVID-19, A potential link to molecular pathophysiology? *Proteomics* **2021**, *21*, e2100133. [CrossRef] [PubMed]
52. Tabara, Y.; Setoh, K.; Kawaguchi, T.; Kosugi, S.; Nakayama, T.; Matsuda, F. Association between serum alpha1-antitrypsin levels and all-cause mortality in the general population: The Nagahama study. *Sci. Rep.* **2021**, *11*, 17241. [CrossRef] [PubMed]
53. Jaimes Campos, M.A.; Andujar, I.; Keller, F.; Mayer, G.; Rossing, P.; Staessen, J.A.; Delles, C.; Beige, J.; Glorieux, G.; Clark, A.L.; et al. Prognosis and Personalized In Silico Prediction of Treatment Efficacy in Cardiovascular and Chronic Kidney Disease: A Proof-of-Concept Study. *Pharmaceuticals* **2023**, *16*, 1298. [CrossRef] [PubMed]

Disclaimer/Publisher's Note: The statements, opinions and data contained in all publications are solely those of the individual author(s) and contributor(s) and not of MDPI and/or the editor(s). MDPI and/or the editor(s) disclaim responsibility for any injury to people or property resulting from any ideas, methods, instructions or products referred to in the content.

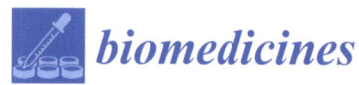 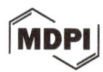

Article

Slow-Paced Breathing Intervention in Healthcare Workers Affected by Long COVID: Effects on Systemic and Dysfunctional Breathing Symptoms, Manual Dexterity and HRV

Marcella Mauro [1,*], Elisa Zulian [1], Nicoletta Bestiaco [1], Maurizio Polano [2] and Francesca Larese Filon [1]

[1] Unit of Occupational Medicine, Department of Medical Sciences, University of Trieste, 34129 Trieste, Italy; larese@units.it (F.L.F.)
[2] Experimental and Clinical Pharmacology Unit, Centro di Riferimento Oncologico di Aviano, Istituto di Ricovero e Cura a Carattere Scientifico, 33081 Aviano, Italy
* Correspondence: mmauro@units.it

Abstract: Background: Many COVID-19 survivors still experience long-term effects of an acute infection, most often characterised by neurological, cognitive and psychiatric sequelae. The treatment of this condition is challenging, and many hypotheses have been proposed. Non-invasive vagus nerve stimulation using slow-paced breathing (SPB) could stimulate both central nervous system areas and parasympathetic autonomic pathways, leading to neuromodulation and a reduction in inflammation. The aim of the present study was to evaluate physical, cognitive, emotional symptoms, executive functions and autonomic cardiac modulation after one month of at-home slow breathing intervention. Methods: 6655 healthcare workers (HCWs) were contacted via a company email in November 2022, of which N = 58 HCWs were enrolled as long COVID (cases) and N = 53 HCWs as controls. A baseline comparison of the two groups was performed. Subsequently each case was instructed on how to perform a resonant SPB using visual heart rate variability (HRV) biofeedback. They were then given a mobile video tutorial breathing protocol and asked to perform it three times a day (morning, early afternoon and before sleep). N = 33 cases completed the FU. At T0 and T1, each subject underwent COVID-related, psychosomatic and dysfunctional breathing questionnaires coupled with heart rate variability and manual dexterity assessments. Results: After one month of home intervention, an overall improvement in long-COVID symptoms was observed: confusion/cognitive impairment, chest pain, asthenia, headache and dizziness decreased significantly, while only a small increase in manual dexterity was found, and no relevant changes in cardiac parasympathetic modulation were observed.

Keywords: long COVID; breathing exercises; autonomic effects; vagus nerve stimulation; clinical trial; Nijmgen questionnaire; medical unexplained symptoms; executive functions; Purdue Pegboard test; heart rate variability

Citation: Mauro, M.; Zulian, E.; Bestiaco, N.; Polano, M.; Larese Filon, F. Slow-Paced Breathing Intervention in Healthcare Workers Affected by Long COVID: Effects on Systemic and Dysfunctional Breathing Symptoms, Manual Dexterity and HRV. *Biomedicines* **2024**, *12*, 2254. https://doi.org/10.3390/biomedicines12102254

Academic Editor: César Fernández-de-las-Peñas

Received: 11 September 2024
Revised: 24 September 2024
Accepted: 29 September 2024
Published: 3 October 2024

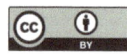

Copyright: © 2024 by the authors. Licensee MDPI, Basel, Switzerland. This article is an open access article distributed under the terms and conditions of the Creative Commons Attribution (CC BY) license (https://creativecommons.org/licenses/by/4.0/).

1. Introduction

Even though the pandemic era is over, many COVID-19 survivors are still experiencing long-lasting effects from an acute infection, with multifaceted symptoms that vary greatly from person to person. A consensus definition of this condition is not fully acknowledged, but the WHO at the end of 2021 defined "long COVID" as the persistence of one or more symptoms over 12+ weeks from the acute infection, which cannot be explained by an alternative diagnosis [1].

The prevalence of this phenomenon is difficult to evaluate due to the differences among studies in case definition, time elapsed since COVID-19, symptoms reported, or confirmed diagnoses, to cite some issues. Morever, a metanalysis of 41 studies estimates the European prevalence of this phenomenon to be around 44% of previously infected subjects [2]. A wide variety of symptoms have been recognised, among which neurological, cognitive and psychiatric ones are commonly the most reported [2–4]. The presence of these symptoms in the majority of these cases does not preclude the possibility of returning to work. However, they do render the performance of one's duties more challenging, particularly in activities that demand both physical and emotional commitment and the caring for others, as is the context of healthcare workers (HCWs) [5,6]. Improving the health condition of these individuals is crucial for multiple reasons, impacting both individual well-being and public health, and to this end, many not mutually exclusive treatments options have been claimed [7,8].

In this regard, while numerous RCTs are aimed at investigating the pharmacological efficacy of various classes of drugs in reducing symptoms (anti-inflammatories, antidepressants, antihistamines, anticlotting, and steroid medication, among others) [9], there is also a growing number of complementary treatments that are currently being evaluating [10]. Such options include physical techniques, supplementation, regenerative treatments and electrical stimulation—to cite some—that can be beneficial as the main options when a patient is unresponsive or has not responded adequately to pharmacological interventions or can be used as concurrent add-on therapies in other circumstances, possibly leading to an enhanced efficacy of the medical treatments.

In long-COVID subjects, autonomic imbalance has been identified as a potential underlying mechanism [11–13]. In the majority of cases, this manifests as a parasympathetic impairment [14,15] and disrupted vagal signalling, particularly following a prolonged course of the acute infection. This is also confirmed by the findings of brain functional MRI studies on adult and paediatric long-COVID subjects, which revealed a decreased metabolism in the central autonomic network (CAN) [16] mainly composed of the limbic system, and also in the brain stem, where the vagus nerve nuclei originate [17,18]. Similarly, deficits in executive functions have been observed in these subjects, as the nature of these processes necessitates a robust exchange of information within the neural network between the cortex and subcortical regions, as well as between the two hemispheres of the brain [19]. Moreover, the persistence of a systemic inflammation could be a consequence of an effectiveness decline in the cholinergic anti-inflammatory pathway (CAP), led by the vagus nerve. In this case, the release of Ach quenches the excess of cytokine release from the mastocytes, which has detrimental effects on the body's recovery after an acute infection [20,21]. For all the aforementioned reasons, vagus nerve stimulation (VNS) has been proposed as a potential treatment option in long-COVID subjects [22,23].

Up to date, few studies have evaluated this approach, mainly though the electrical transcutaneous stimulation of its auricolar branch [24,25], with encouraging results on fatigue and cognitive symptom reduction in a restricted number of individuals. These approaches are minimally invasive yet necessitate the acquisition of a specific device, training duly the patient for its correct utilisation, and has the limitation that it can only stimulate the VN unilaterally.

An alternative, entirely non-invasive method of stimulating this nerve is through breathing modulation (respiratory VN stimulation—rVNS), which is costless and can be performed by the patient at any time and in any location, on the condition that they have received adequate training in its correct and effective execution.

Respiratory VNS is achieved through the slowing down of breathing frequency to six cycles/min (corresponding to the resonant frequency (~0.1 Hz)), which rationally relies on the neurovisceral integration model.

According to this acknowledged theory [26,27], the CNS and autonomic system are bidirectionally connected and can interact with each other both via equally efficient top–down or bottom–up stimuli [28]. In this case, deep breathing at a low respiration rate is the bottom–up trigger and, compared to tVNS, permits a bilateral stimulation of the VN afferent and efferent fibres [29].

When a subject breathes at six cycles/min, projections of central rhythm generator neurons stimulate the nucleus ambiguus (NA), from which a cascading loop activation is established, which is ultimately responsible for the beneficial effects described in the literature. Vagus cardiomotor efferent fibres originate from NA and reach the heart, thereby inducing a bradycardic effect through an enhanced release of Ach. The aortic bulb and carotid wall baroreceptors record an increased cardiac output, which happens with a 5 s delay from the Ach release. Through this delay, the system achieves temporal coherence between respiratory phases, cardiac phases and blood pressure. Moreover, the vagal afferent fibres departing from the baroreceptors stimulate in turn the medullar nucleus of the solitary tract. From this point, the vagal afferent fibres send widespread signals directly to the cingulate and insular cortex and indirectly to the subcortical limbic system in a longer and more powerful way compared to when spontaneous breathing occurs. This activation of interoceptive areas is responsible for the cognitive, emotional, executive and behavioural changes that can be observed [30,31].

The aim of the present study was to evaluate, in a group of healthcare workers affected by long-COVID symptoms, the effects of one-month slow-paced breathing intervention on perceived cognitive functions, cardiac autonomic modulation, and executive functions.

2. Materials and Methods

2.1. Study Design and Ethical Aspects

This interventional study was approved by the FVG's Unite Research Ethics Committee (approval number 245_2023H, ID 17328). All participants signed an informed consent form before being included in the study; the study was conducted in accordance with the principles of the Declaration of Helsinki.

2.2. Participants Enrolment

In early November 2022, all ASUGI employees (n = 6655) were informed via a company email about the nature and purpose of the study. Enrolment was then carried out for each worker who expressed interest in participating in the project and who met the inclusion criteria. Inclusion criteria for the long-COVID HCW group were as follows: previous COVID-19 confirmed by RT-PCR on a nasopharyngeal swab (NPS) and the persistence or new onset of symptoms (1 or more of those listed by [32] beyond 12 weeks after NPS negativisation and still present at baseline). Exclusion criteria were as follows: previous COVID-19 and symptoms still present but less than 12 weeks. Inclusion criteria for the control group of HCWs were as follows: having been regularly tested for SARS-Cov-2 by the NPS in accordance with the hospital safety protocol for the pandemic period and having always been found negative.

2.3. Data Collection

Each participant underwent a series of questionnaires and instrumental assessments, which are described in detail below, in order to assess the following: demographic data, long-COVID symptoms, respiratory dysfunction, manual dexterity and cardiac autonomic modulation.

1. General health and long-COVID symptom questionnaires: Data on age, sex, weight and height, smoking habits, SARS-Cov-2 vaccination status, comorbidities, pharmacotherapy and job descriptors were collected. The symptoms of long-COVID were assessed according to the ones described by the Istituto Superiore di Sanità. [32].
2. Psychosomatic symptoms using the M.U.S. and Distress questionnaires related to autonomic impairment: This tool allows the investigation of "medically unexplained symptoms". It consists of 39 items exploring the physical, psychological, cognitive and emotional domains. Having more than 6 of these symptoms has been associated with low heart rate variability (RMSSD and SDNN values) and an impaired autonomic nervous system [33,34]. Each item can be rated by the patient on a scale from 0 (no symptom) to 10 (highest intensity). The final score is calculated by the sum of the intensity of each item.
3. Dysfunctional breathing symptoms through Nijmegen questionnaire (NQ): Dyspnoea has been described as a common symptom in long-COVID subjects, but it may derive from multiple causes, among which psychological ones may also play a role. This tool

is composed of 16 items, each of which can be scored from 0 to 4 by the participant. It has been used to assess dysfunctional breathing patterns [35].

4. Manual dexterity assessment through Purdue Pegboard test manual dexterity (PPT): After instructions, a short demonstration was delivered to the subject. Subsequently, each participant had the possibility to have a trial before the administration of the evaluated test. The procedure comprises a series of steps that must be carried out in a specific order. The subject must pick up pins placed in a bowl on the corresponding side of the tested hand and try to place as many pins as possible in the prepared holes within 30 s. The task is carried out first with the dominant hand, then with the non-dominant hand, and finally, with both hands at once (three separate tasks). The assembly test is then performed, which is composed of a standardised sequence of assembly of pegs, washers and collars with both hands in one minute. The total score is then calculated adding the 1 to 4 task scores together [36,37].

5. Cardiovascular autonomic function assessment through photoplethysmography (PPG Stress Flow®, BioTekna Co, Italy): This device allows the detection of the digital pulse waves produced by the systolic contractile force of the heart. After 20 min of acclimatisation to the experimental environment (room temperature 22–24 °C; relative humidity 40–60%) while the subjects are seated in a comfortable chair with their forearms resting on the table, the procedure starts. An infrared probe is placed on the II finger of both hands separately, and the acquired optical signal is then processed by means of appropriate algorithms in order to derive the ECG signal. The detailed procedure has been described elsewhere [38]. The equipment used for the study has been authorised by the Italian Ministry of Health (CND Z12040113). Patients underwent the study protocol in the morning. Measurements were taken for 5 min during spontaneous breathing and then for 5 min during slow breathing (6 breaths/min, i.e., 0.1 Hz).

6. Slow-paced breathing protocol: Each long-COVID participant was taught how to perform resonant slow-paced breathing (SPB) during the initial inpatient assessment, a manoeuvre which elicits a cardiovagal modulation. The breathing cycle was the same for all participants and was composed of 2 s. inspiration, 3 s. holding, 2 s. expiration, and 3 s pause (6 breath per minute, i.e., 0.1 Hz), repeated over a 5 min period. This breath frequency is acknowledged to be capable of maximising the temporal coherence between blood pressure, respiratory and cardiac phases, leading to higher cardiac oscillations, which in turn deliver the central and peripherical benefits [30]. The cases were then instructed to perform it three times a day (morning, early afternoon and before bedtime) for one month using a mobile video tutorial. The researchers contacted them once a week to check that they were following the instructions. Figure 1 shows the flowchart of the study.

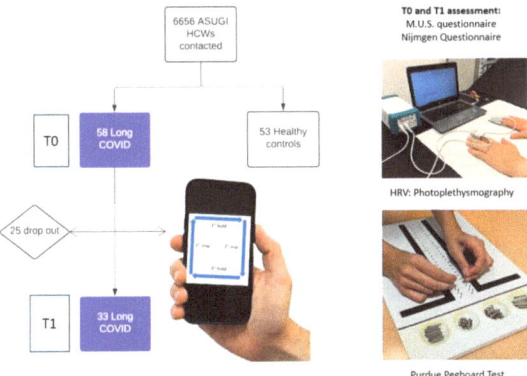

Figure 1. Flow chart of the study, assessment performed and breathing protocol. ASUGI: Azienda Sanitaria Universitaria Giuliano-Isontina.

2.4. Statystical Analysis

The Shapiro–Wilk test was employed to assess the normality of the distributions. Normally distributed continuous data were reported as means (SD) and compared by Student's t-test or the paired t-test if independent or correlated, respectively. Medians (IQR) were used to report not-normally distributed data, which were contrasted by the Wilcoxon Rank sum test or the Wilcoxon Sign Rank test if independent or correlated, respectively. Numbers (percentages) were used to report normally distributed ordinal data, which were compared using the χ^2 test or the McNemar chi-square test if independent or correlated, respectively. Not-normally distributed ordinal data were compared with Fisher's exact test or the McNemar exact test if independent or correlated, respectively. All analyses were conducted using Stata® software version 16 (StataCorp LP, College Station, TX, USA). All *p*-values are two-tailed. Values < 0.05 were considered statistically significant.

3. Results

N = 58 long-COVID subjects were enrolled in the study, out of which N = 33 completed the study and their data were included for the final analysis. N = 53 controls age and sex matched were used as the baseline comparison for MUS and dysfunctional breathing symptoms, HRV and manual dexterity parameters; the results are described elsewhere [37,38]. Moreover, 56% of the cases complained of symptoms for 12+ months, among which cognitive impairment (memory and concentration problems, confusion), a feeling of tightness/anxiety/chest pain, asthenia, dyspnoea and sleep disorders ranked highest (an overall assessment based on questionnaires). None of them had ever been hospitalised for COVID-19 and did not differ significantly from healthy controls in terms of comorbidities (before and after COVID-19) and medication use (for the full results, see [15]). Regarding autonomic symptoms, assessed by M.U.S. and Distress questionnaires (Supplementary Tables S1 and S2), cases showed a significantly higher total number (7.5 (IQR 5-11) vs. 3 (IQR 1-5)) and intensity of symptoms compared to the controls (in 26 out of 38 items (68%)) among physical, cognitive and emotional ones.

After one month of home intervention, N = 33 HCWs completed the FU and received a second inpatient assessment. In total, 63% of them reported that they adhered completely/closely to the protocol, while 36% seldom/never adhered.

The FU population had a median age of 51.5 years (IQR 42-57) and 78% were women. Moreover, one-third were smokers and the median time since the primary infection was 419.5 (IQR 268-730) days.

The prevalence of dysfunctional breathing symptoms was found to have decreased significantly after a one-month intervention, as illustrated in Figure 2. This finding was observed alongside a reduction in the occurrence of other long-COVID symptoms and a decline in the total number of disorders affecting various systems and apparatus (Figure 3a,b and Supplementary Table S3).

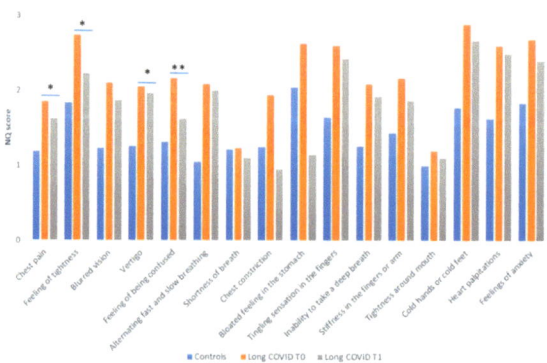

Figure 2. Bar graph of 16-item Nijmegen questionnaire score for control at T0 and long COVID (T0 and T1) who completed the FU. * $p < 0.05$, ** $p \leq 0.01$, for complete results, see Supplementary Table S4.

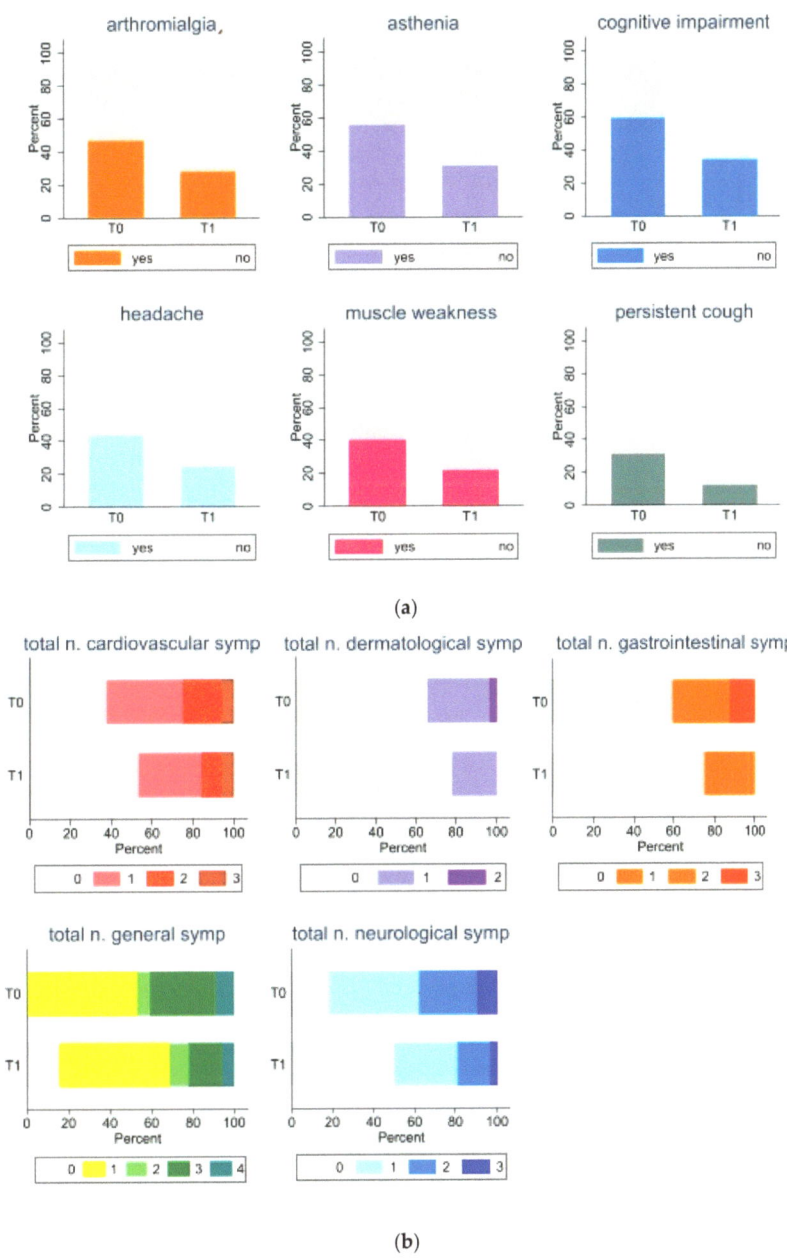

Figure 3. (**a**). Stacked bar graph of long-COVID symptoms, which significantly decreased from T0 to T1. For complete results, see Supplementary Table S2. (**b**). Stacked bar graph of total number of long-COVID symptoms by system/apparatus at T0 and T1. See Supplementary Table S3 for full results.

4. Discussion

Our study evaluated a group of N = 58 healthcare workers affected by long COVID, of whom N = 33 completed one month of the at-home slow breathing programme and received a second out-patient assessment. Each participant has been evaluated before and after the intervention in terms of physical, cognitive and emotional symptom magnitude, cardiac autonomic modulation during vagal stimulation (slow-paced breathing stimulus), and performances in fine manipulative skills.

Our follow-up population consisted of 78% females, with a mean age of 51.8 years (SD 8.8), who had not previously been hospitalised due to COVID-19, evaluated at a relatively long time since an acute infection of 419.5 days (IQR 269-730). Only a small percentage of cases had restrictions on their fit-for-work judgment (such as night shifts or heavy lifting) and most returned to work in the same position as before COVID-19. They were all vaccinated with one or more doses of COVID-19 vaccine (required by law for health workers in Italy at the time prior to the study) and showed a very high antibody titre compared to never-infected but vaccinated controls. There was no excess of newly diagnosed pathologies in the cases, but in 68% of the items investigating psychosomatic disorders (M.U.S. questionnaire), the cases had a significantly higher intensity of impairment than the controls (physical, cognitive, and emotional areas, but not the behavioural one). In addition, 75% of them had a total number of disturbances ≥ 6, a datapoint that has been shown to be associated with low HRV values and RMSSD in particular, an indirect parameter of the parasympathetic autonomic component state of health [33,34].

After one month of the breathing intervention, the results showed a significant reduction in symptoms related to cognitive deterioration, headache, asthenia, chest tightness and dysfunctional breathing,

These findings are consistent with the ones of other studies, which tried to stimulate the VN in different ways.

Badran et al. [24]. and Zheng et al. [27] used electrical transauricular VN stimulation (tVNS), demonstrating a reduction in fatigue and cognitive symptoms in a small group of cases, without any further instrumental evaluation.

Corrado et al. [39] and Polizzi et al. [40] used the respiratory stimulation of the VN (rVNS) like we did, finding a significant reduction in perceived fatigue, autonomic symptoms, breathlessness and an enhancement in the ability to focus, stress control, and quality of life and sleep after the intervention, even if they used a different paced breathing shape. The first study was carried out on a small number of patients (n = 13) at a mean time of 14.7 (SD 5.8) months after acute infection. An assessment was conducted using a Polar watch coupled with a chest strap and a phone application to record HRV variations during SPB and a battery of questionnaires was used to evaluate autonomic imbalance, disability and quality of life (C19-YRSm, COMPASS-31, WHODAS and EQ5D-5L). The second study retrospectively evaluated the subjective effects (self-reported symptoms and well-being on a Likert scale 1 to 5) of a resonant breathing programme (Meo Health) on n = 99 long-COVID anonymous subjects, but no data on the time elapsed since the acute infection were available, nor on drug consumption.

In both cases, the protocol included a 4″: 6″ (inspiration-expiration) breathing pattern, performed twice a day for at least 10 min (up to 30 s in Polizzi) for a total of 1 month, which differed from the breath shape we used (2″3″2″3″, insp., holding, exp., holding, three times a day for one month), but both of them guaranteed a final breathing frequency of six cycles/min.

This particular breathing rate has been used in many other clinical conditions [41] since it is capable of inducing a resonant frequency (~0.1 Hz), which increases cardiac oscillations through the maximisation of the temporal coherence of respiratory, blood pressure, and cardiac phases. Higher cardiac oscillations are then responsible for the peripheral effects, while a longer and stronger stimulation of the limbic system via the afferent fibres of the VN are thought to be at the basis of the cognitive and emotional effects [30].

As regards cardiac autonomic modulation we did not find any relevant change in the intensity of the cardiovagal modulation during slow breathing manoeuvres after the intervention (RMSSD: 33 msn (IQR 23–55) vs. 33 msn (IQR 27–53), pre- and post intervention, respectively, p = 0.84 and LF power: 7.4 (IQR 7–8.3) vs. 7.7 (IQR 7–8.2), pre- and post intervention, respectively, p = 0.91, with the parameters chosen according to [42]), meaning that a cumulative effect and/or an enhancement in the strength of the cardiac parasympathetic stimulation did not happen in our group. This is in contrast with the results of the only other study, to the best of our knowledge, which assessed this point [39], and that found a significant increase in RMSSD at rest after the intervention (RMSSD: 34.2 msn (SD 19.6) vs. 40.9 msn (SD 29.4), pre- and post intervention, respectively, $p = 0.048$).

As regards executive function, which very often worsens in subjects with long COVID [19,43], we found an impairment in fine manipulative skills at baseline [37], which only marginally improved after the intervention. The test used is based on the speed with which the subject can insert a few pins and carry out a simple assembly in a given time. The activities are performed with both hands separately and then with both hands together. This involves understanding, processing and transferring information between both sides of our brain, visual and motor coordination, and lastly, peripheral muscle activation. These deep brain areas probably only partially have been stimulated by the rVNS and need more training with other tools aimed at improving the underlying networking [44]. No other studies, up to date, are available as regards a pre–post evaluation of manipulative skills in long COVID after a VNS intervention.

Given the consistency of the studies in reducing neurological, cognitive, stress-related and respiratory symptoms and the inconclusive results on peripheral autonomic modulation, it can be hypothesised that the efficacy and/or time required for slow controlled breathing to stimulate the VN central afferent fibres and the relative interoceptive brain areas is less than that required to observe effects on the efferent fibres in modulating vagal cardiac function. This finding could be explained by the fact that VN fibres are mixed and unevenly distributed, being made up of 20% efferent fibres and 80% afferent fibres [30,45].

One of the strengths of our study is the relatively bigger number of patients evaluated after a respiratory VN stimulation compared to other studies which have focused on this topic and that subjects received a multidimensional evaluation. Concurrently, this study was initiated as exploratory; thus, its sample size was calculated based on analogous works on this topic, which were scarce at the time. Moreover, we lack a long-COVID control group. This was due to ethical reasons since all 58 long-COVID subjects at the first evaluation were offered access to the breathing protocol, but the 25 dropouts refused to participate in the program and be re-evaluated after a period of time due to personal, time-related or organisational reasons. In particular, shift workers stated that they could not deliberately stop during a shift to perform controlled breathing if it was scheduled at that time of the day. Regardless, we believe that given that 56% of subjects complained of disorders from 12+ months, it is unlikely that the symptoms would have diminished over the course of those month, even without treatment.

5. Conclusions

The results of this study, which evaluated the effects of an at-home vagal stimulation through a six-cycle/min breathing protocol (rVNS), indicated that this approach may be beneficial in reducing the symptoms associated with long COVID. These findings contribute to the expanding body of evidence suggesting that this complementary treatment may be beneficial in alleviating the core symptoms experienced by these individuals, including asthenia, cognitive decline, headaches, and confusion. However, further validation is required to substantiate these findings, ideally through a larger sample size and a randomised controlled trial (RCT) study design with a more extended follow-up period to ascertain the long-term efficacy of the rVNS approach.

Supplementary Materials: The following supporting information can be downloaded at: https://www.mdpi.com/article/10.3390/biomedicines12102254/s1, Table S1. Follow-up results of the Nijmegen questionnaire (NQ); Table S2. Long-COVID symptoms as defined by Istituto Superiore di Sanità [32], assessed at T0 and after one month (T1); Table S3. Heart rate variability (HRV) parameters in long-COVID subjects during slow-paced breathing (SPB) at T0 and T1; Table S4. Medically unexplained symptom (M.U.S.) at T0 and T1; Table S5. Distress symptoms at T0 and T1; Table S6. Manual dexterity assessed through Purdue Pegboard test (PPT) at T0 and T1.

Author Contributions: M.M.: conceptualisation, writing—review and editing; N.B. and E.Z.: investigation, data curation; M.P.: formal analysis, visualisation; F.L.F.: supervision. All authors have read and agreed to the published version of the manuscript.

Funding: This research was funded by Università degli Studi di Trieste (FRA 2022 and FRA 2024).

Institutional Review Board Statement: The study was conducted in accordance with the Declara-tion of Helsinki and approved by the Unite Research Ethics Committee of FVG (protocol code 245_2023H, ID 17328) for studies involving humans.

Informed Consent Statement: Informed consent was obtained from all subjects involved in the study. Written informed consent has been obtained from the patients to publish this paper.

Data Availability Statement: The data presented in this study are available on request from the corresponding author. The data are not publicly available due to privacy restrictions.

Acknowledgments: We thank all of the nursing staff involved in the projects and all the HCWs who joined the project.

Conflicts of Interest: The authors declare no conflicts of interest. The funders had no role in the design of the study; in the collection, analyses, or interpretation of data; in the writing of the manuscript; or in the decision to publish the results.

References

1. WHO Europe. Available online: https://www.who.int/europe/news-room/fact-sheets/item/post-covid-19-condition (accessed on 30 October 2023).
2. Chen, C.; Haupert, S.R.; Zimmermann, L.; Shi, X.; Fritsche, L.G.; Mukherjee, B. Global Prevalence of Post-Coronavirus Disease 2019 (COVID-19) Condition or Long COVID: A Meta-Analysis and Systematic Review. *J. Infect. Dis.* **2022**, *226*, 1593–1607. [CrossRef] [PubMed]
3. Efstathiou, V.; Stefanou, M.I.; Demetriou, M.; Siafakas, N.; Makris, M.; Tsivgoulis, G.; Zoumpourlis, V.; Kympouropoulos, S.P.; Tsoporis, J.N.; Spandidos, D.A.; et al. Long COVID and neuropsychiatric manifestations (Review). *Exp. Ther. Med.* **2022**, *23*, 363. [CrossRef] [PubMed] [PubMed Central]
4. Schou, T.M.; Joca, S.; Wegener, G.; Bay-Richter, C. Psychiatric and neuropsychiatric sequelae of COVID-19-A systematic review. *Brain Behav. Immun.* **2021**, *97*, 328–348. [CrossRef]
5. Mendola, M.; Leoni, M.; Cozzi, Y.; Manzari, A.; Tonelli, F.; Metruccio, F.; Tosti, L.; Battini, V.; Cucchi, I.; Costa, M.C.; et al. Long-term COVID symptoms, work ability and fitness to work in healthcare workers hospitalized for Sars-CoV-2 infection. *Med. Lav.* **2022**, *113*, e2022040. [CrossRef]
6. Cegolon, L.; Mauro, M.; Sansone, D.; Tassinari, A.; Gobba, F.M.; Modenese, A.; Casolari, L.; Liviero, F.; Pavanello, S.; Scapellato, M.L.; et al. A Multi-Center Study Investigating Long COVID-19 in Healthcare Workers from North-Eastern Italy: Prevalence, Risk Factors and the Impact of Pre-Existing Humoral Immunity-ORCHESTRA Project. *Vaccines* **2023**, *11*, 1769. [CrossRef] [PubMed] [PubMed Central]
7. Chee, Y.J.; Fan, B.E.; Young, B.E.; Dalan, R.; Lye, D.C. Clinical trials on the pharmacological treatment of long COVID: A systematic review. *J. Med. Virol.* **2023**, *95*, e28289. [CrossRef] [PubMed] [PubMed Central]
8. Chandan, J.S.; Brown, K.R.; Simms-Williams, N.; Bashir, N.Z.; Camaradou, J.; Heining, D.; Turner, G.M.; Rivera, S.C.; Hotham, R.; Minhas, S.; et al. Non-Pharmacological Therapies for Post-Viral Syndromes, Including Long COVID: A Systematic Review. *Int. J. Environ. Res. Public Health* **2023**, *20*, 3477. [CrossRef] [PubMed] [PubMed Central]
9. Ledford, H. Long-COVID treatments: Why the world is still waiting. *Nature* **2022**, *608*, 258–260. [CrossRef] [PubMed]
10. Motilal, S.; Rampersad, R.; Adams, M.; Goon Lun, S.; Ramdhanie, A.; Ruiz, T.; Shah, A.; Wilkinson, A.; Lewis, J. Randomized Controlled Trials for Post-COVID-19 Conditions: A Systematic Review. *Cureus* **2024**, *16*, e67603. [CrossRef] [PubMed] [PubMed Central]
11. Dani, M.; Dirksen, A.; Taraborrelli, P.; Torocastro, M.; Panagopoulos, D.; Sutton, R.; Lim, P.B. Autonomic dysfunction in 'long COVID': Rationale, physiology and management strategies. *Clin. Med.* **2021**, *21*, e63–e67. [CrossRef] [PubMed] [PubMed Central]
12. Shouman, K.; Vanichkachorn, G.; Cheshire, W.P.; Suarez, M.D.; Shelly, S.; Lamotte, G.J.; Sandroni, P.; Benarroch, E.E.; Berini, S.E.; Cutsforth-Gregory, J.K.; et al. Autonomic dysfunction following COVID-19 infection: An early experience. *Clin. Auton. Res.* **2021**, *31*, 385–394. [CrossRef] [PubMed]
13. DePace, N.L.; Colombo, J. Long-COVID Syndrome and the Cardiovascular System: A Review of Neurocardiologic Effects on Multiple Systems. *Curr. Cardiol. Rep.* **2022**, *24*, 1711–1726. [CrossRef] [PubMed] [PubMed Central]
14. Zanin, A.; Amah, G.; Chakroun, S.; Testard, P.; Faucher, A.; Le, T.Y.V.; Slama, D.; Le Baut, V.; Lozeron, P.; Salmon, D.; et al. Parasympathetic autonomic dysfunction is more often evidenced than sympathetic autonomic dysfunction in fluctuating and polymorphic symptoms of "long-COVID" patients. *Sci. Rep.* **2023**, *13*, 8251. [CrossRef] [PubMed] [PubMed Central]
15. Marques, K.C.; Quaresma, J.A.S.; Falcão, L.F.M. Cardiovascular autonomic dysfunction in "Long COVID": Pathophysiology, heart rate variability, and inflammatory markers. *Front. Cardiovasc. Med.* **2023**, *10*, 1256512. [CrossRef] [PubMed] [PubMed Central]

16. Benarroch, E.E. The central autonomic network: Functional organization, dysfunction and perspective. *Mayo Clin. Proc.* **1993**, *68*, 988–1001. [CrossRef]
17. Hugon, J.; Queneau, M.; Sanchez Ortiz, M.; Msika, E.F.; Farid, K.; Paquet, C. Cognitive decline and brainstem hypometabolism in long COVID: A case series. *Brain Behav.* **2022**, *12*, e2513. [CrossRef]
18. Guedj, E.; Campion, J.Y.; Dudouet, P.; Kaphan, E.; Bregeon, F.; Tissot-Dupont, H.; Guis, S.; Barthelemy, F.; Habert, P.; Ceccaldi, M.; et al. 18F-FDG brain PET hypometabolism in patients with long COVID. *Eur. J. Nucl. Med. Mol. Imaging* **2021**, *48*, 2823–2833. [CrossRef]
19. Velichkovsky, B.B.; Razvaliaeva, A.Y.; Khlebnikova, A.A.; Manukyan, P.A.; Kasatkin, V.N.; Barmin, A.V. Systematic Review and Meta-Analysis of Clinically Relevant Executive Functions Tests Performance after COVID-19. *Behav. Neurol.* **2023**, *2023*, 1094267. [CrossRef] [PubMed] [PubMed Central]
20. Rosas-Ballina, M.; Tracey, K.J. Cholinergic control of inflammation. *J. Intern. Med.* **2009**, *265*, 663–679. [CrossRef] [PubMed] [PubMed Central]
21. Giunta, S.; Giordani, C.; De Luca, M.; Olivieri, F. Long-COVID-19 autonomic dysfunction: An integrated view in the framework of inflammaging. *Mech. Ageing Dev.* **2024**, *218*, 111915. [CrossRef] [PubMed]
22. Azabou, E.; Bao, G.; Bounab, R.; Heming, N.; Annane, D. Vagus Nerve Stimulation: A Potential Adjunct Therapy for COVID-19. *Front. Med.* **2021**, *8*, 625836. [CrossRef] [PubMed] [PubMed Central]
23. Linnhoff, S.; Koehler, L.; Haghikia, A.; Zaehle, T. The therapeutic potential of non-invasive brain stimulation for the treatment of Long-COVID-related cognitive fatigue. *Front. Immunol.* **2023**, *13*, 935614. [CrossRef] [PubMed] [PubMed Central]
24. Badran, B.W.; Huffman, S.M.; Dancy, M.; Austelle, C.W.; Bikson, M.; Kautz, S.A.; George, M.S. A pilot randomized controlled trial of supervised, at-home, self-administered transcutaneous auricular vagus nerve stimulation (taVNS) to manage long COVID symptoms. *Bioelectron. Med.* **2022**, *8*, 13. [CrossRef] [PubMed] [PubMed Central]
25. Zheng, Z.S.; Simonian, N.; Wang, J.; Rosario, E.R. Transcutaneous vagus nerve stimulation improves Long COVID symptoms in a female cohort: A pilot study. *Front. Neurol.* **2024**, *15*, 1393371. [CrossRef] [PubMed] [PubMed Central]
26. Thayer, J.F.; Lane, R.D. A model of neurovisceral integration in emotion regulation and dysregulation. *J. Affect. Disord.* **2000**, *61*, 201–216. [CrossRef] [PubMed]
27. Thayer, J.F.; Loerbroks, A.; Sternberg, E.M. Inflammation and cardiorespiratory control: The role of the vagus nerve. *Respir. Physiol. Neurobiol.* **2011**, *178*, 387–394. [CrossRef] [PubMed]
28. Smith, R.; Thayer, J.F.; Khalsa, S.S.; Lane, R.D. The hierarchical basis of neurovisceral integration. *Neurosci. Biobehav. Rev.* **2017**, *75*, 274–296. [CrossRef] [PubMed]
29. Gerritsen, R.J.S.; Band, G.P.H. Breath of Life: The Respiratory Vagal Stimulation Model of Contemplative Activity. *Front. Hum. Neurosci.* **2018**, *12*, 397. [CrossRef] [PubMed] [PubMed Central]
30. Sevoz-Couche, C.; Laborde, S. Heart rate variability and slow-paced breathing:when coherence meets resonance. *Neurosci. Biobehav. Rev.* **2022**, *135*, 104576. [CrossRef] [PubMed]
31. Colzato, L.; Beste, C. A literature review on the neurophysiological underpinnings and cognitive effects of transcutaneous vagus nerve stimulation: Challenges and future directions. *J. Neurophysiol.* **2020**, *123*, 1739–1755. [CrossRef] [PubMed]
32. Istituto Superiore di Sanità. Special on CoViD-19 Long-CoViD Symptoms. Available online: https://www.iss.it/en/long-covid-sintomi (accessed on 30 October 2022).
33. Chrousos, G.P.; Papadopoulou-Marketou, N.; Bacopoulou, F.; Lucafò, M.; Gallotta, A.; Boschiero, D. Photoplethysmography (PPG)-determined heart rate variability (HRV) and extracellular water (ECW) in the evaluation of chronic stress and in-flammation. *Hormones* **2022**, *21*, 383–390. [CrossRef] [PubMed]
34. Chrousos, G.P.; Boschiero, D. Clinical validation of a non-invasive electrodermal biofeedback device useful for reducing chronic perceived pain and systemic inflammation. *Hormones* **2019**, *18*, 207–213. [CrossRef] [PubMed] [PubMed Central]
35. van Dixhoorn, J.; Folgering, H. The Nijmegen Questionnaire and dysfunctional breathing. *ERJ Open Res.* **2015**, *1*, 00001–02015. [CrossRef] [PubMed] [PubMed Central]
36. Tiffin, J.; Asher, E.J. The Purdue pegboard; norms and studies of reliability and validity. *J. Appl. Psychol.* **1948**, *32*, 234–247. [CrossRef] [PubMed]
37. Mauro, M.; Bestiaco, N.; Zulian, E.; Markežič, M.M.; Bignolin, I.; Sirianni, F.; Larese Filon, F. Manual Dexterity, Tactile Perception and Inflammatory Profile in Hcws Affected by Long Covid: A Case—Control Study. Available online: https://ssrn.com/abstract=4889166 (accessed on 15 September 2024).
38. Mauro, M.; Cegolon, L.; Bestiaco, N.; Zulian, E.; Larese Filon, F. Heart Rate Variability Modulation Through Slow-Paced Breathing in Health Care Workers with Long COVID: A Case-Control Study. *Am. J. Med.* **2024**, in press. [CrossRef] [PubMed]
39. Corrado, J.; Iftekhar, N.; Halpin, S.; Li, M.; Tarrant, R.; Grimaldi, J.; Simms, A.; O'Connor, R.J.; Casson, A.; Sivan, M. HEART Rate Variability Biofeedback for LOng COVID Dysautonomia (HEARTLOC): Results of a Feasibility Study. *Adv. Rehabil. Sci. Pract.* **2024**, *13*, 27536351241227261. [CrossRef] [PubMed] [PubMed Central]
40. Polizzi, J.; Tosto-Mancuso, J.; Tabacof, L.; Wood, J.; Putrino, D. Resonant breathing improves self-reported symptoms and wellbeing in people with Long COVID. *Front. Rehabil. Sci.* **2024**, *5*, 1411344. [CrossRef] [PubMed] [PubMed Central]
41. Fournié, C.; Chouchou, F.; Dalleau, G.; Caderby, T.; Cabrera, Q.; Verkindt, C. Heart rate variability biofeedback in chronic disease management: A systematic review. *Complement. Ther. Med.* **2021**, *60*, 102750. [CrossRef] [PubMed]

42. Laborde, S.; Allen, M.S.; Borges, U.; Dosseville, F.; Hosang, T.J.; Iskra, M.; Mosley, E.; Salvotti, C.; Spolverato, L.; Zammit, N.; et al. Effects of voluntary slow breathing on heart rate and heart rate variability: A systematic review and a meta-analysis. *Neurosci. Biobehav. Rev.* **2022**, *138*, 104711. [CrossRef] [PubMed]
43. Sanal-Hayes, N.E.M.; Hayes, L.D.; Mclaughlin, M.; Berry, E.C.J.; Sculthorpe, N.F. People with Long COVID and ME/CFS Exhibit Similarly Impaired Dexterity and Bimanual Coordination: A Case-Case-Control Study. *Am. J. Med.* **2024**. [CrossRef] [PubMed]
44. Diamond, A. Activities and Programs That Improve Children's Executive Functions. *Curr. Dir. Psychol. Sci.* **2012**, *21*, 335–341. [CrossRef] [PubMed] [PubMed Central]
45. Foley, J.O.; DuBois, F.S. Quantitative studies of the vagus nerve in the cat: I. The ratio of sensory to motor fibers. *J. Nerv. Ment. Dis.* **1937**, *86*, 587. [CrossRef]

Disclaimer/Publisher's Note: The statements, opinions and data contained in all publications are solely those of the individual author(s) and contributor(s) and not of MDPI and/or the editor(s). MDPI and/or the editor(s) disclaim responsibility for any injury to people or property resulting from any ideas, methods, instructions or products referred to in the content.

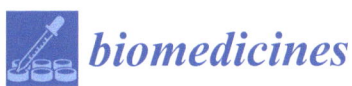

Article

Individualized and Controlled Exercise Training Improves Fatigue and Exercise Capacity in Patients with Long-COVID

Simon Kieffer [1,†], Anna-Lena Krüger [1,2,†], Björn Haiduk [2] and Marijke Grau [1,*]

[1] Institute of Cardiovascular Research and Sports Medicine, Molecular and Cellular Sports Medicine, German Sport University Cologne, 50933 Cologne, Germany
[2] S.P.O.R.T. Institut, Institute of Applied Sports Sciences, 51491 Overath, Germany
* Correspondence: m.grau@dshs-koeln.de
† These authors contributed equally to this work.

Abstract: (1) Background: Long-term health effects after SARS-CoV-2 infections can manifest in a plethora of symptoms, significantly impacting the quality of life of affected individuals. (2) Aim: The present paper aimed to assess the effects of an individualized and controlled exercise intervention on fatigue and exercise capacity among Long-COVID (LC) patients in an ambulatory setting. (3) Methods: Forty-one (n = 41) LC patients performed an exercise protocol with an individualized control of the patients' training intensity during the study period based on the individual's ability to achieve the target criteria. The program was carried out two to three times a week, each session lasted 30 min, and the study parameters were recorded at the beginning of the program, as well as after 6 and 12 weeks, respectively. These included both patient-reported (PCFS questionnaire, FACIT–Fatigue questionnaire) and objective (one-minute sit-to-stand test (1MSTST), workload) outcomes. (4) Results: The exercise training intervention resulted in significant improvements in the FACIT–Fatigue ($F(2, 80) = 18.08$, $p < 0.001$), 1MSTST ($\chi^2(2) = 19.35$, $p < 0.001$) and workload scores ($\chi^2(2) = 62.27$, $p < 0.001$), while the PCFS scores remained unchanged. Changes in the workload scores were dependent on the frequency of the completed exercise sessions and were higher in the LC patients with a moderate Post COVID Syndrome Score (PCS) compared to a severe PCS. (5) Conclusions: The individualized and controlled training approach demonstrated efficacy in reducing fatigue and enhancing exercise capacity among outpatient LC patients. However, for complete regeneration, a longer, possibly indefinite, treatment is required, which in practice would be feasible within the framework of legislation.

Keywords: Long-COVID; Post-COVID; fatigue; exercise capacity; 1MSTST; individualized training

1. Introduction

Sequelae of SARS-CoV-2 infections occur worldwide, with high prevalence and incidence rates in the population, and cause severe health restrictions. Based on current data, a point prevalence of 6–7% can be assumed. Furthermore, the cumulative global incidence of Long-COVID is estimated to affect approximately 400 million individuals, with an anticipated annual economic impact of around $1 trillion, which corresponds to roughly 1% of the global economy [1]. Depending on the time that has passed since the infection, this phenomenon is referred to as Long-COVID or Post-COVID [2]. As an umbrella term, Long-COVID incorporates all long-term health issues that are prevalent more than four weeks after an acute infection, including post-COVID, which describes all symptoms that persist, return, or arise more than twelve weeks after the acute infection [3]. In the following discussion, the term Long-COVID is used to describe the study sample, which includes Post-COVID. The symptoms most frequently reported by those affected by Long-COVID are fatigue, neurological restrictions, and breathlessness [3]. In particular, the main symptom of fatigue, which is defined by a pronounced lack of energy that is not

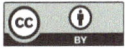

improved by sleep, severely restricts the quality of life for many sufferers and may also lead to the development of accompanying mental illnesses such as depression and anxiety disorders [4,5]. In addition, many sufferers report an intolerance to physical and mental activity, which is associated with an exacerbation of symptoms [6].

Studies that examined the physical and exercise capacity of those affected using functional and performance tests reported below-average test results for most test subjects [7,8]. Furthermore, some authors were able to identify limitations in the heart's response to exercise in some affected individuals, which is also referred to as chronotropic incompetence [7]. The reported limitations not only cause a high burden of disease for affected individuals, reducing their everyday functions and their ability to work [9]. The healthcare system also faces major (financial) challenges in the face of this "new" disease, for which there is (as yet) no monocausal treatment [10,11]. Therefore, there is a need for cost- and time-effective treatment options, which are easy to access for affected individuals.

As no single cause has yet been found for the multitude of symptoms, symptom-oriented treatment involving various specialist disciplines is at the heart of previous recommendations from national and international experts [10,12,13]. The German recommendation guideline for Long-/Post-COVID pointed out the potential benefits of systematic and individualized exercise training for symptom treatment [10]. The effectiveness of exercise training in the treatment of a variety of chronic diseases has already been empirically proven [14–16]. For example, a combination of aerobic and strength training has proven effective in alleviating the symptoms of fatigue in multiple sclerosis and cancer [14,16]. Exercise training has also been shown to increase exercise capacity and quality of life (QoL) across several diseases, including cancer, cardiovascular and musculoskeletal diseases, respiratory conditions, and others [15].

Hence, it can be assumed that exercise training should act as an important cornerstone of rehabilitation in Long- and Post-COVID to counteract both symptom burden and the loss of independence through decreased physical capacity. Initial studies, which investigated the influence of exercise training on the symptoms of those affected by long-term sequelae following a COVID-19 infection also showed positive effects; regular training supervised by appropriately trained exercise professionals and offered with an individualized and collaboratively coordinated increase in intensity reduced the severity of symptoms and increased physical and exercise capacities [17]. However, questions regarding the necessary intensity and frequency of the training as well as the necessary duration of the intervention remain unanswered. In addition, direct differences in the course of the intervention with regard to Long-COVID severity and sex-related differences have not yet been analyzed in detail.

Long-COVID is a new disease which affects a large number of people and can challenge the healthcare system. Affected patients and also health professionals need an empirically tested framework for the time-efficient conceptualization of individualized exercise interventions, which reflects the importance of collaboratively designed training to avoid the deterioration of symptoms by overtraining. Furthermore, professionals working in this field need practical tools to monitor progression during such interventions in Long-COVID patients. This study aims to test such a framework on Long-COVID patients with several objective (one-minute sit-to-stand test (1MSTST), workload) and patient-reported (FACIT–Fatigue score, Post COVID Functional Status scale) outcomes, taking into account the aforementioned aspects.

2. Materials and Methods

2.1. Ethical Approval, Recruitment, and Study Cohort

This study was approved by the ethical review board of the German Sport University Cologne (Reference Number 171/2022). Written informed consent was obtained from all participants. The recruitment was conducted using flyers and advertisements on the homepage of the S.P.O.R.T Institute and the German Sport University Cologne. A U09.9 diagnosis ("Post COVID-19 condition, unspecified") from a medical doctor was required. There was no age limitation. The exclusion criteria included a rating of 4 on the Post COVID Functional Status Scale (PCFS) [18] and a planned inpatient stay within the first six weeks of the intervention.

Sixty-seven participants met the inclusion criteria, with twenty-two withdrawing and data from four missing. A detailed overview of the participants' demographics as well as their medical history and SARS-CoV-2-specific information is illustrated in Table 1. A significant portion (73.2%, n = 30) reported at least one comorbidity, with the most common being endocrine, nutritional, or metabolic diseases (36.6%, n = 15). Analgesics were the most frequently reported medication (51.2%, n = 21). Fatigue-related symptoms (100%, n = 41) were the most common, followed by cognitive/neurological symptoms (87.8%, n = 36). According to the Post COVID Syndrome (PCS) Score [6], 61% (n = 25) were moderately affected and 39% (n = 16) were severely affected.

Table 1. Baseline characteristics.

Variable	Value
Age [years]	48.05 ± 15.15
BMI [kg/m^2]	26.44 ± 5.36
Sex [women]	24 (58.5%)
Comorbidities	
Reported comorbidities [yes]	30 (73.2%)
Endocrine, nutritional, or metabolic diseases	15 (36.6%)
Diseases of the musculoskeletal system and connective tissue	12 (29.3%)
Diseases of the cardiovascular system	9 (21.9%)
Diseases of the respiratory system	8 (19.5%)
Pain disorders/chronic pain syndrome	5 (12.2%)
Neurological diseases	3 (7.3%)
Psychiatric disorders	3 (7.3%)
Others [1]	4 (9.7%)
Medication	
Analgesics	21 (51.2%)
Thyroid medication	9 (21.9%)
Antidepressants	9 (21.9%)
Antihypertensives	8 (19.5%)
Corticosteroids	7 (17.1%)
Anticoagulants	5 (12.2%)
Bronchodilators	4 (9.7%)
Others [2]	9 (21.9%)
SARS-CoV-2 specific information	
Duration between infection and training start [weeks]	51.54 ± 43.10
Vaccination status [yes]	41 (100%)
Received two SARS-CoV-2 vaccinations	7 (17.1%)
Received three SARS-CoV-2 vaccinations	29 (70.7%)
Received four SARS-CoV-2 vaccinations	5 (12.2%)
Inpatient treatment since SARS-CoV-2 infection [yes]	14 (34.1%)

Table 1. Cont.

Variable	Value
Post COVID-19 specific information	
Number of symptom clusters [3] per patient, median	4
Fatigue	41 (100%)
Cognitive/neurological system	36 (87.8%)
Chest symptoms	26 (63.4%)
Musculoskeletal system	24 (58.5%)
Anxiety, depression, or sleep disorders	16 (39%)
Tachycardia	8 (19.5%)
Gastrointestinal symptoms	6 (14.6%)
Flu-like symptoms, chills, or fever	6 (14.6%)
Others [4]	3 (7.3%)
PCS score [5]	23.59 ± 7.33
None/mild	0
Moderate	24 (58.5%)
Severe	17 (41.5%)

[1] Other comorbidities included removal of gallstone (n = 1), infection with the Epstein–Barr virus (n = 1), borreliosis (n = 1), and hyperuricemia (n = 1). [2] Other medications included antipsychotics (n = 1), proton pump inhibitors (n = 1), sedatives (n = 2), alpha blockers (n = 1), anticonvulsants (n = 1), uricostatics (n = 1), TNF (tumor necrosis factor) blockers (n = 1), and non-steroidal anti-inflammatory drugs (n = 1). [3] Symptoms were clustered referring to [3] as follows: fatigue, including fatigue-related symptoms such as a state of exhaustion, reduced exercise tolerance, and prolonged recovery time. Cognitive/neurological symptoms included brain fog, concentration and memory problems, smell or taste distortion, vertigo, dizziness, balance problems, tremor, sound and light sensitivity, headaches/migraines, and vision impairments. Chest symptoms included shortness of breath, chest pain, and wheezing. Musculoskeletal symptoms included muscle and joint pain, paresthesia, muscle cramps, and muscle weakness. Gastrointestinal symptoms included nausea, vomitus, and abdominal pain. Others included lymphoedema and hypotonia. [4] Other symptoms included urinary incontinence (n = 1), lymphoedema (n = 1), and hypotonia under exhaustion (n = 1). [5] The PCS score was calculated according to [6] with thresholds for the PCS score classification of 10.75 and 26.25 for none/mildly, moderately and severely affected participants, respectively.

2.2. Study Design and Intervention

This study followed a single-arm pre-test-post-test design over an initial 12 weeks of the ongoing TRIBAL intervention. The evaluation focuses on time-related outcomes before the commencement of the initial training (T0), after six weeks (T1), and after 12 weeks (T2). Changes in the time-dependent results were also analyzed according to the following: (1) difference in moderate vs. severe LC, (2) difference in the frequency of training sessions, (3) difference in sex.

2.3. Testing Protocol

The testing included patient-reported outcomes (PROs) and objective measurements. The PROs comprised the post-COVID Functional Status (PCFS) scale [18] and the FACIT–Fatigue scale [19]. Objective measurements to assess exercise capacity included the one-minute sit-to-stand test (1MSTST) and workload (average wattage during a 15-minute session with a self-determined pace, derived via the KEISER M Series application) assessment. Vital parameters (blood pressure, heart rate, and oxygen saturation) were controlled during the testing sessions. The rating of perceived exertion (RPE) was gauged using a 10-point visual scale.

2.4. Exercise Intervention

The exercise sessions were supervised by exercise professionals or physiotherapists, specially trained and certified by Long-COVID Network Rhein-Neckar.

The reporting of the intervention was conducted according to the Consensus on Exercise Reporting Template (CERT) checklist [20].

The participants were asked to train at least twice weekly. Each exercise session consisted of 30 min. The *first part* always consisted of 15 min, and the *second part* followed a short break and covered the remaining 10–15 min. Each session was performed in groups of up to three people, with every participant receiving an individualized training regimen.

In the *first* part, the participants were asked to train on the M3i Total Body Trainer (Keiser GmbH, Coburg, Germany). This device was selected due to its medical approval in Germany, which ensures compliance with established health and safety standards. Additionally, it can be calibrated and verified for accuracy, further enhancing its reliability for use in clinical and research settings. The Total Body Trainer (TBT) combines an indoor bike with a cross trainer, which allows both the upper and lower extremities to be simultaneously trained. The primary goal was to train on the TBT for 15 min within a range of 50–60 rounds per minute (RPM). There was no minimum requirement in watts, to avoid overexertion. The initial intensity was estimated based on the individual performance and feedback in the baseline tests and expressed as the gear (resistance) on the TBT. Moderately affected participants started with a medium resistance (e.g., gear 11, where 60 RPM corresponds to about 60 watts), while the more severely affected participants started with a low resistance (e.g., gear 5, where 60 RPM corresponds to about 30 watts).

The progression of the intensity during the study period was based on three criteria: (1) if the participants easily met the time target (15 min) and increased the speed to 60 RPM and beyond within the respective resistance/gear, (2) if the reports of previous sessions did not include the worsening of symptoms, and (3) when the participants reported that they could tolerate a higher intensity. The intensity was then increased by switching up the gear of the TBT, starting with the last two minutes of the exercise session (13–15) and progressing by time during the following exercise sessions (11–15 min, then 7–15 min, and eventually 15 min). The average wattage (workload) of the first part was noted after every single exercise session.

After a short break, in the *second part* (the remaining 10–15 min), the participants were instructed to perform breathing exercises or low-intensity strengthening, stretching, or mobility exercises mainly using their body weight or low-resistance devices (e.g., TotalGym RS Encompass PowerTower (TotalGym Europe B.V, Hoofddorp, The Netherlands), rubber bands, foam rolls, kettlebells, or elastic balls) depending on their capacity and (e.g., orthopedic) demands. In the first weeks of the intervention, breathing and low-intensity stretching or mobility exercises were instructed to increase the participants' body awareness. In the later course of the study, strengthening exercises were applied. To control the intensity and avoid overexertion throughout the *second part*, participants were asked to rate their perceived exertion and not exceed 6 on a 10-point scale. When feeling too exhausted, the participants also had the possibility to receive heat applications (heat therapy) or simply rest for the remaining time.

2.5. Data Analysis

Data analysis was conducted using IBM SPSS Statistics (Version 29). The normality was assessed using the Shapiro–Wilk test, with $p > 0.05$ indicating normally distributed data. The boxplots were visually inspected, and outliers were retained unless attributed to data entry errors. Before running each analysis, the assumptions were tested. Violations prompted corrections (e.g., Greenhouse–Geisser correction) for one-way repeated measures ANOVA [21] or the use of non-parametric alternatives. Significance level for all tests was set at $p < 0.05$.

Given the substantial number of analyses, only statistically significant results will be presented in detail in the results section. Same applies for effect sizes, which are reported only for statistically significant results. Effect sizes are reported as recommended, namely as Cohen's f [22] for (one-way and one-way repeated measures) ANOVA, Kendall's w for the Friedman test, η^2 for the Kruskal Wallis H-test [23], and Cohen's d for independent samples *t*-test [24]. Non-significant findings are briefly summarized with the test results provided in Appendix A.

Statistical analyses encompassed patient-reported and objective outcomes, focusing on time, sex, training sessions, and symptom severity.

(a) Effects of time and sex: Outcome values are reported as mean (SD). A one-way repeated measures ANOVA assessed differences in the FACIT–Fatigue, 1MSTST, and workload scores across three time points (T0, T1, and T2) during the 12-week intervention. Post hoc tests reported the mean differences (M.) with 95% confidence intervals (CI). If the normality was violated or for ordinal outcomes (PCFS), a Friedman test with median (Mdn.) scores was used. To investigate the interaction of time and sex, a two-way mixed ANOVA was employed. (b) PCS score and change scores: Differences in change scores (Δ_2) between moderately and severely affected groups (based on the PCS scores) were analyzed using independent t-tests or Mann–Whitney U tests, with mean differences (M.) and 95% CI reported for t-tests. (c) Completed Training Sessions (CTS) and change scores: Correlation analyses examined the relationship between CTS and change scores (Δ_2) in the FACIT–Fatigue, 1MSTST, and workload scores. Pearson's or Spearman's correlations were applied based on the distribution. Participants were divided into three groups by CTS (<21, 21–24, >24). A one-way ANOVA or Kruskal–Wallis H test assessed differences in outcome changes between the groups. (d) Relationships between the outcomes: Correlations between PCS, PCFS, FACIT–Fatigue, 1MSTST, and workload scores at T0 were analyzed using Pearson's or Spearman's correlations.

3. Results

The summarized results related to the graphs are presented below, and the outcomes that did not reach statistical significance are described in Appendices A and B.

3.1. Effects of Time

The FACIT–Fatigue scores significantly increased from T0 to T1 (M. = −4.56, 95% CI [−7.57, −1.55], $p = 0.002$), from T0 to T2 (M. = −7.41, 95% CI [−11.02, −3.81], $p < 0.001$), and from T1 to T2 (M. = −2.85, 95% CI [−5.49, −0.22], $p = 0.03$). The effect size was large: Cohen's $f = 0.67$ (Figure 1A).

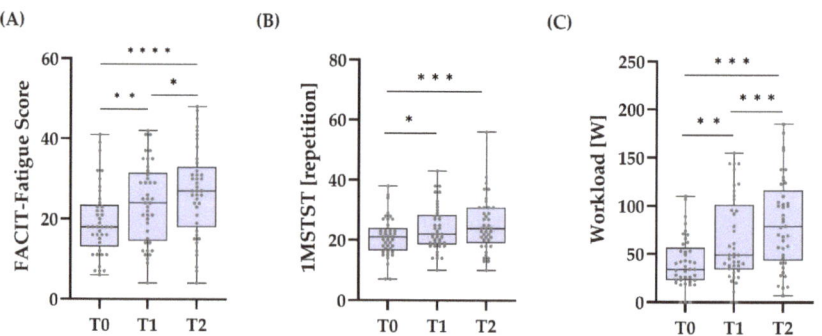

Figure 1. Changes in the Fatigue score and exercise capacity over time. The figure shows boxplots illustrating the distribution of the (**A**) FACIT–Fatigue scores, (**B**) 1MSTST repetitions, and (**C**) workload scores across the three testing sessions (T0, T1, and T2). The results highlight improvements in all three parameters over time. The box represents the interquartile range (IQR), with the median denoted by the horizontal line inside the box. Each dot represents one individual. Whiskers extend from the box to the minimum and maximum values within 1.5 times the IQR. Statistically significant differences between the different time points, as calculated with post hoc pairwise comparisons following the Friedman test, are highlighted with asterisks. * $p < 0.05$; ** $p < 0.01$; *** $p < 0.001$. **** $p < 0.0001$. n = 41.

The 1MSTST scores differed significantly over time: $\chi^2(2) = 19.35$, $p < 0.001$. Effect size was small: Kendall's $w = 0.24$. Median values increased from T0 (Mdn. = 21) to T1 (Mdn. = 22) to T2 (Mdn. = 24). Post hoc tests showed that T0 and T1 ($z = −0.65$, p adjusted = 0.01) and T0 and T2 ($z = −0.93$, p adjusted < 0.001) differed significantly, but T1 and T2 did not (Figure 1B).

Statistical significance was also established in the differences between workload scores: $\chi^2(2) = 62.27$, $p < 0.001$. Effect size of the differences between time points was large:

Kendall's w = 0.76. Median values increased from T0 (Mdn. = 34) to T1 (Mdn. = 49) to T2 (Mdn. = 79). There were statistically significant differences between T0 and T1 (z = −0.829, *p adjusted* = 0.001) and T0 and T2 (z = −1.73, *p adjusted* < 0.001), as well as between T1 and T2 (z = −0.90, *p adjusted* < 0.001) (Figure 1C).

3.2. Effects of Sex

A two-way mixed ANOVA yielded no significant interactions between time and sex, neither for the FACIT–Fatigue nor for 1MSTST or workload scores. Additionally, the main effect of group did only reveal statistically significant differences between males and females for orkload scores (F (1,39) = 4.39, $p = 0.043$, partial $\eta^2 = 0.10$), with males scoring significantly higher than females. The effect size for the main effect of group was medium: Cohen's $f = 0.33$ (Appendix A.1).

3.3. Effects of Training Sessions

Results indicated a significant difference in workload scores across the complete training sessions (CTS) groups, F(2, 40) = 3.96, $p = 0.027$, with significant differences between group 1 (<21 sessions) and group 3 (>24 sessions) (M = −32.03, 95% CI [−60.52, −3.54], $p = 0.025$), emphasizing a significantly greater increase in the workload scores for participants who completed more than 24 compared to those who completed less than 21 training sessions (Figure 2; Appendix A.2 and Appendix Table A2). Analysis further revealed no significant effect between number of CTS and difference in 1MSTST or difference in FACIT–Fatigue score, respectively (Appendix A.2 and Appendix Table A2).

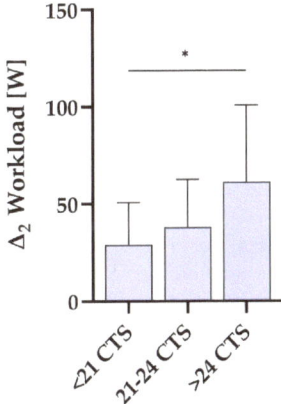

Figure 2. Difference in workload score between 12 weeks and 0 weeks related to number of complete training sessions (CTS). Participants that completed more than 24 CTS showed higher increment in workload score after 12 weeks of training compared to participants that completed less than 21 CTS. * $p < 0.05$. Participant count for groups is as follows: <21 CTS with n = 13, 21–24 CTS with n = 17, and >24 CTS with n = 11.

3.4. Effects of Symptom Severity

3.4.1. Change in PCFS Score After 12 Weeks of Intervention

The median PCFS score (3) did not change significantly during the intervention. Additionally, the distribution of the scores (65.85% scoring 3 pre-intervention and 60.98% scoring 3 post-intervention) indicated moderate functional limitations for the majority of the participants before and after the twelve weeks of the intervention.

3.4.2. Change in Workload, Fatigue Score, and 1MSTST After 12 Weeks Related to Initial PCS Score

The Δ_2 values were examined for moderately and severely affected groups, classified by PCS scores. Analysis revealed significant differences in Δ_2 of workload scores between moderately and severely affected participants (M = −23.60, 95% CI [−5.30, −41.91], t(39) = −2.61, p = 0.013), indicating a larger increase in workload scores for moderately affected participants (Figure 3; Appendix A.3 and Appendix Table A2). The Fatigue score and 1MSTST increased comparably in both groups. The groups did not significantly differ (see Appendix A.3 and Appendix Table A2).

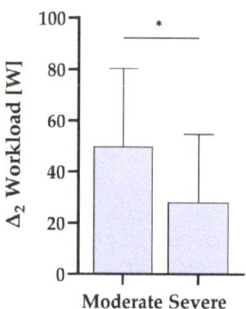

Figure 3. Difference in workload score between 12 weeks and 0 weeks related to PCS score. Statistically significant differences between groups, as calculated by post hoc tests following a one-way ANOVA, are highlighted with an asterisk. * p < 0.05. Participant count for groups is as follows: severe (>26.25) with n = 16, and moderate (10.75–26.25) with n = 25.

3.5. Correlation Analyses

Correlation analyses showed no significant relationships between CTS and Δ_2 for any outcome (Appendix A.3. The results indicated a correlation between lower PCFS scores and higher FACIT–Fatigue scores, as indicated by a moderate negative correlation (r_s = −0.47, p = 0.002). Higher FACIT–Fatigue scores correlated with higher workload scores, as indicated by a moderate positive correlation (r_s = 0.42, p = 0.007), and higher workload scores correlated strongly with higher 1MSTST scores, as indicated by a strong positive correlation (r_s = 0.50, p < 0.001) (Table 2).

Table 2. Correlation matrix of outcome variables at T0.

Variables	1.	2.	3.	4.
1. PCS	-	-	-	-
2. PCFS	0.08	-	-	-
3. Fatigue	−0.23	−0.47 **	-	-
4. 1MSTST	−0.29	−0.27	0.13	-
5. WL	−0.25	−0.30	0.42 **	0.50 ***

PCS = Post COVID Syndrome Score; PCFS = Post COVID Functional Status Scale; 1MSTST = one minute sit to stand test; WL = workload; ** p < 0.01, *** p < 0.001.

4. Discussion

Twelve weeks of individualized and controlled exercise training, combining one part of endurance training on a stationary Total Body Trainer with another part of mixed breathing, stretching, and/or strengthening exercises, led to significant improvements in exercise capacity (as measured by 1MSTST and workload test) and fatigue (as measured by FACIT–Fatigue scale) in male and female ambulatory Long-COVID patients. The controlled approach of the supervision by exercise professionals and a criteria-based collaborative progression of the intensity led to improvement rates of 95.1% in the workload and 82.9%

in both the FACIT–Fatigue score and 1MSTST over twelve weeks, showing the success of the program for most of the participants.

4.1. Main Effect of Time

These results are in line with prior investigations examining the influence of exercise training on fatigue and exercise capacity in several other chronic conditions including cancer and multiple sclerosis [14,16]. The current study, furthermore, adds evidence to early empirical works finding reduced fatigue and enhanced exercise capacity after different exercise training regimens in Long-COVID patients [25].

The sample analyzed in the present study presented with a high symptom and fatigue burden as well as restrictions in exercise capacity and daily functioning. More precisely, almost half of the participants (41.5%) were classified as severely affected according to the PCS score, and mean FACIT–Fatigue scores were below a value of 30 and thus clinically relevant across all time points [6,26,27]. Moreover, the mean 1MSTST score was lower and the median PCFS scores were higher compared to a previous study in Long-COVID patients [17].

Regarding fatigue symptomatology, every single participant investigated in this study reported fatigue-related symptoms prior to the intervention. Furthermore, despite a clinically important mean change by 7.42 points in the FACIT–Fatigue scores over the course of the intervention, the mean score remained clinically elevated after the twelve weeks (26.80 points), considering an increase by three to five points and a cut-off score of ≤ 30 as clinically relevant [27,28]. For comparison, another study which also used the FACIT–Fatigue score in a cross-sectional investigation of symptomatic individuals nine months after the acute infection reported a mean score of 39.2 points [26]. The finding that fatigue symptoms were still in a clinically relevant range after the twelve-week program despite the participants improving significantly suggests that the training needs to be continued to bring the values into line with a healthy reference group.

The impact of the symptom burden was also expressed in the second patient-reported outcome, that was assessed in this study, the PCFS score. The median PCFS score (3) did not change significantly during the intervention. Additionally, the distribution of the scores as reported in Section 3.4.1 indicated moderate functional limitations for the majority of the participants before and after the twelve weeks of the intervention. While the improvement in fatigue is in line with previous studies investigating the effect of exercise training in Long-COVID patients, the stagnation in the PCFS scores might contrast to previous findings [17]. However, in one study cited by Sick & König [17], reported improvements were expressed as means [29], while the present study statistically analyzed median values as recommended for ordinal scales such as the PCFS scale [18]. Another study by the same author derived improvements in PCFS scores by comparing the number of participants presenting with a score of <2 before and after the intervention [30]. Another study reported an improvement in the median PCFS score over six weeks [31]. The different findings in this study could be explained by two reasons: First, the concerned study investigated a multidisciplinary outpatient rehabilitation, including nutritional education and psychosocial counseling besides structured exercise training. Second, the baseline median score was 2 in the examination of Nopp et al. [31], indicating fewer functional limitations compared to the sample analyzed in this study (median of 3) and thus possibly indicating a better prognosis with regard to the potential improvements during the intervention related to the initial impairments.

The differences between the studies regarding the severity of the functional limitation are also reflected in the lower exercise capacity of the patients examined in the present study. While Nopp et al. [31] reported a mean of 33.3 repetitions at baseline testing in the 1MSTST, the sample of this study performed a mean of 20.98 repetitions before and 25.07 repetitions after twelve weeks. Although the score increased by a mean of 4.10 repetitions, which exceeds the minimal important difference (≥ 3 repetitions) according to [32], it remained comparably low. This finding adds to the results previously reported for the FACIT–Fatigue scores and implicates restrictions in exercise capacity.

As a second outcome depicting exercise capacity, workload scores improved significantly over time, with a mean increase of 24.50 watts in the first six weeks and of 43.03 watts over the twelve weeks. The workload scores derived in this study are hardly comparable to other investigations of exercise interventions since the assessment is not standardized as in questionnaires (like the FACIT–Fatigue) or standardized tests like the 1MSTST. The present study defined workload as the average wattage of 15 min on the Total Body Trainer, which allowed the simultaneous training of the lower and upper extremities and therefore differs from exercise training on a stationary bicycle ergometer by involved muscles and metabolic demands. Comparable studies did either not specify which device was used for endurance training [29–31] or reported the use of a bicycle ergometer [25]. Additionally, studies mentioning workload as an outcome either did not specify training time at all [31] or differed in training time (e.g., in [25], participants were asked to train for 18 min). The use of different devices and different definitions to assess the workload hinders their comparability with the present study.

However, the improvements in workload are in line with the improvements in FACIT–Fatigue score and 1MSTST and therefore reflect the general trainability of Long-COVID patients and the positive influence of training on one of the main symptoms in Long-COVID patients, fatigue, as well as exercise capacity. These findings complement previous studies reporting an amelioration of symptoms as well as physical performance parameters [17].

Based on these results, it could be hypothesized that ongoing training exceeding the twelve weeks, which have been investigated in this study, would lead to further improvements in fatigue symptomatology as well as in exercise capacity, which eventually would also reduce functional restrictions in daily living (PCFS score). The development of improvements, which does not only present in the mean scores but also in the proportion of the participants experiencing ameliorations (of at least one point) after six weeks (78% in FACIT–Fatigue, 70.7% in 1MSTST, 87.8% in workload score, and 4.9% in PCFS score) and after twelve weeks (82.9% in FACIT–Fatigue, 82.9% in 1MSTST, 95.1% in workload score, and 14.6% in PCFS score) supports this hypothesis. This hypothesis is further supported by previous investigations which showed improvements in several outcomes but were limited to a total duration of four to twelve weeks [17].

Further, it should be noted that 14.6% (n = 6) of the participants in the analyzed sample showed decreased FACIT–Fatigue scores, 17.07% (n = 7) showed reductions in 1MSTST, and 4.9% (n = 2) showed reductions in workload scores after twelve weeks. Following the line of basic training principles [33], one might suggest that the participants that showed a worsening in the previously stated scores did not set sufficient training stimuli for (physiological or psychological) adaptations or that the total duration of the intervention was not long enough. To support this assumption, individual analyses revealed that the two participants showing reductions in their workload scores after 12 weeks only completed 15 and 24 training sessions, respectively. The individuals showing decreased FACIT–Fatigue scores completed less than 21 (n = 3) or between 21 and 24 (n = 3) training sessions. And, finally, n = 4 participants with CTS between 21-24 and n = 3 participants with CTS > 24 showed reduced 1MSTST scores. Yet, because the highest increment in the workload score was achieved by a number of participants with CTS > 24, it is concluded that Long-COVID patients benefit from regular training with two to three training sessions per week.

However, the low number of CTS cannot completely explain the described findings, as further explained below. Previous studies reported that a substantial number of Long-COVID patients share symptoms with ME/CFS, in particular post-exertional malaise (PEM), which describes the deterioration of symptoms after (physical or mental) activity [34,35]. It could be hypothesized that some of the participants might also fit the clinical definition of ME/CFS, but the presence of ME/CFS was not systematically assessed. However, since the same participants did not consistently show the reductions mentioned, a more detailed analysis is required here, which also includes other factors.

4.2. The Effect of Sex

Although a "sex bias" is discussed in the literature, higher prevalence rates and higher symptom severity have been reported in women [3,36]. Based on the findings of this study, this bias does not translate into any differences in trainability between both sexes, as indicated by the absence of interaction effects in the two-way mixed ANOVA. This is in line with Mooren et al. [25] who did not find a different response to training with respect to sex. It can be stated that both sexes did benefit similarly from the individualized training approach conducted in this study. Therefore, sex is not a characteristic that requires differentiation in training management. However, it should be noted that the present study included a small sample size. Future investigations including more participants should further validate these findings.

The only statistical difference that was found between the sexes was in the mean workload score, which was higher in males than in females when averaged across all testing sessions. This result is in line with a study in cardiorespiratory outpatient rehabilitation that showed a reduced VO_2 peak in females compared to males, both before and after exercise training [37], but this was not related to Long-COVID or the training applied herein. The (biological) mechanisms which are discussed to be responsible for the differences in mean workload production between males and females are beyond the scope of this investigation and are therefore not further discussed.

4.3. The Influence of Symptom Severity

To date and knowledge of the authors, this is the first study implementing the PCS score in an investigation of exercise training. At baseline, 41.5% of the participants were classified as severely affected, which adds to the previously discussed evidence of a comparably high disease burden in the present sample. For comparison, Bahmer et al. [6] found 13–20% of Long-COVID patients to be severely affected in the initial study, in which the PCS score was introduced. Furthermore, none of the participants investigated in this study were classified as only mildly influenced.

The investigation of differences between moderately and severely affected participants showed significant differences for the development of the workload, yet the scores did improve in both groups, namely by a relative mean of 77.8% in severely affected and of 113.6% in moderately affected participants. Furthermore, FACIT–Fatigue and 1MSTST scores developed comparably in both groups, showing increments in the mean scores over the course of the intervention. These findings indicate that, despite the difference in workload scores, both groups were trainable and experienced ameliorations in fatigue symptomatology and exercise capacity. As discussed previously in comparing male and female participants, it appears that both moderately and severely affected PCS patients improve through exercise training.

It was beyond the scope of this analysis to systematically assess which characteristics could be responsible for the differing workload production in severely affected Long-COVID patients. Since this is the first study comparing the results for Long-COVID patients based on a symptom severity score, the results remain preliminary. It would be of high clinical relevance to clarify the findings of this study with a reasonable sample size to further evaluate if there are differences in the adaption between patient groups differing in symptom severity.

However, deducing practical considerations for training management in Long-COVID patients from the findings of this study, it appears most important to adhere to the basic training principle of individualization in order to reflect the conditions of patients with varying degrees of severity and to be able to address these in training planning [33]. The principle of individualization is in line with the recommendations as well as the prior investigations of exercise training in this cohort [10,17].

4.4. The Influence of Completed Training Sessions

The number of completed training sessions (CTS) did influence the change scores only in one comparison in the workload, showing no consistent dose–response relationship between the training frequency and adaptions in fatigue symptomatology or exercise capacity in the studied Long-COVID sample. Consistent with this finding, Mooren et al. [25] did not find an effect of overall training sessions on outcomes.

The finding of a differing change in workload scores between the group with the most training sessions compared to the group with the least training sessions could be explained by a more pronounced cardiovascular response in relation to a higher number of training sessions. However, the positive mean in change scores across the different ranges of the training sessions in fatigue and exercise capacity (refer to Appendix B, Table A2) points to the assumption that the health benefits experienced by the participants of this study were mostly independent of the training frequency. Nevertheless, according to the principles of training science, it should be taken into account that a certain number of training stimuli are necessary to achieve optimal adaptations [33].

While previous studies have recommended that participants train three to five times per week, with investigation periods of four to twelve weeks [17], the present study recommends at least two training sessions per week, which was met only by 26.8% of the participants (n = 11). Furthermore, the range of the completed training sessions (15–36 CTS) over the twelve weeks indicated a high variability in the adherence to the recommendations. The participant with the most training sessions trained three times per week, while a mean of 1.25 sessions per week accounted for the participant with the least training sessions. The main self-reported reasons for the lower numbers of attended training sessions included scheduling problems, personal problems (job/family), illness, or other.

To summarize, finding no consistent dose–response relationship, training frequency does not appear to be the sole limiting factor for the positive effects observed across the different ranges of CTS across the twelve weeks investigated in this study.

4.5. Relationships of Outcomes

The findings of correlation analyses offer valuable insights into the baseline dynamics of Long-COVID patients undergoing exercise training. The negative correlation between the PCFS and FACIT–Fatigue scores suggests that patients with a lower functional status may experience lower levels of fatigue, underscoring the intricate relationship between functionality and subjective well-being which has already been stated in previous investigations [38,39].

The positive correlation between the FACIT–Fatigue and workload scores implies that patients being less fatigued may be capable of more demanding exercise training. This finding appears to be in line with the finding of the present study that the FACIT–Fatigue and workload scores both increased significantly across the different testing sessions. Contrary to this assumption, a relationship between the workload and 1MSTST scores was found which was not expressed as an equal improvement in both values: while the workload differed significantly between all three time points in the time-related analyses, 1MSTST scores did not increase significantly between six and twelve weeks.

The 1MSTST primarily measures lower limb strength endurance (quadriceps, hamstrings, and gluteal muscles) during a functional task (sit-to-stand) and progressively increases cardiovascular demands through elevated heart rate and oxygen consumption (VO_2max), engaging both aerobic and anaerobic systems. In contrast, the workload measurement used in this study emphasizes aerobic capacity and involves whole-body coordination, requiring simultaneous alternating movements of the arms and legs. It could be assumed that the workload measure may be more sensitive to exercise-induced changes in aerobic capacity, as the 1MSTST improvements between 6 and 12 weeks were not statistically significant. However, as summarized by Sick & König [17], most of the studies investigating exercise training in Long-COVID patients report improvements in physical performance (including several versions of the sit-to-stand test) as well as fatigue measures.

5. Conclusions

This study demonstrates that the twelve-week individualized and controlled exercise program, combining endurance training with breathing, stretching, and strengthening exercises, demonstrated significant improvements in fatigue and exercise capacity among ambulatory Long-COVID patients. The intervention's controlled approach, supervised by exercise professionals, yielded high improvement rates in the workload (95.1%) and both the FACIT–Fatigue and 1MSTST (82.9%) scores. Despite improvements, fatigue symptoms remained clinically relevant, emphasizing the need for continued training. This study explored sex differences, indicating a similar trainability for both sexes, and considered the influence of symptom severity, showing positive outcomes for both moderately and severely affected Long-COVID patients. Overall, this study contributes valuable insights into the effectiveness of individualized exercise interventions for Long-COVID patients and highlights areas for future exploration and refinement in the management of Long-COVID symptoms including the need for longer-term interventions to fully assess the potential benefits of exercise on recovery outcomes. Further research should give attention to factors influencing the adherence and individual responses to training in terms of symptom severity and include monitoring of other common symptoms.

Author Contributions: Conceptualization, M.G. and B.H.; methodology, M.G., B.H. and A.-L.K.; validation, S.K., A.-L.K., M.G. and B.H.; formal analysis, S.K.; investigation, S.K. and A.-L.K.; resources, B.H.; data curation, A.-L.K., S.K., M.G. and B.H.; writing—original draft preparation, S.K.; writing—review and editing, M.G., A.-L.K. and B.H.; visualization, M.G.; supervision, M.G. and B.H.; project administration, B.H. and M.G. All authors have read and agreed to the published version of the manuscript.

Funding: This research received no external funding.

Institutional Review Board Statement: This study was conducted in accordance with the Declaration of Helsinki and approved by approved by the ethical review board of the German Sport University Cologne (Reference Number 171/2022).

Informed Consent Statement: Informed consent was obtained from all subjects involved in the study.

Data Availability Statement: The data that support the findings of this study are available upon reasonable request from the corresponding author. The data are not publicly available due to privacy or ethical restrictions.

Conflicts of Interest: The authors declare no conflicts of interest. The funders had no role in the design of the study, in the collection, analyses, or interpretation of data, or in the decision to publish the results, but they edited the manuscript.

Appendix A

Appendix A.1. Interaction Effects of Time and Sex

FACIT–Fatigue scores:
There was no statistically significant interaction between sex and time in the FACIT Fatigue scores, $F(2, 78) = 0.83$, $p = 0.441$, partial $\eta^2 = 0.02$. The main effect of the group showed that there was no statistically significant difference in the FACIT Fatigue scores between the sexes, $F(1, 39) = 0.22$, $p = 0.643$, partial $\eta^2 = 0.01$.

1MSTST scores:
There was no statistically significant interaction between sex and time in the STS scores, $F(1.598, 62.334) = 0.43$, $p = 0.608$, partial $\eta^2 = 0.01$, $\varepsilon = 0.80$. The main effect of the group showed that there was no statistically significant difference in the STS scores between the sexes, $F(1,39) = 0.14$, $p = 0.714$, partial $\eta^2 = 0.003$.

Workload (WL) scores:
There was no statistically significant interaction between sex and time in the WL scores, $F(1.531, 59.707) = 1.99$, $p = 0.156$, partial $\eta^2 = 0.048$, $\varepsilon = 0.76$. The main group effect showed that there was a statistically significant difference in mean WL scores between men

and women, $F(1, 39) = 4.392$, $p = 0.043$, partial $\eta^2 = 0.101$. The effect size for the group differences was medium: Cohen's $f = 0.33$.

Appendix A.2. Completed Training Sessions (CTS) and Change Scores

Appendix A.2.1. Relationship Analyses

Spearman's rank–order correlation indicated that the number of CTS did not correlate significantly with any of the outcomes, neither with the Δ_2 of the FACIT–Fatigue scores, $r_s = -0.05$, $p = 0.597$, n = 41, nor with the Δ_2 of the 1MSTST scores, $r_s = -0.30$, $p = 0.052$, n = 41, nor with the Δ_2 of the WL scores, $r_s = 0.29$, $p = 0.069$, n = 41.

Appendix A.2.2. Difference Analyses Related to Number of CTS

FACIT–Fatigue scores:

The mean rank of the FACIT–Fatigue change scores was not statistically significantly different between the groups < 21 CTS, 21–24 CTS, and >24CTS, $\chi_2(2) = 1.21$, $p = 0.546$ (two-sided).

1MSTST scores:

There were no statistically significant differences in the 1MSTST scores between the groups < 21 CTS, 21–24 CTS, and >24 CTS, $F(2, 40) = 1.07$, $p = 0.51$.

Appendix A.3. Interaction Effects of PCS Score and Change Scores

FACIT–Fatigue scores:

There was no statistical significant difference in the Fatigue score changes between the groups, M. = -0.206, 95%CI [-6.198, 5.786], $t(39) = -0.07$, $p = 0.945$ (two-sided).

1MSTST scores:

The distributions of the change in the 1MSTST scores for the moderately and severely affected patients were similar. The median change in the 1MSTST scores was not statistically significantly different between the groups, U = 169.5, $z = -0.92$, $p = 0.360$.

Appendix A.4. Relationships between Outcomes

Spearman's rank–order correlation found a statistically significant moderate negative correlation between the PCFS scale scores and FACIT–Fatigue scores ($r_s = -0.47$, $p = 0.002$), a moderate positive correlation between WL scores and FACIT–Fatigue scores ($r_s = 0.42$, $p = 0.007$), and a strong positive correlation between the WL scores and 1MSTST scores ($r_s = 0.50$, $p < 0.001$). Except for these, there were no statistically significant correlations.

The PCS scores did not correlate significantly with the PCFS scores ($r_s = 0.08$, $p = 0.638$), FACIT–Fatigue scores ($r_p = -0.23$, $p = 0.154$), 1MSTST scores ($r_p = -0.29$, $p = 0.061$), or WL scores ($r_s = -0.25$, $p = 0.119$). The PCFS scores did not correlate significantly with the 1MSTST scores ($r_s = -0.27$, $p = 0.087$) or WL scores ($r_s = -0.30$, $p = 0.057$). The FACIT–Fatigue scores did not correlate significantly with the 1MSTST scores ($r_s = -0.13$, $p = 0.399$).

Appendix B

Table A1. Overview of outcomes at time-related testing sessions.

	PCFS	Fatigue	1MSTST	WL
T0	3	19.39 (8.72) **,***	20.98 (6.59) *,***	41.29 (26.47) **,***
T1	3	23.95 (9.92) **,*	23.83 (7.59) *	64.98 (43.88) **,***
T2	3	26.80 (11.11) ***,*	25.07 (9.02) ***	82.76 (46.97) ***,***

This table shows the median for the PCFS and the mean (standard deviation) for the other outcomes pre-intervention (T0), at six weeks (T1), and at twelve weeks (T2). PCFS = Post COVID Functional Status Scale; 1MSTST = one-minute sit-to-stand test; WL = workload. Statistical significance is highlighted with asterisks, with * $p < 0.05$; ** $p < 0.01$; and *** $p < 0.001$. A comma (,) after the first asterisk indicates more than one statistically significant comparison; e.g., in the third column, the FACIT–Fatigue scores differed significantly in the following comparisons: T0 vs. T1 **, T0 vs. T2 ***, and T1 vs. T2 *.

Table A2. Overview of Δ_2 of outcomes for the three groups of CTS and two groups of PCS.

	n	Δ_2 Fatigue	Δ_2 1MSTST	Δ_2 WL
CTS, Group 1	13	7.62 (12.57)	5.69 (6.57)	29.15 (21.57) *
CTS, Group 2	17	6.41 (7.48)	4.00 (5.61)	38.12 (24.46)
CTS, Group 3	11	8.73 (7.59)	2.36 (3.85)	61.18 (39.67) *
PCS, moderate	24	7.50 (8.68)	3.96 (7.06)	51.25 (30.38) *
PCS, severe	17	7.29 (10.22)	4.29 (2.39)	27.65 (25.71) *

Overview of participants and means (standard deviations) of Δ_2 (T2-T0) values for the three groups of CTS and the two groups of PCS. CTS = completed training sessions; CTS group 1: <21 CTS; group 2: 21–24 CTS; 3: >24 CTS; PCS = Post COVID Syndrome Score; 1MSTST = one-minute sit-to-stand test; WL = workload. Statistical significance is highlighted with asterisks, with * $p < 0.05$.

References

1. Al-Aly, Z.; Davis, H.; McCorkell, L.; Soares, L.; Wulf-Hanson, S.; Iwasaki, A.; Topol, E.J. Long COVID Science, Research and Policy. *Nat. Med.* **2024**, *30*, 2148–2164. [CrossRef] [PubMed]
2. Gloeckl, R.; Leitl, D.; Schneeberger, T.; Jarosch, I.; Koczulla, A.R. Rehabilitative Interventions in Patients with Persistent Post COVID-19 Symptoms—A Review of Recent Advances and Future Perspectives. *Eur. Arch. Psychiatry Clin. Neurosci.* **2023**. [CrossRef] [PubMed]
3. Robert Koch Institut. Long COVID. 2023. Available online: https://www.rki.de/SharedDocs/FAQ/NCOV2019/FAQ_Liste_Gesundheitliche_Langzeitfolgen.html (accessed on 22 August 2023).
4. Peter, R.S.; Nieters, A.; Kräusslich, H.-G.; Brockmann, S.O.; Göpel, S.; Kindle, G.; Merle, U.; Steinacker, J.M.; Rothenbacher, D.; Kern, W.V. Post-Acute Sequelae of COVID-19 Six to 12 Months after Infection: Population Based Study. *BMJ* **2022**, *379*, e071050. [CrossRef]
5. Alkodaymi, M.S.; Omrani, O.A.; Fawzy, N.A.; Shaar, B.A.; Almamlouk, R.; Riaz, M.; Obeidat, M.; Obeidat, Y.; Gerberi, D.; Taha, R.M.; et al. Prevalence of Post-Acute COVID-19 Syndrome Symptoms at Different Follow-up Periods: A Systematic Review and Meta-Analysis. *Clin. Microbiol. Infect.* **2022**, *28*, 657–666. [CrossRef]
6. Michelen, M.; Manoharan, L.; Elkheir, N.; Cheng, V.; Dagens, A.; Hastie, C.; O'Hara, M.; Suett, J.; Dahmash, D.; Bugaeva, P.; et al. Characterising Long COVID: A Living Systematic Review. *BMJ Glob. Health* **2021**, *6*, e005427. [CrossRef]
7. Bahmer, T.; Borzikowsky, C.; Lieb, W.; Horn, A.; Krist, L.; Fricke, J.; Scheibenbogen, C.; Rabe, K.F.; Maetzler, W.; Maetzler, C.; et al. Severity, Predictors and Clinical Correlates of Post-COVID Syndrome (PCS) in Germany: A Prospective, Multi-Centre, Population-Based Cohort Study. *eClinicalMedicine* **2022**, *51*, 101549. [CrossRef]
8. Durstenfeld, M.S.; Peluso, M.J.; Kaveti, P.; Hill, C.; Li, D.; Sander, E.; Swaminathan, S.; Arechiga, V.M.; Lu, S.; Goldberg, S.A.; et al. Reduced Exercise Capacity, Chronotropic Incompetence, and Early Systemic Inflammation in Cardiopulmonary Phenotype Long Coronavirus Disease 2019. *J. Infect. Dis.* **2023**, *228*, 542–554. [CrossRef]
9. Yelin, D.; Levi, R.; Babu, C.; Moshe, R.; Shitenberg, D.; Atamna, A.; Tishler, O.; Babich, T.; Shapira-Lichter, I.; Abecasis, D.; et al. Assessment of Exercise Capacity of Individuals with Long COVID: A Cross-Sectional Study. *Isr. Med. Assoc. J.* **2023**, *25*, 83–87.
10. Wright, J.; Astill, S.; Sivan, M. The Relationship between Physical Activity and Long COVID: A Cross-Sectional Study. *Int. J. Environ. Res. Public Health* **2022**, *19*, 5093. [CrossRef]
11. Koczulla, A.R.; Ankermann, T.; Behrends, U.; Berlit, P.; Berner, R.; Böing, S.; Brinkmann, F.; Frank, U.; Franke, C.; Glöckl, R.; et al. S1-Leitlinie Long-/Post-COVID. *Pneumologie* **2022**, *76*, 855–907. [CrossRef]
12. Walter, N.; Rupp, M.; Lang, S.; Leinberger, B.; Alt, V.; Hinterberger, T.; Loew, T. A Comprehensive Report of German Nationwide Inpatient Data on the Post-COVID-19 Syndrome Including Annual Direct Healthcare Costs. *Viruses* **2022**, *14*, 2600. [CrossRef] [PubMed]
13. Kluge, H.H.P.; Muscat, N.A.; Mishra, S.; Nielsen, S.; Tille, F.; Pfeifer, D.; COVID Europe, L.; Sivan, M. Call for Action: Health Services in the European Region Must Adopt Integrated Care Models to Manage Post-COVID-19 Condition. *Lancet Reg. Health Eur.* **2022**, *18*, 100435. [CrossRef] [PubMed]
14. National Institute for Health and Care Excellence. COVID-19 Rapid Guideline: Managing the Long-Term Effects of COVID-19. [NICE Guideline No. 188]. 2024. Available online: https://www.nice.org.uk/guidance/ng188 (accessed on 18 October 2024).
15. Dong, B.; Qi, Y.; Lin, L.; Liu, T.; Wang, S.; Zhang, Y.; Yuan, Y.; Cheng, H.; Chen, Q.; Fang, Q.; et al. Which Exercise Approaches Work for Relieving Cancer-Related Fatigue? A Network Meta-Analysis. *J. Orthop. Sports Phys. Ther.* **2023**, *53*, 343–352. [CrossRef]
16. Posadzki, P.; Pieper, D.; Bajpai, R.; Makaruk, H.; Könsgen, N.; Neuhaus, A.L.; Semwal, M. Exercise/Physical Activity and Health Outcomes: An Overview of Cochrane Systematic Reviews. *BMC Public. Health* **2020**, *20*, 1724. [CrossRef]
17. Torres-Costoso, A.; Martínez-Vizcaíno, V.; Reina-Gutiérrez, S.; Álvarez-Bueno, C.; Guzmán-Pavón, M.J.; Pozuelo-Carrascosa, D.P.; Fernández-Rodríguez, R.; Sanchez-López, M.; Cavero-Redondo, I. Effect of Exercise on Fatigue in Multiple Sclerosis: A Network Meta-Analysis Comparing Different Types of Exercise. *Arch. Phys. Med. Rehabil.* **2022**, *103*, 970–987.e18. [CrossRef]
18. Sick, J.; König, D. Exercise Training in Non-Hospitalized Patients with Post-COVID-19 Syndrome—A Narrative Review. *Healthcare* **2023**, *11*, 2277. [CrossRef]

19. Klok, F.A.; Boon, G.J.A.M.; Barco, S.; Endres, M.; Geelhoed, J.J.M.; Knauss, S.; Rezek, S.A.; Spruit, M.A.; Vehreschild, J.; Siegerink, B. The Post-COVID-19 Functional Status Scale: A Tool to Measure Functional Status over Time after COVID-19. *Eur. Respir. J.* **2020**, *56*, 2001494. [CrossRef]
20. FACIT-Group. (n.d.). FACIT-Fatigue. Assessment of Chronic Illness Therapy-Fatigue Scale. Available online: https://www.facit.org/measures/facit-fatigue (accessed on 25 January 2024).
21. Gradidge, P.J.-L.; Torres, G.; Constantinou, D.; Zanwar, P.P.; Pinto, S.M.; Negm, A.; Heyn, P.C. Exercise Reporting Template for Long COVID Patients: A Rehabilitation Practitioner Guide. *Arch. Phys. Med. Rehabil.* **2023**, *104*, 991–995. [CrossRef]
22. Greenhouse, S.W.; Geisser, S. On Methods in the Analysis of Profile Data. *Psychometrika* **1959**, *24*, 95–112. [CrossRef]
23. Cohen, J. Statistical Power Analysis. *Curr. Dir. Psychol. Sci.* **1992**, *1*, 98–101. [CrossRef]
24. Sawilowsky, S.S. New Effect Size Rules of Thumb. *J. Mod. App. Stat. Meth.* **2009**, *8*, 597–599. [CrossRef]
25. Tomczak, M.; Tomczak, E. The Need to Report Effect Size Estimates Revisited. An Overview of Some Recommended Measures of Effect Si. *Trends Sport Sci.* **2014**, *1*, 19–25.
26. Mooren, J.M.; Garbsch, R.; Schäfer, H.; Kotewitsch, M.; Waranski, M.; Teschler, M.; Schmitz, B.; Mooren, F.C. Medical Rehabilitation of Patients with Post-COVID-19 Syn-Drome—A Comparison of Aerobic Interval and Continuous Training. *J. Clin. Med.* **2023**, *12*, 6739. [CrossRef] [PubMed]
27. Hartung, T.J.; Neumann, C.; Bahmer, T.; Chaplinskaya-Sobol, I.; Endres, M.; Geritz, J.; Haeusler, K.G.; Heuschmann, P.U.; Hildesheim, H.; Hinz, A.; et al. Fatigue and Cognitive Impairment after COVID-19: A Prospective Multicentre Study. *eClinicalMedicine* **2022**, *53*, 101651. [CrossRef]
28. Piper, B.F.; Cella, D. Cancer-Related Fatigue: Definitions and Clinical Subtypes. *J. Natl. Compr. Canc. Netw.* **2010**, *8*, 958–966. [CrossRef]
29. Cella, D.; Johansson, P.; Ueda, Y.; Tomazos, I.; Gustovic, P.; Wang, A.; Patel, A.S.; Schrezenmeier, H. Clinically Important Change for the FACIT-Fatigue Scale in Paroxysmal Nocturnal Hemoglobinuria: A Derivation from International PNH Registry Patient Data. *J. Patient Rep. Outcomes* **2023**, *7*, 63. [CrossRef]
30. Jimeno-Almazán, A.; Franco-López, F.; Buendía-Romero, Á.; Martínez-Cava, A.; Sánchez-Agar, J.A.; Sánchez-Alcaraz Martínez, B.J.; Courel-Ibáñez, J.; Pallarés, J.G. Rehabilitation for Post-COVID-19 Condition through a Supervised Exercise Intervention: A Randomized Controlled Trial. *Scand. Med. Sci. Sports* **2022**, *32*, 1791–1801. [CrossRef]
31. Jimeno-Almazán, A.; Buendía-Romero, Á.; Martínez-Cava, A.; Franco-López, F.; Sánchez-Alcaraz, B.J.; Courel-Ibáñez, J.; Pallarés, J.G. Effects of a Concurrent Training, Respiratory Muscle Exercise, and Self-Management Recommendations on Recovery from Post-COVID-19 Conditions: The RECOVE Trial. *J. Appl. Physiol.* **2023**, *134*, 95–104. [CrossRef]
32. Nopp, S.; Moik, F.; Klok, F.A.; Gattinger, D.; Petrovic, M.; Vonbank, K.; Koczulla, A.R.; Ay, C.; Zwick, R.H. Outpatient Pulmonary Rehabilitation in Patients with Long COVID Improves Exercise Capacity, Functional Status, Dyspnea, Fatigue, and Quality of Life. *Respiration* **2022**, *101*, 593–601. [CrossRef]
33. Vaidya, T.; De Bisschop, C.; Beaumont, M.; Ouksel, H.; Jean, V.; Dessables, F.; Chambellan, A. Is the 1-Minute Sit-to-Stand Test a Good Tool for the Evaluation of the Impact of Pulmonary Rehabilitation? Determination of the Minimal Important Difference in COPD. *COPD* **2016**, *11*, 2609–2616. [CrossRef]
34. Kasper, K. Sports Training Principles. *Curr. Sports Med. Rep.* **2019**, *18*, 95–96. [CrossRef] [PubMed]
35. Renz-Polster, H.; Scheibenbogen, C. Post-COVID-Syndrom mit Fatigue und Belastungsintoleranz: Myalgische Enzephalomyelitis bzw. Chronisches Fatigue-Syndrom. *Inn. Med.* **2022**, *63*, 830–839. [CrossRef] [PubMed]
36. Vernon, S.D.; Hartle, M.; Sullivan, K.; Bell, J.; Abbaszadeh, S.; Unutmaz, D.; Bateman, L. Post-Exertional Malaise among People with Long COVID Compared to Myalgic Encephalomyelitis/Chronic Fatigue Syndrome (ME/CFS). *WOR* **2023**, *74*, 1179–1186. [CrossRef] [PubMed]
37. Kostev, K.; Smith, L.; Koyanagi, A.; Jacob, L. Prevalence of and Factors Associated with Post-Coronavirus Disease 2019 (COVID-19) Condition in the 12 Months After the Diagnosis of COVID-19 in Adults Followed in General Practices in Germany. *Open Forum Infect. Dis.* **2022**, *9*, ofac333. [CrossRef] [PubMed]
38. Smith, J.R.; Thomas, R.J.; Bonikowske, A.R.; Hammer, S.M.; Olson, T.P. Sex Differences in Cardiac Rehabilitation Outcomes. *Circ. Res.* **2022**, *130*, 552–565. [CrossRef]
39. Machado, F.V.C.; Meys, R.; Delbressine, J.M.; Vaes, A.W.; Goërtz, Y.M.J.; Van Herck, M.; Houben-Wilke, S.; Boon, G.J.A.M.; Barco, S.; Burtin, C.; et al. Construct Validity of the Post-COVID-19 Functional Status Scale in Adult Subjects with COVID-19. *Health Qual. Life Outcomes* **2021**, *19*, 40. [CrossRef]

Disclaimer/Publisher's Note: The statements, opinions and data contained in all publications are solely those of the individual author(s) and contributor(s) and not of MDPI and/or the editor(s). MDPI and/or the editor(s) disclaim responsibility for any injury to people or property resulting from any ideas, methods, instructions or products referred to in the content.

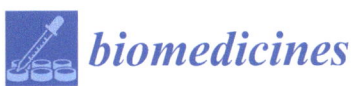

Article

The Progression of Symptoms in Post COVID-19 Patients: A Multicentre, Prospective, Observational Cohort Study

Merel E. B. Cornelissen [1,2,3,*], Myrthe M. Haarman [1], Jos W. R. Twisk [4], Laura Houweling [1,2,3,5], Nadia Baalbaki [1,2,3], Brigitte Sondermeijer [6], Rosanne J. H. C. G. Beijers [7], Debbie Gach [7], Lizan D. Bloemsma [1,2,3] and Anke H. Maitland-van der Zee [1,2,3] on behalf of the P4O2 Consortium

[1] Department of Pulmonary Medicine, Amsterdam UMC, University of Amsterdam, de Boelelaan 1117, 1081 HV Amsterdam, The Netherlands; a.h.maitland@amsterdamumc.nl (A.H.M.-v.d.Z.)
[2] Amsterdam Institute for Infection and Immunity, de Boelelaan 1117, 1081 HV Amsterdam, The Netherlands
[3] Amsterdam Public Health, de Boelelaan 1117, 1081 HV Amsterdam, The Netherlands
[4] Department of Epidemiology and Data Science, Amsterdam University Medical Centers, Van der Boechorststraat 7, 1081 BT Amsterdam, The Netherlands
[5] Department of Environmental Epidemiology, Institute for Risk Assessment Sciences (IRAS), Utrecht University, Yalelaan 2, 3584 CM Utrecht, The Netherlands
[6] Department of Pulmonology, Spaarne Hospital, Spaarnepoort 1, 2134 TM Hoofddorp, The Netherlands
[7] Department of Respiratory Medicine, NUTRIM Institute of Nutrition and Translational Research in Metabolism, Maastricht University Medical Centre+, Universiteitssingel 50, 6229 ER Maastricht, The Netherlands
* Correspondence: m.e.b.cornelissen@amsterdamumc.nl

Abstract: Background: Although the coronavirus disease 2019 (COVID-19) pandemic is no longer a public health emergency of international concern, 30% of COVID-19 patients still have long-term complaints. A better understanding of the progression of symptoms after COVID-19 is needed to reduce the burden of the post COVID-19 condition. Objective: This study aims to investigate the progression of symptoms, identify patterns of symptom progression, and assess their associations with patient characteristics. Methods: Within the P4O2 COVID-19 study, patients aged 40–65 years were recruited from five Dutch hospitals. At 3–6 and 12–18 months post COVID-19, medical data were collected, and pulmonary function tests were performed. In between, symptoms were assessed monthly with a questionnaire. Latent class mixed modelling was used to identify symptom progression patterns over time, with multinomial logistic regression to examine associations with patient characteristics. Results: Eighty-eight patients (aged 54.4 years, 48.9% males) were included. Three trajectories were identified for fatigue and dyspnoea: decreasing, high persistent, and low persistent. The odds of "decreasing fatigue" was higher for never smokers and participants in the lifestyle intervention and lower for those having a comorbidity. The odds of "decreasing dyspnoea" was higher for moderate COVID-19 patients and lifestyle intervention participants and lower for males, mild COVID-19 patients, and those with a higher age. Conclusions: Three distinct trajectories were identified for fatigue and dyspnoea, delineating patterns of symptom persistence following COVID-19. Sex, age, smoking status, participation in lifestyle interventions and COVID-19 severity were associated with the likelihood of belonging to different trajectories. These findings highlight the heterogeneity of the long-term symptoms experienced by post COVID-19 patients and emphasise the importance of personalised treatment strategies.

Keywords: post COVID-19 condition; symptom progression; trajectories; dyspnoea; fatigue

1. Introduction

Severe acute respiratory syndrome coronavirus 2 (SARS-CoV-2) has led to a major pandemic, resulting in substantial mortality and morbidity worldwide. Since the outbreak, more than 700 million coronavirus disease 2019 (COVID-19) cases and almost seven million deaths have been reported [1]. The average recovery time from acute COVID-19 is

2–3 weeks, depending on the symptom severity [2]. However, some cases may exhibit symptoms that are still present three months after the infection, last for at least two months and cannot be explained by an alternative diagnosis, referred to as the post COVID-19 condition by the World Health Organization (WHO) Delphi consensus definition [3]. Post COVID-19 condition has a significant social and economic impact. It leads to lower quality of life, and more people may need healthcare support in the near future, which could overburden the healthcare system [4,5].

Several studies have been conducted on symptoms associated with post COVID-19 condition. The results of recent systematic reviews [6–8] show that post COVID-19 symptoms are present in 30–45% of hospitalised and non-hospitalised ex-COVID-19 patients after four months [8]. These patients exhibit at least one post COVID-19 symptom for more than 30 days after the onset of infection, where fatigue and dyspnoea were the most prevalent [7]. Next to these symptoms, psychological symptoms were also frequently mentioned, like problems with concentration and sleeping, and difficulty finding words [9]. After one year, fatigue and dyspnoea were still reported by, respectively, 41% and 31% of the post COVID-19 patients [6], and, after two years, 30% of the patients still experienced symptoms [7]. It is still under debate in the literature whether the persistence of symptoms increases or decreases over time, as Ong et al. found a decrease in the number of patients with persistent symptoms from 30 to 90 days and a slight increase in this number from 90 to 180 days [10]. While previous studies have documented post-COVID-19 symptoms at specific time points, the progression of these symptoms over time remains largely unexplored.

Risk factors for the development of post COVID-19 condition and the persistence of symptoms are presented in several studies but are not always consistent. Frequently mentioned risk factors are age, sex, body mass index (BMI), smoking, comorbidities and the severity of acute COVID-19. According to these studies, women have an increased risk of developing post COVID-19 condition compared to men [11–13]. A higher BMI, smoking or former smoking and different comorbidities are also associated with a greater risk of post COVID-19 condition [13,14]. Frequently mentioned comorbidities are diabetes, hypertension, cardiovascular disease (CVD) and chronic obstructive pulmonary disease (COPD) [6,12–14]. Furthermore, age > 65 years and more severe acute COVID-19 increase the chance of having persistent symptoms of post COVID-19 condition [6,10,15–17].

A better understanding of the progression of symptoms after acute COVID-19 over time and its associations with patient characteristics are needed to create therapeutic strategies, to reduce the burden of post COVID-19 condition and to lower the social and economic impact. Therefore, the primary aim of this study is to investigate the progression of symptoms within the first twelve to eighteen months after acute SARS-CoV-2 infection in the Precision Medicine for more Oxygen (P4O2) COVID-19 cohort. The second aim is to identify trajectories of symptom progression for the most prevalent post COVID-19 symptoms. The third aim is to assess the associations between patient characteristics and these trajectories of symptom progression.

2. Materials and Methods

2.1. Study Design and Population

The P4O2 COVID-19 study is a multicentre, prospective, observational cohort study in the Netherlands and is approved by the ethical board of the Amsterdam University Medical Centre (UMC) (ref. no. NL74701.018.20). Details of the study design have been described by Baalbaki et al. [18]. In brief, 95 ex-COVID-19 patients were recruited between May 2021 and September 2022 at post COVID-19 outpatient clinics in five Dutch hospitals. Patients visited the post COVID-19 outpatient clinic 3–6 months after hospitalisation or, if not hospitalised, were referred to the outpatient clinic by their general practitioner three months after their positive polymerase chain reaction (PCR) test. Inclusion criteria were a confirmed SARS-CoV-2 infection (by PCR, serology tests or a COVID-19 Reporting and Data System (CO-RADS) score of 4 or 5), the ability to provide informed consent, aged 40–65 years, access to the internet and an understanding of the Dutch language. Exclusion criteria were the inability to provide informed consent, a terminal illness and participation in another study involving investigational or marketed products concomitantly or within four weeks prior to study entry or during the study. All participants were invited to two study visits: at 3–6 and 12–18 months after hospitalisation or positive PCR test. In between, patients completed monthly questionnaires at home and were invited to participate in a lifestyle intervention, consisting of personalised counselling on dietary quality and physical activity. Further detailed information of the lifestyle intervention is described by Baalbaki et al. [18]. The total duration of the study per participant was 9–12 months.

2.2. Data Collection

Written informed consent was obtained during the first study visit, and baseline characteristics concerning the patient's health status prior to and during COVID-19 were obtained from electronic patient files. During both study visits, pulmonary function tests (spirometry and diffusion capacity) were executed, and several questionnaires were administered. One of these questionnaires (Disease Progression and Adverse Events) contained questions on the frequency of pulmonary and extra-pulmonary symptoms (Supplementary Material S1). This questionnaire was developed in collaboration with post COVID-19 outpatient clinic physicians. Patients were asked to complete this questionnaire at home every month. This "monthly questionnaire" assessed whether a patient experienced different symptoms in the past two weeks and, if they did, how frequently they experienced them. The first monthly questionnaire was completed during the first study visit and the last questionnaire during the second study visit.

2.3. Outcome

The outcome of the study was the progression of symptoms after COVID-19. The symptoms that were assessed by the monthly questionnaire were fatigue, headache, chest pressure, dyspnoea, loss of smell and taste, abdominal pain, diarrhoea and obstipation. On the monthly questionnaire, patients were asked whether they had experienced each symptom (yes vs. no) in the past two weeks, and, if yes, whether this was daily or weekly. When the answer was "weekly", the patient was subsequently asked how many times a week they experienced this symptom. We created a new variable to describe the weekly frequency (in days per week) that the patient experienced per symptom. When the patient's answer was "daily", the new variable was coded as "7". When the answer was "weekly", the patient subsequently stated how many times a week they experienced this symptom, and the new variable was given this number.

2.4. Patient Characteristics

In this study, the patient characteristics included age (in years), sex, BMI (in kg/m^2), smoking status (current and ex-smoker vs. never smoker), COVID-19 severity (mild, moderate, or severe), diffusion capacity of carbon monoxide (DLCO) (in % predicted) and having a comorbidity (yes vs. no). COVID-19 severity was defined according to the WHO Clinical Progression Scale, based on oxygen supplementation during the infection [19]. Comorbidities that were assessed were COPD, asthma, interstitial lung disease (ILD), thrombosis, heart failure, renal failure, hepatic disease, diabetes, cancer, rheumatic diseases, CVD and neurological diseases.

2.5. Data Analysis

First, exploratory analyses were conducted. Patients who completed less than two monthly questionnaires were excluded from this study. Histograms were generated for each symptom to assess the mean weekly frequency at each time point. Fatigue and dyspnoea were selected for further trajectory analysis, since these symptoms were most frequently mentioned in the literature [6,7].

Second, to investigate patterns of symptom progression over time, latent class mixed modelling (LCMM) was performed (with R package LCMM) [20], which can divide the heterogeneity of symptom progression into more homogeneous trajectories of symptom progression. The model can handle missing data, meaning that it does not need the same number of measurements per time point or per participant. Two models were constructed: for the first model, fatigue was the dependent variable, and, for the second model, dyspnoea was the dependent variable. The time in months since acute infection was the independent variable for both models. Trajectories were added one by one to capture the underlying variability in symptom progression patterns. Model selection was based on the Akaike Information Criterion (AIC) and the Bayesian Information Criterion (BIC), with lower values indicating a better fit. Participants were divided over the trajectories based on probability scores, where the highest probability score indicated in which trajectory they belonged. Additionally, the best-fitting models were visually inspected by creating plots to ensure that the identified patterns aligned with our expectations of fatigue and dyspnoea progression. Furthermore, the assumption of normality of the residuals was checked.

Finally, to assess the associations between patient characteristics and the trajectories of symptom progression for fatigue and dyspnoea, first, univariable multinomial logistic regression analyses were performed for each patient characteristic separately; second, a multivariable multinomial logistic regression analysis was performed, including all significant patient characteristics ($p < 0.05$) from the univariable analyses.

Statistical analyses were performed using the R software, version 4.2.1.

3. Results

3.1. Baseline Characteristics

In total, 88 patients completed at least two monthly questionnaires and were included in this study. Their mean age was 54.4 ± 6.1 years and 48.9% were male (Table 1). The mean BMI was 30.5 ± 5.4 kg/m^2 and 63.2% of the patients had at least one comorbidity. Of all patients, 88.6% were hospitalised, with a median duration of eight days, and most of the patients (63.6%) had moderate severity of COVID-19. There were 761 monthly questionnaires collected, with a median of 9.0 (25–75th percentile: 8.0–10.3) questionnaires per patient.

Table 1. Patient characteristics (n = 88).

	Mean ± SD, Median (25th–75th Percentile) or n (%)
Age, in years	54.4 ± 6.1
Male sex	44 (48.9)
Ethnicity	
Caucasian	67/84 (79.8)
Other	17/84 (20.2)
BMI, in kg/m^2	30.5 ± 5.4
Smoking status	
Current	4 (4.6)
Ex	47 (53.4)
Never	37 (42.1)
At least one comorbidity [a]	55/87 (63.2)
Comorbidities	
Heart failure	5/87 (5.8)
Renal failure	6/85 (7.1)
Diabetes	13/87 (14.9)
COPD	6/87 (6.9)
Asthma	16/87 (18.4)
Cardiovascular disease	22/86 (25.6)
Hospitalised	78 (88.6)

Table 1. *Cont.*

	Mean ± SD, Median (25th–75th Percentile) or n (%)
Hospital duration, in days	8.0 (4.0–15.5)
COVID-19 severity [b]	
Mild	10 (11.4)
Moderate	56 (63.6)
Severe	22 (25.0)
Number of monthly questionnaires completed	9.0 (8.0–10.3)
Participated in lifestyle intervention	42 (47.7)

BMI: body mass index, COPD: chronic obstructive pulmonary disease, DLCO: diffusion capacity for carbon monoxide, SD: standard deviation. [a] At least one of the following comorbidities: COPD, asthma, interstitial lung disease, thrombosis, heart failure, renal failure, hepatic disease, diabetes, cancer, rheumatic disease, CVD and neurological disease. [b] According to the WHO Clinical Progression Scale.

3.2. Symptom Progression

The mean weekly frequency (in days per week) of all eight symptoms was calculated for each month (Figure S1). The mean weekly frequency of fatigue declined from 5.2 days at four months to 3.6 days at eighteen months after the infection. Similarly, dyspnoea showed a decrease from 4.4 days at four months to 3.2 days at eighteen months after the infection. For chest pressure, the mean weekly frequency decreased from 1.8 days at four months to 0.1 days at eighteen months after the infection. The reported frequency of headache remained relatively stable throughout the study period, from 1.3 days per week at four months to 2.1 days at eighteen months after the infection. Loss of smell and taste, abdominal pain, diarrhoea and constipation showed consistently low scores throughout the study period.

3.3. Identified Trajectories of Fatigue

With LCMM, three trajectories were identified for fatigue (Figure 1). Trajectory one ("decreasing fatigue", n = 23) contained patients whose weekly frequency decreased over time, trajectory two ("high persistent fatigue", n = 39) consisted of patients whose weekly frequency remained high, and trajectory three ("low persistent fatigue", n = 26) consisted of patients whose weekly frequency remained low over the study period. The AIC, BIC and probability scores per participant can be found in Table S1. Differences in patient characteristics between the three trajectories are shown in Table S2.

Multinomial logistic regression analyses, with "high persistent fatigue" as reference category, were performed for each patient characteristic separately (Table S3). Thereafter, a multivariable analysis was performed with all significant patient characteristics (Table 2). The odds of "decreasing fatigue" was lower for patients with at least one comorbidity (odds ratio (OR) [95% confidence interval (CI)]: 0.54 [0.37, 0.80]), while it was higher for never smokers (1.90 [1.30, 2.78]) and participants in the lifestyle intervention (1.58 [1.07, 2.32]). The odds of "low persistent fatigue" was lower for mild COVID-19 patients (0.41 [0.18, 0.95]) and for patients with at least one comorbidity (0.63 [0.43, 0.93]), while it was higher for males (2.09 [1.38, 3.17]).

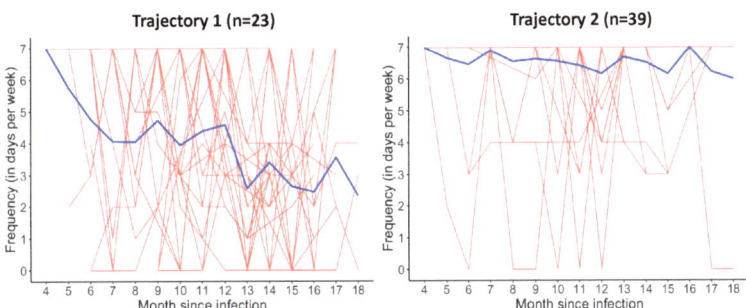

Figure 1. *Cont.*

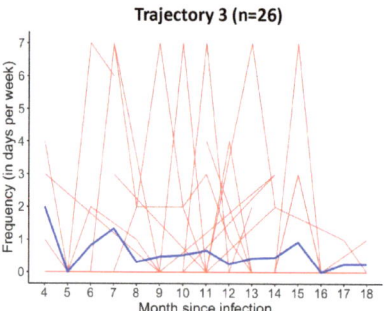

Figure 1. Three trajectories based on the weekly frequency of fatigue from month 4 to month 18 after SARS-CoV-2 infection. Each red line represents a patient and each blue line represents a trajectory.

Table 2. Multivariable associations between patient characteristics and the different trajectories for fatigue.

	OR (95% CI) for Belonging to Trajectory 1 "Decreasing Fatigue" (n = 23)	OR (95% CI) for Belonging to Trajectory 3 "Low Persistent Fatigue" (n = 26)
Age [a]	0.96 (0.93, 1.00)	1.03 (0.99, 1.06)
Male sex	0.73 (0.48, 1.11)	**2.09 (1.38, 3.17)**
BMI [a]	0.96 (0.92, 1.00)	0.98 (0.94, 1.01)
Never smoker [b]	**1.90 (1.30, 2.78)**	1.19 (0.81, 1.75)
Moderate COVID-19 [c]	1.38 (0.87, 2.17)	0.91 (0.60, 1.36)
Mild COVID-19 [c]	0.55 (0.26, 1.17)	**0.41 (0.18, 0.95)**
At least one comorbidity [d]	**0.54 (0.37, 0.80)**	**0.63 (0.43, 0.93)**
Lifestyle intervention	**1.58 (1.07, 2.32)**	0.98 (0.67, 1.43)

BMI: body mass index, CI: confidence interval, OR: odds ratio. ORs were obtained by comparing the trajectories with the reference category trajectory 2 "high persistent fatigue". The significant ORs are marked in bold. [a] OR is per unit increase in age (years) or BMI (kg/m^2). [b] Reference category is current and ex-smoker. [c] According to the WHO Clinical Progression Scale. Reference category is severe COVID-19. [d] At least one of the following comorbidities: COPD, asthma, interstitial lung disease, thrombosis, heart failure, renal failure, hepatic disease, diabetes, cancer, rheumatic disease, CVD and neurological disease.

3.4. Identified Trajectories of Dyspnoea

Just like for fatigue, three trajectories were identified for dyspnoea (Figure 2): trajectory one ("decreasing dyspnoea", n = 22), trajectory two ("high persistent dyspnoea", n = 29) and trajectory three ("low persistent dyspnoea", n = 37). The AIC, BIC and probability scores per participant can be found in Table S4. Differences in patient characteristics between the three trajectories are shown in Table S5.

For dyspnoea, the same univariable analyses were performed as for fatigue (Table S6). When performing the multivariable analysis, the odds of "decreasing dyspnoea" was lower for patients with a higher age (OR [95% CI]: 0.88 [0.84, 0.92]), males (0.37 [0.22, 0.61]) and mild COVID-19 patients (0.12 [0.05, 0.31]), while it was higher for moderate COVID-19 patients (1.73 [1.05, 2.85]) and participants in the lifestyle intervention (2.21 [1.39, 3.53]) (Table 3). The odds of "low persistent dyspnoea" was lower for patients with a higher BMI (0.90 [0.86, 0.94]), patients with at least one comorbidity (0.56 [0.37, 0.84]) and mild COVID-19 patients (0.08 [0.03, 0.18]), while it was higher for males (1.66 [1.08, 2.55]) and patients with a higher DLCO % predicted (1.05 [1.04, 1.07]).

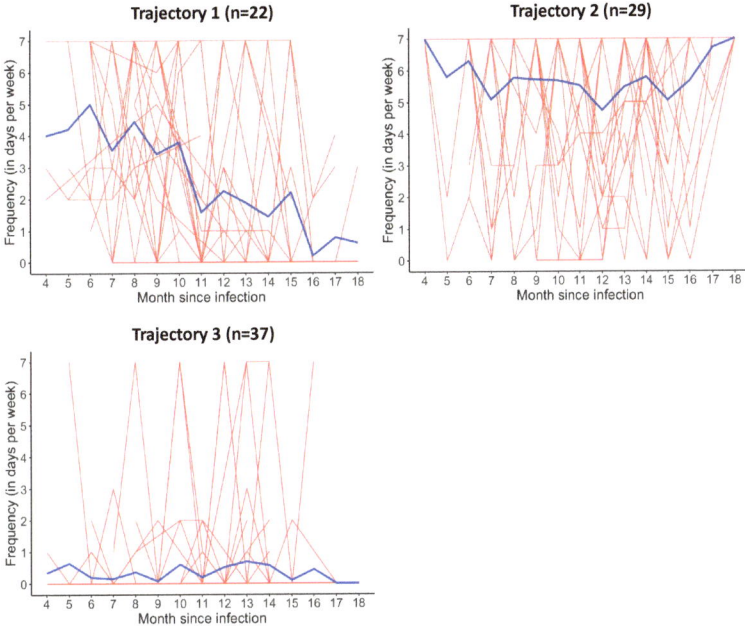

Figure 2. Three trajectories based on the weekly frequency of dyspnoea from month 4 to month 18 after SARS-CoV-2 infection. Each red line represents a patient and each blue line represents a trajectory.

Table 3. Multivariable associations between patient characteristics and the different trajectories for dyspnoea.

	OR (95% CI) for Belonging to Trajectory 1 "Decreasing Dyspnoea" (n = 22)	OR (95% CI) for Belonging to Trajectory 3 "Low Persistent Dyspnoea" (n = 37)
Age [a]	**0.88 (0.84, 0.92)**	0.97 (0.94, 1.01)
Male sex	**0.37 (0.22, 0.61)**	**1.66 (1.08, 2.55)**
BMI [a]	0.98 (0.94, 1.02)	**0.90 (0.86, 0.94)**
Moderate COVID-19 [b]	**1.73 (1.05, 2.85)**	1.17 (0.75, 1.81)
Mild COVID-19 [b]	**0.12 (0.05, 0.31)**	**0.08 (0.03, 0.18)**
DLCO [a]	1.00 (0.99, 1.02)	**1.05 (1.04, 1.07)**
At least 1 comorbidity [c]	1.42 (0.88, 2.28)	**0.56 (0.37, 0.84)**
Lifestyle intervention	**2.21 (1.39, 3.53)**	0.77 (0.51, 1.14)

BMI: body mass index, CI: confidence interval, OR: odds ratio. ORs were obtained by comparing the trajectories with the reference category trajectory 2 "high persistent dyspnoea". The significant ORs are marked in bold. [a] OR is per unit increase in age (years), BMI (kg/m^2) or DLCO (% predicted). [b] According to the WHO Clinical Progression Scale. Reference category is severe COVID-19. [c] At least one of the following comorbidities: COPD, asthma, interstitial lung disease, thrombosis, heart failure, renal failure, hepatic disease, diabetes, cancer, rheumatic disease, CVD and neurological disease.

4. Discussion

This study showed an overall decline in the mean weekly frequency of fatigue, dyspnoea and chest pressure over the course of eighteen months after SARS-CoV-2 infection. Fatigue and dyspnoea demonstrated variability in symptom progression among three distinct trajectories: decreasing fatigue/dyspnoea, high persistent fatigue/dyspnoea, and low persistent fatigue/dyspnoea. Multinomial logistic regression analyses highlighted the significance of different patient characteristics in predicting the likelihood of belonging to different trajectories. The odds of "decreasing fatigue" was higher for never smokers and participants in the lifestyle intervention, while the odds of "low persistent fatigue" was higher for males. The odds of "decreasing dyspnoea" was higher for moderate COVID-19 patients and participants in the lifestyle intervention, and the odds of "low persistent dyspnoea" was higher for males and patients with a higher DLCO % predicted.

This study showed that the most reported persistent symptoms were fatigue, headache and dyspnoea, whereas diarrhoea, constipation and abdominal pain were less commonly reported. This is consistent with previous studies on symptoms after COVID-19, although these studies had a shorter follow-up period [21–24]. Brinkley et al. [25] found that the most reported symptoms by US adults were fatigue, headache, decreased smell and taste and cough. Symptoms that did not persist for a longer period were gastrointestinal symptoms (nausea, vomiting and diarrhoea). However, their follow-up period was only 28 days, whereas, in this study, symptoms were measured for between four and eighteen months. A longitudinal German study with a follow-up period of 12 months reported that the most likely symptoms to persist were reduced exercise capacity, fatigue and dyspnoea [9]. In our study, we found that approximately 40% of the patients experienced headache, with a weekly frequency ranging from 1.3 days to 2.1 days. In other studies, headache was found to be a persistent symptom in 18–22% of post COVID-19 patients [26–28]. In our study, the weekly frequencies of headache did not change considerably over time, so we were unable to create trajectories for this symptom. For future research, it could be of interest to study headache, since its prevalence is relatively high.

Factors associated with a high frequency of fatigue during the entire study period included female sex, (ex-)smoking, not being hospitalised, mild COVID-19 and the presence of comorbidities. The characteristics for a high frequency of dyspnoea were a higher age, female sex, a higher BMI, not being hospitalised, mild COVID-19 and a lower DLCO % predicted. These findings align with the existing literature reporting a higher age [14,21], higher BMI [25] and comorbidities [14,15] as risk factors for persistent symptoms after COVID-19. We found that females were more likely to experience persistent symptoms than males, which is in line with the studies by Bai et al. [29], who found female sex to be independently associated with a higher risk of post COVID-19 condition, and Onieva et al. [30], who found that females had a higher risk of persistent symptoms after infection. Furthermore, a study conducted in Suriname found female sex as a predictor of persistent symptoms at 3–4 months after COVID-19 [31]. Kamal et al. [15] also identified severe COVID-19 as a risk factor for the persistence of symptoms. This is in contrast with the results of this study, since mild COVID-19 was found to be associated with the persistence of symptoms. Notably, the study of Kamal et al. did not specify the time point of symptom assessment and used all symptoms together, instead of focussing on specific symptoms. When comparing the results of this study with those of a longitudinal study in a Dutch population [32], similar results were found. In their study, they found that slower recovery from dyspnoea was associated with a higher age, and slower recovery from fatigue was associated with having comorbidities.

Furthermore, a lifestyle intervention seems to influence fatigue and dyspnoea, since the odds of decreasing fatigue and decreasing dyspnoea were higher compared to high persistent fatigue and high persistent dyspnoea. This is in line with previous research, where it was found that a physically active lifestyle is important to overcome persistent symptoms and reduce the risk of post COVID-19 condition [33,34]. Detailed quantitative as well as qualitative analyses of the effects and experiences of participating in the lifestyle intervention are ongoing and will be further elaborated in future manuscripts.

Only one previous study was found that used trajectory analysis to find different patterns in persistent symptoms during the first year after SARS-CoV-2 infection [35]. This French cohort study, which used the Long COVID Symptom Tool to assess 53 symptoms, identified three trajectories, "highly persistent symptoms", "rapidly decreasing symptoms" and "slowly decreasing symptoms", and compared the patient characteristics between these trajectories. They also found that patients with highly persistent symptoms were older. However, contrary to the findings of this study, the authors did not observe associations with BMI or hospitalisation. This discrepancy might be because this study focused on the trajectories of fatigue and dyspnoea, whereas the French study created trajectories based on all symptoms together.

Strengths and Limitations

This study has several strengths. First, the study had a prospective design, which offered the best overview of the symptoms that patients experienced at that moment. In addition, the questionnaire was administered every month, which provided longitudinal data and a detailed overview of the progression of symptoms over time. Second, in this study LCMM was used. This type of model can handle missing data points in longitudinal datasets and therefore prevented the exclusion of numerous cases that would have otherwise been eliminated due to incomplete data. Another strength is that the trajectories of fatigue and dyspnoea were created separately, instead of using all symptoms, so the symptoms could be treated more specifically.

This study also had some limitations. First, the questionnaire that was used to assess the frequency of symptoms was not a validated questionnaire. However, the questionnaire was developed in collaboration with post-COVID-19 outpatient clinic physicians, and the questions were very specific and easy to understand and interpret. Second, by only including patients who completed the monthly questionnaire at least twice, there was a risk of selection bias. Patients who completed fewer than two questionnaires might have been more likely to have experienced symptom resolution, or, on the contrary, patients experiencing a high disease burden may have been unable to complete the questionnaires. Third, there was no information on the health status prior to COVID-19, which made it challenging to obtain conclusions on whether the reported symptoms were caused by the SARS-CoV-2 infection. Although the study included information on comorbidities, which provided some insight into participants' health profiles, a comprehensive understanding of their pre-existing conditions would have strengthened the interpretation of symptom presentation. Fourth, there was no control group (i.e., persons without post COVID-19 condition), which made it difficult to determine whether the observed symptoms were specific to post COVID-19 condition or could be attributed to other factors. Including a control group would have enhanced the study's validity and enabled a more nuanced understanding of post COVID-19 condition's symptomatology. Lastly, the sample size was small, which makes it difficult to generalise the findings to all post COVID-19 patients. Increasing the sample size in future studies would enhance the reliability, validity and generalisability of these findings.

5. Conclusions

Three distinct trajectories were identified for fatigue and dyspnoea, delineating patterns of symptom persistence in post COVID-19 patients. Sex, age, smoking status, participation in a lifestyle intervention and COVID-19 severity were associated with the likelihood of belonging to different trajectories. These findings highlight the heterogeneity of the long-term symptoms experienced by post COVID-19 patients and emphasise the importance of personalised treatment strategies. Future research should focus on validating these findings in larger cohorts with a longer follow-up time and exploring treatments targeting modifiable risk factors to improve the long-term outcomes in COVID-19 survivors.

Supplementary Materials: The following supporting information can be downloaded at: https://www.mdpi.com/article/10.3390/biomedicines12112493/s1, Supplementary Material S1. Questionnaire on disease progression and adverse events. Figure S1. Mean weekly frequency per symptom per month; Table S1. Selection criteria for weekly frequency of fatigue trajectories; Table S2. Patient characteristics per fatigue trajectory; Table S3. Univariable associations between patient characteristics and the different trajectories for fatigue; Table S4. Selection criteria weekly for frequency of dyspnoea trajectories; Table S5. Patient characteristics per dyspnoea trajectory; Table S6. Univariable associations between patient characteristics and the different trajectories for dyspnoea.

Author Contributions: Conceptualisation, M.E.B.C., L.D.B. and A.H.M.-v.d.Z.; Methodology, M.E.B.C., L.D.B. and A.H.M.-v.d.Z.; Software, M.E.B.C. and J.W.R.T.; Formal Analysis, M.E.B.C. and J.W.R.T.; Investigation, M.E.B.C., M.M.H., L.H., N.B. and D.G.; Data Curation, M.E.B.C.; Writing—Original Draft Preparation, M.E.B.C. and M.M.H.; Writing—Review and Editing, J.W.R.T., M.M.H., L.H., N.B., D.G., L.D.B., B.S., R.J.H.C.G.B. and A.H.M.-v.d.Z.; Visualisation, M.E.B.C.; Supervision, L.D.B. and A.H.M.-v.d.Z.; Project Administration, M.E.B.C. All authors have read and agreed to the published version of the manuscript.

Funding: Partners in the Precision Medicine for more Oxygen (P4O2) consortium are the Amsterdam UMC, Leiden University Medical Center, Maastricht UMC+, Maastricht University, UMC Groningen, UMC Utrecht, Utrecht University, TNO, Abbvie, Aparito, Boehringer Ingelheim, Breathomix, Clear, Danone Nutricia Research, Fluidda, Ncardia, Olive, Ortec Logiqcare, Philips, Proefdiervrij, Quantib-U, RespiQ, Roche, Smartfish, SODAQ, Thirona, TopMD, Lung Alliance Netherlands (LAN) and the Lung Foundation Netherlands (Longfonds). The consortium is additionally funded by the PPP Allowance made available by Health~Holland, Top Sector Life Sciences & Health (LSHM20104; LSHM20068), to stimulate public-private partnerships, and by Novartis.

Institutional Review Board Statement: This study was conducted according to the guidelines of the Declaration of Helsinki and approved by the Institutional Review Board (or Ethics Committee) of Amsterdam University Medical Centre (UMC) (reference number NL74701.018.20).

Informed Consent Statement: Informed consent was obtained from all subjects involved in the study.

Data Availability Statement: The datasets generated and/or analysed during the current study are not publicly available due to agreements made by the consortium, which only allow access by each consortium partner to specific data that answers their pre-specified research questions, but they are available from the corresponding author on reasonable request. A request for access to the data by organisations outside of the consortium can be submitted to the P4O2 Data Committee (via p4o2@amsterdamumc.nl) and the research will need to be performed in collaboration with one of the P4O2 consortium partners.

Conflicts of Interest: MMH, JWRT and BS—the authors declare no conflict of interest. MEBC, LH, NB, RJHCGB, DG and LDB—public and private partners in the P4O2 consortium, as listed under 'Funding'. AHM—PI of a public private consortium (P4O2 (Precision Medicine for More Oxygen)) sponsored by Health Holland, involving many private partners that contribute in cash and/or in kind (AbbVie. Boehringer Ingelheim, Breathomix, Clear, Fluidda, Ortec Logiqcare, Olive, Philips, Quantib-U, Smartfish, Clear, SODAQ, Thirona, Roche, TopMD, Novartis, RespiQ); received unrestricted research grants from GSK and Boehringer Ingelheim; received Vertex Innovation Award grant; honoraria paid to Institution from Boehringer Ingelheim, Astra Zeneca and GSK; chair of a DSMB of a study on BPD in neonates.

Abbreviations

AIC	Akaike Information Criterion
BIC	Bayesian Information Criterion
BMI	Body mass index
CVD	Cardiovascular disease
CI	Confidence interval
COPD	Chronic obstructive pulmonary disease
COVID-19	Coronavirus disease 2019
DLCO	Diffusion capacity of carbon monoxide
ILD	Interstitial lung disease
LCMM	Latent class mixed modelling
OR	Odds ratio
P4O2	Precision Medicine for more Oxygen
SARS-CoV-2	Severe acute respiratory syndrome coronavirus 2
UMC	University Medical Centre

References

1. World Health Organization. WHO Coronavirus (COVID-19) Dashboard. 2022. Available online: https://covid19.who.int/ (accessed on 19 April 2024).
2. Daher, A.; Balfanz, P.; Cornelissen, C.; Muller, A.; Bergs, I.; Marx, N.; Muller-Wieland, D.; Hartmann, B.; Dreher, M.; Muller, T. Follow up of patients with severe coronavirus disease 2019 (COVID-19): Pulmonary and extrapulmonary disease sequelae. *Respir. Med.* 2020, *174*, 106197. [CrossRef] [PubMed]
3. World Health Organization. *A Clinical Case Definition of Post COVID-19 Condition by a Delphi Consensus, 6 October 2021*; World Health Organization: Geneva, Switzerland, 2021.
4. Liska, D.; Liptakova, E.; Babicova, A.; Batalik, L.; Banarova, P.S.; Dobrodenkova, S. What is the quality of life in patients with long COVID compared to a healthy control group? *Front. Public Health* 2022, *10*, 975992. [CrossRef] [PubMed]
5. Raveendran, A.V.; Jayadevan, R.; Sashidharan, S. Long COVID: An overview. *Diabetes Metab. Syndr.* 2021, *15*, 869–875. [CrossRef] [PubMed]
6. Alkodaymi, M.S.; Omrani, O.A.; Fawzy, N.A.; Shaar, B.A.; Almamlouk, R.; Riaz, M.; Obeidat, M.; Obeidat, Y.; Gerberi, D.; Taha, R.M.; et al. Prevalence of post-acute COVID-19 syndrome symptoms at different follow-up periods: A systematic review and meta-analysis. *Clin. Microbiol. Infect.* 2022, *28*, 657–666. [CrossRef]
7. Fernandez-de-Las-Penas, C.; Notarte, K.I.; Macasaet, R.; Velasco, J.V.; Catahay, J.A.; Ver, A.T.; Chung, W.; Valera-Calero, J.A.; Navarro-Santana, M. Persistence of post-COVID symptoms in the general population two years after SARS-CoV-2 infection: A systematic review and meta-analysis. *J. Infect.* 2024, *88*, 77–88. [CrossRef]
8. O'Mahoney, L.L.; Routen, A.; Gillies, C.; Ekezie, W.; Welford, A.; Zhang, A.; Karamchandani, U.; Simms-Williams, N.; Cassambai, S.; Ardavani, A.; et al. The prevalence and long-term health effects of Long Covid among hospitalised and non-hospitalised populations: A systematic review and meta-analysis. *EClinicalMedicine* 2023, *55*, 101762. [CrossRef]
9. Seessle, J.; Waterboer, T.; Hippchen, T.; Simon, J.; Kirchner, M.; Lim, A.; Muller, B.; Merle, U. Persistent Symptoms in Adult Patients 1 Year After Coronavirus Disease 2019 (COVID-19): A Prospective Cohort Study. *Clin. Infect. Dis.* 2022, *74*, 1191–1198. [CrossRef]
10. Ong, S.W.X.; Fong, S.W.; Young, B.E.; Chan, Y.H.; Lee, B.; Amrun, S.N.; Chee, R.S.; Yeo, N.K.; Tambyah, P.; Pada, S.; et al. Persistent Symptoms and Association With Inflammatory Cytokine Signatures in Recovered Coronavirus Disease 2019 Patients. *Open Forum Infect. Dis.* 2021, *8*, ofab156. [CrossRef]
11. Asadi-Pooya, A.A.; Akbari, A.; Emami, A.; Lotfi, M.; Rostamihosseinkhani, M.; Nemati, H.; Barzegar, Z.; Kabiri, M.; Zeraatpisheh, Z.; Farjoud-Kouhanjani, M.; et al. Risk Factors Associated with Long COVID Syndrome: A Retrospective Study. *Iran. J. Med. Sci.* 2021, *46*, 428–436.
12. Davis, H.E.; McCorkell, L.; Vogel, J.M.; Topol, E.J. Long COVID: Major findings, mechanisms and recommendations. *Nat. Rev. Microbiol.* 2023, *21*, 133–146. [CrossRef]
13. Subramanian, A.; Nirantharakumar, K.; Hughes, S.; Myles, P.; Williams, T.; Gokhale, K.M.; Taverner, T.; Chandan, J.S.; Brown, K.; Simms-Williams, N.; et al. Symptoms and risk factors for long COVID in non-hospitalized adults. *Nat. Med.* 2022, *28*, 1706–1714. [CrossRef]
14. Tenforde, M.W.; Kim, S.S.; Lindsell, C.J.; Billig Rose, E.; Shapiro, N.I.; Files, D.C.; Gibbs, K.W.; Erickson, H.L.; Steingrub, J.S.; Smithline, H.A.; et al. Symptom Duration and Risk Factors for Delayed Return to Usual Health Among Outpatients with COVID-19 in a Multistate Health Care Systems Network—United States, March-June 2020. *MMWR Morb. Mortal. Wkly. Rep.* 2020, *69*, 993–998. [CrossRef] [PubMed]
15. Kamal, M.; Abo Omirah, M.; Hussein, A.; Saeed, H. Assessment and characterisation of post-COVID-19 manifestations. *Int. J. Clin. Pract.* 2021, *75*, e13746. [CrossRef] [PubMed]
16. Moreno-Perez, O.; Merino, E.; Leon-Ramirez, J.M.; Andres, M.; Ramos, J.M.; Arenas-Jimenez, J.; Asensio, S.; Sanchez, R.; Ruiz-Torregrosa, P.; Galan, I.; et al. Post-acute COVID-19 syndrome. Incidence and risk factors: A Mediterranean cohort study. *J. Infect.* 2021, *82*, 378–383. [CrossRef] [PubMed]
17. Sudre, C.H.; Murray, B.; Varsavsky, T.; Graham, M.S.; Penfold, R.S.; Bowyer, R.C.; Pujol, J.C.; Klaser, K.; Antonelli, M.; Canas, L.S.; et al. Attributes and predictors of long COVID. *Nat. Med.* 2021, *27*, 626–631. [CrossRef]
18. Baalbaki, N.; Blankestijn, J.M.; Abdel-Aziz, M.I.; de Backer, J.; Bazdar, S.; Beekers, I.; Beijers, R.; van den Bergh, J.P.; Bloemsma, L.D.; Bogaard, H.J.; et al. Precision Medicine for More Oxygen (P4O2)-Study Design and First Results of the Long COVID-19 Extension. *J. Pers. Med.* 2023, *13*, 1060. [CrossRef]
19. W.H.O. Working Group. A minimal common outcome measure set for COVID-19 clinical research. *Lancet Infect. Dis.* 2020, *20*, e192–e197. [CrossRef]
20. Lennon, H.; Kelly, S.; Sperrin, M.; Buchan, I.; Cross, A.J.; Leitzmann, M.; Cook, M.B.; Renehan, A.G. Framework to construct and interpret latent class trajectory modelling. *BMJ Open* 2018, *8*, e020683. [CrossRef]
21. Abdelrahman, M.M.; Abd-Elrahman, N.M.; Bakheet, T.M. Persistence of symptoms after improvement of acute COVID-19 infection, a longitudinal study. *J. Med. Virol.* 2021, *93*, 5942–5946. [CrossRef]
22. Davis, H.E.; Assaf, G.S.; McCorkell, L.; Wei, H.; Low, R.J.; Re'em, Y.; Redfield, S.; Austin, J.P.; Akrami, A. Characterizing long COVID in an international cohort: 7 months of symptoms and their impact. *EClinicalMedicine* 2021, *38*, 101019. [CrossRef]

23. Nehme, M.; Braillard, O.; Chappuis, F.; Courvoisier, D.S.; Guessous, I.; CoviCare Study, T. Prevalence of Symptoms More Than Seven Months After Diagnosis of Symptomatic COVID-19 in an Outpatient Setting. *Ann. Intern. Med.* **2021**, *174*, 1252–1260. [CrossRef] [PubMed]
24. Tran, V.T.; Porcher, R.; Pane, I.; Ravaud, P. Course of post COVID-19 disease symptoms over time in the ComPaRe long COVID prospective e-cohort. *Nat. Commun.* **2022**, *13*, 1812. [CrossRef] [PubMed]
25. Brinkley, E.; Knuth, K.; Kwon, T.; Mack, C.; Leister-Tebbe, H.; Bao, W.; Reynolds, M.W.; Dreyer, N. Daily COVID-19 symptom assessment over 28 days—Findings from a daily direct-to-patient registry of COVID-19 positive patients. *J. Patient Rep. Outcomes* **2023**, *7*, 128. [CrossRef] [PubMed]
26. Caronna, E.; Ballve, A.; Llaurado, A.; Gallardo, V.J.; Ariton, D.M.; Lallana, S.; Lopez Maza, S.; Olive Gadea, M.; Quibus, L.; Restrepo, J.L.; et al. Headache: A striking prodromal and persistent symptom, predictive of COVID-19 clinical evolution. *Cephalalgia* **2020**, *40*, 1410–1421. [CrossRef]
27. Sampaio Rocha-Filho, P.A.; Magalhaes, J.E.; Fernandes Silva, D.; Carvalho Soares, M.; Marenga Arruda Buarque, L.; Dandara Pereira Gama, M.; Oliveira, F.A.A. Neurological manifestations as prognostic factors in COVID-19: A retrospective cohort study. *Acta Neurol. Belg.* **2022**, *122*, 725–733. [CrossRef]
28. Tana, C.; Bentivegna, E.; Cho, S.J.; Harriott, A.M.; Garcia-Azorin, D.; Labastida-Ramirez, A.; Ornello, R.; Raffaelli, B.; Beltran, E.R.; Ruscheweyh, R.; et al. Long COVID headache. *J. Headache Pain.* **2022**, *23*, 93. [CrossRef]
29. Bai, F.; Tomasoni, D.; Falcinella, C.; Barbanotti, D.; Castoldi, R.; Mule, G.; Augello, M.; Mondatore, D.; Allegrini, M.; Cona, A.; et al. Female gender is associated with long COVID syndrome: A prospective cohort study. *Clin. Microbiol. Infect.* **2022**, *28*, 611.e9–611.e16. [CrossRef]
30. Onieva, A.R.; Castro, C.S.; Morales, V.G.; Vacas, M.A.; Requena, A.H. Long COVID: Factors influencing persistent symptoms and the impact of gender. *Med. Fam. SEMERGEN* **2024**, *50*, 102208. [CrossRef]
31. Krishnadath, I.; Harkisoen, S.; Gopie, F.; van der Hilst, K.; Hollum, M.; Woittiez, L.; Baldew, S.S. Prevalence of persistent symptoms after having COVID-19 in a cohort in Suriname. *Rev. Panam. Salud Publica* **2023**, *47*, e79. [CrossRef]
32. Wynberg, E.; van Willigen, H.D.G.; Dijkstra, M.; Boyd, A.; Kootstra, N.A.; van den Aardweg, J.G.; van Gils, M.J.; Matser, A.; de Wit, M.R.; Leenstra, T.; et al. Evolution of Coronavirus Disease 2019 (COVID-19) Symptoms During the First 12 Months After Illness Onset. *Clin. Infect. Dis.* **2022**, *75*, e482–e490. [CrossRef]
33. Centorbi, M.; Di Martino, G.; Della Valle, C.; Iuliano, E.; Di Claudio, G.; Mascioli, A.; Calcagno, G.; di Cagno, A.; Buonsenso, A.; Fiorilli, G. Regular Physical Activity Can Counteract LONG COVID Symptoms in Adults over 40. *J. Funct. Morphol. Kinesiol.* **2024**, *9*, 119. [CrossRef] [PubMed]
34. Feter, N.; Caputo, E.L.; Delpino, F.M.; Leite, J.S.; da Silva, L.S.; de Almeida Paz, I.; Santos Rocha, J.Q.; Vieira, Y.P.; Schroeder, N.; da Silva, C.N.; et al. Physical activity and long COVID: Findings from the Prospective Study About Mental and Physical Health in Adults cohort. *Public Health* **2023**, *220*, 148–154. [CrossRef] [PubMed]
35. Servier, C.; Porcher, R.; Pane, I.; Ravaud, P.; Tran, V.T. Trajectories of the evolution of post-COVID-19 condition, up to two years after symptoms onset. *Int. J. Infect. Dis.* **2023**, *133*, 67–74. [CrossRef] [PubMed]

Disclaimer/Publisher's Note: The statements, opinions and data contained in all publications are solely those of the individual author(s) and contributor(s) and not of MDPI and/or the editor(s). MDPI and/or the editor(s) disclaim responsibility for any injury to people or property resulting from any ideas, methods, instructions or products referred to in the content.

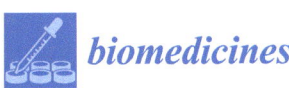

Systematic Review

Pathophysiological, Neuropsychological, and Psychosocial Influences on Neurological and Neuropsychiatric Symptoms of Post-Acute COVID-19 Syndrome: Impacts on Recovery and Symptom Persistence

Alex Malioukis *, R Sterling Snead, Julia Marczika and Radha Ambalavanan

Self Research Institute, Broken Arrow, OK 18452, USA
* Correspondence: alex@selfresearch.org

Abstract: Although the impact of post-acute COVID-19 syndrome (PACS) on patients and public health is undeniably significant, its etiology remains largely unclear. Much research has been conducted on the pathophysiology, shedding light on various aspects; however, due to the multitude of symptoms and clinical conditions that directly or indirectly define PACS, it is challenging to establish definitive causations. In this exploration, through systematically reviewing the latest pathophysiological findings related to the neurological symptoms of the syndrome, we aim to examine how psychosocial and neuropsychological symptoms may overlap with neurological ones, and how they may not only serve as risk factors but also contribute to the persistence of some primary symptoms of the disorder. Findings from our synthesis suggest that psychological and psychosocial factors, such as anxiety, depression, and loneliness, may interact with neurological symptoms in a self-reinforcing feedback loop. This cycle seems to be affecting both physical and psychological distress, potentially increasing the persistence and severity of PACS symptoms. By pointing out this interaction, in this review study, we attempt to offer a new perspective on the interconnected nature of psychological, psychosocial, and neurological factors, emphasizing the importance of integrated treatment approaches to disrupt this cycle and improve outcomes when possible.

Keywords: post-acute COVID syndrome; long COVID; pathophysiology; neurological symptoms; cognitive dysfunction; psychological; neuropsychological; psychosocial

1. Introduction

PACS refers to a spectrum of symptoms and conditions that persist following the acute phase of infection caused by the severe acute respiratory syndrome coronavirus-2 (SARS-CoV-2) [1]. The terminology surrounding this condition is extensive, with various names such as long-haul COVID-19, post-COVID-19 conditions (PCCs), or post-acute sequelae of SARS-CoV-2 infection (PASC) often used interchangeably. In this review, we adopt the term post-acute COVID-19 syndrome (PACS) to describe the symptomatology under investigation. As noted by Ezpeleta et al., this term is preferable as it carries fewer negative implications compared to the alternatives that suggest SARS-CoV-2 may linger in the body for extended periods, a claim unsupported by the current evidence [2].

It is estimated that PACS has impacted nearly 400 million individuals since the start of the pandemic [3]. Although still the subject of extensive global research, this condition is recognized as an intricate, multisystemic disorder that can influence almost every organ system, including the nervous, cardiovascular, gastrointestinal, and endocrine systems [3–5]. While certain individuals, such as older adults, females, those with lower socioeconomic status, and individuals with pre-existing health conditions or mental health disorders, are most at risk for developing long-lasting symptoms after a COVID-19 infection, the syndrome can affect people across all age groups, including children and older adults,

Citation: Malioukis, A.; Snead, R.S.; Marczika, J.; Ambalavanan, R. Pathophysiological, Neuropsychological, and Psychosocial Influences on Neurological and Neuropsychiatric Symptoms of Post-Acute COVID-19 Syndrome: Impacts on Recovery and Symptom Persistence. *Biomedicines* **2024**, *12*, 2831. https://doi.org/10.3390/biomedicines12122831

Academic Editor: César Fernández-de-las-Peñas

Received: 2 December 2024
Revised: 9 December 2024
Accepted: 11 December 2024
Published: 13 December 2024

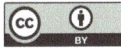

Copyright: © 2024 by the authors. Licensee MDPI, Basel, Switzerland. This article is an open access article distributed under the terms and conditions of the Creative Commons Attribution (CC BY) license (https://creativecommons.org/licenses/by/4.0/).

and across diverse races, ethnicities, genders, and health backgrounds. Importantly, PACS has been documented following both severe and mild cases of acute COVID-19 [6,7]. The commonly reported symptoms include fatigue, shortness of breath, and brain fog, but they can also extend to joint pain, dizziness, chest discomfort, sleep disturbances, and altered senses of smell or taste. Additional symptoms may involve headaches, gastrointestinal issues, and psychological impacts such as anxiety and depression [8]. The symptoms persist for more than 12 weeks following the onset of COVID-19 and cannot be explained by any alternative diagnosis. The condition is identified through clinical evaluation, as there is currently no definitive biomarker to confirm its presence [9,10].

In this study, we will primarily focus on the neurological, neuropsychological, and neuropsychiatric symptoms of PACS. Our review presents a new angle on PACS by exploring the complex interactions between psychological, psychosocial, and neurobiological factors, which, to the best of our knowledge, have not been thoroughly explored in previous studies. By examining how these interconnected symptoms may create a feedback loop, where the physical and psychological conditions exacerbate one another, we aim to offer a more holistic perspective on the disorder. This integrated approach, which includes psychosocial and psychological dimensions, offers new insights into the persistence and complexity of PACS, going beyond typical studies focused mainly on the pathophysiological aspects.

2. Methods

2.1. Search Strategy

An online search of the existing published literature was conducted to identify studies examining the multifactorial causes of PACS, covering the period from 2020 to 2024. This study was registered in the OSF; registration DOI https://doi.org/10.17605/OSF.IO/RCGH2. We used the PRISMA guidelines as a general framework to guide our review [11]. In doing so, five scientific literature databases—namely, Google Scholar, Scopus, PubMed, PsycINFO, and the ACM Digital Library—were electronically searched. To ensure a comprehensive retrieval of related articles, we employed a strong set of keywords covering essential and supporting terms related to PACS, its physiological and psychological causes, and treatment strategies (see Table 1). The search for relevant articles was conducted between 5 September 2024 and 15 November 2024, and was limited to English-language publications.

Table 1. List of keywords used in database searches.

Keywords
Post-Acute COVID-19 Syndrome, PACS, PASC, Long COVID, Post-COVID, Pathology, Neuroinflammation, Brain Imaging, Brain Fog, Cognitive Dysfunction, Memory Impairment, Executive Function, Neuropsychiatric Symptoms, Neuropsychological Deficits, Quarantine Impact, Psychological Stress, Social Isolation, Loneliness, Mental Health, Fatigue, Headache, Insomnia, Depression, Immune Response, Autonomic Dysfunction, Viral Persistence

Thematic and keyword search results were then manually screened for relevance to PACS and its underlying mechanisms. Each study was carefully examined, with particular attention to recent findings on the neuropathology of PACS, as well as the neuropsychological and psychosocial factors affecting the disorder.

2.2. Eligibility Criteria

The inclusion criteria for this review were peer-reviewed journal articles, conference papers, and review articles presenting empirical findings, theoretical frameworks, or innovative methodologies related to PACS or post-COVID-19 conditions, published in English between 2020 and 2024. Studies focused specifically on PACS or post-COVID-19 symptoms were included. The exclusion criteria included studies that focused on populations without a PACS diagnosis, such as healthy controls or individuals with unrelated comorbidities. Studies that did not address PACS-related neurological, neuropsychological, or psychosocial outcomes were excluded. Additionally, studies focused on disorders unrelated to PACS, such as general neurological diseases not linked to COVID-19, were excluded.

2.3. Data Synthesis

The authors performed an independent screening of this article based on the inclusion and exclusion criteria described previously. Initially, a total of 10,879 articles were retrieved from keyword searches conducted across the databases mentioned above. By limiting our selection to peer-reviewed journal articles published in English, for which full texts were available, and by removing duplicates, the total was reduced to 2576 articles. In conducting this review, the first batch of retrieved publications served as the basis for screening to choose those that fulfilled our set criteria. In the first phase, all articles underwent an initial screening based on their titles to ensure consistency and relevance to our research goals. Following this initial screening, 981 were selected for further evaluation. The second step in preliminary coding involved the reviewing of abstracts, keywords, and, when necessary, introductory sections of the articles with an aim to determining which had close relevance to our current research focus. This narrowed down our selection to a subset of 244 articles. Lastly, in the final stage of screening, the articles that were remaining were thoroughly read through with an objective of determining their applicability and relevance within the scope of our study. Accordingly, a final set of 115 articles that substantially contributed to our research objectives and met the set inclusion criteria was identified and retained. The process for article retrieval, screening, and selection is shown in Figure 1.

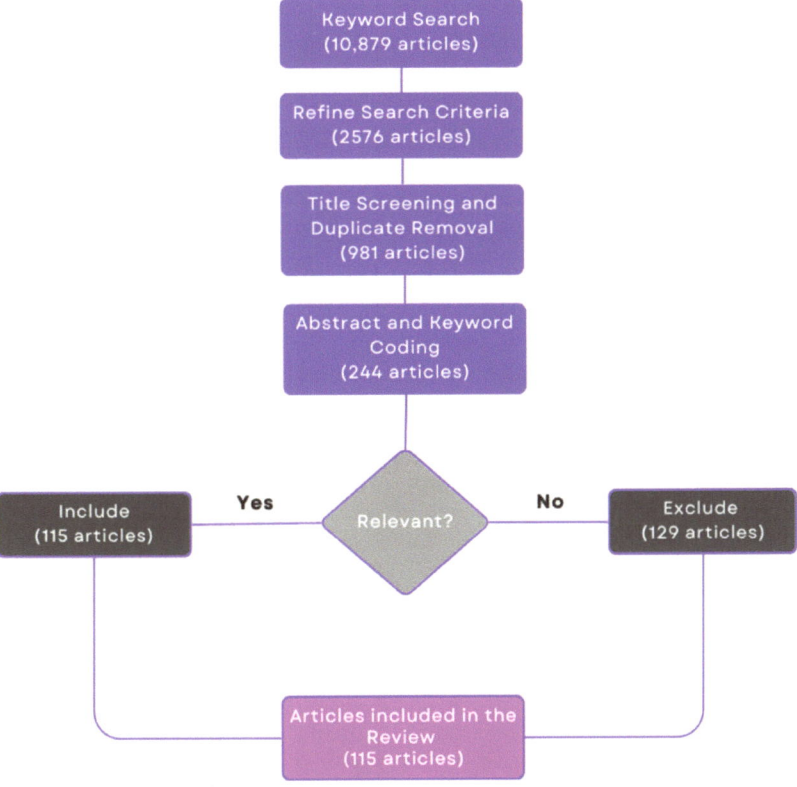

Figure 1. Flow diagram of literature search and selection process.

3. Neurological, Neurocognitive, and Neuropsychiatric Symptomatology of PACS

While COVID-19 is primarily recognized as a respiratory illness, it is also closely linked to a variety of neurological and neuropsychiatric manifestations due to its impact on both the central nervous system (CNS) and peripheral nervous system (PNS). In the context of PACS, the extensive range of symptoms, including numerous neurological and neuropsychological issues, has led clinicians worldwide to suggest that it resembles a neurological disorder in many respects [12].

3.1. Neurological Symptoms

PACS manifests a wide range of neurological and neuropsychological symptoms, highlighting the intricate relationship between the CNS and the PNS after a SARS-CoV-2 infection 9 (see Table 2). Notably, many of these neurological symptoms often overlap with issues impacting various organ systems. Furthermore, some nonspecific symptoms that we will examine may indicate secondary effects arising from underlying conditions in the endocrine, autoimmune, or psychiatric and psychological areas.

Table 2. Prevalence of neurological symptoms in PACS.

Neurological Symptom	Percentage of Affected Patients
Fatigue	Up to 58%
Sleep disturbances	Up to 30%
Headaches	Up to 44%
Dizziness and Vertigo	Up to 5%
POTS	Up to 14%
ME/CFS	Up to 51%
Gastrointestinal disturbances	Up to 22%

One of the most severe and persistent symptoms reported in the literature is fatigue. This condition affects a considerable proportion of PACS patients, with evidence indicating that up to 58% experience long-lasting fatigue, which can negatively influence daily functioning and overall well-being [13,14]. Sleep disturbances, particularly insomnia, are also prevalent among PACS patients and are closely associated with cognitive impairments and emotional distress. Insomnia affects up to 30% of this population, with these disruptions in sleep quality potentially exacerbating fatigue and affecting cognitive performance [15,16].

Headaches are another commonly documented symptom, with varying severity and frequency. Observational studies report that up to 44% of patients continue to experience headaches months post-infection. These headaches are often resistant to standard treatment and are associated with other symptoms, such as concentration problems and heightened sensory sensitivities [17,18].

In addition, symptoms of dizziness and vertigo are also frequently observed, affecting up to 5% of PACS patients, and can present as episodes of lightheadedness and balance impairment, which can have a negative impact on mobility and quality of life. These symptoms may be indicative of autonomic dysfunction, which is commonly reported in PACS. More specifically, it has been observed that post-COVID-19, up to 14% of patients present with postural orthostatic tachycardia syndrome (POTS), a manifestation of autonomic dysfunction, which is characterized by symptoms such as increased heart rate upon standing, palpitations, chest pain, lightheadedness, and fainting episodes, illustrating the widespread autonomic impact of SARS-CoV-2 infection. As with many other symptoms of the disorder, it is still unclear whether POTS is a direct symptom of PACS or if COVID-19 infection acts as a trigger in individuals who may already be predisposed to developing dysautonomia. In these cases, COVID-19 might not directly cause dysautonomia but instead exacerbates or activates an underlying susceptibility [19,20].

Another syndrome that overlaps with PACS, and shares similarities with POTS, is myalgic encephalitis/chronic fatigue syndrome (ME/CFS). Common ME/CFS-like symptoms, experienced by up to 51% of patients, include severe muscle weakness, joint pain, dizziness, and cognitive dysfunction, often occurring alongside unrefreshing sleep. These findings suggest a potential shared pathophysiology between PACS and ME/CFS, contributing to the complexity of symptom management and quality of life deterioration [21].

Finally, other common symptoms, while not entirely neurological and also frequently observed in neuropsychiatric and psychological disorders, are gastrointestinal (GI) disturbances. We chose to explore these symptoms further because they have become a notable area of focus, partly due to recent studies suggesting the involvement of the gut–brain axis and the bidirectional relationship between the CNS and the gut [22–24]. GI symptoms are reported in a significant portion of PACS patients, with a systematic review and meta-analysis revealing that 22% experience GI issues—nearly double the 12% observed during the acute infection phase. Common symptoms include abdominal pain, nausea, vomiting, loss of appetite, loss of taste, diarrhea, dyspepsia, and irritable bowel syndrome (IBS). These GI symptoms often occur alongside systemic and neuropsychiatric issues; for instance, gut dysbiosis in PACS patients has been associated with fatigue, cognitive impairments, and neuropsychiatric symptoms such as anxiety and depression [25–28].

3.2. Neurocognitive and Neuropsychological Symptoms

Building on the neurological symptoms discussed in the previous section, neurocognitive symptoms in PACS reflect the complex interplay between the neurological, neuropsychological, and psychological factors. The emerging literature over the past four years has begun to shed light on how these symptoms affect cognitive processes, including attention, memory, and executive functioning (see Table 3). In this chapter, we will review the current research to better understand these cognitive challenges and their impact on daily life.

Table 3. Prevalence of neurocognitive symptoms in PACS.

Neurocognitive Symptom	Percentage of Affected Patients
Cognitive Impairment	Up to 65%
Persistent Fatigue	Up to 46.6%
Brain Fog	Up to 31.9%
Attention Deficits	Up to 55%
Memory Impairment	Up to 40%
Executive Function Deficits	Up to 59%
Language Difficulties	Up to 93%

Regarding the prevalence of the symptoms, a systematic review by Tavares-Júnior et al. found that cognitive impairment was observed in 21% to 65% of COVID-19 survivors who had been hospitalized, with assessments conducted 12 weeks or more after the initial infection [29].

Following COVID-19 infection, numerous studies have documented a range of cognitive challenges reported by patients months post-recovery. Common complaints, from up to 47% of patients, include persistent fatigue as well as brain fog, and difficulties with attention and memory [30–32]. The results from neuropsychological testing indicate that individuals with a recent SARS-CoV-2 infection often exhibit impaired global cognitive function, leading to notable challenges in concentration and sustained attention, among other difficulties [33]. The research has consistently shown that memory problems, including deficits in working memory, verbal memory, and visual memory, are also prevalent among those recovering from COVID-19, affecting up to 40% of PACS patients [34–36].

Additionally, studies indicate that up to 59% of individuals with PACS demonstrate executive function deficits and slowed information processing speed, factors which can also complicate everyday functioning and well-being [37,38]. Language difficulties are also frequently reported among adults with PACS, with studies showing poorer performance in areas such as discourse informativeness, verbal recall, and fluency. Cummings, for instance, found that while adults with PACS can produce grammatically correct speech, their discourse often lacks informativeness, a problem linked to executive dysfunctions like impaired planning. Memory deficits further contribute to reduced informativeness, as seen in significant recall challenges among participants. Additionally, the same study indicates that word-finding difficulty is a common complaint, affecting 93% of surveyed adults, despite normal naming task performance. Verbal fluency tasks reveal further deficits, especially in letter and category fluency, which when coupled with the other language difficulties, highlight the cognitive–communication disruptions experienced by individuals with PACS [39].

Brain fog, a term frequently discussed in studies on PACS, encompasses a combination of the aforementioned symptoms along with other psychological phenomena [40]. More specifically, in post-COVID-19 syndromes, brain fog is recognized as a symptom cluster characterized by fatigue, headaches, word-finding difficulties, memory impairment, inattention, short-term memory loss, and reduced mental acuity. This cluster significantly affects cognition, concentration, and sleep and is associated with adverse psychological and psychomotor outcomes [41,42].

These findings, among others, indicate that cognitive challenges such as attention, memory, and executive dysfunction are not merely isolated symptoms but instead reflect the broader neurological substructures affected, either directly or indirectly, by the virus.

3.3. Neuropsychiatric Symptoms

While examining the literature on psychiatric symptoms after COVID-19 infection, we cannot overlook the overlapping nature of these symptoms with other domains and the role they play in the complex interactions of PACS. Once again, the research suggests that the psychiatric symptoms in PACS are not isolated occurrences but are deeply interwoven with both neurological and psychosocial variables, influencing the broader spectrum of symptoms experienced (see Table 4).

Table 4. Prevalence of neuropsychiatric symptoms in PACS.

Neuropsychiatric Symptom	Percentage of Affected Patients
Anxiety	Up to 29.6%
Depression	Up to 35%
PTSD	Up to 16%
Psychotic Symptoms	Up to 4%

Anxiety and depression emerge as some of the most frequently reported psychiatric symptoms, with studies highlighting that these issues can persist for extended periods post-infection, affecting up to 29.6% and 35% of individuals, respectively. The symptoms often linger for weeks to months and show higher prevalence among females and those with a history of psychiatric disorders, suggesting that COVID-19 may act as a trigger or an exacerbating factor for pre-existing mental health vulnerabilities. This persistent presence of anxiety and depression contributes to the complexity of PACS, as these symptoms interact with other cognitive and physical challenges, potentially increasing the overall burden on patients [43,44].

PTSD, too, is a prominent psychiatric concern in the context of PACS, with multiple studies noting substantial rates of PTSD symptoms among COVID-19 survivors. Although prevalence estimates vary, with up to 16% of patients experiencing symptoms of the disorder, the high occurrence of PTSD could reflect the significant psychological distress that individuals may experience following severe or life-threatening COVID-19 infections.

Factors such as hospitalization, prolonged isolation, and the psychological toll of the pandemic itself may also contribute to the persistence of these symptoms [45–48].

Sleep disturbances—observed both in the context of neurological symptoms and from a psychiatric perspective—also constitute a common complaint among patients. Mekhael et al. utilized wearable health devices to examine the impact of PACS on sleep quality and found that individuals with a history of COVID-19 infection exhibited significant alterations in sleep architecture. Specifically, these patients experienced reduced total sleep duration and less deep sleep compared to matched controls, irrespective of demographic factors and symptom severity [49]. Insomnia and hypersomnia frequently appear as prevalent symptoms, with disrupted sleep potentially acting as both a direct response to the virus and as a secondary effect of co-occurring psychiatric conditions, such as anxiety or depression. Notably, sleep problems are often among the most pervasive symptoms of PACS, impacting mental health, cognitive function, and overall well-being [50–52]. Interestingly, in their recent paper, Schilling et al. concluded that disturbed sleep patterns could even potentially predict an increased risk of developing post-acute sequelae of COVID-19 [53].

The recent research highlights another dimension of psychiatric disorders related to COVID-19, specifically psychotic symptomatology. These may include delusions, hallucinations, disorganized thoughts, and confusion and can affect up to 4% of the patients. Cases vary in duration, lasting from a few days to several weeks, with some extending up to 90 days [54,55]. Studies by Ferrando et al. and Smith et al. have documented symptoms such as paranoia, megalomania, mystical beliefs, and catatonia, affecting predominantly male patients with a mean onset age of 43.9 years. Long-term symptoms were also noted in some patients months after initial infection [54,56,57].

In conclusion, the psychiatric symptoms of the syndrome are complex and interconnected with other neurological and psychological factors. Of these, anxiety, depression, and PTSD are the most frequent and often aggravate the cognitive and physical difficulties, creating a vicious circle that further escalates the severity of both mental and physical suffering. Moreover, common sleep disturbances also interact with these psychiatric symptoms, increasing the overall burden of PACS. These overlapping domains seem to contribute to the multifaceted nature of PACS, where certain psychiatric manifestations are not merely symptoms themselves but also potential risk factors for the development or exacerbation of other symptoms. In the following sections, we will explore the neurobiology and psychological aspects of these symptoms and how they may contribute to the broader challenges of PACS.

4. Pathophysiology

The pathophysiological and neurophysiological mechanisms underlying the resulting neurological, neuropsychological, and neuropsychiatric symptomatology are under active investigation. The extant literature puts forward a variety of neurobiological mechanisms that could be implicated in these symptoms, and it may well be that an interplay among these processes could drive the diverse manifestations seen thus far.

4.1. Immune–Inflammatory Signaling and Cytokine Response

According to the low-grade inflammation theory, the pathogenesis of PACS is promoted by a persistent, low-level inflammatory responses rather than the intense hyperinflammation usually seen in acute COVID-19 cases. This chronic, mild immune activation subtly seems to perturb cellular and systemic functions, contributing to the diversity of symptoms in PACS, such as fatigue, cognitive dysfunction, and mood disturbances. In contrast to the acute and life-threatening inflammation presented during the initial phases of infection, persistent low-grade inflammation is similar to para-inflammatory mechanisms observed in chronic viral infections and post-infectious syndromes. Manifestation of this dysregulation of immune response may lead to the sustained activation of microglia and release of cytokines, thereby providing grounds for the development of neuropsychiatric symptoms, especially through changes in susceptible brain areas, such as the limbic system [58,59].

Cytokines such as TNF-α (tumor necrosis factor), IL-6 (interleukin-6), and IL-1β are implicated not only in the inflammatory response to COVID-19 but also in the development of conditions like major depressive disorder and Alzheimer's disease. Such cytokines may contribute to dysregulated stress responses, mood changes, and cognitive dysfunction in post-infection individuals. The fact that elevated levels of these cytokines are often seen in COVID-19 patients suggests that inflammation could play a significant role in the cognitive and emotional disturbances observed in PACS [51].

Further supporting this hypothesis, one narrative review article underlines some neuropsychiatric manifestations related to immune–inflammatory signaling in COVID-19, suggesting that systemic inflammation per se can cause psychiatric presentations even in the absence of direct viral CNS invasion [48]. Indeed, significant correlations exist between levels of TNF-α, IL-6, IL-1β, IL-10, IFN-γ, and CCL2 with cognitive and behavioral changes in COVID-19 patients, thus showing generalized neuroinflammation. This dysregulation, especially the pro-inflammatory cytokines, can affect the integrity of the blood–brain barrier by allowing immune cells to penetrate the central nervous system, which impairs neurotransmission. Accordingly, such immune-mediated alterations may subsequently give rise to neuropsychiatric manifestations of depression, anxiety, and cognitive dysfunction [60,61]. The immune response against COVID-19 is thought to result in a high-degree inflammatory response by the release of both Th1 and Th2 cytokines. This excessive response could lead to an exaggerated state of inflammation in the body, hence facilitating different kinds of organ injuries. Within the central nervous system, this can lead to immune-mediated disorders characterized by delirium, cognitive dysfunction, and changes in mood [62]. Indeed, elevated levels of pro-inflammatory biomarkers, like IL-6 and CCL2, have been found to relate to changes in cerebral activity, particularly in those regions—such as the sub-genual cingulate cortex—critical for maintaining mood [63].

4.2. Prolonged Neuroinflammation and Psychiatric and Neurocognitive Symptoms

Some studies have suggested that rather than being a mere residue of the acute infection, many psychiatric symptoms in PACS may appear and increase post-infection as a consequence of neuroinflammation persisting for long periods [64,65]. Such an effect might depend importantly on the activation of microglia and reactive astrogliosis. The mentioned glial cell responses can disrupt glutamate signaling and elevate the risk of both new-onset psychiatric disorders and exacerbation of pre-existing conditions. This ongoing neuroinflammatory response possibly indicates a complicated way in which COVID-19 maintains its effects on brain function even long after infection. Speculations are that this greatly contributes to the cognitive and emotional symptoms seen in patients with PACS [66].

4.3. Viral Pathways to the CNS and Brainstem Dysfunction

COVID-19's impact on the CNS may also be linked to direct or indirect viral entry. While the olfactory bulb has been identified as a potential entry point for the virus, autopsy findings have shown the presence of viral RNA in the brainstem, a region with high ACE2 receptor expression. This suggests that SARS-CoV-2 may infect the brainstem and, thus, may be involved in neurodegenerative processes. Not all cases, however, show detectable viral RNA in the brainstem, for which reason, researchers also believe that neurological damage is largely immune-mediated rather than via the direct infection of brain tissue. This notion receives further support from the fact that symptoms related to PACS, including tiredness and cognitive confusion, are in line with symptoms of chronic fatigue syndrome, in which abnormalities in the brain stem are often observed [67,68].

4.4. Neuroimaging Findings

Several recent neuroimaging studies have indeed underlined the long-term neurological burden of COVID-19 and showed both structural and functional alterations in the brain. Indeed, several studies using different imaging modalities, such as FDG-PET and MRI (see Figure 2), have suggested that COVID-19 may induce frontoparietal hypometabolism and a reduced gray matter volume of the orbitofrontal cortex and the parahippocampal gyrus. These findings resonate with the cognitive and emotional disturbances noted in patients suffering from PACS, which frequently manifest as challenges in attention, memory, and the regulation of mood [69–71].

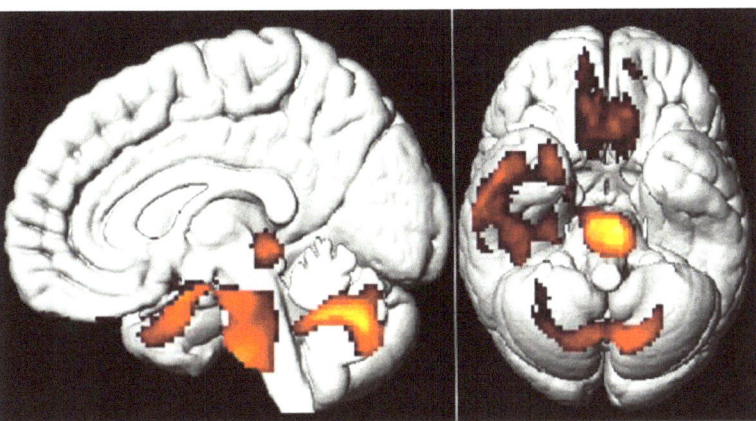

Figure 2. The 18F-FDG PET demonstrating hypometabolism in the bilateral rectal/orbital gyrus, the right temporal lobe, the bilateral pons/medulla brainstem, and the bilateral cerebellum in patients with PACS. Reproduced with permission from reference Guedj et al. [72].

Researchers have therefore speculated that dysfunction here might be contributing to the chronic fatigue and brain fog commonly reported by patients with PACS, which somewhat echoes related studies into chronic fatigue syndrome where the brainstem has also been implicated. This association of cognitive symptoms with brainstem dysfunction is further supported by the diffusion-weighted (DWI) studies which have shown microstructural changes in the thalamus, another region implicated in CFS [72,73].

Various neuroimaging studies have also invariably pointed to changes not only in the brainstem and thalamus but also in different white matter tracts connecting far-reaching cortical regions. These include the corona radiata, corticospinal tract, corpus callosum, and arcuate fasciculus, among others. These white matter changes imply an interruption to communicating streams across different brain regions; these, in turn, can be considered responsible for the cognitive–affective symptoms constituting PACS [70].

Supporting these structural findings, the recent narrative review by Theofilis et al. summarized important neurophysiological findings with significant changes in the functional and structural features of the brains of subjects affected by PACS [74]. In a longitudinal EEG study, patients recovering from COVID-19 presented increases in regional current density and connectivity in the delta band, associated with executive function impairment two months post hospitalization [75]. Further neuroimaging studies have also been able to show frontoparietal hypometabolism, possible dysfunction in the locus coeruleus, gray matter reduction in the orbitofrontal cortex and parahippocampal gyrus, alongside global brain volume loss, following COVID-19 infection. This would suggest that COVID-19 infection may result in long-lasting structural changes to those parts of the brain involved in cognitive and emotional processing [69,76].

4.5. Gut-Brain Axis

The emerging research has suggested that the gut–brain axis may also play a role in the neuropsychopathology of PACS. SARS-CoV-2 can disrupt the gut microbiome, leading to neuroimmune interactions that potentially contribute to prolonged cognitive and mood disturbances. The virus uses ACE2 receptors, found abundantly in both the gut lining and the brain's blood vessels, to gain entry into these regions. This interaction could facilitate the disruption of the blood–brain barrier, allowing inflammatory and neurotoxic molecules to cross into the brain and facilitate symptoms such as memory deficits and mood swings. The gut–brain axis research has determined that the permeability of the gut is increased due to stress and illness, a condition popularly called "leaky gut", through which toxins may enter the bloodstream. These products, once in the brain, can further increase cognitive symptoms like brain fog and amnesia, and even influence mood. Moreover, gut dysbiosis, or an imbalance in the gut microbiota, may result in chronic inflammation and immune activation, further promoting neuropsychiatric symptoms in PACS. The gut–brain axis disruption model contrasts with the hypothesis of direct viral entry into the brain and thus offers an indirect route for neurocognitive symptoms associated with PACS [77,78].

4.6. Impact of Viral Variants and Vaccination on PACS

To further explore the variability in post-COVID-19 presentations, it could also be helpful to consider the influence that different viral variants may have on the severity and persistence of symptoms in PACS patients.

Investigations have indicated that variants of SARS-CoV-2 may also affect the presentation and likelihood of PACS. An analysis contrasting individuals infected with the wild-type virus (March–December 2020) with those infected by the Alpha variant (January–April 2021) uncovered a change in symptomatology, especially within the neurological and cognitive/emotional areas. Despite this diversity, persistent fatigue and breathlessness continued to be the symptoms most often reported. These data therefore support the concept that a switch in tropism and/or other viral properties could partially explain the phenotypic differences among post-COVID-19 symptoms [79].

In a similar manner, another study analyzed the relationship between SARS-CoV-2 variant and PACS risk in 7699 hospitalized patients from six centers. Researchers found that patients infected with the wild-type virus exhibited the highest prevalence of symptoms, with fatigue, brain fog, and respiratory symptoms as the most common manifestations. Interestingly, Omicron had a lower risk compared to the variants from the earlier period, Alpha and Delta. The mediation analyses showed that part of the decrease in the risk was mediated through the weaker severity of acute disease with lower rates of ICU admission [80]. Further research has identified symptom clusters with distinct variants. For example, an unsupervised analysis of post-COVID-19 profiles revealed three primary symptom clusters—cardiorespiratory, central neurological, and severe multi-organ dysfunction. The frequency and severity of these clusters were variant-dependent. For instance, the Delta variant elicited severe symptoms of multi-organ dysfunction, whereas neurological symptoms, including altered mental status and seizures, were more frequent in infections attributed to Omicron [81]. In addition, large-scale studies have indeed corroborated the fact that the incidence of PACS was highest among those infected with the original virus type but has gradually declined in its succeeding variants, including Omicron. But even so, fatigue seemed to remain the most common symptom in all variants, followed by pain, and then cognitive impairment [82].

Finally, cohort studies among pediatric populations have already shown differences among variants with respect to symptomatology. In fact, during the Omicron period, the respiratory and gastrointestinal manifestations significantly decreased in comparison to the period of previous variants, while increased severe neurological manifestations were recorded during this period. More specifically, there was an increase in altered mental status and seizures that were significantly higher in the Omicron period than in the non-variant and Alpha and Delta periods [83].

It is important to note that some contradictions exist across studies regarding the prevalence, severity, and types of PACS symptoms associated with different variants. These might have a biological underpinning, including but not limited to differences in virus–host interaction and immune response, and the psychosocial matters regarding the experience of the illness and perhaps the stress of living through the pandemic itself. Such complexities underscore the need for further research to reconcile these differences and provide a more comprehensive understanding of the factors shaping post-COVID-19 conditions.

4.7. Impact of Vaccination on PACS

Although the relationship between vaccination and PACS remains to be more deeply investigated in order to understand the underlying mechanisms, a portion of the literature has explored its protective effects. Specifically, statistics show that the probability of developing PACS is considerably lower among vaccinated people compared to unvaccinated people. One case, for example, identified vaccination to decrease the risk by about 29%, particularly after two vaccine doses. Another study found that only 8% of the vaccinated experienced post infection symptoms, compared with 27% of the unvaccinated [84,85].

Vaccination appears to protect against the severity of the symptoms, as well. Vaccinated persons report fewer severe respiratory symptoms, including shortness of breath, with overall alleviation of these symptoms with time. The protection may occur irrespective of whether vaccination has occurred before or after the SARS-CoV-2 infection, underlining the broad importance of vaccination in lowering the risk of post-COVID-19 conditions. Large population studies seem to support these findings. For example, a study in the UK showed that vaccinated people had a lower incidence of PACS symptoms, emphasizing the role of vaccination in lessening its impact. Interestingly, some patients with chronic symptoms also reported improvement after being vaccinated. All these disclosures underline the immense importance of vaccination, not only in the prevention of severe and acute cases of COVID-19, but also possibly in the alleviation of its long-term consequences [85,86].

5. The Psychological Dimensions of PACS

So far, based on a very careful review of the literature available on this topic, we have been able to cover most of the symptomatology and psychopathology of the neurological profile of patients with PACS. In this chapter, we will examine these symptoms from both a psychological and psychosocial lens, taking into consideration not only the way in which these factors influence the course and experience of PACS but also the way in which they may be shaped by the condition itself (see Figure 3).

First of all, although a considerable portion of the current literature suggests that psychological factors contribute not only to the development but also to the ongoing maintenance of PACS, the influence of these psychological mechanisms is some-times overlooked or even dismissed—possibly due to concerns that acknowledging psychological factors could be perceived as diminishing the severity of the disease [87–90]. Within the academic community, the term "psychological" is often misinterpreted as something distinct from biological processes. However, in this review, we agree with the view almost collectively accepted within modern cognitive neuroscience, that psychological mechanisms are inherently brain-based and fundamentally integrated within the biological domain. In that sense, acknowledging the role of psychological factors does not imply a dismissal of the physiological complexities of PACS, but rather an expanded understanding of its multifaceted nature.

The research on persistent somatic symptoms and chronic medical conditions has highlighted the substantial role of psychological factors in these conditions. Given that PACS is often characterized by persistent somatic symptoms, these psychological mechanisms are likely relevant to this condition as well. Interestingly, health anxiety, negative expectations, and psychological distress frequently play a more critical role in reducing quality of life than the severity of somatic symptoms themselves. Other than depression and anxiety, cognitive perceptual factors such as selected attention, somatosensory amplification, and cognitive distortions—like catastrophizing—may further perpetuate symptom continuity [91–93].

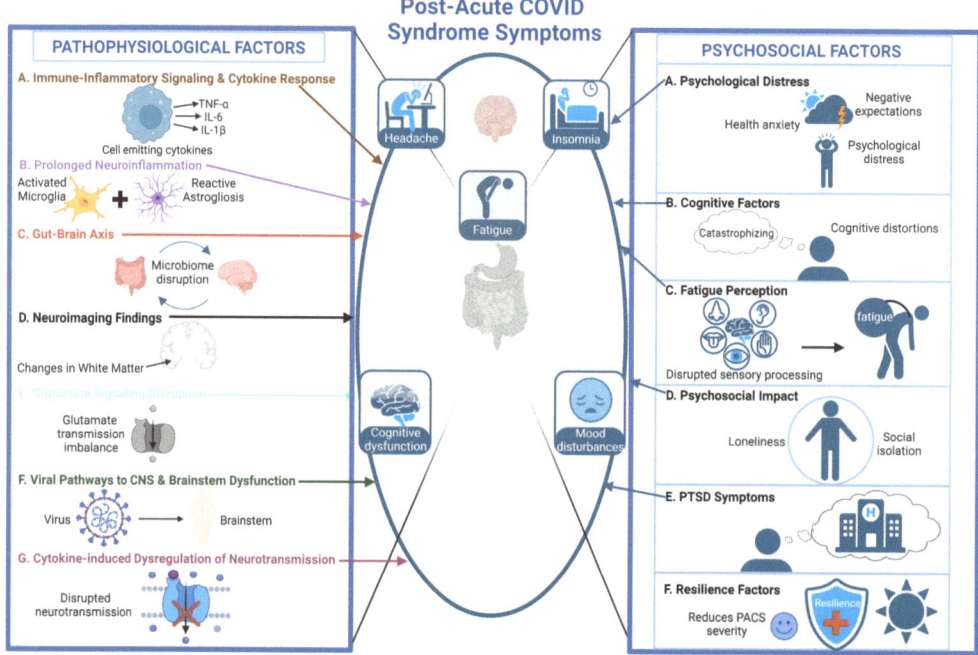

Figure 3. Integrative model of pathophysiological and psychosocial factors contributing to neurological symptoms in PACS (TNF-α: tumor necrosis factor-alpha; IL-6: interleukin-6; IL-1β: interleukin-1 beta; CNS: central nervous system; PACS: post-acute COVID-19 syndrome; PTSD: post-traumatic stress disorder).

As in many other chronic and somatic diseases, in PACS as well, it is presumed that psychological distress is not only a symptom but also a risk factor [44,94,95]. Other studies have found that psychological distress measured at the start of the pandemic was associated with increased risk of developing lasting symptoms among individuals who later became infected with SARS-CoV-2. Another interesting finding in the literature shows that in some cases, the expectation of COVID-19 symptoms and self-reported history of infection have been found to be stronger predictors of worsening somatic symptom burden compared to a laboratory-confirmed COVID-19 infection [96–98].

The intersection of somatic and psychological factors has recently driven Hüsing et al. to develop the PSY-PSS framework, a model designed to systematically examine psychological influences on the etiology of persistent somatic symptoms (PSSs). This framework provides a structured set of psychological variables that appear to aggravate symptomatology in individuals with PSSs. Key mechanisms include behavioral avoidance, where patients avoid situations that physically challenge the body, leading to inactivity and subsequent physical deconditioning. Cognitive factors, such as persistent rumination on physical complaints and a self-concept of bodily vulnerability, further contribute to symptom perpetuation. Additionally, affective traits—negative affectivity, anger linked to somatic experiences, and deficits in emotional regulation, particularly alexithymia—are central components in the PSY-PSS model. Without underestimating other physiological mechanisms, we can see the relevance of this psychological framework in understanding persistent somatic symptoms related to COVID-19 [92,93].

As we have seen thus far, fatigue is a common and disabling symptom in PACS, having a significant impact on daily functioning. Among other common factors, a model that could provide a valuable framework to further understand this persistent fatigue is what has been called the sensory attenuation model [99]. Under normal conditions, the brain suppresses self-generated sensory inputs—such as sensations from our own movements—to minimize unnecessary "noise" in perception, conserving energy and making physical tasks more efficient. This model does, however, suggest that once this mechanism is disrupted even simple movements could be more effortful and give rise to a sustained sense of fatigue. Indeed, the studies are suggesting that individuals with PACS could be experiencing disruption in the sensory process, thus giving them an increased sense of the feeling of effort and exhaustion in everyday tasks [100]. Unlike physical exhaustion alone, this is a type of fatigue that is produced by the changed way the brain handles the afferent input, which raises the perceived effort.

Arguably, fatigue is a symptom influenced by a variety of factors, and it can simultaneously contribute to the development of new symptoms. The positive feedback loop commonly observed in chronic diseases, where psychological and somatic manifestations interact and exacerbate each other, seems highly relevant to PACS as well. In this case, a vicious cycle is somewhat evident, as a somatic symptom triggers a psychological response, which in turn worsens the physical symptom or creates a new one, and so on. Interestingly, the cycle could also begin with a psychological trigger. Whatever the point of initiation of the circle is, however, it becomes clear that psychological symptoms could be powerful modifiers of the course of PACS. For instance, regarding the perception of fatigue in PACS, one study showed that patients who self-reportedly felt fatigued did not show additional objective fatigability compared to a control group without post-COVID-19 symptoms [101]. This could suggest that at least in some cases, the perception of fatigue in PACS may be more influenced by psychological factors than by objective measures of physical fatigue.

An interesting model that seems to align with the feedback loop mechanism described above was suggested by Scharfenberg et al. [102]. In this framework, the authors proposed that the SARS-CoV-2 infection may first induce symptoms like tiredness. Then, this could act as a central node, triggering a cascade of connected symptoms, via feedback loops within the network of symptoms. Next, the tiredness might lead to disturbed sleep, which could enhance the feelings of exhaustion. This persistent exhaustion may impair intellectual functioning, manifesting as difficulties with concentration, slowed processing speed, and a general sense of brain fog. These neuropsychological impairments may then enhance emotional suffering, which in turn increases symptoms like depression or anxiety. These neuropsychiatric symptoms could then feed back into the system, potentially escalating sleep disturbance and perpetuating the fatigue—thus completing a self-reinforcing cycle. The authors point out that this is merely one example of how symptoms could be interacting together, since these networks are very individualized and may vary quite a bit from person to person.

As we have seen in detail so far, the neuropsychological and neuropsychiatric consequences of COVID-19, particularly in the context of PACS, appear driven by a complex interplay of factors. These include the direct effects of the virus on the brain, as well as other indirect physiological influences. In the indirect pathway, we have already seen the psychological mechanisms that shape the course of the disorder. Beyond that, numerous studies have underlined the considerable psychosocial impact of the pandemic. Loneliness and social isolation, as well as the imposed restrictions during the pandemic, have been strongly associated with increasing levels of anxiety, depression, and other negative emotions, which could also increase the prevalence and severity of psychiatric symptoms among PACS patients [103–106]. Anxiety linked to the pandemic does not involve only the people who became infected with SARS-CoV-2. Anxiety disorders in the general population have also been found to present with similar physical symptoms to those of PACS, which, independent of the infection, would suggest that psychological distress may be implicated in symptom reporting [107]. On the contrary, higher personal resilience levels were linked to lower levels of PACS severity, therefore underlining the potential role of psychosocial factors in modulating symptom experience and recovery trajectories [89,108]. Similarly, neuropsychological problems, for instance, have been observed as persisting in the majority of cases, although other individuals seem to show higher rates of recovery, again pointing out that a combination of psychosocial and neuropsychological factors is at play [109,110].

A multitude of studies have shown that the gut–brain axis is critical in influencing and possibly precipitating the development of psychiatric and psychological disorders [111,112]. Furthermore, in our study, the hypothesis was highlighted that the gut–brain axis might also play a significant role in the pathogenesis of PACS itself. At this point, we interrupted the cycle to examine how stress can impact the gut–brain axis through its intricate bidirectional relationship. Sustained or severe stress can disrupt the activity of the vagus nerve—a key component of the gut–brain connection that regulates the parasympathetic nervous system. Decreased vagal tone, a reflection of the activity of the vagus nerve, can impair the ability of the body to recover from stress, maintain calmness, and support gastrointestinal and cardiovascular health. This disruption has the potential to impair gut function, leading to dysbiosis, and further exacerbating the dysfunction of the gut–brain axis, thus creating a feedback loop of physiological and psychological consequences of stress [113,114].

Finally, we have already highlighted that symptoms of PTSD, such as intrusive thoughts and hypervigilance, are common in PACS subjects. The symptomatology seems, for the most part, to be linked to the trauma of serious illness, hospitalization, the loss of a family member due to COVID-19, or even the fear of contracting the disease. The feedback loops persist in this domain as well, as the residual effects of PTSD, coupled with increased anxiety, seem to lead to sleep disturbances. About 26% of the PACS cases presented with prolonged sleep symptoms, including nightmares, which mapped the intensity of psychological stress onto nightly rest. Oneiric activity is consistent with the studies that have described patterns of dreams during the pandemic, suggesting continuity between wakeful and sleep mental activity [115–117].

6. Future Directions

At this point, we want to emphasize that the purpose of this study is not to underestimate the role of specific neurophysiological aspects in the course of PACS, as these are undeniably critical. Instead, the aim is to highlight the role of psychological and psychosocial factors—both in how they influence and are influenced by the disorder. For example, linking stress to worse outcomes in certain autoimmune conditions, such as rheumatoid arthritis, does not imply that the disease itself is psychogenic. In the same vein, acknowledging the influence of psychological elements such as anxiety or depression on PACS outcomes does not lessen the syndrome's neurobiological reality but could add a new dimension to it that the healthcare community could utilize therapeutically.

6.1. The Role of Neuropsychological Assessments and Standardized Protocols

Throughout this review, it has become clear that the direct effects of the virus on the brain are, sometimes, very difficult to distinguish from the psychological and emotional repercussions of PACS. Neuropsychological assessments could play an essential role in navigating this complexity. While these evaluations cannot independently identify the underlying neuropathology of PACS, when combined with clinical expertise, they can contribute to a more comprehensive understanding of the condition. This combination could then allow clinicians to manage the neurological symptoms more effectively by also addressing the psychological and emotional toll of the disease.

Along these lines, a standardized approach to assessing the psychological aspects of PACS is also crucial. Utilizing a core set of neuropsychological and psychological instruments could improve the understanding of the relationship between psychological, biomedical, and social factors in the disease. Such tests could reveal the modifiable psychological processes, such as stress, cognitive distortions, and mood disorders, which are important targets for treatment strategies. Addressing these facets can enable healthcare providers to enhance the effectiveness of treatment and quality of life for the patients.

6.2. Psychological Interventions

The recent literature has determined the efficacy of psychological interventions, especially Cognitive Behavioral Therapy (CBT), to help patients with PACS manage some of their symptoms. One CBT protocol, modified for inpatient use, has shown promise in addressing psychological distress and persistent somatic symptoms associated with PACS. Those models commonly include structured group-therapy sessions focusing on cognitive restructuring, stress management, and illness-related coping strategies that are engaging psychophysiological mechanisms underlying somatic distress, with secondary attention to anxiety and depression, common comorbidities of PACS [118,119].

Expanding beyond traditional CBT approaches, interventions incorporating complementary techniques have shown promise in managing PACS-related psychological challenges. For example, combining CBT with mindfulness-based therapies, relaxation training, or eye movement desensitization and reprocessing has yielded additional advantages, especially in reducing emotional as well as somatic complaints. Dialectical behavioral therapy, focused on enhancing the regulation of emotions, has also proved to be useful for patients with PACS [120].

Another intervention that has shown positive results in the management of PACS is acceptance and commitment therapy, which focuses on enhancing psychological flexibility and acceptance. The studies have indicated that this kind of treatment may thus contribute to improving resilience and health-related quality of life in PACS patients, with the effects remaining up to several months after the treatment [121]. These findings, among others, show us the necessity of adaptive coping strategies when dealing with the complex psychological difficulties arising in patients with PACS.

Interpersonal and relational therapies, like interpersonal therapy and emotion-focused approaches, further provide frameworks for addressing the relational and emotional aspects of psychological suffering. These include relaxational interventions such as mindfulness and breathing to reduce anxiety and improve emotional resilience. Psychoeducation along with social support, meditation practices, therapies ranging from music therapy to narrative exposure therapy, and positive psychology interventions represent newer forms of therapy that have also been utilized in intervention strategies [122–124].

While these interventions have improved several symptoms in patients, more randomized controlled trials are much needed to establish the effectiveness of these treatments and for the optimization of their application in all aspects of diverse PACS.

6.3. Multidisciplinary and Patient-Centered Approaches

As we already mentioned, a portion of the current literature emphasizes the critical need for accessible, patient-centered, multidisciplinary healthcare provision. From healthcare professionals to family members and friends, ensuring that people with PACS are listened to and their experiences validated is paramount. Addressing the psychosocial aspects, which, as we saw, play a significant role in the prevalence of symptomatology, those responsible for healthcare policy and delivery should prioritize supporting individuals with PACS in adapting their work, social, and physical activities to align with their health capabilities. Helping them maintain or redefine their social functions and identities could be enormously beneficial as part of tailored occupational health programs. Finally, the impact of PACS on participation in social activities emphasizes the potentially huge value that tailored community groups and social prescribing hold, provided the programs are underpinned by ongoing research and evaluation to confirm their appropriateness and effectiveness.

6.4. The Role of AI in PACS Management

In light of the complexities involved in treating PACS, we already explored how a multidisciplinary approach is essential. Psychological support should be integrated into a comprehensive care model that also includes neurological treatments and cognitive rehabilitation. Integration of therapies such as CBT, together with cognitive rehabilitation and acceptance and commitment therapy, might provide comprehensive care that will address the psychological and cognitive impairments attributed to PACS. Symptom-matched and severity-matched interventions within a symptom management therapeutic model may enhance this care further in those patients whose symptoms remained in the mild category but were persistent enough to impact quality of life. Since we are living in the age of AI, its potential could provide valuable opportunities to enhance the management of PACS and its complexities. By integrating diverse data sources—such as electronic health records (EHRs), imaging, wearable sensors, and patient-reported outcomes—AI might support the development of more precise monitoring and intervention systems. Additionally, AI could contribute to more personalized care by leveraging data-driven insights to guide interventions tailored to each patient's unique needs.

7. Discussion

The main goal of this review study was to explore the role of psychological, psychosocial, and neurobiological factors in the symptomatology of PACS. We have attempted to review the most recent neuropathological findings that lie behind the neurological and neuropsychiatric symptoms associated with PACS, in the context of how these might be modulated by psychological and psychosocial factors, which could in turn affect the severity and persistence of symptoms. By pointing out such complex interactions, we aim to contribute to the debate about how the development of an integrated treatment focused on neurobiological and psychological dimensions of PACS can be furthered.

Our findings suggest that psychological factors, such as stress, anxiety, and depression, along with psychosocial challenges arising from the aftereffects of quarantine measures, the isolation and loneliness experienced during the pandemic, and the pervasive fear and uncertainty surrounding health and recovery, are common among individuals with PACS. These factors appear to interact with the somatic manifestations of PACS in a way that creates a self-reinforcing cycle, where physical symptoms exacerbate psychological distress, which in turn worsens the physical symptoms. While this cycle is challenging to address, even small-scale interventions regarding psychological distress—such as CBT or supportive therapies—could help interrupt this loop. The partial interruption of this cycle could provide considerable relief and improvement in mental and physical health outcomes among affected individuals.

These findings seem to be compatible with a portion of the existing literature supporting the role of psychological distress in the exacerbation of symptoms of chronic diseases, especially those with a neurological component, including autoimmune diseases. However, the present study points out the need for a broader perspective. While much emphasis has been placed on the neurobiological aspects of PACS, we believe that psychological and psychosocial elements should be incorporated into treatment interventions in an attempt to possibly enhance holistic care. While further research is required to ascertain the effectiveness of these combined approaches, the evidence points to a promising direction for the development of PACS treatment.

In this context, we indicate the requirement for a multidisciplinary approach to PACS, in which psychological treatment strategies are considered along with neurobiological ones. Further research should focus on psychological interventions that reduce stress and anxiety in order to understand their potential in mitigating the exacerbation of symptoms. Longitudinal studies will further help in specifying the long-term effects of the interventions on neurological as well as psychological symptoms. Furthermore, it would be of value to identify how health care systems can support the development of models of care that address both the psychological and physical dimensions of PACS. Finally, newer technologies, such as artificial intelligence, could help in the identification of patterns and also support tailored intervention strategies.

Although this study may provide valuable insights, there are several limitations that must be stated. As in all research endeavors, there is always the possibility that some aspects of the literature may have been overlooked or that methodological flaws could create certain biased outcomes. Nevertheless, we believe this study represents a significant advance in understanding the complexities of PACS and indicating future research avenues. First of all, as previously mentioned, we spotted variability and sometimes conflicting results across different studies regarding the underlying causes of PACS and the effectiveness of various interventions. These inconsistencies may reflect differences in study design, population characteristics, or the evolving understanding of the condition. Second, the short duration since PACS has been identified as a distinct condition contributes to the difficulties in identifying absolute causal pathways or associations; much of the existing research is based on cross-sectional or early longitudinal data that may not fully capture the extended course of PACS or provide a comprehensive view of its long-term outcomes. Furthermore, the feedback loop created by psychosocial and pathophysiological elements, as has been elucidated in this paper, makes it sometimes difficult to have clear and conclusive endpoints. With that in mind, in this paper, it is acknowledged that our understanding of PACS is still evolving. However, the aim of our work is not to draw final conclusions but to add to the accumulation of knowledge about PACS and to discuss actionable strategies for harm reduction and improvements in patient outcomes. Further research must be defined into the diagnostic criteria, causal mechanisms, and optimal management strategies as more evidence comes in.

8. Conclusions

PACS is a complex disease with important health implications for patients and the medical infrastructure. Our review describes the complex combination of neurological, neuropsychological, and psychosocial influences on the longevity and complexity of PACS symptoms. It is clear that psychological stress, anxiety, and depression—as well as psychosocial difficulties like loneliness and uncertainty—can meld with neurobiological symptoms in a feedback loop to add an extra burden to both the physical and psychological suffering. While the understanding of PACS is still evolving, we want to highlight the importance of integrated, multidisciplinary approaches that address both biological and psychological dimensions. Among the promising areas for intervention are psychological interventions and holistic treatments, that attempt to break the cycle of symptom persistence. Although challenges remain, including variability and contradictions in research findings and the limitations of short-term data, in this work, the aim was to improve our knowledge of PACS and its management. Future research should prioritize longitudinal studies, refined diagnostic criteria, and innovative therapeutic strategies, contributing to a more comprehensive approach to PACS care and improving patient outcomes.

Author Contributions: Conceptualization, A.M. and R.S.S.; validation, R.S.S.; formal analysis, A.M. and R.S.S.; investigation, A.M. and R.S.S.; data curation, A.M. and R.S.S.; writing—original draft preparation, A.M.; writing—review and editing, A.M., J.M., R.A. and R.S.S.; visualization, A.M.; supervision, R.S.S. All authors have read and agreed to the published version of the manuscript.

Funding: The authors received no financial support for this article's research, authorship, and/or publication.

Conflicts of Interest: The authors declare no conflicts of interest.

References

1. Chen, X.; Laurent, S.; Onur, O.A.; Kleineberg, N.N.; Fink, G.R.; Schweitzer, F.; Warnke, C. A systematic review of neurological symptoms and complications of COVID-19. *J. Neurol.* **2020**, *268*, 392–402. [CrossRef] [PubMed]
2. Ezpeleta, D.; García-Azorín, D. Post–COVID-19 neurological symptoms. *Neurol. Perspect.* **2021**, *1*, S1–S3. [CrossRef] [PubMed]

3. Al-Aly, Z.; Davis, H.; McCorkell, L.; Soares, L.; Wulf-Hanson, S.; Iwasaki, A.; Topol, E.J. Long COVID science, research and policy. *Nat. Med.* **2024**, *30*, 2148–2164. [CrossRef] [PubMed]
4. Davis, H.E.; McCorkell, L.; Vogel, J.M.; Topol, E.J. Author Correction: Long COVID: Major findings, mechanisms and recommendations. *Nat. Rev. Microbiol.* **2023**, *21*, 408. [CrossRef]
5. Xu, E.; Xie, Y.; Al-Aly, Z. Long-term neurologic outcomes of COVID-19. *Nat. Med.* **2022**, *28*, 2406–2415. [CrossRef] [PubMed]
6. Astin, R.; Banerjee, A.; Baker, M.R.; Dani, M.; Ford, E.; Hull, J.H.; Lim, P.B.; McNarry, M.; Morten, K.; O'Sullivan, O.; et al. Long COVID: Mechanisms, risk factors and recovery. *Exp. Physiol.* **2022**, *108*, 12–27. [CrossRef] [PubMed]
7. Van Kessel, S.A.M.; Hartman, T.C.O.; Lucassen, P.L.B.J.; Van Jaarsveld, C.H.M. Post-acute and long-COVID-19 symptoms in patients with mild diseases: A systematic review. *Fam. Pract.* **2021**, *39*, 159–167. [CrossRef] [PubMed]
8. Lopez-Leon, S.; Wegman-Ostrosky, T.; Perelman, C.; Sepulveda, R.; Rebolledo, P.A.; Cuapio, A.; Villapol, S. More than 50 long-term effects of COVID-19: A systematic review and meta-analysis. *Sci. Rep.* **2021**, *11*, 16144. [CrossRef] [PubMed]
9. Woodrow, M.; Carey, C.; Ziauddeen, N.; Thomas, R.; Akrami, A.; Lutje, V.; Greenwood, D.C.; Alwan, N.A. Systematic Review of the Prevalence of Long COVID. *Open Forum Infect. Dis.* **2023**, *10*, ofad233. [CrossRef] [PubMed]
10. Erlandson, K.M.; Geng, L.N.; Selvaggi, C.A.; Thaweethai, T.; Chen, P.; Erdmann, N.B.; Goldman, J.D.; Henrich, T.J.; Hornig, M.; Karlson, E.W.; et al. Differentiation of Prior SARS-CoV-2 Infection and Postacute Sequelae by Standard Clinical Laboratory Measurements in the RECOVER Cohort. *Ann. Intern. Med.* **2024**, *177*, 1209–1221. [CrossRef]
11. Page, M.J.; Moher, D.; Bossuyt, P.M.; Boutron, I.; Hoffmann, T.C.; Mulrow, C.D.; Shamseer, L.; Tetzlaff, J.M.; Akl, E.A.; Brennan, S.E.; et al. PRISMA 2020 explanation and elaboration: Updated guidance and exemplars for reporting systematic reviews. *BMJ* **2021**, *372*, n160. [CrossRef] [PubMed]
12. Teodoro, T.; Chen, J.; Gelauff, J.; Edwards, M.J. Functional neurological disorder in people with long COVID: A systematic review. *Eur. J. Neurol.* **2023**, *30*, 1505–1514. [CrossRef]
13. Vélez-Santamaría, R.; Fernández-Solana, J.; Méndez-López, F.; Domínguez-García, M.; González-Bernal, J.J.; Magallón-Botaya, R.; Oliván-Blázquez, B.; González-Santos, J.; Santamaría-Peláez, M. Functionality, physical activity, fatigue and quality of life in patients with acute COVID-19 and Long COVID infection. *Sci. Rep.* **2023**, *13*, 19907. [CrossRef]
14. Thomas, B.; Pattinson, R.; Edwards, D.; Dale, C.; Jenkins, B.; Lande, H.; Bundy, C.; Davies, J.L. Definitions and measures of long COVID fatigue in adults: A scoping review protocol. *JBI Evid. Synth.* **2023**, *22*, 481–488. [CrossRef] [PubMed]
15. Tedjasukmana, R.; Budikayanti, A.; Islamiyah, W.R.; Witjaksono, A.M.A.L.; Hakim, M. Sleep disturbance in post COVID-19 conditions: Prevalence and quality of life. *Front. Neurol.* **2023**, *13*, 1095606. [CrossRef]
16. Tan'ski, W.; Tomasiewicz, A.; Jankowska-Polańska, B. Sleep Disturbances as a Consequence of Long COVID-19: Insights from Actigraphy and Clinimetric Examinations—An Uncontrolled Prospective Observational Pilot Study. *J. Clin. Med.* **2024**, *13*, 839. [CrossRef] [PubMed]
17. Rodrigues, A.N.; Dias, A.R.N.; Paranhos, A.C.M.; Silva, C.C.; Da Rocha Bastos, T.; De Brito, B.B.; Da Silva, N.M.; De Jesus Soares De Sousa, E.; Quaresma, J.A.S.; Falcão, L.F.M. Headache in long COVID as disabling condition: A clinical approach. *Front. Neurol.* **2023**, *14*, 1149294. [CrossRef] [PubMed]
18. Rueb, M.; Ruzicka, M.; Fonseca, G.J.I.; Valdinoci, E.; Benesch, C.; Pernpruner, A.; Von Baum, M.; Remi, J.; Jebrini, T.; Schöberl, F.; et al. Headache severity in patients with post COVID-19 condition: A case-control study. *Eur. Arch. Psychiatry Clin. Neurosci.* **2024**, *274*, 1935–1943. [CrossRef]
19. Seeley, M.-C.; Gallagher, C.; Ong, E.; Langdon, A.; Chieng, J.; Bailey, D.; Page, A.; Lim, H.S.; Lau, D.H. High Incidence of Autonomic Dysfunction and Postural Orthostatic Tachycardia Syndrome in Patients with Long COVID: Implications for Management and Health Care Planning. *Am. J. Med.* **2023**. [CrossRef]
20. Cantrell, C.; Reid, C.; Walker, C.S.; Tidd, S.J.S.; Zhang, R.; Wilson, R. Post-COVID postural orthostatic tachycardia syndrome (POTS): A new phenomenon. *Front. Neurol.* **2024**, *15*, 1297964. [CrossRef]
21. Wong, T.L.; Weitzer, D.J. Long COVID and Myalgic Encephalomyelitis/Chronic Fatigue Syndrome (ME/CFS)—A Systemic Review and Comparison of Clinical Presentation and Symptomatology. *Medicina* **2021**, *57*, 418. [CrossRef] [PubMed]
22. Riggott, C.; Ford, A.C.; Gracie, D.J. Review article: The role of the gut–brain axis in inflammatory bowel disease and its therapeutic implications. *Aliment. Pharmacol. Ther.* **2024**, *60*, 1200–1214. [CrossRef] [PubMed]
23. Zamani, M.; Ebrahimtabar, F.; Alizadeh-Tabari, S.; Kasner, S.E.; Elkind, M.S.V.; Ananthakrishnan, A.N.; Choden, T.; Rubin, D.T.; Malekzadeh, R. Risk of Common Neurological Disorders in Adult Patients with Inflammatory Bowel Disease: A Systematic Review and Meta-analysis. *Inflamm. Bowel Dis.* **2024**, *30*, 2195–2204. [CrossRef] [PubMed]
24. Goudman, L.; Demuyser, T.; Pilitsis, J.G.; Billot, M.; Roulaud, M.; Rigoard, P.; Moens, M. Gut dysbiosis in patients with chronic pain: A systematic review and meta-analysis. *Front. Immunol.* **2024**, *15*, 1342833. [CrossRef] [PubMed]
25. ZhZhang, D.; Zhou, Y.; Ma, Y.; Chen, P.; Tang, J.; Yang, B.; Li, H.; Liang, M.; Xue, Y.; Liu, Y.; et al. Gut Microbiota Dysbiosis Correlates With Long COVID-19 at One-Year After Discharge. *J. Korean Med. Sci.* **2023**, *38*, e120. [CrossRef]
26. Liu, Q.; Mak, J.W.Y.; Su, Q.; Yeoh, Y.K.; Lui, G.C.-Y.; Ng, S.S.S.; Zhang, F.; Li, A.Y.L.; Lu, W.; Hui, D.S.-C.; et al. Gut microbiota dynamics in a prospective cohort of patients with post-acute COVID-19 syndrome. *Gut* **2022**, *71*, 544–552. [CrossRef]
27. Vakili, K.; Fathi, M.; Yaghoobpoor, S.; Sayehmiri, F.; Nazerian, Y.; Nazerian, A.; Mohamadkhani, A.; Khodabakhsh, P.; Réus, G.Z.; Hajibeygi, R.; et al. The contribution of gut-brain axis to development of neurological symptoms in COVID-19 recovered patients: A hypothesis and review of literature. *Front. Cell. Infect. Microbiol.* **2022**, *12*, 983089. [CrossRef]

28. Choudhury, A.; Tariq, R.; Jena, A.; Vesely, E.K.; Singh, S.; Khanna, S.; Sharma, V. Gastrointestinal manifestations of long COVID: A systematic review and meta-analysis. *Ther. Adv. Gastroenterol.* **2022**, *15*, 175628482211184. [CrossRef]
29. Tavares-Júnior, J.W.L.; De Souza, A.C.C.; Borges, J.W.P.; Oliveira, D.N.; Siqueira-Neto, J.I.; Sobreira-Neto, M.A.; Braga-Neto, P. COVID-19 associated cognitive impairment: A systematic review. *Cortex* **2022**, *152*, 77–97. [CrossRef]
30. Megari, K.; Thomaidou, E.; Chatzidimitriou, E. Highlighting the Neuropsychological Consequences of COVID-19: Evidence From a Narrative Review. *INQUIRY J. Health Care Organ. Provis. Financ.* **2024**, *61*. [CrossRef] [PubMed]
31. Shariff, S.; Uwishema, O.; Mizero, J.; Thambi, V.D.; Nazir, A.; Mahmoud, A.; Kaushik, I.; Khayat, S.; Maigoro, A.Y.; Awde, S.; et al. Long-term cognitive dysfunction after the COVID-19 pandemic: A narrative review. *Ann. Med. Surg.* **2023**, *85*, 5504–5510. [CrossRef] [PubMed]
32. Delgado-Alonso, C.; Díez-Cirarda, M.; Pagán, J.; Pérez-Izquierdo, C.; Oliver-Mas, S.; Fernández-Romero, L.; Martínez-Petit, Á.; Valles-Salgado, M.; Gil-Moreno, M.J.; Yus, M.; et al. Unraveling brain fog in post-COVID syndrome: Relationship between subjective cognitive complaints and cognitive function, fatigue, and neuropsychiatric symptoms. *Eur. J. Neurol.* **2023**, *32*, e16084. [CrossRef] [PubMed]
33. Daroische, R.; Hemminghyth, M.S.; Eilertsen, T.H.; Breitve, M.H.; Chwiszczuk, L.J. Cognitive Impairment After COVID-19—A Review on Objective Test Data. *Front. Neurol.* **2021**, *12*, 699582. [CrossRef]
34. Baseler, H.A.; Aksoy, M.; Salawu, A.; Green, A.; Asghar, A.U.R. The negative impact of COVID-19 on working memory revealed using a rapid online quiz. *PLoS ONE* **2022**, *17*, e0269353. [CrossRef]
35. Cui, R.; Gao, B.; Ge, R.; Li, M.; Li, M.; Lu, X.; Jiang, S. The effects of COVID-19 infection on working memory: A systematic review. *Curr. Med. Res. Opin.* **2023**, *40*, 217–227. [CrossRef] [PubMed]
36. Llana, T.; Zorzo, C.; Mendez-Lopez, M.; Mendez, M. Memory alterations after COVID-19 infection: A systematic review. *Appl. Neuropsychol. Adult* **2022**, *31*, 292–305. [CrossRef] [PubMed]
37. Prabhakaran, D.; Day, G.S.; Munipalli, B.; Rush, B.K.; Pudalov, L.; Niazi, S.K.; Brennan, E.; Powers, H.R.; Durvasula, R.; Athreya, A.; et al. Neurophenotypes of COVID-19: Risk factors and recovery outcomes. *Res. Sq.* **2023**, *30*, 100648. [CrossRef]
38. Kozik, V.; Reuken, P.; Utech, I.; Gramlich, J.; Stallmach, Z.; Demeyere, N.; Rakers, F.; Schwab, M.; Stallmach, A.; Finke, K. Characterization of neurocognitive deficits in patients with post-COVID-19 syndrome: Persistence, patients' complaints, and clinical predictors. *Front. Psychol.* **2023**, *14*, 1233144. [CrossRef]
39. Cummings, L. Long COVID: The impact on language and cognition. *Lang. Health* **2023**, *1*, 2–9. [CrossRef]
40. McWhirter, L.; Smyth, H.; Hoeritzauer, I.; Couturier, A.; Stone, J.; Carson, A.J. What is brain fog? *J. Neurol. Neurosurg. Psychiatry* **2022**, *94*, 321–325. [CrossRef]
41. Bulla, R.; Rossi, L.; Furlanis, G.; Agostinis, C.; Toffoli, M.; Balduit, A.; Mangogna, A.; Liccari, M.; Morosini, G.; Kishore, U.; et al. A likely association between low mannan-binding lectin level and brain fog onset in long COVID patients. *Front. Immunol.* **2023**, *14*, 1191083. [CrossRef] [PubMed]
42. Jennings, G.; Monaghan, A.; Xue, F.; Duggan, E.; Romero-Ortuño, R. Comprehensive Clinical Characterisation of Brain Fog in Adults Reporting Long COVID Symptoms. *J. Clin. Med.* **2022**, *11*, 3440. [CrossRef]
43. Sampogna, G.; Di Vincenzo, M.; Giallonardo, V.; Perris, F.; Volpicelli, A.; Del Vecchio, V.; Luciano, M.; Fiorillo, A. The Psychiatric Consequences of Long-COVID: A Scoping Review. *J. Pers. Med.* **2022**, *12*, 1767. [CrossRef] [PubMed]
44. Zakia, H.; Pradana, K.; Iskandar, S. Risk factors for psychiatric symptoms in patients with long COVID: A systematic review. *PLoS ONE* **2023**, *18*, e0284075. [CrossRef] [PubMed]
45. Huang, L.; Xu, X.; Zhang, L.; Zheng, D.; Liu, Y.; Feng, B.; Hu, J.; Lin, Q.; Xi, X.; Wang, Q.; et al. Post-traumatic Stress Disorder Symptoms and Quality of Life of COVID-19 Survivors at 6-Month Follow-Up: A Cross-Sectional Observational Study. *Front. Psychiatry* **2022**, *12*, 782478. [CrossRef] [PubMed]
46. Houben-Wilke, S.; Goërtz, Y.M.; Delbressine, J.M.; Vaes, A.W.; Meys, R.; Machado, F.V.; van Herck, M.; Burtin, C.; Posthuma, R.; Franssen, F.M.; et al. The Impact of Long COVID-19 on Mental Health: Observational 6-Month Follow-Up Study. *JMIR Ment. Health* **2022**, *9*, e33704. [CrossRef]
47. Vo, H.T.; Dao, T.D.; Van Duong, T.; Nguyen, T.T.; Do, B.N.; Do, T.X.; Pham, K.M.; Vu, V.H.; Van Pham, L.; Nguyen, L.T.H.; et al. Impact of long COVID-19 on posttraumatic stress disorder as modified by health literacy: An observational study in Vietnam. *Osong Public Health Res. Perspect.* **2024**, *15*, 33–44. [CrossRef]
48. Thye, A.Y.-K.; Law, J.W.-F.; Tan, L.T.-H.; Pusparajah, P.; Ser, H.-L.; Thurairajasingam, S.; Letchumanan, V.; Lee, L.-H. Psychological Symptoms in COVID-19 Patients: In-sights into Pathophysiology and Risk Factors of Long COVID-19. *Biology* **2022**, *11*, 61. [CrossRef]
49. Mekhael, M.; Lim, C.H.; El Hajjar, A.H.; Noujaim, C.; Pottle, C.; Makan, N.; Dagher, L.; Zhang, Y.; Chouman, N.; Li, D.L.; et al. Studying the Effect of Long COVID-19 Infection on Sleep Quality Using Wearable Health Devices: Observational Study. *J. Med. Internet Res.* **2022**, *24*, e38000. [CrossRef]
50. Sunada, N.; Nakano, Y.; Otsuka, Y.; Tokumasu, K.; Honda, H.; Sakurada, Y.; Matsuda, Y.; Hasegawa, T.; Omura, D.; Ochi, K.; et al. Characteristics of Sleep Disturbance in Patients with Long COVID: A Retrospective Observational Study in Japan. *J. Clin. Med.* **2022**, *11*, 7332. [CrossRef]
51. Titze-De-Almeida, R.; Lacerda, P.H.A.; de Oliveira, E.P.; de Oliveira, M.E.F.; Vianna, Y.S.S.; Costa, A.M.; dos Santos, E.P.; Guérard, L.M.C.; Ferreira, M.A.d.M.; dos Santos, I.C.R.; et al. Sleep and memory complaints in long COVID: An insight into clustered psychological phenotypes. *PeerJ* **2024**, *12*, e16669. [CrossRef] [PubMed]

52. Lee, E.K.; Auger, R.R. Sleep and Long COVID—A Review and Exploration of Sleep Disturbances in Post Acute Sequelae of SARS-CoV-2 (PASC) and Therapeutic Possibilities. *Curr. Sleep Med. Rep.* **2024**, *10*, 169–180. [CrossRef]
53. Schilling, C.; Nieters, A.; Schredl, M.; Peter, R.S.; Rothenbacher, D.; Brockmann, S.O.; Göpel, S.; Kindle, G.; Merle, U.; Steinacker, J.M.; et al. Pre-existing sleep problems as a predictor of post-acute sequelae of COVID-19. *J. Sleep Res.* **2023**, *33*, e13949. [CrossRef] [PubMed]
54. Smith, C.M.; Gilbert, E.B.; Riordan, P.A.; Helmke, N.; Von Isenburg, M.; Kincaid, B.R.; Shirey, K.G. COVID-19-associated psychosis: A systematic review of case reports. *Gen. Hosp. Psychiatry* **2021**, *73*, 84–100. [CrossRef] [PubMed]
55. Costa, P.; Pinto, I.; Branco, P. COVID-19 induced psychosis. Should we be concerned? *Eur. Psychiatry* **2022**, *65* (Suppl. S1), S201–S202. [CrossRef]
56. Păunescu, R.L.; Micluţia, I.V.; Verișezan, O.R.; Crecan-Suciu, B.D. Acute and long-term psychiatric symptoms associated with COVID-19 (Review). *Biomed. Rep.* **2022**, *18*, 4. [CrossRef] [PubMed]
57. Ferrando, S.J.; Klepacz, L.; Lynch, S.; Tavakkoli, M.; Dornbush, R.; Baharani, R.; Smolin, Y.; Bartell, A. COVID-19 Psychosis: A Potential New Neuropsychiatric Condition Triggered by Novel Coronavirus Infection and the Inflammatory Response? *Psychosomatics* **2020**, *61*, 551–555. [CrossRef] [PubMed]
58. Gusev, E.; Sarapultsev, A. Exploring the Pathophysiology of Long COVID: The Central Role of Low-Grade Inflammation and Multisystem Involvement. *Int. J. Mol. Sci.* **2024**, *25*, 6389. [CrossRef] [PubMed]
59. Bayat, A.-H.; Azimi, H.; Moghaddam, M.H.; Ebrahimi, V.; Fathi, M.; Vakili, K.; Mahmoudiasl, G.-R.; Forouzesh, M.; Boroujeni, M.E.; Nariman, Z.; et al. COVID-19 causes neuronal degeneration and reduces neurogenesis in human hippocampus. *APOPTOSIS* **2022**, *27*, 852–868. [CrossRef] [PubMed]
60. Aziz, M.; Fatima, R.; Assaly, R. Elevated interleukin-6 and severe COVID-19: A meta-analysis. *J. Med. Virol.* **2020**, *92*, 2283–2285. [CrossRef]
61. Zhu, J.; Pang, J.; Ji, P.; Zhong, Z.; Li, H.; Li, B.; Zhang, J. Elevated interleukin-6 is associated with severity of COVID-19: A meta-analysis. *J. Med. Virol.* **2020**, *93*, 35–37. [CrossRef]
62. Kumar, S.; Veldhuis, A.; Malhotra, T. Neuropsychiatric and Cognitive Sequelae of COVID-19. *Front. Psychol.* **2021**, *12*, 577529. [CrossRef]
63. Mazza, M.G.; Palladini, M.; De Lorenzo, R.; Magnaghi, C.; Poletti, S.; Furlan, R.; Ciceri, F.; Rovere-Querini, P.; Benedetti, F. Persistent psychopathology and neurocognitive impairment in COVID-19 survivors: Effect of inflammatory biomarkers at three-month follow-up. *Brain Behav. Immun.* **2021**, *94*, 138–147. [CrossRef] [PubMed]
64. Saikarthik, J.; Saraswathi, I.; Alarifi, A.; Al-Atram, A.A.; Mickeymaray, S.; Paramasivam, A.; Shaikh, S.; Jeraud, M.; Alothaim, A.S. Role of neuroinflammation mediated potential alterations in adult neurogenesis as a factor for neuropsychiatric symptoms in Post-Acute COVID-19 syndrome—A narrative review. *PeerJ* **2022**, *10*, e14227. [CrossRef] [PubMed]
65. VanElzakker, M.B.; Bues, H.F.; Brusaferri, L.; Kim, M.; Saadi, D.; Ratai, E.-M.; Dougherty, D.D.; Loggia, M.L. Neuroinflammation in post-acute sequelae of COVID-19 (PASC) as assessed by [11C]PBR28 PET correlates with vascular disease measures. *Brain Behav. Immun.* **2024**, *119*, 713–723. [CrossRef]
66. Colizzi, M.; Peghin, M.; De Martino, M.; Bontempo, G.; Gerussi, V.; Palese, A.; Isola, M.; Tascini, C.; Balestrieri, M. Mental health symptoms one year after acute COVID-19 infection: Prevalence and risk factors. *Rev. Psiquiatr. Y Salud Ment.* **2022**, *16*, 38–46. [CrossRef] [PubMed]
67. Manca, R.; De Marco, M.; Ince, P.G.; Venneri, A. Heterogeneity in Regional Damage Detected by Neuroimaging and Neuropathological Studies in Older Adults With COVID-19: A Cognitive-Neuroscience Systematic Review to Inform the Long-Term Impact of the Virus on Neurocognitive Trajectories. *Front. Aging Neurosci.* **2021**, *13*, 646908. [CrossRef] [PubMed]
68. Orrù, G.; Conversano, C.; Malloggi, E.; Francesconi, F.; Ciacchini, R.; Gemignani, A. Neurological Complications of COVID-19 and Possible Neuroinvasion Pathways: A Systematic Review. *Int. J. Environ. Res. Public Health* **2020**, *17*, 6688. [CrossRef]
69. Hugon, J.; Queneau, M.; Ortiz, M.S.; Msika, E.F.; Farid, K.; Paquet, C. Cognitive decline and brainstem hypometabolism in long COVID: A case series. *Brain Behav.* **2022**, *12*, e2513. [CrossRef]
70. Shan, D.; Li, S.; Xu, R.; Nie, G.; Xie, Y.; Han, J.; Gao, X.; Zheng, Y.; Xu, Z.; Dai, Z. Post-COVID-19 human memory impairment: A PRISMA-based systematic review of evidence from brain imaging studies. *Front. Aging Neurosci.* **2022**, *14*, 1077384. [CrossRef] [PubMed]
71. Meyer, P.T.; Hellwig, S.; Blazhenets, G.; Hosp, J.A. Molecular Imaging Findings on Acute and Long-Term Effects of COVID-19 on the Brain: A Systematic review. *J. Nucl. Med.* **2022**, *63*, 971–980. [CrossRef]
72. Guedj, E.; Campion, J.Y.; Dudouet, P.; Kaphan, E.; Bregeon, F.; Tissot-Dupont, H.; Guis, S.; Barthelemy, F.; Habert, P.; Ceccaldi, M.; et al. 18F-FDG brain PET hypometabolism in patients with long COVID. *Eur. J. Nucl. Med. Mol. Imaging* **2021**, *48*, 2823–2833. [CrossRef] [PubMed]
73. Cull, O.; Qadi, L.A.; Stadler, J.; Martin, M.; Helou, A.E.; Wagner, J.; Maillet, D.; Chamard-Witkowski, L. Radiological markers of neurological manifestations of post-acute sequelae of SARS-CoV-2 infection: A mini-review. *Front. Neurol.* **2023**, *14*, 1233079. [CrossRef] [PubMed]
74. Theofilis, P.; Oikonomou, E.; Vasileiadou, M.; Tousoulis, D. A Narrative Review on Prolonged Neuropsychiatric Consequences of COVID-19: A Serious Concern. *Heart Mind* **2024**, *8*, 177–183. [CrossRef]
75. Cecchetti, G.; Agosta, F.; Canu, E.; Basaia, S.; Barbieri, A.; Cardamone, R.; Bernasconi, M.P.; Castelnovo, V.; Cividini, C.; Cursi, M.; et al. Cognitive, EEG, and MRI features of COVID-19 survivors: A 10-month study. *J. Neurol.* **2022**, *269*, 3400–3412. [CrossRef]

76. Douaud, G.; Lee, S.; Alfaro-Almagro, F.; Arthofer, C.; Wang, C.; McCarthy, P.; Lange, F.; Andersson, J.L.R.; Griffanti, L.; Duff, E.; et al. SARS-CoV-2 is associated with changes in brain structure in UK Biobank. *Nature* **2022**, *604*, 697–707. [CrossRef] [PubMed]
77. Plummer, A.M.; Matos, Y.L.; Lin, H.C.; Ryman, S.G.; Birg, A.; Quinn, D.K.; Parada, A.N.; Vakhtin, A.A. Gut-brain pathogenesis of post-acute COVID-19 neurocognitive symptoms. *Front. Neurosci.* **2023**, *17*, 1232480. [CrossRef]
78. Tizenberg, B.N.; Brenner, L.A.; Lowry, C.A.; Okusaga, O.O.; Benavides, D.R.; Hoisington, A.J.; Benros, M.E.; Stiller, J.W.; Kessler, R.C.; Postolache, T.T. Biological and Psychological Factors Determining Neuropsychiatric Outcomes in COVID-19. *Curr. Psychiatry Rep.* **2021**, *23*, 68. [CrossRef] [PubMed]
79. Spinicci, M.; Graziani, L.; Tilli, M.; Nkurunziza, J.; Vellere, I.; Borchi, B.; Mencarini, J.; Campolmi, I.; Gori, L.; Giovannoni, L.; et al. Infection with SARS-CoV-2 Variants Is Associated with Different Long COVID Phenotypes. *Viruses* **2022**, *14*, 2367. [CrossRef]
80. Bai, F.; Santoro, A.; Hedberg, P.; Tavelli, A.; De Benedittis, S.; De Morais Caporali, J.F.; Marinho, C.C.; Leite, A.S.; Santoro, M.M.; Silberstein, F.C.; et al. The Omicron Variant Is Associated with a Reduced Risk of the Post COVID-19 Condition and Its Main Phenotypes Compared to the Wild-Type Virus: Results from the EuCARE-POSTCOVID-19 Study. *Viruses* **2024**, *16*, 1500. [CrossRef]
81. Canas, L.S.; Molteni, E.; Deng, J.; Sudre, C.H.; Murray, B.; Kerfoot, E.; Antonelli, M.; Rjoob, K.; Pujol, J.C.; Polidori, L.; et al. Profiling post-COVID-19 condition across different variants of SARS-CoV-2: A prospective longitudinal study in unvaccinated wild-type, unvaccinated alpha-variant, and vaccinated delta-variant populations. *Lancet Digit. Health* **2023**, *5*, e421–e434. [CrossRef]
82. Fernández-De-Las-Peñas, C.; Notarte, K.I.; Peligro, P.J.; Velasco, J.V.; Ocampo, M.J.; Henry, B.M.; Arendt-Nielsen, L.; Torres-Macho, J.; Plaza-Manzano, G. Long-COVID Symptoms in Individuals Infected with Different SARS-CoV-2 Variants of Concern: A Systematic Review of the Literature. *Viruses* **2022**, *14*, 2629. [CrossRef] [PubMed]
83. Sahin, A.; Karadag-Oncel, E.; Buyuksen, O.; Ekemen-Keles, Y.; Ustundag, G.; Elvan-Tuz, A.; Tasar, S.; Didinmez-Taskirdi, E.; Baykan, M.; Kara-Aksay, A.; et al. The diversity in the clinical features of children hospitalized with COVID-19 during the nonvariant, Alpha (B.1.1.7), Delta (B.1.617.2), and Omicron (B.1.1.529) variant periods of SARS CoV-2: Caution for neurological symptoms in Omicron variant. *J. Med. Virol.* **2023**, *95*, e28628. [CrossRef]
84. Gao, P.; Liu, J.; Liu, M. Effect of COVID-19 Vaccines on Reducing the Risk of Long COVID in the Real World: A Systematic Review and Meta-Analysis. *Int. J. Environ. Res. Public Health* **2022**, *19*, 12422. [CrossRef]
85. Maier, H.E.; Kowalski-Dobson, T.; Eckard, A.; Gherasim, C.; Manthei, D.; Meyers, A.; Davis, D.; Bakker, K.; Lindsey, K.; Chu, Z.; et al. Reduction in long-COVID symptoms and symptom severity in vaccinated compared to unvaccinated adults. *Open Forum Infect. Dis.* **2024**, *11*, ofae039. [CrossRef]
86. Ayoubkhani, D.; Bermingham, C.; Pouwels, K.B.; Glickman, M.; Nafilyan, V.; Zaccardi, F.; Khunti, K.; Alwan, N.A.; Walker, A.S. Trajectory of long covid symptoms after covid-19 vaccination: Community based cohort study. *BMJ* **2022**, *377*, e069676. [CrossRef]
87. Engelmann, P.; Reinke, M.; Stein, C.; Salzmann, S.; Löwe, B.; Toussaint, A.; Shedden-Mora, M. Psychological factors associated with Long COVID: A systematic review and meta-analysis. *EClinicalMedicine* **2024**, *74*, 102756. [CrossRef]
88. Engelmann, P.; Büchel, C.; Frommhold, J.; Klose, H.F.E.; Lohse, A.W.; Maehder, K.; Nestoriuc, Y.; Scherer, M.; Suling, A.; Toussaint, A.; et al. Psychological risk factors for Long COVID and their modification: Study protocol of a three-arm, randomised controlled trial (SOMA.COV). *BJPsych Open* **2023**, *9*, e207. [CrossRef] [PubMed]
89. Milde, C.; Glombiewski, J.A.; Wilhelm, M.; Schemer, L. Psychological Factors Predict Higher Odds and Impairment of Post-COVID Symptoms: A Prospective Study. *Psychosom. Med.* **2023**, *85*, 479–487. [CrossRef] [PubMed]
90. Bravo, R.G.; Infanti, A.; Billieux, J.; Ritzen, M.; Vögele, C.; Benoy, C. The psychological syndrome associated with Long-COVID: A study protocol. *Front. Epidemiol.* **2023**, *3*, 1193369. [CrossRef]
91. Engelmann, P.; Löwe, B.; Brehm, T.T.; Weigel, A.; Ullrich, F.; Addo, M.M.; Wiesch, J.S.Z.; Lohse, A.W.; Toussaint, A. Risk factors for worsening of somatic symptom burden in a prospective cohort during the COVID-19 pandemic. *Front. Psychol.* **2022**, *13*, 1022203. [CrossRef]
92. Hüsing, P.; Smakowski, A.; Löwe, B.; Kleinstäuber, M.; Toussaint, A.; Shedden-Mora, M.C. The framework for systematic reviews on psychological risk factors for persistent somatic symptoms and related syndromes and disorders (PSY-PSS). *Front. Psychiatry* **2023**, *14*, 1142484. [CrossRef] [PubMed]
93. Kube, T.; Rozenkrantz, L.; Rief, W.; Barsky, A. Understanding persistent physical symptoms: Conceptual integration of psychological expectation models and predictive processing accounts. *Clin. Psychol. Rev.* **2020**, *76*, 101829. [CrossRef] [PubMed]
94. Molero, P.; Reina, G.; Blom, J.D.; Martínez-González, M.Á.; Reinken, A.; De Kloet, E.R.; Molendijk, M.L. COVID-19 risk, course and outcome in people with mental disorders: A systematic review and meta-analyses. *Epidemiol. Psychiatr. Sci.* **2023**, *32*, e61. [CrossRef] [PubMed]
95. Oppenauer, C.; Burghardt, J.; Kaiser, E.; Riffer, F.; Sprung, M. Psychological Distress During the COVID-19 Pandemic in Patients With Mental or Physical Diseases. *Front. Psychol.* **2021**, *12*, 703488. [CrossRef]
96. Mulchandani, R.; Taylor-Philips, S.; Jones, H.E.; Ades, A.; Borrow, R.; Linley, E.; Kirwan, P.D.; Stewart, R.; Moore, P.; Boyes, J.; et al. Self assessment overestimates historical COVID-19 disease relative to sensitive serological assays: Cross-sectional study in UK key workers. *MedRxiv* **2020**, *22*, 2020–2108. [CrossRef]
97. Matta, J.; Wiernik, E.; Robineau, O.; Carrat, F.; Touvier, M.; Severi, G.; De Lamballerie, X.; Blanché, H.; Deleuze, J.-F.; Gouraud, C.; et al. Association of Self-reported COVID-19 Infection and SARS-CoV-2 Serology Test Results With Persistent Physical Symptoms Among French Adults During the COVID-19 Pandemic. *JAMA Intern. Med.* **2021**, *182*, 19. [CrossRef]

98. Ayling, K.; Jia, R.; Coupland, C.; Chalder, T.; Massey, A.; Broadbent, E.; Vedhara, K. Psychological Predictors of Self-reported COVID-19 Outcomes: Results From a Prospective Cohort Study. *Ann. Behav. Med.* **2022**, *56*, 484–497. [CrossRef]
99. Kuppuswamy, A. The Neurobiology of Pathological Fatigue: New Models, New Questions. *Neurosci.* **2021**, *28*, 238–253. [CrossRef]
100. Thomas, B.; Pattinson, R.; Bundy, C.; Davies, J.L. Somatosensory processing in long COVID fatigue and its relations with physiological and psychological factors. *Exp. Physiol.* **2024**, *109*, 1637–1649. [CrossRef]
101. Fietsam, A.C.; Bryant, A.D.; Rudroff, T. Fatigue and perceived fatigability, not objective fatigability, are prevalent in people with post-COVID-19. *Exp. Brain Res.* **2022**, *241*, 211–219. [CrossRef]
102. Scharfenberg, D.; Schild, A.-K.; Warnke, C.; Maier, F. A network perspective on neuropsychiatric and cognitive symptoms of the post-COVID syndrome. *Eur. J. Psychol.* **2022**, *18*, 350–356. [CrossRef]
103. Benke, C.; Autenrieth, L.K.; Asselmann, E.; Pané-Farré, C.A. Lockdown, quarantine measures, and social distancing: Associations with depression, anxiety and distress at the beginning of the COVID-19 pandemic among adults from Germany. *Psychiatry Res.* **2020**, *293*, 113462. [CrossRef]
104. Loades, M.E.; Chatburn, E.; Higson-Sweeney, N.; Reynolds, S.; Shafran, R.; Brigden, A.; Linney, C.; McManus, M.N.; Borwick, C.; Crawley, E. Rapid Systematic Review: The Impact of Social Isolation and Loneliness on the Mental Health of Children and Adolescents in the Context of COVID-19. *J. Am. Acad. Child Adolesc. Psychiatry* **2020**, *59*, 1218–1239.e3. [CrossRef]
105. Banerjee, D.; Vaishnav, M.; Rao, T.S.; Raju, M.; Dalal, P.K.; Javed, A.; Saha, G.; Mishra, K.K.; Kumar, V.; Jagiwala, M.P. Impact of the COVID-19 pandemic on psychosocial health and well-being in South-Asian (World Psychiatric Association zone 16) countries: A systematic and advocacy review from the Indian Psychiatric Society. *Indian J. Psychiatry* **2020**, *62*, 343. [CrossRef]
106. Dubey, S.; Biswas, P.; Ghosh, R.; Chatterjee, S.; Dubey, M.J.; Chatterjee, S.; Lahiri, D.; Lavie, C.J. Psychosocial impact of COVID-19. *Diabetes Metab. Syndr. Clin. Res. Rev.* **2020**, *14*, 779–788. [CrossRef] [PubMed]
107. Xiong, J.; Lipsitz, O.; Nasri, F.; Lui, L.M.W.; Gill, H.; Phan, L.; Chen-Li, D.; Iacobucci, M.; Ho, R.; Majeed, A.; et al. Impact of COVID-19 pandemic on mental health in the general population: A systematic review. *J. Affect. Disord.* **2020**, *277*, 55–64. [CrossRef] [PubMed]
108. Riepenhausen, A.; Veer, I.M.; Wackerhagen, C.; Reppmann, Z.C.; Köber, G.; Ayuso-Mateos, J.L.; Bögemann, S.A.; Corrao, G.; Felez-Nobrega, M.; Abad, J.M.H.; et al. Coping with COVID: Risk and resilience factors for mental health in a German representative panel study. *Psychol. Med.* **2022**, *53*, 3897–3907. [CrossRef]
109. Grunden, N.; Calabria, M.; García-Sánchez, C.; Pons, C.; Arroyo, J.A.; Gómez-Ansón, B.; Del Carmen Estévez-García, M.; Belvís, R.; Morollón, N.; Cordero-Carcedo, M.; et al. Evolving trends in neuropsychological profiles of post COVID-19 condition: A 1-year follow-up in individuals with cognitive complaints. *PLoS ONE* **2024**, *19*, e0302415. [CrossRef] [PubMed]
110. Braga, L.W.; Oliveira, S.B.; Moreira, A.S.; Pereira, M.E.M.d.S.M.; Serio, A.S.S.; Carneiro, V.d.S.; Freitas, L.d.F.P.; Souza, L.M.D.N. Long COVID neuropsychological follow-up: Is cognitive rehabilitation relevant? *Neurorehabilitation* **2023**, *53*, 517–534. [CrossRef]
111. Arneth, B.M. Gut–brain axis biochemical signalling from the gastrointestinal tract to the central nervous system: Gut dysbiosis and altered brain function. *Postgrad. Med. J.* **2018**, *94*, 446–452. [CrossRef]
112. Chen, P.; Zhang, L.; Feng, Y.; Liu, Y.-F.; Si, T.L.; Su, Z.; Cheung, T.; Ungvari, G.S.; Ng, C.H.; Xiang, Y.-T. Brain-gut axis and psychiatric disorders: A perspective from bibliometric and visual analysis. *Front. Immunol.* **2022**, *13*, 1047007. [CrossRef]
113. Bonaz, B.; Bazin, T.; Pellissier, S. The Vagus Nerve at the Interface of the Microbiota-Gut-Brain Axis. *Front. Neurosci.* **2018**, *12*, 49. [CrossRef] [PubMed]
114. Breit, S.; Kupferberg, A.; Rogler, G.; Hasler, G. Vagus Nerve as Modulator of the Brain–Gut Axis in Psychiatric and Inflammatory Disorders. *Front. Psychiatry* **2018**, *9*, 44. [CrossRef]
115. Scarpelli, S.; De Santis, A.; Alfonsi, V.; Gorgoni, M.; Morin, C.M.; Espie, C.; Merikanto, I.; Chung, F.; Penzel, T.; Bjorvatn, B.; et al. The role of sleep and dreams in long-COVID. *J. Sleep Res.* **2022**, *32*, e13789. [CrossRef]
116. Scarpelli, S.; Gorgoni, M.; Alfonsi, V.; Annarumma, L.; Di Natale, V.; Pezza, E.; De Gennaro, L. The impact of the end of COVID confinement on pandemic dreams, as assessed by a weekly sleep diary: A longitudinal investigation in Italy. *J. Sleep Res.* **2021**, *31*, e13429. [CrossRef] [PubMed]
117. Davis, H.E.; Assaf, G.S.; McCorkell, L.; Wei, H.; Low, R.J.; Re'em, Y.; Redfield, S.; 1064 Austin, J.P.; Akrami, A. Characterizing long COVID in an international cohort: 7 months of symptoms and their impact. *EClinicalMedicine* **2021**, *38*, 101019. [CrossRef] [PubMed]
118. Huth, D.; Bräscher, A.-K.; Tholl, S.; Fiess, J.; Birke, G.; Herrmann, C.; Jöbges, M.; Mier, D.; Witthöft, M. Cognitive-behavioral therapy for patients with post-COVID-19 condition (CBT-PCC): A feasibility trial. *Psychol. Med.* **2023**, *54*, 1122–1132. [CrossRef] [PubMed]
119. Kuut, T.A.; Müller, F.; Csorba, I.; Braamse, A.; Aldenkamp, A.; Appelman, B.; Assmann-Schuilwerve, E.; Geerlings, S.E.; Gibney, K.B.; Kanaan, R.; et al. Efficacy of Cognitive-Behavioral Therapy Targeting Severe Fatigue Following Coronavirus Disease 2019: Results of a Randomized Controlled Trial. *Clin. Infect. Dis.* **2023**, *77*, 687–695. [CrossRef] [PubMed]
120. Martínez-Borba, V.; Martínez-García, L.; Peris-Baquero, Ó.; Osma, J.; Del Corral-Beamonte, E. Guiding future research on psychological interventions in people with COVID-19 and post COVID syndrome and comorbid emotional disorders based on a systematic review. *Front. Public Health* **2024**, *11*, 1305463. [CrossRef] [PubMed]
121. Nikrah, N.; Bahari, F.; Shiri, A. Effectiveness of the acceptance and commitment therapy on resilience and quality of life in patients with post-acute COVID-19 syndrome. *Appl. Nurs. Res.* **2023**, *73*, 151723. [CrossRef] [PubMed]

122. Samad, F.D.A.; Pereira, X.V.; Chong, S.K.; Latif, M.H.B.A. Interpersonal psychotherapy for traumatic grief following a loss due to COVID-19: A case report. *Front. Psychiatry* **2023**, *14*, 1218715. [CrossRef]
123. Mahendru, K.; Pandit, A.; Singh, V.; Choudhary, N.; Mohan, A.; Bhatnagar, S. Effect of Meditation and Breathing Exercises on the Well-being of Patients with SARS-CoV-2 Infection under Institutional Isolation: A Randomized Control Trial. *Indian J. Palliat. Care* **2021**, *27*, 490–494. [CrossRef] [PubMed]
124. Situmorang, D.D.B. "When the first session may be the last!": A case report of the implementation of "rapid tele-psychotherapy" with single-session music therapy in the COVID-19 outbreak. *Palliat. Support. Care* **2021**, *20*, 290–295. [CrossRef]

Disclaimer/Publisher's Note: The statements, opinions and data contained in all publications are solely those of the individual author(s) and contributor(s) and not of MDPI and/or the editor(s). MDPI and/or the editor(s) disclaim responsibility for any injury to people or property resulting from any ideas, methods, instructions or products referred to in the content.

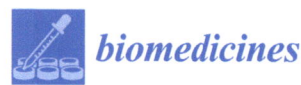 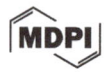

Article

Overlapping Systemic Proteins in COVID-19 and Lung Fibrosis Associated with Tissue Remodeling and Inflammation

Barbora Svobodová [1], Anna Löfdahl [1], Annika Nybom [1], Jenny Wigén [1], Gabriel Hirdman [2,3,4], Franziska Olm [2,3,4], Hans Brunnström [4], Sandra Lindstedt [2,3,4], Gunilla Westergren-Thorsson [1] and Linda Elowsson [1,*]

[1] Lung Biology Unit, Department of Experimental Medical Science, Lund University, 221 84 Lund, Sweden; barbora.svobodova@med.lu.se (B.S.); jenny.wigen@med.lu.se (J.W.); gunilla.westergren-thorsson@med.lu.se (G.W.-T.)
[2] Department of Cardiothoracic Surgery and Transplantation, Skåne University Hospital, 222 42 Lund, Sweden; gabriel.hirdman@med.lu.se (G.H.); franziska.olm@med.lu.se (F.O.); sandra.lindstedt@med.lu.se (S.L.)
[3] Wallenberg Center for Molecular Medicine, Lund University, 221 84 Lund, Sweden
[4] Department of Clinical Sciences, Lund University, 221 84 Lund, Sweden; hans.brunnstrom@med.lu.se
* Correspondence: linda.elowsson@med.lu.se; Tel.: +46-46-2228596

Abstract: Background/Objectives: A novel patient group with chronic pulmonary fibrosis is emerging post COVID-19. To identify patients at risk of developing post-COVID-19 lung fibrosis, we here aimed to identify systemic proteins that overlap with fibrotic markers identified in patients with idiopathic pulmonary fibrosis (IPF) and may predict COVID-19-induced lung fibrosis. **Methods:** Ninety-two proteins were measured in plasma samples from hospitalized patients with moderate and severe COVID-19 in Sweden, before the introduction of the vaccination program, as well as from healthy individuals. These measurements were conducted using proximity extension assay (PEA) technology with a panel including inflammatory and remodeling proteins. Histopathological alterations were evaluated in explanted lung tissue. **Results:** Connecting to IPF pathology, several proteins including decorin (DCN), tumor necrosis factor receptor superfamily member 12A (TNFRSF12A) and chemokine (C-X-C motif) ligand 13 (CXCL13) were elevated in COVID-19 patients compared to healthy subjects. Moreover, we found incrementing expression of monocyte chemotactic protein-3 (MCP-3) and hepatocyte growth factor (HGF) when comparing moderate to severe COVID-19. **Conclusions:** Both extracellular matrix- and inflammation-associated proteins were identified as overlapping with pulmonary fibrosis, where we found DCN, TNFRSF12A, CXCL13, CXCL9, MCP-3 and HGF to be of particular interest to follow up on for the prediction of disease severity.

Keywords: COVID-19; fibrosis; IPF; biomarkers; DCN; TNFRSF12A; MCP-3; HGF

Citation: Svobodová, B.; Löfdahl, A.; Nybom, A.; Wigén, J.; Hirdman, G.; Olm, F.; Brunnström, H.; Lindstedt, S.; Westergren-Thorsson, G.; Elowsson, L. Overlapping Systemic Proteins in COVID-19 and Lung Fibrosis Associated with Tissue Remodeling and Inflammation. *Biomedicines* **2024**, *12*, 2893. https://doi.org/10.3390/biomedicines12122893

Academic Editors: Jun Lu and César Fernández-de-las-Peñas

Received: 14 November 2024
Revised: 9 December 2024
Accepted: 17 December 2024
Published: 19 December 2024

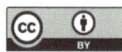

Copyright: © 2024 by the authors. Licensee MDPI, Basel, Switzerland. This article is an open access article distributed under the terms and conditions of the Creative Commons Attribution (CC BY) license (https://creativecommons.org/licenses/by/4.0/).

1. Introduction

The COVID-19 pandemic has caused severe aftermaths, with pulmonary fibrosis being considered an emerging problem. Around 20% of COVID-19 patients have developed severe symptoms, usually appearing after a week of an initial sick period, where about 5% of these patients have presented with critical conditions such as acute respiratory distress syndrome (ARDS). These conditions result from the massive immune response involving a cytokine storm [1], leading to an imbalance of the renin–angiotensin system (RAS) and the dysregulation of various cytokines [2,3]. RAS is primarily known for its role in regulating blood pressure and fluid balance, implicated in COVID-19 patients with common complications of coagulopathy [4] and endotheliopathy [5]. In addition, the cytokine storm contains an excess of pro-inflammatory markers including interleukins, monocyte attractant factors and tumor necrosis factor (TNF) [6,7], several factors that have been described in chronic interstitial lung diseases such as idiopathic pulmonary fibrosis (IPF). IPF is thought to be the result of repeated microinjuries of the epithelium, leading to a dysregulated epithelial–mesenchymal crosstalk that in turn results in an aberrant wound healing response [8,9].

We and others have demonstrated in vitro how a distorted microenvironment promotes the progression of disease [10]. Severe cases of COVID-19 typically exhibit diffuse alveolar damage (DAD) characterized by fibrin exudates, hyaline membrane formation, hyperplasia and a loss of alveolar type II cells, the disruption of the basement membrane and thickened alveolar walls. These changes can result in alveolar collapse, edema, inflammation and fatal dyspnea [11,12]. In IPF, fibroblasts are thought to be the main effector cell contributing to the accumulation of excessive extracellular matrices (ECMs) in the lungs, activated by pathways including TNF and transforming growth factor beta (TGF-β) and by epithelial-to-mesenchymal transition (EMT). Additional studies have implicated monocyte chemotactic protein-3 (MCP-3) and Chemokine (C-X-C motif) ligand 13 (CXCL13) as biomarkers for the pathogenesis of IPF, suggesting their roles in fibroblast recruitment and activation [7,13,14]. ECM-associated proteins such as decorin (DCN) and periostin (POSTN) are both involved in tissue remodeling, DCN in fibrillogenesis and POSTN in fibroblast activation and collagen deposition. The long-term risk of developing pulmonary fibrosis increases with the severity of initial diseases including ARDS and has been seen to be more pronounced in patients who have been subjected to mechanical ventilation [15]. Ravaglia et al. recently reported on histological patterns in patients with persistent symptoms after COVID-19 infection. Classified into three clusters, two were related to chronic fibrosing and different grades of lung injury for usual interstitial pneumonia (UIP) and DAD [16].

Identifying patients at risk of developing chronic pulmonary fibrosis is important for managing and intervening with the underlying pathological pathways [3,7,9,12,17]. Smoking, identified as a risk factor in the onset of lung fibrosis [18] has also been noted as a contributing factor to all-cause mortality in COVID-19 infections [19]. We hypothesized that early alterations in systemic cytokines and ECM components associated with remodeling may be indicative of the risk of developing chronic manifestations of pulmonary fibrosis. In this study we identified potential biomarkers in hospitalized COVID-19 patients, included prior to the vaccination program, with both moderate and severe symptoms, that overlap with previous findings linked to pulmonary fibrosis. The biomarkers were found to be associated with both inflammation and tissue remodeling. Among the identified proteins, we found elevated systemic levels of remodeling proteins decorin (DCN), tumor necrosis factor receptor superfamily member 12A (TNFRSF12A) and hepatocyte growth factor (HGF), and chemoattractant factors MCP-3 and CXCL13 in pre-vaccine plasma samples from COVID-19 patients, which supports previous findings of these molecules in patients with IPF and pulmonary fibrosis post COVID-19 [20–24].

2. Materials and Methods

2.1. Study Design

Plasma samples collected from hospitalized pre-vaccine COVID-19 patients were analyzed and divided into two groups: severe and moderate. The two groups were compared to healthy subjects that were age- and gender-matched. Selected proteins of interest were further analyzed by histology and immunohistochemistry in explanted lung tissue from COVID-19 patients and compared to IPF patients and healthy subjects. Supplementary Table S1 presents patient and healthy control characteristics.

2.2. Plasma from COVID-19 Patients and Controls

Plasma samples were collected (in EDTA tubes) two weeks after hospital admission during 2020 prior to the initiation of COVID-19 vaccination programs. Patients with severe COVID-19 and ARDS were treated via mechanical ventilation (n = 8), and patients with moderate symptoms (n = 8) were treated with supplemental oxygen. Patients treated via mechanical ventilation had a PaO_2/FiO_2 ratio between 80 and 200 at the time of blood sample collection, equal to severe-to-moderate ARDS using the Berlin definition of ARDS [25]. None of the patients on mechanical ventilation had any CO_2 retention. Patients treated with oxygen support other than mechanical ventilation had a P/F ratio above 200 but below 300 at the time of blood sample collection, equal to mild ARDS using the Berlin definition of ARDS. None of the patients had any CO_2 retention. As the control group, plasma samples from age- and gender-matched healthy subjects were used (n = 7). The plasma samples were analyzed in an immuno-oncology panel (encompassing inflammatory and remodeling proteins) of 92 proteins using proximity extension assay (PEA) technology (Olink AB, Uppsala, Sweden). PEA is a highly sensitive method that uses antibody pairs with DNA tags to detect and quantify multiple proteins simultaneously via qPCR. The panel used in this study was chosen to match the one employed in our previous biomarker research on IPF.

2.3. Explanted Human Lung Tissue

Explanted distal lung tissue specimens derived from post-COVID-19 patients, IPF patients and lung donors were used for histological evaluation. Specimens from explanted lungs were collected from three post-COVID-19 patients (male n = 1, age 61; female n = 2, age = 63, and 64; all ex-smokers). One of the post-COVID-19 patients was treated with extracorporeal membrane oxygenation for 5 months before the lung transplantation. The other two patients developed interstitial lung disease, out of which one of them had symptoms of COPD. The two IPF patients included in this study (female n = 1, age 65; male n = 1, age 57; both ex-smokers) were diagnosed based on ATS and ERS criteria [26]. Three healthy lungs from organ donors were included (males n = 3, age 62, 66 and 68) out of which two were ex-smokers and one had never smoked.

2.4. Histology and Immunohistochemistry

Formalin-fixed paraffin-embedded distal lung tissue with 1–3 tissue blocks per individual were antibody-labeled with HRP-DAB immunohistochemistry for periostin (POSTN) and decorin (DCN), with corresponding tissue sections stained with hematoxylin and eosin (HE) for the visualization of tissue morphology and pathological features. In short, following deparaffinization, sections were treated with heat-induced antigen retrieval at a low pH, using Flex target retrieval solution (cat no. K8005, Agilent Dako, Santa Clara, CA, USA). The sections were stained with primary antibodies for DCN (1:1000, cat no. HPA003315, Atlas antibodies, Bromma, Sweden) and POSTN (1:1000, ab79946, Abcam, Cambridge, UK) together with Envision dual link system-HRP (DAB) (cat no. K4065, Dako) and counterstained with hematoxylin before dehydration and mounting with Pertex. The sections were scanned with the VS120 virtual microscopy slide scanning system (VS120-L100-FL080, Olympus, Tokyo, Japan). Representative images were acquired using the OlyVIA software 3.3 (Olympus) Qupath 0.3.0 (The University of Edinburgh, UK) [27] and ImageJ 1.53j (National Institutes of Health, Bethesda, MD, USA). The morphology of tissue sections was assessed by using the modified Russell–Movat pentachrome stain kit (cat. No. KSC-L53PIA-1, Nordic Biosite, Täby, Sweden) according to the manufacturer's protocol.

2.5. Statistical Analysis

The data from the PEA of the plasma samples were presented as normalized protein expression (NPX) values for each protein on a log2 scale, i.e., a difference of 1 NPX between proteins equals a doubling of protein concentration. In the analyzed samples, six proteins with a detectability lower than 67% (>33% of limit of detection per protein) were excluded (IL13, IL-1α, IL-2, IL33, CD28, IL4), resulting in the inclusion of 86 proteins (93.5%) to be evaluated. One-way ANOVA with Tukey's multiple comparisons test with a cut-off at a mean group difference >1 NPX was used to analyze statistical differences between groups. We categorized the proteins, as described in Kalafatis et al. (2021) [28], according to three main biological functions related to inflammation and chemotaxis (I), tissue remodeling (R) or proteins with overlapping functions (O).

3. Results

3.1. Altered Proteins in Plasma Samples from COVID-19 Patients and Healthy Controls

The majority of included COVID-19 patients were men in both the severe and moderate group, of which two died during their hospital visit. The healthy controls were age- and gender- matched (Table 1); however, smoking status for most of the patients with severe COVID-19 was not available.

Table 1. Patient characteristics of plasma cohorts.

	Moderate COVID-19 (n = 8)	Severe COVID-19 (n = 8)	Healthy Subjects (n = 7)
Age (Mean ± SD)	57.1 ± 6.7	64.9 ± 13.8	55.1 ± 12.8
Male/female (n, %)	5/3 (62.5%/37.5%)	7/1 (87.5%/12.5%)	5/2 (71%/29%)
Smoking history			
Never smoked (n, %)	6 (75%)	2 (25%)	3 (42.9%)
Ex-smokers (n, %)	2 (25%)	-	2 (28.6%)
Current smokers (n, %)	-	1 (12.5%)	2 (28.6%)
Unknown (n, %)		5 (62.5%)	
Death during hospital visit (n, %)	0 (0%)	2 (25%)	NA

Comparing plasma samples from patients with severe COVID-19 with those from healthy controls revealed 42 significantly altered proteins with a >1 NPX mean difference. Out of these, 23 proteins were also significantly elevated in patients with moderate COVID-19 in comparison to healthy controls. Fifteen proteins were significantly increased in the severe group in comparison to healthy controls, of which pleiotrophin (PTN), adhesion G protein-coupled receptor G1 (ADGRG1) and C-C motif chemokine ligand 19 (CCL19) were the top three proteins most elevated in patients with severe COVID-19 (Table 2). As seen in our previous studies on lung fibrosis (5, 8), DCN was elevated in severe COVID-19 patients (Table 2, Figure 1).

Table 2. Altered plasma protein expression in patients with moderate and severe COVID-19 versus healthy subjects.

Protein	Mean Difference (NPX)	SE of Mean Difference	p-Value	Biological Process
Severe vs Healthy				
CCL19	1.512	0.5816	0.0433	I
LAG3	1.330	0.3436	0.0026	I
LAMP-3	1.259	0.3815	0.0095	I
KLRD1	1.185	0.3737	0.0127	I
IL15	1.179	0.2884	0.0016	I
CD70	1.045	0.2492	0.0012	I
GAL-9	1.099	0.2206	0.0002	I
ADGRG1	1.705	0.5260	0.0093	R
CAIX	1.404	0.4422	0.0127	R
PGF	1.284	0.3599	0.0052	R
DCN	1.065	0.1967	<0.0001	R
PDGFB	−1.683	0.5761	0.0220	R
TNF	1.110	0.3078	0.0280	O
PTN	2.107	0.5692	0.0039	O
MCP-1	1.451	0.3251	0.0007	O

Table 2. *Cont.*

Protein	Mean Difference (NPX)	SE of Mean Difference	*p*-Value	Biological Process
		Severe vs Moderate		
CXCL9	1.525	0.5082	0.0185	I
MCP-3	1.468	0.3895	0.0033	I
CXCL13	1.204	0.3540	0.0076	I
HGF	1.388	0.4436	0.0140	R
ADGRG1	1.167	0.5082	0.0719	R
PTN	1.108	0.5499	0.0030	R
TNFRSF12A	1.663	0.3250	0.0001	O
		Moderate vs Healthy		
CD40	−1.882	0.3263	<0.0001	I
PD-L1	−1.752	0.3044	<0.0001	I
CD4	−1.077	0.3336	0.0112	I
TWEAK	−1.144	0.2957	0.0026	O

Significantly altered protein levels with ≥1 NPX mean difference (normalized protein expression, NPX), categorized according to biological function: I = inflammation/chemotaxis, R = tissue remodeling and O = overlapping functions. Standard error (SE) of difference in means.

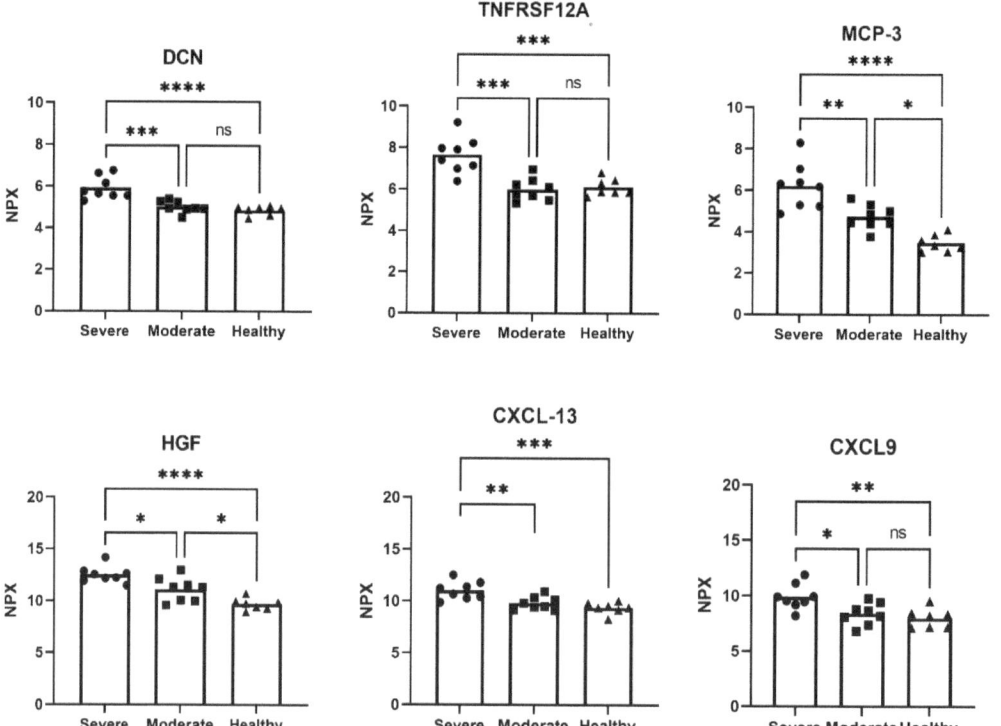

Figure 1. Elevated protein amount of DCN, TNFRSF12A, MCP-3, HGF, CXCL13 and CXCL9 in plasma from patients with moderate and severe COVID-19 in comparison to healthy subjects. NPX = normalized protein expression. Patients with moderate (n = 8) and severe (n = 8) COVID-19; healthy individuals (n = 7). One-way ANOVA with Tukey's multiple comparison test. * $p < 0.05$, ** $p < 0.01$, *** $p < 0.001$, **** $p < 0.0001$, ns = not significant.

In patients with moderate COVID-19, but not with severe illness, four proteins involved in inflammatory and chemotactic processes were significantly reduced in comparison to healthy controls (Table 2). Distinguishing patients with severe and moderate COVID-19, seven proteins were significantly altered (>1 NPX mean difference) (Table 2) including CXCL13 and C-X-C motif chemokine ligand 9 (CXCL9), where TNF receptor superfamily member 12A (TNFRSF12A) was the most increased (Figure 1), highlighting the involvement of the TNF-a pathway. MCP-3 and HGF were significantly increased (>1 NPX mean difference) in all patient groups, incrementing from healthy to moderate to severe COVID-19 (Figure 1). All significantly altered proteins with a >1 NPX mean difference between COVID-19 groups and healthy controls are shown in Supplementary Table S2. It is noteworthy that two patients with severe COVID-19 who died during their hospital visit exhibited additional elevated plasma levels of CCL19, placenta growth factor (PGF) and carbonic anhydrase IX (CAIX), proteins mainly involved in tissue remodeling processes (Supplement Figure S2).

3.2. Tissue Morphology and Protein Expression in Distal Lung in Severe Post-COVID-19 and IPF

Tissue sections from post-COVID-19 and IPF patients demonstrated an accumulation of dense connective tissue rich in collagens, proteoglycans and disrupted parenchymal structures with inflammatory cell infiltrates (Supplement Figure S2). The airways and alveolar structures were filled with mucus and inflammatory cells (in particular macrophages). Furthermore, fibroblast foci formation in IPF and the accumulation of fibroblasts and myofibroblasts in post-COVID-19 resembling the IPF fibroblast foci as well as possible alveolar edema and alveolar type II hyperplasia were observed. With computed tomography, one of the patients with COVID-19 showed consolidated parenchymal changes in their lungs with severe ARDS and fibrotic development (Supplement Figure S3). Decorin, known for its role in collagen fibrillogenesis, showed increased expression with clear localization to the subepithelial regions of bronchioles (Figure 2), consistent with previous findings in IPF lung tissue [10]. Similarly, periostin, which is involved in fibroblast recruitment at active fibrotic sites, also exhibited elevated expression in the subepithelial regions of bronchioles. Moreover, periostin was localized to fibroblastic foci in IPF lungs and in similar structures within post-COVID-19 lung tissue (Figure 2G–J). A shared spatial expression pattern of DCN was seen in both post-COVID-19 and IPF with elevated staining intensity, corresponding to the increased deposition of extracellular matrices. DCN was detected in the vascular adventitia (Figure 2K–L), and both DCN and POSTN were highly expressed in the visceral pleura, where DCN was also expressed in mesothelial cells (Figure 2N–P, Supplementary Figure S5). In heavily remodeled areas with dense connective tissue and cell infiltration in post-COVID-19, DCN was seen to be embedded in the ECM with fiber-like formation, while in IPF, DCN appeared more fragmented. DCN and POSTN were also found in regions of honeycomb cysts, a typical pathological pulmonary feature in IPF (Supplementary Figure S4).

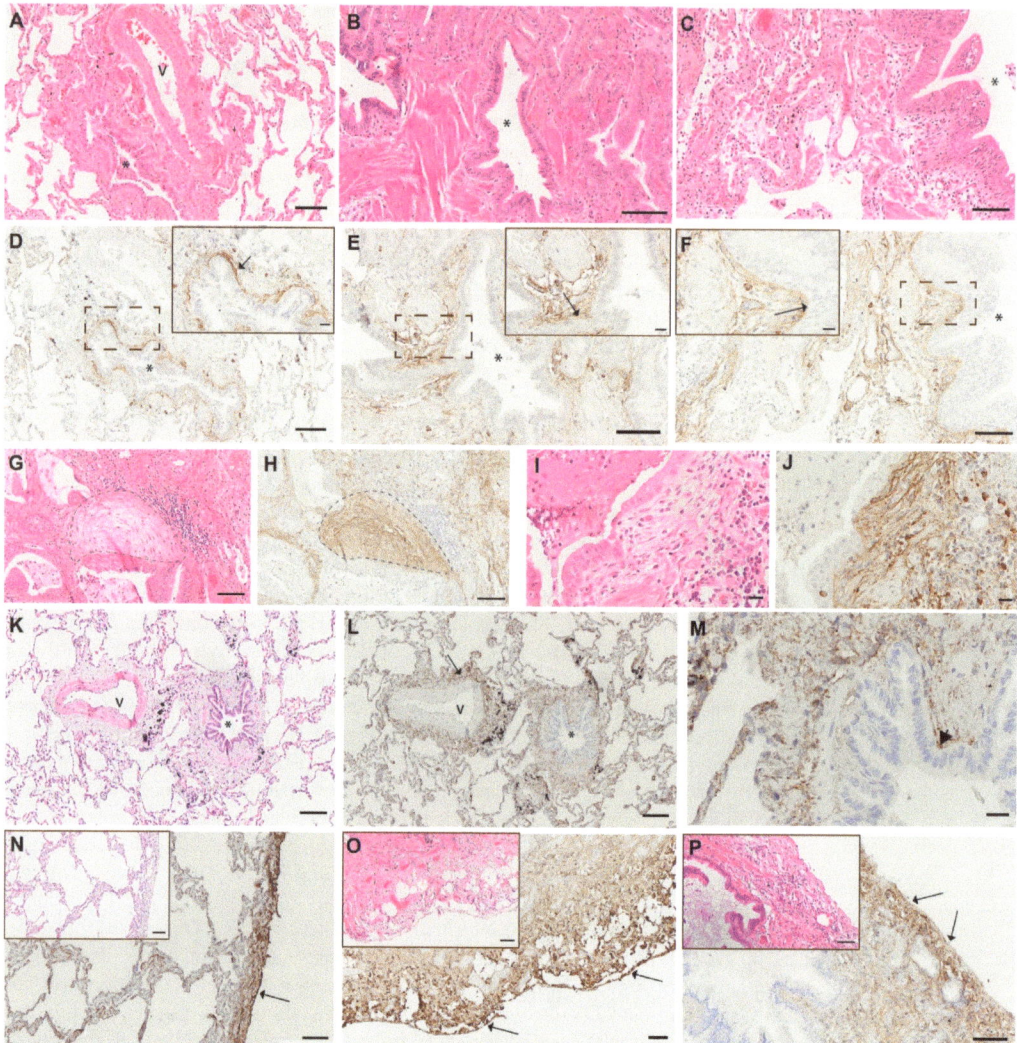

Figure 2. The overlapping protein patterns of DCN and POSTN in post-COVID-19 and IPF. In distal lung tissue, the expression of POSTN was mainly localized to the subepithelial regions of bronchioles in healthy (**A**,**D**), post-COVID-19 (**B**,**E**) and IPF (**C**,**F**) patients, enclosed upon magnification in the basement membrane zone (arrow). POSTN was highly expressed in fibroblastic foci in IPF (**G**,**H**, encircled area) and in similar structures in post-COVID-19 patients (**I**,**J**). Similarly, DCN was found to be intensely expressed in the subepithelial regions of bronchioles (arrowhead) and in vascular adventitia (arrow) (healthy, **K**–**M**). Increased DCN expression was also seen in pleura (arrows) and subpleural regions in healthy (**N**, including HE staining), post-COVID-19 (**O**, including HE staining) and IPF (**P**, including HE staining) patients. Scale bar: 500 µm (**N**–**P**); 100 µm (**A**–**F**, **K**–**M**; enlargements **N**–**P**); 20 µm (enlargement (**D**–**F**), **G**–**J**). * = bronchiole; v = vessel.

4. Discussion

The immune response of COVID-19-affected lungs results not only in inflammatory activity but also in long-term structural changes in the lung tissue. The differentially expressed proteins identified in our study are involved in various signaling pathways that contribute to pulmonary fibrosis by influencing inflammation, ECM remodeling, angiogenesis and fibroblast activation. Remodeling processes are often driven by pro-fibrotic factors released during inflammation, which can promote the excessive production of extracellular matrix proteins and scarring. In most cases, it is resolved, but there is an emerging post-COVID-19 group that is at risk of developing chronic pulmonary fibrosis. This study focuses on severely affected COVID-19 patients from the early phase of the pandemic, a group in which additional risk factors, such as advanced age and smoking, may have heightened inflammatory responses and influenced tissue remodeling, mirroring the patterns observed in IPF. The study's limitations include missing data on risk factors for some individuals and a small sample size, impacting statistical power. However, the unvaccinated status of this cohort offers essential insights into inflammatory and remodeling responses which are valuable for understanding potential outcomes in future pandemics. Guided by the hypothesis that chronic pulmonary diseases propagate through remodeling processes closely associated with inflammatory mechanisms, this analysis of unique early pandemic cases in Sweden reveals several markers overlapping with established IPF biomarkers. Markers found to be significantly elevated in COVID-19 compared to control samples included CCL19, CXCL-13, MCP-3, PGF, HGF and TNF. Of interest, DCN and TNFRSF12A were distinctly elevated in severe COVID-19, separating severe disease from moderate, while MCP-3 and HGF were found to increment with disease severity. Notably, 32 proteins were found to be significantly altered in the IPF cohort compared to healthy controls in our previous study but were not significantly altered in the COVID-19 study group. Among these were IL6 and angiopoietin-2 (ANGPT2), two proteins recognized as potential biomarkers for IPF.

The TNFRSF12A signaling pathway has been identified in IPF to accelerate collagen synthesis through the regulation of matrix metalloproteinase 9 (MMP9), which has been suggested as a therapeutic target in several lung diseases [29]. In a previous study, we discovered that TNFRSF12A was significantly elevated in IPF serum compared to healthy subjects and strongly correlated to disease progression [28]. Interestingly, in moderate COVID-19, the ligand to TNFRSF12A, TWEAK, was significantly reduced compared to in controls (Table 2), and although this was not significant, it was also reduced in the ICU group. This finding indicates that TNF signaling is increased in severe disease compared to moderate. While TNF signaling is crucial for tissue repair and the recruitment of cells such as fibroblasts, excessive or prolonged signaling is thought to contribute to fibrosis [30]. In a recent study by Iosef et al., patients with long COVID were found to have elevated plasma levels of TNF, TGF-β1 and MMP9 along with increased levels of angiogenic factors such as vascular endothelial growth factor A (VEGFA) and angiopoietin 1 (ANGPT1), indicating activated TNF-α pathway signaling and sustained involvement of the vascular system [31]. The inflammatory role of TNF in IPF has long been investigated [8]. In a study by Oikonomou et al., the link between TNF signaling and TGF-β1 expression was investigated, and the results demonstrated its involvement in fibrosis [30]. Thus, it is conceivable that the previously reported cytokine storm in severe COVID-19 predisposes for lung fibrosis [2,6], as we found the TNF-α pathway to be involved through TNFRSF12A.

Extracellular proteins linked to tissue remodeling, namely POSTN and DCN [20,32], along with chemokine CXCL13 [22], have all been proposed as prognostic biomarkers for IPF. Interestingly, all of these were altered in the COVID-19 patients compared to the healthy subjects. DCN was upregulated in the plasma from patients with severe COVID-19, differentiating them from patients with moderate COVID-19. In its soluble form, DCN has been proposed to prevent lung fibrosis in severe COVID-19 by engaging the receptor of interferon regulatory factors (IRFs), thereby protecting epithelial cells from apoptosis and also neutralizing TGF-β, a strong fibrosis mediator [14,32]. Meanwhile, ECM-incorporated DCN plays an important role in collagen fibrillogenesis. POSTN, on the other hand, a crucial factor for fibroblast activation, was found to be elevated in patients with both severe and moderate COVID-19 compared to controls, which has been shown by others as well to be associated with critical illness [33] and has been suggested as a potential therapeutic target in IPF [24]. Factors frequently discussed in IPF research including MMP7, MMP12,

VEGFA and ANGPT2 did not show a significant change compared to control samples in our study.

We also found increased levels of CXCL13, a chemokine expressed by a subset of T helper cells upon antigen presentation and proposed as a biomarker for IPF [34]. We recently demonstrated in a previous study that the fibrotic environment of an IPF lung triggered a profibrotic response in healthy cells, where the chemokine CXCL13 was significantly elevated compared to cells cultured in a healthy lung microenvironment [10]. The combined increased levels of CXCL13 and HGF were shown in a large Swiss study to be the best predictor of COVID-19 admission to the intensive care unit (ICU) [35]. HGF, fundamentally involved in tissue regeneration, is likely to be upregulated to counteract the cyto/chemokine storm, including CXCL13, in an attempt to counteract fibrotic signals by interfering with TGF-β signaling. Further, the angiogenic factor PGF, correlated in one study to in-hospital mortality in COVID-19 [36], was, along with CCL19, GAL-9 and DCN, significantly elevated in patients with severe COVID-19 in comparison to healthy controls, as in our IPF ex vivo model and in IPF serum [28]. Interestingly, the two patients that died in hospital in our cohort had higher levels of CCL19 and PGF compared to the rest in the severe COVID-19 group. Furthermore, several monocyte attractant chemokines have been reported to be associated with disease severity in both COVID-19 and IPF patients. In our data, MCP-3 was an indicator of disease severity, which is in line with Yang et al.'s study [23] showing that there is a sustained high level of MCP-3 in the lung tissue in fatal cases even after the viral infection is gone. Taken together, these data emphasize the common pathways in IPF and severe COVID-19, which may explain the increased severity of COVID-19 infection in IPF patients [37]. In line with this, in patients with severe COVID-19, alveolar macrophages primarily interact with fibroblasts via the TNFSF12-TNFRSF12A signaling pathway, which drives fibroblast proliferation and the production of fibrotic factors [38]. TNFa, which is increased during severe COVID-19 infection, induces CXCL13, a predictor of IPF severity, in alveolar macrophages [39]. Based on our data, we therefore conclude that IPF patients are at risk of adverse outcome from COVID-19 infection.

5. Conclusions

Herein, we describe shared histopathological findings in explanted lung tissue from post-COVID-19 and IPF patients linked to ECM remodeling. Blood samples collected two weeks post-hospitalization from pre-vaccine COVID-19 patients exhibited elevated plasma levels of proteins associated with both tissue remodeling and inflammation that overlap with markers found in IPF, processes that are tightly connected. With time, hospitalization due to COVID-19 infection has decreased and only a few individuals have required transplantation in Sweden so far. However, there is an emerging subset of post-COVID-19 cases experiencing lung complications [40]. We found the combination of the following factors to be of most interest to follow up on in a larger cohort of post-COVID-19 patients: CXCL13, DCN, HGF, MCP-3 and TNFRSF12A. Notably, we lacked smoking status data for most of the severely affected COVID-19 patients, which may have influenced their inflammatory response. Although the direct link between COVID-19 and the development of IPF remains unestablished and is a subject of ongoing debate, these proteins may serve as critical biomarkers for identifying patients at risk of pulmonary fibrosis. This potential role underscores the importance of investigating their expression in larger, more diverse cohorts to validate their utility and relevance.

Supplementary Materials: The following supporting information can be downloaded at https://www.mdpi.com/article/10.3390/biomedicines12122893/s1: Table S1. Patient characteristics including laboratory measurements. Table S2. Proteins with >1 NPX mean difference between COVID-19 groups and healthy group. Figure S1: Elevated protein amount of CCL19, PGF and CAIX in plasma from patients with severe COVID-19 that died during hospital visit; Figure S2: Lung tissue remodeling and shared histopathological features in COVID-19 and IPF; Figure S3: HRCT image of consolidated parenchymal changes; Figure S4: Pulmonary expression of DCN and POSTN in COVID-19 and IPF. Figure S5: Pulmonary expression of DCN and PSTN in another COVID-19 patient.

Author Contributions: Conceptualization and design: A.L., B.S., S.L., G.W.-T. and L.E.; data acquisition and analysis: A.L., B.S., A.N., G.H., F.O., H.B. and L.E.; interpretation of data: A.L., B.S., J.W., H.B., S.L., G.W.-T. and L.E.; funding acquisition: S.L., G.W.-T. and L.E.; writing—review and editing: A.L., B.S., A.N., J.W., G.H., F.O., H.B., S.L., G.W.-T. and L.E. All authors have read and agreed to the published version of the manuscript.

Funding: This research was funded by the Swedish Research Council in Medicine and Health (2020-01375), the Swedish Heart–Lung Foundation (20200330, 20210086, 20210289), the Royal Physiographical Society in Lund, the Medical Faculty of Lund University, and The Åke and Inger Bergkvist, Evy and Gunnar Sandberg, Greta and John Kock, Alfred Österlund, Crafoord, the Foundation of Lars Hiertas Minne, Mats Kleberg and Consul Thure Bergh foundations. The APC was funded by Lund University, ALF Grants Region Skåne, the Wallenberg Centre for Molecular Medicine and the Swedish Foundation for Strategic Research SBE13-0130.

Institutional Review Board Statement: This study was conducted in accordance with the Declaration of Helsinki and approved by the Institutional Review Board (or Ethics Committee) in Lund, Sweden for studies involving human lung tissues and plasma samples. Dnr 2008/431 (2022-00947-02), Dnr 2018/129 (2018/380, 2020-01864), Dnr 2017/396 (2018/386), Dnr 413/2008 (2022-01221-02) and Gothenburg Dnr 1026-15.

Informed Consent Statement: Informed consent was obtained from all subjects involved in this study or their closest relative.

Data Availability Statement: The data that support the findings of this study are available on request from the corresponding author. The data are not publicly available due to privacy or ethical restrictions.

Acknowledgments: We thank Göran Dellgren (Dpt of Cardiothoracic Surgery and Transplant Institute, Sahlgrenska University Hospital, Gothenburg, Sweden) and Sofia Lundin (AstraZeneca, Gothenburg, Sweden) for the important collaboration in receiving the human lung tissue. We acknowledge the collaboration with Leif Bjermer (Dpt of Respiratory Medicine and Allergology, Skåne University Hospital, Lund University) and Ellen Tufvesson (Dpt of Clinical Sciences, Lund University, Lund, Sweden) in receiving the healthy cohort plasma samples. We thank Magnus Sköld and Dimitrios Kalafatis (Dpt of Medicine Solna and Center for Molecular Medicine, Karolinska Institutet, Stockholm, Sweden) for their outstanding collaboration in the investigation of fibrotic biomarkers in IPF.

Conflicts of Interest: GWT reports grants from the Swedish Heart and Lung foundation, The Swedish Research Council and Lund University, and governmental funding for clinical research within the National Health Service (project 097). The other authors declare no conflicts of interest.

List of Abbreviations

ADGRG1	adhesion G protein-coupled receptor G1
ANGPT1	angiopoietin 1
ARDS	acute respiratory distress syndrome
CAIX	carbonic anhydrase IX
CCL19	C-C motif chemokine ligand 19
CXCL13	chemokine (C-X-C motif) ligand 13
CXCL9	C-X-C motif chemokine ligand 9
DAD	diffuse alveolar damage
DCN	decorin
ECM	extracellular matrix
EMT	epithelial-to-mesenchymal transition
HE	hematoxylin and eosin
HGF	hepatocyte growth factor
I	inflammation- and chemotaxis-related proteins
ICU	intensive care unit
IPF	idiopathic pulmonary fibrosis
IRFs	interferon regulatory factors
MCP-3	monocyte chemotactic protein-3
MMP9	matrix metalloproteinase 9
NPX	normalized protein expression

O	proteins with overlapping functions
PEA	proximity extension assay
PGF	placenta growth factor
POSTN	periostin
PTN	pleiotrophin
R	tissue remodeling-related proteins
RAS	renin–angiotensin system
TGF-β	transforming growth factor beta
TNF	tumor necrosis factor
TNFRSF12A	TNF receptor superfamily member 12A
UIP	usual interstitial pneumonia
VEGFA	vascular endothelial growth factor A

References

1. Sun, X.; Wang, T.; Cai, D.; Hu, Z.; Chen, J.; Liao, H.; Zhi, L.; Wei, H.; Zhang, Z.; Qiu, Y.; et al. Cytokine storm intervention in the early stages of COVID-19 pneumonia. *Cytokine Growth Factor. Rev.* 2020, 53, 38–42. [CrossRef] [PubMed]
2. Hrenak, J.; Simko, F. Renin-Angiotensin System: An Important Player in the Pathogenesis of Acute Respiratory Distress Syndrome. *Int. J. Mol. Sci.* 2020, 21, 8038. [CrossRef] [PubMed]
3. Wang, J.; Chen, L.; Chen, B.; Meliton, A.; Liu, S.Q.; Shi, Y.; Liu, T.; Deb, D.K.; Solway, J.; Li, Y.C. Chronic Activation of the Renin-Angiotensin System Induces Lung Fibrosis. *Sci. Rep.* 2015, 5, 15561. [CrossRef] [PubMed]
4. Connors, J.M.; Levy, J.H. COVID-19 and its implications for thrombosis and anticoagulation. *Blood* 2020, 135, 2033–2040. [CrossRef]
5. Smadja, D.M.; Mentzer, S.J.; Fontenay, M.; Laffan, M.A.; Ackermann, M.; Helms, J.; Jonigk, D.; Chocron, R.; Pier, G.B.; Gendron, N.; et al. COVID-19 is a systemic vascular hemopathy: Insight for mechanistic and clinical aspects. *Angiogenesis* 2021, 24, 755–788. [CrossRef] [PubMed]
6. Mohd Zawawi, Z.; Kalyanasundram, J.; Mohd Zain, R.; Thayan, R.; Basri, D.F.; Yap, W.B. Prospective Roles of Tumor Necrosis Factor-Alpha (TNF-alpha) in COVID-19: Prognosis, Therapeutic and Management. *Int. J. Mol. Sci.* 2023, 24, 6142. [CrossRef]
7. Hirawat, R.; Jain, N.; Aslam Saifi, M.; Rachamalla, M.; Godugu, C. Lung fibrosis: Post-COVID-19 complications and evidences. *Int. Immunopharmacol.* 2023, 116, 109418. [CrossRef]
8. Shenderov, K.; Collins, S.L.; Powell, J.D.; Horton, M.R. Immune dysregulation as a driver of idiopathic pulmonary fibrosis. *J. Clin. Investig.* 2021, 131, e143226. [CrossRef]
9. Wigen, J.; Lofdahl, A.; Bjermer, L.; Elowsson-Rendin, L.; Westergren-Thorsson, G. Converging pathways in pulmonary fibrosis and COVID-19—The fibrotic link to disease severity. *Respir. Med. X* 2020, 2, 100023. [CrossRef]
10. Elowsson Rendin, L.; Lofdahl, A.; Ahrman, E.; Muller, C.; Notermans, T.; Michalikova, B.; Rosmark, O.; Zhou, X.H.; Dellgren, G.; Silverborn, M.; et al. Matrisome Properties of Scaffolds Direct Fibroblasts in Idiopathic Pulmonary Fibrosis. *Int. J. Mol. Sci.* 2019, 20, 4013. [CrossRef] [PubMed]
11. Lee, J.H.; Koh, J.; Jeon, Y.K.; Goo, J.M.; Yoon, S.H. An Integrated Radiologic-Pathologic Understanding of COVID-19 Pneumonia. *Radiology* 2023, 306, e222600. [CrossRef] [PubMed]
12. Perez-Mies, B.; Caniego-Casas, T.; Bardi, T.; Carretero-Barrio, I.; Benito, A.; Garcia-Cosio, M.; Gonzalez-Garcia, I.; Pizarro, D.; Rosas, M.; Cristobal, E.; et al. Progression to lung fibrosis in severe COVID-19 patients: A morphological and transcriptomic study in postmortem samples. *Front. Med.* 2022, 9, 976759. [CrossRef]
13. Tsukui, T.; Sun, K.H.; Wetter, J.B.; Wilson-Kanamori, J.R.; Hazelwood, L.A.; Henderson, N.C.; Adams, T.S.; Schupp, J.C.; Poli, S.D.; Rosas, I.O.; et al. Collagen-producing lung cell atlas identifies multiple subsets with distinct localization and relevance to fibrosis. *Nat. Commun.* 2020, 11, 1920. [CrossRef] [PubMed]
14. Chanda, D.; Otoupalova, E.; Smith, S.R.; Volckaert, T.; De Langhe, S.P.; Thannickal, V.J. Developmental pathways in the pathogenesis of lung fibrosis. *Mol. Asp. Med.* 2019, 65, 56–69. [CrossRef] [PubMed]
15. Shen, H.; Zhang, N.; Liu, Y.; Yang, X.; He, Y.; Li, Q.; Shen, X.; Zhu, Y.; Yang, Y. The Interaction Between Pulmonary Fibrosis and COVID-19 and the Application of Related Anti-Fibrotic Drugs. *Front. Pharmacol.* 2021, 12, 805535. [CrossRef]
16. Ravaglia, C.; Doglioni, C.; Chilosi, M.; Piciucchi, S.; Dubini, A.; Rossi, G.; Pedica, F.; Puglisi, S.; Donati, L.; Tomassetti, S.; et al. Clinical, radiological and pathological findings in patients with persistent lung disease following SARS-CoV-2 infection. *Eur. Respir. J.* 2022, 60, 2102411. [CrossRef]
17. Mulet, A.; Tarraso, J.; Rodriguez-Borja, E.; Carbonell-Asins, J.A.; Lope-Martinez, A.; Marti-Martinez, A.; Murria, R.; Safont, B.; Fernandez-Fabrellas, E.; Ros, J.A.; et al. Fibrosis Biomarkers in a Cohort of COVID-19 Patients One Year after Hospital Discharge. *Am. J. Respir. Cell Mol. Biol.* 2023, 69, 321–327. [CrossRef] [PubMed]
18. Baumgartner, K.B.; Samet, J.M.; Stidley, C.A.; Colby, T.V.; Waldron, J.A. Cigarette smoking: A risk factor for idiopathic pulmonary fibrosis. *Am. J. Respir. Crit. Care Med.* 1997, 155, 242–248. [CrossRef]
19. Gao, M.; Aveyard, P.; Lindson, N.; Hartmann-Boyce, J.; Watkinson, P.; Young, D.; Coupland, C.; Clift, A.K.; Harrison, D.; Gould, D.; et al. Association between smoking, e-cigarette use and severe COVID-19: A cohort study. *Int. J. Epidemiol.* 2022, 51, 1062–1072. [CrossRef]

20. Nikaido, T.; Tanino, Y.; Wang, X.; Sato, Y.; Togawa, R.; Kikuchi, M.; Misa, K.; Saito, K.; Fukuhara, N.; Kawamata, T.; et al. Serum decorin is a potential prognostic biomarker in patients with acute exacerbation of idiopathic pulmonary fibrosis. *J. Thorac. Dis.* **2018**, *10*, 5346–5358. [CrossRef]
21. Perreau, M.; Suffiotti, M.; Marques-Vidal, P.; Wiedemann, A.; Levy, Y.; Laouenan, C.; Ghosn, J.; Fenwick, C.; Comte, D.; Roger, T.; et al. The cytokines HGF and CXCL13 predict the severity and the mortality in COVID-19 patients. *Nat. Commun.* **2021**, *12*, 4888. [CrossRef]
22. Vuga, L.J.; Tedrow, J.R.; Pandit, K.V.; Tan, J.; Kass, D.J.; Xue, J.; Chandra, D.; Leader, J.K.; Gibson, K.F.; Kaminski, N.; et al. C-X-C motif chemokine 13 (CXCL13) is a prognostic biomarker of idiopathic pulmonary fibrosis. *Am. J. Respir. Crit. Care Med.* **2014**, *189*, 966–974. [CrossRef]
23. Yang, Y.; Shen, C.; Li, J.; Yuan, J.; Wei, J.; Huang, F.; Wang, F.; Li, G.; Li, Y.; Xing, L.; et al. Plasma IP-10 and MCP-3 levels are highly associated with disease severity and predict the progression of COVID-19. *J. Allergy Clin. Immunol.* **2020**, *146*, 119–127.e4. [CrossRef] [PubMed]
24. Neighbors, M.; Cabanski, C.R.; Ramalingam, T.R.; Sheng, X.R.; Tew, G.W.; Gu, C.; Jia, G.; Peng, K.; Ray, J.M.; Ley, B.; et al. Prognostic and predictive biomarkers for patients with idiopathic pulmonary fibrosis treated with pirfenidone: Post-hoc assessment of the CAPACITY and ASCEND trials. *Lancet Respir. Med.* **2018**, *6*, 615–626. [CrossRef]
25. Force, A.D.T.; Ranieri, V.M.; Rubenfeld, G.D.; Thompson, B.T.; Ferguson, N.D.; Caldwell, E.; Fan, E.; Camporota, L.; Slutsky, A.S. Acute respiratory distress syndrome: The Berlin Definition. *JAMA* **2012**, *307*, 2526–2533. [CrossRef]
26. Raghu, G.; Rochwerg, B.; Zhang, Y.; Garcia, C.A.; Azuma, A.; Behr, J.; Brozek, J.L.; Collard, H.R.; Cunningham, W.; Homma, S.; et al. An Official ATS/ERS/JRS/ALAT Clinical Practice Guideline: Treatment of Idiopathic Pulmonary Fibrosis. An Update of the 2011 Clinical Practice Guideline. *Am. J. Respir. Crit. Care Med.* **2015**, *192*, e3–e19. [CrossRef]
27. Bankhead, P.; Loughrey, M.B.; Fernandez, J.A.; Dombrowski, Y.; McArt, D.G.; Dunne, P.D.; McQuaid, S.; Gray, R.T.; Murray, L.J.; Coleman, H.G.; et al. QuPath: Open source software for digital pathology image analysis. *Sci. Rep.* **2017**, *7*, 16878. [CrossRef] [PubMed]
28. Kalafatis, D.; Lofdahl, A.; Nasman, P.; Dellgren, G.; Wheelock, A.M.; Elowsson Rendin, L.; Skold, M.; Westergren-Thorsson, G. Distal Lung Microenvironment Triggers Release of Mediators Recognized as Potential Systemic Biomarkers for Idiopathic Pulmonary Fibrosis. *Int. J. Mol. Sci.* **2021**, *22*, 3421. [CrossRef] [PubMed]
29. Todd, J.L.; Vinisko, R.; Liu, Y.; Neely, M.L.; Overton, R.; Flaherty, K.R.; Noth, I.; Newby, L.K.; Lasky, J.A.; Olman, M.A.; et al. Circulating matrix metalloproteinases and tissue metalloproteinase inhibitors in patients with idiopathic pulmonary fibrosis in the multicenter IPF-PRO Registry cohort. *BMC Pulm. Med.* **2020**, *20*, 64. [CrossRef]
30. Oikonomou, N.; Harokopos, V.; Zalevsky, J.; Valavanis, C.; Kotanidou, A.; Szymkowski, D.E.; Kollias, G.; Aidinis, V. Soluble TNF mediates the transition from pulmonary inflammation to fibrosis. *PLoS ONE* **2006**, *1*, e108. [CrossRef] [PubMed]
31. Iosef, C.; Knauer, M.J.; Nicholson, M.; Van Nynatten, L.R.; Cepinskas, G.; Draghici, S.; Han, V.K.M.; Fraser, D.D. Plasma proteome of Long-COVID patients indicates HIF-mediated vasculo-proliferative disease with impact on brain and heart function. *J. Transl. Med.* **2023**, *21*, 377. [CrossRef]
32. Nanri, Y.; Nunomura, S.; Terasaki, Y.; Yoshihara, T.; Hirano, Y.; Yokosaki, Y.; Yamaguchi, Y.; Feghali-Bostwick, C.; Ajito, K.; Murakami, S.; et al. Cross-Talk between Transforming Growth Factor-beta and Periostin Can Be Targeted for Pulmonary Fibrosis. *Am. J. Respir. Cell Mol. Biol.* **2020**, *62*, 204–216. [CrossRef] [PubMed]
33. Zeng, H.L.; Chen, D.; Yan, J.; Yang, Q.; Han, Q.Q.; Li, S.S.; Cheng, L. Proteomic characteristics of bronchoalveolar lavage fluid in critical COVID-19 patients. *FEBS J.* **2021**, *288*, 5190–5200. [CrossRef] [PubMed]
34. Deng, L.; Huang, T.; Zhang, L. T cells in idiopathic pulmonary fibrosis: Crucial but controversial. *Cell Death Discov.* **2023**, *9*, 62. [CrossRef] [PubMed]
35. Perrotta, F.; Matera, M.G.; Cazzola, M.; Bianco, A. Severe respiratory SARS-CoV2 infection: Does ACE2 receptor matter? *Respir. Med.* **2020**, *168*, 105996. [CrossRef] [PubMed]
36. Smadja, D.M.; Philippe, A.; Bory, O.; Gendron, N.; Beauvais, A.; Gruest, M.; Peron, N.; Khider, L.; Guerin, C.L.; Goudot, G.; et al. Placental growth factor level in plasma predicts COVID-19 severity and in-hospital mortality. *J. Thromb. Haemost.* **2021**, *19*, 1823–1830. [CrossRef] [PubMed]
37. Cilli, A.; Hanta, I.; Uzer, F.; Coskun, F.; Sevinc, C.; Deniz, P.P.; Parlak, M.; Altunok, E.; Tertemiz, K.C.; Ursavas, A. Characteristics and outcomes of COVID-19 patients with IPF: A multi-center retrospective study. *Respir. Med. Res.* **2022**, *81*, 100900. [CrossRef]
38. Guo, L.; Chen, Q.; Xu, M.; Huang, J.; Ye, H. Communication between alveolar macrophages and fibroblasts via the TNFSF12-TNFRSF12A pathway promotes pulmonary fibrosis in severe COVID-19 patients. *J. Transl. Med.* **2024**, *22*, 698. [CrossRef]
39. Bellamri, N.; Viel, R.; Morzadec, C.; Lecureur, V.; Joannes, A.; de Latour, B.; Llamas-Gutierrez, F.; Wollin, L.; Jouneau, S.; Vernhet, L. TNF-alpha and IL-10 Control CXCL13 Expression in Human Macrophages. *J. Immunol.* **2020**, *204*, 2492–2502. [CrossRef]
40. Stewart, I.; Jacob, J.; George, P.M.; Molyneaux, P.L.; Porter, J.C.; Allen, R.J.; Aslani, S.; Baillie, J.K.; Barratt, S.L.; Beirne, P.; et al. Residual Lung Abnormalities after COVID-19 Hospitalization: Interim Analysis of the UKILD Post-COVID-19 Study. *Am. J. Respir. Crit. Care Med.* **2023**, *207*, 693–703. [CrossRef] [PubMed]

Disclaimer/Publisher's Note: The statements, opinions and data contained in all publications are solely those of the individual author(s) and contributor(s) and not of MDPI and/or the editor(s). MDPI and/or the editor(s) disclaim responsibility for any injury to people or property resulting from any ideas, methods, instructions or products referred to in the content.

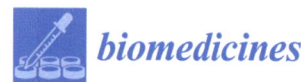

Article

Persistent Health and Cognitive Impairments up to Four Years Post-COVID-19 in Young Students: The Impact of Virus Variants and Vaccination Timing

Ashkan Latifi and Jaroslav Flegr *

Laboratory of Evolutionary Biology, Department of Philosophy and History of Sciences, Faculty of Science, Charles University, Viničná 7, 128 00 Prague, Czech Republic; ashkan.latify@gmail.com
* Correspondence: flegr@cesnet.cz

Abstract: Background: The long-term consequences of COVID-19 infection are becoming increasingly evident in recent studies. This repeated cross-sectional study aimed to explore the long-term health and cognitive effects of COVID-19, focusing on how virus variants, vaccination, illness severity, and time since infection impact post-COVID-19 outcomes. **Methods:** We examined three cohorts of university students ($N = 584$) and used non-parametric methods to assess correlations of various health and cognitive variables with SARS-CoV-2 infection, COVID-19 severity, vaccination status, time since infection, time since vaccination, and virus variants. **Results:** Our results suggest that some health and cognitive impairments may persist, with some even appearing to progressively worsen—particularly fatigue in women and memory in men—up to four years post-infection. The data further indicate that the ancestral SARS-CoV-2 variant may have the most significant long-term impact, while the Omicron variant appears to have the least. Interestingly, the severity of the acute illness was not correlated with the variant of SARS-CoV-2. The analysis also revealed that individuals who contracted COVID-19 after vaccination had better health and cognitive outcomes compared to those infected before vaccination. **Conclusions**: Overall, our results indicate that even in young individuals who predominantly experienced only mild forms of the infection, a gradual decline in health and fitness can occur over a span of four years post-infection. Notably, some negative trends—at least in men—only began to stabilize or even reverse during the fourth year, whereas in women, these trends showed no such improvement. These findings suggest that the long-term public health impacts of COVID-19 may be more severe and affect a much broader population than is commonly assumed.

Keywords: SARS-CoV-2; cognition; mental health; long-term effects; long COVID

1. Introduction

The start of COVID-19, associated with a new coronavirus (SARS-CoV-2) found in Wuhan, China, occurred in late 2019, resulting in a worldwide pandemic [1,2]. While the acute effects of the virus were extensively studied in earlier phases of the pandemic, increasing evidence now highlights the potential for long-term impacts even after recovery. These impacts, commonly known as 'long COVID' or post-acute sequelae of SARS-CoV-2 infection, can manifest as a range of physical, neurological, and psychological symptoms [3,4]. Research has indicated that certain individuals may suffer a decrease in lung function or develop pulmonary fibrosis following recovery from COVID-19 [5]. In this respect, a study investigating the post-recovery results of 587,330 patients admitted to hospitals in the United States, of whom 257,075 had COVID-19 and 330,255 were not infected with the virus, found that among the patients, there were 10,979 cases of heart failure within a 367-day period after discharge. COVID-19 hospitalization led to a 45% increased risk of developing heart failure, particularly in younger patients, white individuals, and those with a prior history of heart conditions [6]. Similarly, a recent study of healthcare workers in Italy identified the severity of acute COVID-19, early pandemic waves (ancestral SARS-CoV-2 and Alpha variants), and prolonged viral shedding time as significant risk factors for long COVID-19. This study also highlighted that the prevalence of long COVID-19 decreased with subsequent infections and was lower during the Omicron wave, likely due to increased immunity and milder strains [7].

In a community-based cross-sectional study in China, researchers presented results for 1000 individuals who survived COVID-19 20 months after being diagnosed. These COVID-19 survivors were recruited from the communities in Hongshan district, Wuhan City, Hubei Province, from 12 October to 19 November 2021. The most commonly reported symptoms were aspecific (fatigue, joint pain, hair loss, sweating, myalgia, skin rash, and chill) (60.7%), mental (48.3%), cardio-pulmonary (39.8%), neurological (37.1%, including cognitive impairment in 15.6% of cases), and digestive (19.1%) symptoms [8]. A meta-analysis of 29 peer-reviewed studies and 4 preprints, published up until 20 March 2021, encompassing a sample of 15,244 hospitalized and 9011 non-hospitalized patients, revealed that 63.2%, 71.9%, and 45.9% of the sample exhibited at least one post-COVID-19 symptom 30, 60, or 90 days after the onset of illness or hospitalization. The most prevalent symptoms were fatigue and dyspnea. Additional reported post-COVID-19 symptoms included cough (20–25%), anosmia (10–20%), ageusia (15–20%), and joint pain (15–20%). Time trend analysis showed a decrease in symptom prevalence measured on day 30, followed by an increase measured on day 60 [9]. In this respect, a recent study, which conducted an online survey in South Korea between January and May 2022, surveyed 111 COVID-19 and 189 non-COVID-19 patients aged over 55, using tools like PRMQ, SMCQ, ISI (ISI-K), and WHOQOL-BREF (YLP-BREF). COVID-19 significantly impacted memory, physical activity, diet, depression, insomnia, and quality of life, but not anxiety, COVID-19 fear, or activity participation, highlighting critical differences between the groups [10].

Post-COVID-19 symptoms also encompass cognitive impairment and mental health deterioration. For instance, a large online survey of 4445 participants investigating the impact of SARS-CoV-2 infection, COVID-19 severity, and vaccination on health and cognition found that both infection with and the severity of COVID-19 had negative effects on patients' health. Additionally, a correlation was observed between COVID-19 severity and various cognitive functions. Specifically, the severity of COVID-19 negatively impacted health and fatigue at the time of the study and had a significant adverse effect on intelligence and negative trends with memory, precision, and performance on the Stroop test [11]. A large-scale study of 81,337 participants in Britain also reported that individuals recovered from COVID-19, regardless of symptom presence, showed significant cognitive deficits in domains such as reasoning, problem solving, spatial planning, and target detection compared to controls after adjusting for various demographic and health factors. Hospitalized patients ($N = 192$) exhibited substantial deficits, as did non-hospitalized individuals with confirmed infections ($N = 326$). Analysis indicated that these cognitive differences were not pre-existing [12]. Another study, recruiting 475 participants (mean age 58.26) who were followed 2–3 years post-hospitalization, indicated that cognitive scores were significantly lower than expected across all domains assessed by the Montreal Cognitive Assessment—memory, executive functioning, attention, language, visuospatial skills, and orientation—with most participants reporting mild to severe depression, anxiety, fatigue, or cognitive decline. Symptoms worsened over time, and severity at 6 months strongly predicted outcomes at 2–3 years. Occupational changes were reported by 26.9% of participants, largely due to health issues, and were closely linked to cognitive deficits [13]. A recent systematic review of 16 studies (from 502 retrieved) examining COVID-19's impact on working memory in patients without prior cognitive impairment also showed 22.5–55% experienced acute-phase impairment, with 6.2–10% still affected at six months. Factors influencing impairment included age, time since infection, and severity. Neuroinflammation, viral invasiveness, and brain structural changes were implicated, and concomitant symptoms often persisted long-term [14]

The effects of COVID-19 on young individuals after recovery can also include physical, cognitive, and psychological symptoms. Research indicates that some young subjects experience lingering symptoms which can include fatigue, cognitive difficulties, and respiratory issues even months after recovery [15]. A study of individuals from the Swedish birth cohort BAMSE (average age: 26.5 years) investigated post-COVID-19 symptoms, defined as those persisting for at least 2 months following confirmed infection. Altered smell and taste were the most frequent post-COVID-19 symptoms, followed by dyspnea and fatigue [16]. Another recent study assessing COVID-19's effects on the physical and mental health, fatigue, and cognitive skills of a sample of 214 students averaging 21.8 years old showed that contracting COVID-19 was associated with a higher frequency of fatigue reports [17]. In addition, the disease's impact on physical health, mental well-being, fatigue, and reaction time was moderated by severity. In the first 24 months following the infection, improvements in both physical and mental well-being were observed, along with a reduction in the frequency of errors in attention-demanding tests. However, there was a tendency towards a decline in reaction time and fatigue. By the second year, physical health and error rates improved, but fatigue and reaction times continued their ongoing decline, and mental health began to deteriorate.

More importantly, a meta-analysis of 55 studies involving 1,139,299 participants provided a broader view of post-COVID-19 conditions. This study found more than two hundred symptoms linked to this condition, with gastrointestinal issues, headaches, cough, and fever being the most common, respectively. From these studies, 21 symptoms reported in 11 studies were identified as suitable for inclusion in the meta-analysis, and their subsequent analysis revealed significantly higher pooled estimates for symptoms such as altered or lost smell or taste, dyspnea, fatigue, and myalgia in children and young people who had confirmed SARS-CoV-2 infections. The meta-analysis concluded that many children and young people experience persistent symptoms after SARS-CoV-2 infection [18]. Nonetheless, it should be noted that some studies suggest that ongoing symptoms and impairments in post-COVID-19 conditions may be influenced by factors beyond the virus itself, particularly psychosocial aspects of pre-existing psychological conditions [19]. For example, a study highlighted that pre-existing psychological conditions, such as depression and anxiety, are significant risk factors for persistent symptoms, including psychiatric and neurological complaints, as well as reduced work ability long after COVID-19 recovery [20].

It should be noted that many earlier studies have focused on a limited timeframe shortly after recovery from COVID-19 or overlooked the specific variant involved (see [21–23]). Extending the duration of observation, however, allows researchers to better track the potential long-term effects of post-COVID-19 infection on health and performance. The current article aimed to address these gaps along with the other objectives listed below.

Aims and Scope of This Study

The primary aim of this study was to determine whether the trends observed in a previous, smaller-scale study (which included a sample size three times smaller and covered a shorter duration post-COVID-19 infection, specifically up to 39 months) continued into the fourth year after the initial illness (covering up to 54 months post-infection). The second objective was to rule out the possibility that the observed correlations between certain health- and performance-related variables and the time since infection were merely artifacts of the different virus variants, which emerged in distinct waves before the start of this study. The third aim of this study was to obtain a sufficiently large sample size to allow for the analysis of not only the impact of COVID-19 but also the effects of vaccination against COVID-19 and the duration since vaccination on health- and performance-related variables. A large sample size was essential to ensure adequate representation of the unvaccinated minority, comprising only about 5% of the student population, allowing for meaningful comparisons between vaccinated and unvaccinated groups.

To achieve these objectives in our cross-sectional study, we conducted tests on nearly 300 participants enrolled in an undergraduate evolutionary biology course each year for three consecutive years, consistently during the same month (January). The same panel of performance tests was administered, and data on current health status, details about their COVID-19 illness, and vaccination history were collected through a consistent electronic questionnaire. The collected data were analyzed using multivariate non-parametric methods, a choice informed by the statistical characteristics of the data. The findings, including those that may seem counterintuitive, are discussed considering the specifics of cross-sectional studies.

2. Materials and Methods

2.1. Study Participants

Over three consecutive years (2022, 2023, and 2024), always in the second week of January, all students enrolled in the basic course in evolutionary biology were invited to take part in an anonymous online study. However, it should be noted that the questionnaires were designed during the summer of 2021, and the protocol was approved by the IRB in the fall of 2021. This timing relatively limited the scope of the questions in accordance with the knowledge of COVID-19's probable long-term effects available at that time. Before beginning the survey, participants were informed about the general goals of this study—examining specific hypotheses in evolutionary psychology and investigating the influence of various factors on cognitive performance. We included all students who provided their age and sex at birth, answered questions related to COVID-19 and health, and completed at least one of the cognition tests. The questionnaire distribution method excluded individuals who did not provide informed consent to participate in this study by clicking the appropriate button on the electronic form, as well as students who did not have proficiency in the Czech language.

The students were assured that their participation was voluntary and that the data would be used solely for scientific purposes, with no means of identifying individual participants. They were also informed that they could withdraw from this study at any time simply by closing the survey page.

Both the examination and the subsequent survey were conducted separately on the Qualtrics platform. After completing the exam, students were notified of their scores, specifically the number of correct answers, and were asked to report this number in the anonymous survey.

This study adhered to the ethical guidelines relevant to research involving human participants. The project's protocol, participant recruitment methods, including the scope and generality of information provided to participants before this study, and the method of obtaining informed consent (achieved by clicking a designated button on the screen), received approval from the Institutional Review Board of the Faculty of Science at Charles University (No. 2021/19).

2.2. Questionnaires and Tests

In this survey, we assessed participants' intelligence using the Cattell 16PF test (Variant A, Scale B) [24]. Memory abilities, including free recall and recognition memory, were evaluated using a modified Meili test [25,26]. Psychomotor skills, particularly reaction time and precision, were measured using the Choice Reaction Time Test and the Stroop Test, with both reaction time and accuracy recorded. Detailed descriptions of these tests are available elsewhere [17]. The 'Reading Time' variable was calculated as the average Z-score of the times taken to read instructions for the included tests. For each individual, the 'Accuracy Score' was calculated as the mean of the Z-scores of the number of correct answers in the four tests: Evolutionary Biology, IQ, Choice Reaction Time, and Stroop test. The 'Reaction Time Score' was determined as the mean Z-score of Reading Time and reaction times recorded during the Choice Reaction Time test and Stroop test, while the 'Memory Score' was calculated as the mean Z-score of the two memory tests.

In the anamnestic section of the questionnaire, participants answered 21 questions regarding their physical health. These questions addressed the frequency of conditions such as allergies, skin disorders, cardiovascular diseases, digestive tract disorders, metabolic disorders, common infectious diseases, orthopedic disorders, neurological disorders, headaches, physical pains, and other chronic physical issues. Participants also provided information on how often they had taken antibiotics in the previous three years, their frequency of visits to a general practitioner, and the number of times they had been hospitalized for more than a week in the past five years. Responses to these questions were recorded on a 6-point Likert scale ranging from 'never' to 'daily or more frequently'. Additionally, they reported the number of non-mental health medications currently prescribed by a doctor, with options ranging from 0 to 7, where 7 indicated six or more medications. At the start and end of the questionnaire, participants rated their current and usual physical well-being using 6-point scales. Finally, participants were asked to estimate their life expectancy, with six response options ranging from 'more than 99 years' to 'less than 60 years'. They also provided information on their usual blood pressure, selecting from five options ('very low', 'rather low', 'normal", 'rather high', and 'very high'). No participant selected 'very high', so we used these responses to calculate two binary variables: low blood pressure and high blood pressure. For the exact wording of all questions, refer to the questionnaire text attached to the pre-registration form (https://doi.org/10.17605/OSF.IO/M5FYC, accessed on 27 December 2024).

For health-related questions, certain responses were reversed so that higher scores consistently indicated poorer health, allowing for a standardized interpretation of the results. Then, a physical sickness index score was calculated using the mean Z-scores of all relevant questions [27]. Similarly, a mental sickness score was derived from questions related to nine variables, including frequencies of depression, anxiety, other mental health issues, the number of prescribed mental health medications, and assessments of the participant's current and usual mental states. The latter two questions were posed at both the beginning and end of the questionnaire.

Participants were also asked to rate the frequency of fatigue using a 6-point scale ranging from 'never' to 'daily or several times a day', resulting in the variable Fatigue. Additionally, the survey collected demographic and medical history data, including participants' age and official sex as listed on their birth certificates (with men coded as 1 and women as 0). At the end of the questionnaire, participants were queried about their history of SARS-CoV-2 infection. Responses to COVID-19 status were categorized as follows: 'not yet', 'no but I was in quarantine', 'yes, I was diagnosed with COVID-19', 'probably yes, but I was not diagnosed with COVID-19', and 'I am waiting for the result of a diagnostic test'.

Those who confirmed a COVID-19 diagnosis were asked to rate the severity of their illness on a 6-point scale, with 1 being 'no symptoms' and 6 being 'I was in ICU'.

All participants provided information about their vaccination status, the date of their most severe COVID-19 episode, and the date of their last vaccination. These dates were used to calculate the time since the onset of COVID-19, the time since the last vaccination, and the binary variable COVID-19 after vaccination. Based on the dates of the waves of COVID-19 outbreaks in Czechia (see [28]) and the participants' date of infection, the likely variant of SARS-CoV-2 was estimated for most participants and encoded into four binary dummy variables: ancestral SARS-CoV-2 variant, Alpha, Delta, and Omicron (for more information on the codes see Supplementary Table S1).

2.3. Data Analysis

To mitigate potential complications arising from the irregular distribution of some dependent variables and partly to avoid some of the issues associated with an imbalanced dataset—with a two-to-one ratio of women to men and vaccinated individuals outnumbering unvaccinated ones by more than tenfold—we employed a non-parametric multivariate analytical method, specifically the partial Kendall correlation controlled for age, sex, and survey year, to examine the relationships between variables related to COVID-19 (such as infection status, severity of COVID-19 infection, time elapsed since infection, vaccination status, time since the last vaccination, and occurrences of COVID-19 post-vaccination) and health and cognitive performance indicators. In analyses specific to sex, only age and survey year were controlled. The partial Kendall correlation offers several advantages that make it particularly suitable for this study. Being an exact test, it enables precise significance calculations even in cases where some groups contain very few observations, such as unvaccinated men. Additionally, its ability to analyze associations between binary, ordinal, and continuous variables simplifies the analytical process. This avoids the need for multiple distinct methods, thereby enhancing the clarity and consistency of the results presentation.

Furthermore, the partial Kendall correlation can control for the effects of virtually any number of covariates of various types (nominal categorical via dummy coding, ordinal as ranks, and continuous variables directly) if a sufficiently powerful computational setup is available. While the test is theoretically less sensitive than parametric methods due to its reliance on variable ranks rather than raw values, it performs comparably well with real-world biological data, which seldom adhere to a Gaussian distribution. This combination of precision, versatility, and robust performance with non-normally distributed data makes partial Kendall correlation an optimal choice for addressing the analytical challenges posed by our dataset.

The correlational analysis was conducted using the Explorer v. 1.0 R script [29], leveraging the ppcor R package v. 1.1 [30].

To correct for multiple comparisons, we applied the Benjamini–Hochberg correction for multiple testing with a false discovery rate (FDR) set at 0.10 [31]. This correction was performed only for the main seven variables (physical health issues, mental health issues, fatigue, intelligence, memory, reactions, accuracy), not for post hoc tests exploring the sources of observed associations. In addition, due to the issue of normality, we employed the Wilcoxon rank-sum test to compare the frequency, age, and the time elapsed since infection between men and women in the dataset. The dataset for this study is publicly accessible on Figshare 10.6084/m9.figshare.27618876 [32].

Technical Notes: In this article, the term 'effect' is used in its statistical sense, referring to the difference between the true population parameter and the null hypothesis value. Causal interpretations are only discussed in the Discussion section. Given the exploratory nature of a large part of this study, we also consider trends that did not reach statistical significance.

3. Results

3.1. Descriptive Statistics

The initial dataset comprised 724 individuals, 520 women (71.8%, average age = 21.54, SD = 2.36) and 204 men (28.2%; average age = 21.50; SD = 2.13). Among the women, 169 (36.18%) reported not having been diagnosed with COVID-19, 210 (45.0%) had a confirmed laboratory diagnosis of COVID-19, 52 (11.1%) believed they had contracted the virus but lacked laboratory confirmation, and 36 (7.7%) reported not having COVID-19 but were quarantined. Among the men, 61 (32.4%) reported not having been diagnosed with COVID-19, 85 (45.2%) had a confirmed laboratory diagnosis, 19 (10.1%) believed they had contracted the virus but lacked laboratory confirmation, and 23 (12.2%) reported not having COVID-19 but were quarantined. No students reported awaiting test results.

From the final dataset, we excluded 52 individuals who stated they might have had COVID-19 but lacked laboratory confirmation, 156 individuals who did not respond to COVID-19-related questions, and 4 individuals who provided unreliable data, such as reporting an age over 90 or giving identical responses to most questions. The final sample included 584 participants: 415 women (49.4% COVID-19-negative, 50.6% COVID-19-positive) and 169 men (49.7% COVID-19-negative, 50.3% COVID-19-positive). There was no significant difference in the incidence of COVID-19 between men and women ($Chi^2_{(1)}$ = 0.004; p = 0.946). The ages of the women and men were similar (21.58, SD 2.36 vs. 21.51, SD 2.02; W = 33945; p = 0.624). Similarly, there was no significant age difference between uninfected and infected individuals (21.59, SD 1.99 vs. 21.53 SD 2.51; W = 44699; p = 0.200).

A significant majority of the students were vaccinated against COVID-19, with the last vaccination occurring on average 12.38 months prior and at most 50.8 months prior. Among 409 women who responded to this question, 34 (8.3%) were not vaccinated; among 165 men, only 7 (4.2%) were unvaccinated; however, this difference was not statistically significant ($Chi^2_{(1)}$ = 2.93; p = 0.086). Of the 100 vaccinated women who had COVID-19, 29 (29.0%) contracted the virus after their last vaccination; among 49 men, this was the case for 17 (34.7%), ($Chi^2_{(1)}$ = 0.499; p = 0.479).

On average, women contracted COVID-19 24.39 months prior (SD = 14.32; maximum 54.58), and men 21.68 months prior (SD 13.97; maximum = 52.61). In this respect, there was no significant difference between these two groups (W = 0.5368; p = 0.261). Among the 282 individuals diagnosed with COVID-19, 26 (9.22%) reported 'No symptoms', 94 (33.33%) described it as 'Like mild flu', another 106 (37.58%) as 'Like normal flu', and 52 (18.44%) as 'Like severe flu'; 4 (1.41%) were hospitalized. None reported being treated in the Intensive Care Unit (ICU). The distribution of responses regarding the severity of COVID-19 did not differ between men and women ($Chi^2_{(4)}$ = 1.47; p = 0.831). In contrast, the long-term impact of COVID-19 on health and performance, particularly the dynamics of these changes over time, differed by sex (see below). Accordingly, all relevant analyses were stratified by sex, and descriptive statistics (Table 1 and Supplementary Table S1) were presented separately for men and women.

Table 1. Descriptive statistics of health and cognitive performance-related indices by sex.

	Mean		N		Standard Deviation	
	Women	Men	Women	Men	Women	Men
Physical Health Issues	0.05	−0.13	415	169	0.45	0.39
Mental Health Issues	0.08	−0.20	415	169	0.67	0.60
Fatigue	4.56	4.23	412	166	1.11	1.23
Intelligence	9.28	9.63	405	164	1.47	1.38

Table 1. Cont.

	Mean		N		Standard Deviation	
	Women	Men	Women	Men	Women	Men
Memory	−0.02	−0.30	413	168	1.03	0.95
Reactions	0.00	0.00	415	169	0.65	0.64
Accuracy	−0.03	0.08	415	169	0.57	0.50

Except for fatigue and intelligence, other indices were calculated as mean Z-scores.

3.2. Confirmation Statistics—Associations of COVID-19-Related Variables with Health and Cognition Issues

In the confirmatory part of the study, we aimed to test the following H_0 hypotheses:

H1: *Trends in health and cognitive performance impairments do not persist into the fourth year after infection.*

H2: *The observed trends over time are artifacts caused by the gradual replacement of more virulent strains with less and less virulent variants of SARS-CoV-2.*

H3: *There is no difference in health and cognitive performance between individuals vaccinated before or after contracting COVID-19.*

H4: *Neither the health nor cognitive performance of participants changes with the time elapsed since vaccination.*

Age and especially sex significantly impacted some health- and performance-related variables. Consequently, we used a partial Kendall correlation, controlling for age, sex, and the survey year, to investigate the effects of COVID-19-related variables on health and performance outcomes (Table 2). The partial correlations between health and performance outcomes associated with different variants of SARS-CoV-2 are presented separately (Table 3).

Table 2. Correlations between health- and performance-related variables and COVID-19-related variables controlled for age, sex, and survey year (all subjects).

	Infected	Course	Months Since Infection	Vaccination	Months Since Vaccination	COVID-19 After Vaccination	Age	Sex
Physical Health Issues	0.012	**0.211**	0.013	**0.062**	0.013	−0.012	0.012	**0.163**
Mental Health Issues	−0.049	0.066	−0.045	0.048	−0.015	−0.025	0.036	**0.162**
Fatigue	−0.042	**0.093**	0.044	**0.089**	0.036	−0.005	−0.005	**0.097**
Intelligence	0.021	−0.057	−0.071	−0.044	0.005	**0.171**	−0.021	**−0.099**
Memory	0.045	−0.010	−0.053	−0.039	−0.011	0.029	**−0.055**	**0.111**
Reactions	0.029	0.029	0.036	**−0.075**	0.027	−0.067	−0.009	0.020
Accuracy	0.001	**−0.082**	−0.025	−0.015	0.051	**0.194**	−0.053	**−0.096**
				p-values				
Physical Health Issues	0.655	0.000	0.769	0.026	0.707	0.828	0.672	0.000
Mental Health Issues	0.079	0.101	0.298	0.084	0.670	0.653	0.191	0.000
Fatigue	0.128	0.021	0.313	0.002	0.314	0.931	0.846	0.001
Intelligence	0.451	0.161	0.106	0.122	0.887	0.002	0.451	0.000
Memory	0.108	0.809	0.227	0.167	0.757	0.612	0.048	0.000
Reactions	0.302	0.473	0.411	0.007	0.444	0.230	0.744	0.467
Accuracy	0.973	0.041	0.566	0.587	0.145	0.001	0.057	0.001

Significant correlations (Kendall Tau) are presented in bold. The *p*-values that were significant after the application of the Benjamini–Hochberg correction for multiple testing (with FDR set at 0.1) are underlined.

Table 3. Correlations between health- and performance-related variables and SARS-CoV-2 variants controlled for age, sex, and survey year (all subjects).

	Ancestral	Alpha	Delta	Omicron
Physical Health Issues	0.050	−0.024	0.001	−0.029
Mental Health Issues	−0.051	0.018	−0.023	0.052
Fatigue	**0.126**	**−0.103**	−0.062	−0.007
Intelligence	**−0.099**	−0.076	0.018	**0.172**
Memory	**−0.119**	−0.035	0.065	0.068
Reactions	**0.097**	**−0.095**	−0.025	−0.024
Accuracy	−0.023	−0.073	0.010	0.075
	p-values			
Physical Health Issues	0.251	0.585	0.988	0.510
Mental Health Issues	0.245	0.675	0.601	0.237
Fatigue	0.004	0.018	0.159	0.881
Intelligence	0.024	0.083	0.676	0.000
Memory	0.007	0.428	0.141	0.119
Reactions	0.027	0.030	0.565	0.584
Accuracy	0.599	0.093	0.812	0.088

Significant correlations (Kendall Tau) are presented in bold. The *p*-values that were significant after the application of the Benjamini–Hochberg correction for multiple testing (with FDR set at 0.1) are underlined.

Our analysis showed that the severity of COVID-19 was significantly associated with worse physical health, fatigue, and a lower cognitive accuracy. After applying the Benjamini–Hochberg (BH) correction for multiple testing, all of these associations remained significant. COVID-19 vaccination was associated with poorer physical health and increased fatigue but with improved (shorter) reaction times in vaccinated students compared to unvaccinated ones. All of these associations remained significant even after the BH correction. Subjects who contracted COVID-19 after receiving the vaccine showed significantly higher intelligence and accuracy scores than those who contracted COVID-19 before receiving the vaccine. These also remained significant after the BH correction. The analysis of the effects of virus variants revealed that the ancestral SARS-CoV-2 variant had the most adverse effects compared to other variants. This variant correlated with lower scores in the subjects' intelligence and memory and higher scores in their reaction times, which mean worse cognitive performance, and was associated with higher levels of fatigue. These associations remained significant even after applying the BH correction. The Alpha variant demonstrated significant negative associations with fatigue and reaction times, indicating lower levels of fatigue and also shorter (better) reaction times compared to other variants. The Omicron variant exhibited a significant positive association with the subjects' intelligence scores, indicating higher intelligence scores in those infected with this variant. The Delta variant did not have any significantly negative or positive associations with any of these seven variables.

There were no significant associations between the seven index variables and COVID-19 infection, the time elapsed since COVID-19 infection, or the time elapsed since receiving COVID-19 vaccination (see Table 2). The results of separate analyses for women and men are shown in Supplementary Tables S2–S5.

When we included the variable representing the SARS-CoV-2 variant in the model (coded ordinally, with 1 for the earliest variant, the ancestral SARS-CoV-2 variant, and 4 for the most recent variant, Omicron), the results remained unchanged (see Supplementary Tables S6 and S7). This result suggests that the observed patterns of effects and trends and the absence of trends among the predictors were not simply artifacts caused by the replacement of more virulent variants with progressively less virulent ones throughout the course of the pandemic.

Our analyses of the trajectories of the index variables over the time elapsed since COVID-19 infection (almost 54 months) for all participants, and also separately for men and women, indicated that the first-degree linear models had smaller Bayesian Information Criterion (BIC) coefficients compared to those of higher-degree polynomial models. Accordingly, the following section discusses the results based on our first-degree linear models.

The results for all participants showed a noticeable, relatively small decline in memory performance over the time elapsed since infection. In contrast, trends of marginal improvement in mental health issues, accuracy, and intelligence were observed. Fatigue showed the largest increase over the time elapsed since infection. Marginal trends of deterioration in reaction times and physical health were also present (see Figure 1 and Table 2). The results of separate analyses for women and men are shown in Supplementary Figures S1 and S2 and Supplementary Tables S2–S5.

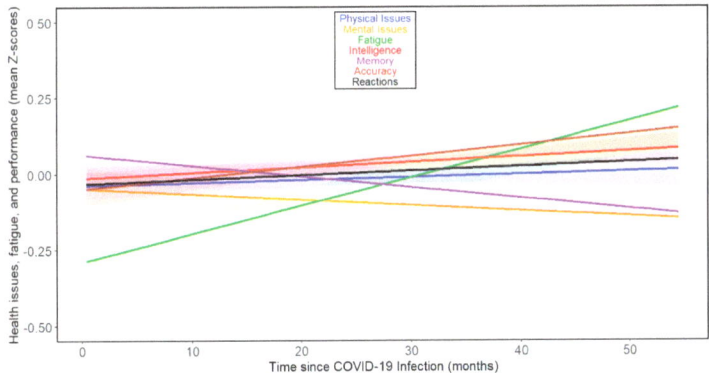

Figure 1. Changes in health- and performance-related variables with time since COVID-19 infection—all participants. Based on the comparison of BIC values, all observed dependencies were best approximated by a first-degree polynomial (a straight line). The shaded areas around the lines indicate 60% confidence intervals. It should be noted that the slopes of the lines on the graph cannot be directly compared with the (more accurate) Tau values calculated using the non-parametric partial Kendall test, which is less sensitive to the presence of outliers and additionally controlled for the influence of 3 confounding variables (sex, age, and year of survey).

The results of the previous study [17] suggested that the direction and rate of changes over time varied during the first two years after infection but likely increased thereafter. Therefore, we repeated the analyses for 111 subjects from 24 months post-infection onwards. Figure 2 and Supplementary Tables S8–S13 show that there were negative associations between months since infection and physical health, mental health, fatigue, intelligence, memory, reaction times, and accuracy during the fourth year after infection in this group, among which the correlation between intelligence and months since infection was significant. Based on the binomial distribution, the probability of obtaining seven correlations indicating adverse relationships out of seven would be 0.008. See Figures S3 and S4 for separate analyses of the trajectories of the seven index variables over time beyond 24 months post-infection for women and men, respectively. When fifty-one participants who were infected at least 36 months before this study were analyzed, the results were more complex (Supplementary Tables S14 and S15). In the whole population, we saw a relative decrease in intelligence (Tau = −0.072), and worsening of reaction times (Tau = 0.093); however, we also saw a clear improvement in accuracy (Tau = 0.125). Analyses split by sex showed that in women, all health- and cognitive performance-related variables except accuracy (Tau = 0.144) and memory (Tau = 0.038) were impaired (physical issues: Tau = 0.077; mental issues: Tau = 0.213; fatigue: Tau = 0.083; intelligence: Tau = −0.079; and reactions: Tau = 0.054). In contrast, in men, all changes except worsening in reaction times (Tau = 0.350) were improvements (physical issues: Tau = −0.328; mental issues: Tau = −0.414; fatigue: Tau = −0.159; intelligence: Tau = 0.129; memory: Tau = 0.314; and accuracy: Tau = 0.060). It must be noted, however, that none of the trends observed in participants infected more than three years ago were statistically significant, and only 15 participants were included in the subset of men (for the correlational analyses split by sex, see Supplementary Tables S16 and S17 for women and S18 and S19 for men, respectively).

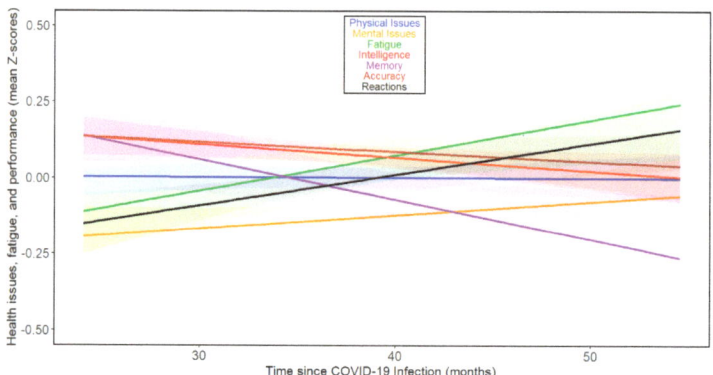

Figure 2. Changes in health- and performance-related variables with time since COVID-19 beyond 24 months post-infection in all participants. For the legend, refer to Figure 1.

When we analyzed the effect of time since vaccination, as opposed to time since COVID-19 infection, we observed rather distinct results (Figure 3). The comparison of results in columns 3 and 5 of Table 2 shows that correlations with time since vaccination were consistently weaker than those with time since COVID-19. In the case of accuracy and intelligence, the correlations even shifted from negative (indicating worsening performance over time) to positive. None of the correlations came anywhere close to the threshold for statistical significance (that is, $p < 0.05$). See Figures S5 and S6 for separate analyses of the trajectories of the seven index variables over the months following vaccination for women and men, respectively.

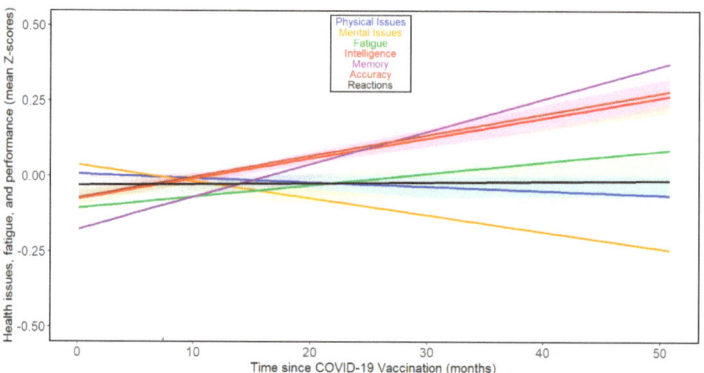

Figure 3. Changes in health- and performance-related variables with time since COVID-19 vaccination in all participants. For the legend, refer to Figure 1.

A summary of the results of the confirmatory part of this study is provided below.

We rejected hypotheses H1 and H3, but we could not reject hypotheses H2 and H4. In other words, our data suggest the following:

(1) The deterioration of certain health and cognitive functions continues even during the fourth year after COVID-19. However, the direction of nonsignificant trends in the subset of 15 men more than three years post-COVID-19 suggested that the deterioration may stop and potentially even reverse, except for intelligence and reaction times, at least in men.

(2) To test hypothesis H2, we also included the confounding factor 'COVID-19 variant' in the model. The results showed that the lack of significant correlations between the outcome variables and the time since infection persisted, even with this factor in the model. However, all nonsignificant trends were markedly weaker when the confounding variable of the virus variant was controlled. In several cases, the corresponding trend even reversed direction. For example, the Tau value characterizing memory decline shifted from -0.053 to 0.006, and in the case of intelligence, from -0.071 to 0.012 (see Supplementary Tables S6 and S7 and compare with Supplementary Tables S20 and S21). Thus, based on our data, we cannot refute hypothesis H2, which posits that the observed nonsignificant trends (the intensification of certain symptoms of impaired health or cognition over time since infection) are artifacts caused by the gradual replacement of more virulent strains with progressively less virulent variants of SARS-CoV-2.

(3) Additionally, individuals who were vaccinated before contracting COVID-19 are in better health and have better cognitive performance than those who received the vaccination only after recovering from COVID-19.

(4) Finally, neither the health nor the cognitive performance of participants changed with the time elapsed since vaccination.

3.3. Exploration Statistics—Association of COVID-19-Related Variables with Primary Health- and Cognition-Related Variables

In this exploratory part of this study, we did not apply corrections for multiple testing [33].

3.3.1. All Participants

Generally, the severity of COVID-19 (course of COVID-19) showed strong, statistically significant positive associations with worse health outcomes and lower cognitive test performance; see Supplementary Tables S20 and S21. These included lower precision in Stroop test performance, higher levels of allergies, skin conditions, digestive issues, infections, neurological problems, headaches, recurrent health issues, overall physical pain, depression, overall psychological problems, higher consumption of psychotropic medication, higher rates of doctor visits, higher use of other types of medication, greater antibiotic intake over the past three years, more frequent hospitalizations in the past five years, and shorter life expectancy.

In contrast, the associations of health and performance with merely having contracted COVID-19 were much less frequent and generally weaker and nonsignificant. Exceptions included a significant negative association with usually feeling mentally miserable, and positive associations with recognition memory, neurological disorders, infections, and the frequency of antibiotic use in the past three years. The last two variables included COVID-19 and the treatment of associated bacterial infections, making their correlation with contracting COVID-19 inevitable. Individuals who had contracted COVID-19 reported generally feeling mentally well.

COVID-19 vaccination demonstrated positive associations with allergies, digestive problems, cardiovascular issues, headaches, recurrent health problems, medication intake, and usually feeling mentally miserable. However, it was associated with shorter (better) simple reaction times.

Individuals who contracted COVID-19 after vaccination exhibited higher scores on the evolutionary biology exam and better Stroop test precision. They also had higher rates of skin conditions, elevated blood pressure, and reported a longer life expectancy compared to those infected before vaccination.

To assess the differences in the effects of various virus variants, we studied the correlations of the output variables with four dummy variables, each indicating whether a person was infected with a specific variant (coded as 1) compared with other variants (coded as 0). Investigating the correlations of the output variables with these dummy variables showed that infection with the ancestral SARS-CoV-2 variant was negatively associated with memory (it had negative associations with both free-recall memory and recognition memory). It was also linked to higher rates of recurrent health problems. Infection with the Alpha variant was associated with worse precision in simple reaction time tests, lower instances of infections, higher rates of orthopedic issues, and a higher tendency to feel mentally miserable. The Delta variant did not show significant associations with the output variables, while the Omicron variant was linked to higher levels of depression and anxiety.

Associations between the studied output variables and the time since infection were weak and sparse, and even weaker were corresponding associations between these variables and time since vaccination.

Results of all analyses remained nearly the same when we also controlled for the time elapsed since infection in addition to age, sex, and survey year (see Supplementary Tables S22 and S23), showcasing that the associations of virus variants with health and cognition were not confounded by this variable.

3.3.2. Women

Investigating the results for women and men separately revealed several statistically significant associations. A comprehensive set of results is presented in Supplementary Tables S2 and S4.

In the female group, the long-term effects of COVID-19 infection were evident in higher rates of allergies, higher susceptibility to infections, a higher number of doctor visits, and an elevated rate of antibiotic consumption over the past three years. Conversely, they expressed lower psychological distress, as indicated by a reduced tendency to usually feel mentally miserable, along with higher memory and word recognition scores. More critically, the severity of COVID-19 was associated with a greater incidence of allergies, skin conditions, digestive issues, infections, neurological problems, and headaches. It also correlated with more frequent physical problems, a higher number of doctor visits, and higher rates of antibiotic use during the past three years, as well as greater medication consumption for both mental and physical health concerns. The analysis for this group also showed that there were negative associations between the time elapsed since infection and both the utilization of psychotropic medications and the number of doctor visits.

COVID-19 vaccination was associated with better performance in simple reaction times tests, higher rates of allergies, cardiovascular issues, orthopedic problems, headaches, medication consumption, a tendency to feel mentally miserable, and shorter life expectancy in the female group. Additionally, there was a positive correlation between the time elapsed since COVID-19 vaccination and higher precision on the Stroop test. Those who contracted COVID-19 after vaccination had higher scores on the evolutionary biology exam and better precision on the Stroop test. They also reported higher rates of skin conditions, infections, neurological problems, and feeling physically miserable, but reported a longer life expectancy.

We also investigated the associations between the four variants of the SARS-CoV-2 virus and the output variables. The analysis showed that infection with the ancestral SARS-CoV-2 variant was associated with more frequent orthopedic problems, overall physical pains, and recurrent health issues. Infection with the Alpha variant was associated with lower simple reaction time precision, lower precision on the Stroop test, fewer skin conditions, lower rates of infections, and reduced levels of medication consumption. Infection with the Delta variant was associated with higher rates of metabolic problems but lower levels of anxiety. And finally, infection with the Omicron variant was associated with lower scores on the evolutionary biology exam, better performance on the Stroop test, lower orthopedic issues, higher levels of depression, higher levels of anxiety, and higher rates of the utilization of medication for mental issue purposes.

3.3.3. Men

Despite the small sample size of men, COVID-19 was significantly associated with worse reading time and more frequent hospitalization over the past five years but lower levels of medication use for mental purposes and overall less frequent other psychological problems. More importantly, the severity of COVID-19 was associated with higher rates of allergies, metabolic problems, recurrent health conditions, overall other physical pains, overall other psychological problems, higher utilization of medications for mental health purposes, a larger number of doctor visits, higher overall medication consumption, higher incidents of hospitalization during the past five years, and worse precision on the Stroop test. The time elapsed since infection did not show any significant correlations with the output variables, but the time since vaccination was associated with reduced levels of depression and lower mental distress at the time of the survey. Those who had contracted COVID-19 after vaccination in this group had lower levels of feeling physically miserable now than those who had contracted COVID-19 before vaccination. COVID-19 vaccination was associated with higher rates of infections, headaches, lower incidents of hospitalizations during the past five years, and lower blood pressure.

Investigating the effects of the four variants of the SARS-CoV-2 virus indicated that infection with the ancestral SARS-CoV-2 variant was associated with worse performance in both memory tests, lower orthopedic issues, and lower anxiety. Infection with Alpha variant was associated with worse performance in the recognition memory task, shorter reading times, higher cardiovascular problems, more orthopedic issues, more headaches, higher rates of doctor visits, and longer life expectancies. Infection with the Delta variant was associated with better performance in both memory tests, lower doctor visits, and lower consumption of medications. Infection with the Omicron variant was associated with better performance on the evolutionary biology exam, lower levels of feeling mentally miserable now, and a negative association with low blood pressure. The aforementioned results concerning the long-term consequences of COVID-19 infection differed from those related to the acute phase of the illness. Supplementary Tables S6 and S7 show that no effect of any SARS-CoV-2 variant on the reported severity of acute COVID-19 was detected.

4. Discussion

The current study employed a design and technical execution similar to our previous research [17]. However, it differed in that the data for this study were collected from participants of a basic-level course in evolutionary biology, which had twice the number of students compared to the advanced course used in the previous study. This larger student population allowed for a more robust sample size. Data collection occurred each time in January instead of May and spanned the years 2022, 2023, and 2024, whereas the previous study was limited to 2022 and 2023. Additionally, the questionnaire used in this study differed slightly from the previous one, with most changes affecting questions unrelated to the core objectives of either study. The current study aimed to determine whether the health and performance trends observed over 39 months post-infection in the previous study persisted mainly in the following 12 months. Furthermore, the current study sought to determine whether these trends were due to increasing time since infection or merely because the time since infection closely correlated with the virus variant a person was infected with. Lastly, the nearly threefold increase in respondents in the new study (584 vs. 214) allowed for the analysis of the impact of vaccination, which only a small number of students had not received (8.3% of women and 4.2% of men).

4.1. Trends in Health and Performance Post-COVID-19

The results showed that some trends reversed, with health and performance parameters beginning to improve, although some negative trends persisted even 51 months post-COVID-19. This was particularly evident in the higher levels of fatigue among both men and women. At least in men, there was a continued decline in physical health. While previous data from a smaller dataset suggested that the direction of ongoing changes varied over time, the new, more extensive data indicated that the trends were likely linear, as the relevant data points were best fitted by a first-degree polynomial, a straight line. Even so, beyond three years post-COVID-19 infection, mental health, memory, intelligence, fatigue, reaction times, and accuracy deteriorated further; however, physical health remained relatively constant. When men who had been infected more than 3 years prior were analyzed separately, it appeared that the negative trends were finally beginning to reverse. However, given the small number of these men (15), this result should be interpreted with caution, and it will certainly need to be confirmed in a larger sample.

In our study, we interpreted the observed trends of performance decline over time since infection as either a result of the gradual accumulation of the infection's negative effects or, alternatively, as the replacement of more virulent strains by less virulent ones over the course of the epidemic. However, due to the design of this study, all participants were approximately 21.5 years old. As a result, the time since infection negatively correlated with the age at which each participant contracted COVID-19. It is therefore possible that the poorer health and cognitive performance in individuals who had COVID-19 longer ago could be related to the fact that they were younger at the time of infection, and their bodies, particularly their brains, were more susceptible to the negative effects of the illness. Recent studies in part corroborate this suggestion and warrant further research [34,35].

4.2. Impact of SARS-CoV-2 Variants

Our study confirmed that the SARS-CoV-2 variant affected the variables studied, similar to findings by [36,37]. Similar to the study by Cegelon et al. [7], our study also demonstrated that the ancestral SARS-CoV-2 variant had the most severe long-term consequences, while the Omicron variant had the mildest. However, these studies focused mainly on physical health variables or case fatality rates, whereas our research examined a broader range of health and cognitive outcomes. Specifically, Torabi et al. almost exclusively focused on physical health variables such as myalgia, cough, taste/smell disorder, diarrhea, etc., and investigated the personal characteristics, symptoms, and underlying conditions of individuals infected with different variants of SARS-CoV-2 over a period of two years, while Xia et al. concentrated on the case fatality rates of the variants of this virus during the epidemic periods by continents. In our study, the observed associations between the studied dependent variables and the dummy variables representing the different virus variants did not change when the time since infection was included as a covariate in Kendall's partial correlation tests, save for the removal of the effects of the ancestral SARS-CoV-2 variant on the three variables related to intelligence, reactions, and memory. This indicates that the observed differences are primarily driven by the specific virus variant present at the time of infection, rather than the time elapsed since infection. Conversely, the noticeable changes in the model outputs after controlling for the ordinal virus variant variable suggest that the trends—namely, the weakening or intensifying of symptoms over time since infection—could be driven by differences in the virulence levels of the virus variants contracted at different times.

Our data do not clarify whether the more pronounced symptoms associated with the ancestral SARS-CoV-2 variant are due to its inherent properties or the fact that, during its spread, there was no vaccine available in the Czech Republic, leading to all patients infected with this variant being unvaccinated. However, the absence of vaccination cannot fully account for these differences, as most students infected with the Alpha variant also had not been vaccinated, given that the vaccination of young, low-risk individuals in the Czech Republic began only in the summer months of 2021, i.e., after the Alpha variant wave had passed. This suggests that factors beyond vaccination status likely contributed to the differences in symptoms between the ancestral SARS-CoV-2 variant and other variants. An unexpected result of this study is that the observed differences between the virus variants were limited to the long-term consequences of COVID-19 and had no measurable effect on the severity of the acute phase of the illness.

When discussing the varying effects of different virus variants, it is important to reiterate that our study was conducted on a young student population, where the illness generally presented mildly, as evidenced by the fact that only four students (0.7%) required hospitalization due to COVID-19. It is possible, and indeed likely, that the impact of different virus variants on individuals in older age groups, particularly those who experienced severe or very severe illness, would differ significantly from our observations.

4.3. Impact of Sex

We did not observe any differences in the risk of infection or the severity of COVID-19 between men and women. However, men and women differed significantly in physical and mental health, as well as in cognition-related variables. With the exception of memory and reaction times, women scored significantly worse on all seven focal variables (see Supplementary Table S7). This was the primary reason for controlling for sex in the confirmatory part of this study and for analyzing the effects of COVID-19-related variables on health and cognition separately for men and women in the main exploratory analysis. This approach, however, did not allow for formal testing of the effect of the interaction between sex and COVID-19-related variables on health and performance. Nevertheless, visual inspection of Supplementary Figures S1 and S2 suggests notable trends. Among individuals who had recovered from COVID-19, men reported significantly better physical and mental health immediately after infection. Over time, however, these measures showed substantial declines. In contrast, women's physical health remained relatively stable throughout the observation period, while their mental health gradually improved.

Men reported lower fatigue levels than women shortly after infection, but fatigue in men progressively worsened over time. In women, fatigue levels also worsened, but at a faster rate, resulting in a pronounced difference between the sexes by the end of the study period. Intelligence in men was slightly higher shortly after infection but gradually declined, while intelligence in women showed a slight increase over time, eventually surpassing that of men by the end of the observation period.

Memory was markedly poorer in men immediately after infection and declined at a much faster rate, leading to a difference between men and women that was twice as large at the end of the study period compared to its beginning. In contrast, accuracy in cognitive performance tests was slightly higher in men immediately post-infection and increased markedly more over time than in women, leading to a notable advantage for men by the end of the study. Reaction times were initially slightly better in men and gradually worsened at a similar rate to those in women.

The most pronounced differences emerged during the fourth year post-infection. While women continued to experience declines in health and cognitive performance (except for memory and accuracy in cognitive tests), men showed improvement in all parameters except reaction times. However, it is important to note that the dataset included only 15 men who had been infected more than three years prior, which limits the generalizability of these observations.

4.4. Role of Vaccination in Health and Performance

As previously mentioned, individuals who had been vaccinated showed poorer health outcomes in some aspects compared to unvaccinated individuals. As suggested in earlier studies [11,17], the most probable explanation for this phenomenon is that individuals with poorer health were more likely to opt for vaccination as a precaution during the pandemic. This explanation is substantiated by a number of studies showing that the elderly and those at risk held more positive attitudes towards vaccination [38,39]. In our study, we further supported this hypothesis by finding no significant correlations between health- and performance-related variables and the time elapsed since vaccination. Even when nonsignificant trends were present, they were generally much weaker than those related to the time since COVID-19 infection. It is also important to note that, in contrast to the frequent adverse correlations with time since COVID-19, nearly all correlations with time since vaccination were beneficial.

Our data corroborate earlier findings that the experience of having had COVID-19 has a relatively weak impact on the health status and cognitive performance of young individuals [11,17,40]. On average, those who had been infected demonstrated slightly better health and performed better on performance tests. The most pronounced and often significant negative symptoms were observed in individuals previously infected with the ancestral SARS-CoV-2 variant, while those infected with the Omicron variant showed the least severe symptoms. However, even in our sample of young individuals, the severity of the illness had a strong impact. The intensity of symptoms associated with worsening health generally changed only slowly with time since COVID-19 illness (mostly showing nonsignificant trends). *Vaccinated individuals generally exhibited poorer health compared to unvaccinated individuals. However, the difference in their health and performance did not change significantly with time since vaccination, which does not support the existence of a causal relationship between vaccination and poorer health. Most importantly, individuals vaccinated before contracting COVID-19 demonstrated superior performance on cognitive tests and often exhibited significantly (or nonsignificantly) better health parameters compared to those vaccinated after recovering from COVID-19.* Of course, the difference in health between these two subgroups (individuals vaccinated before and after contracting COVID-19) could have existed prior to vaccination, as high-risk individuals were prioritized for vaccination during the early phases of the pandemic, unlike low-risk individuals. However, if this were the case, we would expect those in worse health to have been vaccinated before, not after, contracting COVID-19.

The relatively weak impacts of having had COVID-19, as well as the observed negative association between vaccination and health status, can be attributed to the design of this study. Since this was an observational cross-sectional study, individuals were not randomly assigned to groups such as infected vs. uninfected, vaccinated vs. unvaccinated, or vaccinated before vs. after contracting COVID-19. Previous studies have shown that individuals with better health were more likely to contract COVID-19, as they took fewer precautions against infection, compared to those with chronic health issues [41,42]. Indeed, this inverse relationship between long-term health conditions and the likelihood of contracting the infection was statistically confirmed [11,43]. A study that separately tracked long-term and current health statuses showed a nonsignificant negative association between prior health issues and contracting COVID-19 and a significant positive association between contracting COVID-19 and current health problems [11]. The same study revealed a nonsignificant negative association between vaccination and current health issues and a significant positive association with long-term health problems. Unlike the present study, the earlier study included 4445 individuals from a general internet population. This population was much more age-diverse, allowing for the study of age effects. As expected, age was much more strongly correlated with health and cognitive performance than in our highly age-homogeneous sample. The study showed that younger individuals were more likely to contract COVID-19 and less likely to be vaccinated compared to older individuals, who were generally more at risk. The positive association between long-term poor health and the willingness to get vaccinated persisted even after controlling for age, suggesting that the reported link between vaccination willingness and age is not mediated by age itself, but by age-related health issues.

For a precise examination of the impact of COVID-19 and vaccination on health status and cognitive performance, data from randomized experimental studies would be necessary. However, these studies are not feasible, except in rare cases, due to ethical constraints. A potential solution is to monitor the severity of the illness, the time elapsed since infection, and the time elapsed since vaccination, as we did in this and our previous study [17]. Additionally, prospective observational studies can provide important information regarding the causality of observed associations. However, prospective studies are more demanding to conduct, require large sample sizes, and involve repeated assessments of the same individuals before and after illness or vaccination. A prospective study conducted on 30,000 Czech internet users, of whom 5164 participated repeatedly, showed that having COVID-19 had a strong impact on physical health (partial Tau = 0.25) and a weaker yet still highly significant impact (partial Tau = 0.04, $p < 0.001$) on mental health [43]. Data collection for this study was completed by the end of March 2021, so the study could not assess the impact of vaccines on health status.

4.5. Strength and Limitations

The present study has several strengths and limitations. One of its main strengths, compared to similar studies, is the rigorous implementation of all available measures to limit selection bias and reduce distortions arising from subjective opinions on the topic. More than 80% of course participants volunteered for this study. Given the strong polarization within Czech society regarding the effects of COVID-19 and vaccination on health, steps were taken to avoid potential bias stemming from participants' personal beliefs. For example, students were informed that this study would investigate the impact of various 'biological factors' on health, but they were not explicitly told that COVID-19 infection would be one of these factors. Additionally, relevant questions about COVID-19 and vaccination were placed at the end of the questionnaire, ensuring that participants answered health-related questions and completed performance tests without being given any indication that this study might relate to COVID-19.

However, this study also had some limitations. The first is an inherent limitation of all cross-sectional observational studies: the observed statistical associations do not establish causality and cannot discern what is cause and what is effect. The basic design of our study was a serial cross-sectional study. This design allows for the identification of statistical associations between dependent and independent variables. However, without supplementary information from other studies, it does not allow for conclusions about causality.

For example, the observed better health status of individuals who had experienced COVID-19 could be explained in two ways: either that contracting COVID-19 had a positive effect on health or that individuals in better health were less cautious in protecting themselves from SARS-CoV-2 infection during the first year of the pandemic, prior to the availability of vaccines, and thus were more likely to contract COVID-19. Similarly, the observed associations between health, cognitive performance, and vaccination could be interpreted in dramatically different ways.

To assess which interpretation of the observed associations is more plausible, we applied the established Bradford Hill criteria for causality in epidemiology [39]. Specifically, we focused on the following:

Strength of Association (Criterion 1): The more severe a case of COVID-19 a student experienced, the poorer their health status and cognitive performance at the time of the study.

Temporality (Criterion 4): Individuals exhibited better health and cognitive performance if they were vaccinated before contracting COVID-19 compared to those vaccinated after contracting the virus.

Plausibility (Criterion 6): It is more likely that SARS-CoV-2 infection worsens health rather than improves it.

It is important to emphasize, however, that these criteria are merely heuristic tools. A definitive answer to questions of causality can only be provided by experimental studies—which, in the case of COVID-19, are not ethically feasible. Accordingly, we have maintained a moderate tone in the causal interpretation of our findings. Furthermore, we acknowledge that some of the purported health or performance effects associated with long COVID may not stem solely from COVID-19-induced complications but could also arise from other factors such as psychological issues or individual vulnerabilities to health problems that may or may not be related to COVID-19. Nevertheless, the design of our study and the associations identified at the sample level suggest that these effects are more likely attributable to long COVID rather than to individual vulnerabilities unrelated to the effects of COVID-19.

Another limitation of this study was that the assessment of participants' health relied on their self-reported information. To minimize the subjectivity inherent in self-assessment, we required participants to answer 30 questions addressing specific aspects of their health (e.g., the number of different prescription medications they were currently taking, the number of hospitalizations lasting more than a week in the past five years, and similar metrics). Based on their responses to these questions, we calculated indices of physical and mental health. Cognitive performance, on the other hand, was directly measured as part of this study.

In this study, we controlled for only three variables: age, survey year, and sex. Naturally, both health and cognitive performance are influenced by numerous additional confounding factors that were not examined or included in our statistical models. It is important to emphasize that the population of the Czech Republic, and particularly the participants in this study, is exceptionally homogeneous. Nearly all participants resided in Prague, all shared a Caucasian European racial background, and all belonged to a similar age group. They also had comparable educational qualifications as undergraduate biology students enrolled in an elective course on evolutionary biology, likely driven by similar motivations and interests. This high degree of homogeneity significantly minimized variability that could introduce confounding effects. However, it simultaneously limits the generalizability of the findings.

A further limitation was technical: the questionnaire asked participants for the date of their last vaccination, which, along with the date of their most severe COVID-19 episode, was used to determine the binary variable 'COVID-19 before or after vaccination.' In reality, some participants with a longer time since their last COVID-19 infection than since their last vaccination had their first vaccination before contracting COVID-19. The presence of such misclassified individuals in the dataset likely skewed the results, specifically diminishing the measured effects of the binary variable vaccination before COVID-19 and increasing the risk of failing to detect an existing effect (but not risk of detecting a non-existent effect).

The questionnaire, developed in mid-2021, did not track how many times respondents contracted COVID-19 or how many doses and types of vaccines they received. These variables inevitably contribute to variability in the results and increase the risk of failing to detect existing associations in statistical tests.

5. Conclusions

Our study suggests that contracting COVID-19, especially when accompanied by severe symptoms, may negatively affect health and cognitive performance. It also indicates that even among young individuals, who mostly experienced relatively mild cases of COVID-19, some symptoms (such as frequent fatigue, impaired memory, and certain health issues) could persist for up to four years. Notably, while these symptoms tend to worsen for everyone over the first three years, they may continue to worsen in women even during the fourth year after infection. In contrast, neither participants' health nor cognition correlated significantly with the time elapsed since vaccination, and nearly all nonsignificant trends (except for the levels of fatigue) were beneficial. SARS-CoV-2 variants differ in the severity and nature of their long-term impacts on health and cognitive performance. The ancestral SARS-CoV-2 variant had the most severe long-term consequences, followed by the Alpha variant, with the Delta variant showing intermediate effects. The Omicron variant had the mildest impact on physical health and cognition, though it may have a relatively stronger effect on mental health. These differences do not appear to be strongly related to variations in the clinical course of the original acute illness or the time elapsed since COVID-19. Individuals who contracted COVID-19 after being vaccinated tend to fare better in terms of health and cognition compared to those who contracted it before vaccination. However, it is important to emphasize that future research controlling for additional factors such as the number of infections, antibody levels, vaccine types, the number of doses received, and probable pre-COVID-19 infection differences among subjects can provide greater insight into these findings.

This study also highlighted the need for caution when interpreting the results of cross-sectional studies. The likelihood of infection and adherence to preventive measures, including vaccination, often correlate with an individual's overall health status and their perception of the risks associated with the illness. As a result, observational studies may occasionally find that unvaccinated individuals who were infected show better health in certain parameters compared to vaccinated individuals who were not infected. Given that randomized experimental studies are rarely ethically permissible in human medicine to assess the impact of infection or vaccination on health, prospective case–control studies should be prioritized. In observational studies, it is essential to consider the Bradford Hill criteria for causality [44], a set of principles that help assess whether observed associations are likely to be causal [45]. In particular, the dose–response criterion highlights the need to examine correlations between health outcomes and both the severity of illness and the time elapsed since illness or vaccination.

Supplementary Materials: The following supporting information can be downloaded at https://www.mdpi.com/article/10.3390/biomedicines13010069/s1: Table S1: Distribution of data for the levels of ordinal variables. Table S2: Correlations between health- and performance-related variables and COVID-19-related variables controlled for age, sex, and survey year (women). Table S3: p-values of the correlations between health- and performance-related variables and COVID-19-related variables controlled for age, sex, and survey year (women). Table S4: Correlations between health- and performance-related variables and COVID-19-related variables controlled for age, sex, and survey year (men). Table S5: p-values of the correlations between health- and performance-related variables and COVID-19-related variables controlled for age, sex, and survey year (men). Table S6: Correlations between health and performance-related variables and COVID-related variables controlled for age, sex, survey year, and SARS-CoV-2 variants- All subjects. Table S7: p-values of the correlations between health- and performance-related variables and COVID-19-related variables controlled for age, sex, survey year, and SARS-CoV-2 variant (all subjects). Table S8: Correlations between health- and performance-related variables and COVID-19-related variables controlled for age, sex, and survey year (all subjects beyond 24 months post-infection). Table S9: p-values of the correlations between health- and performance-related variables and COVID-19-related variables controlled for age, sex, and survey year (all subjects beyond 24 months post-infection). Table S10: Correlations between health- and performance-related variables and COVID-19-related variables controlled for age, sex, and survey year (women beyond 24 months post-infection). Table S11: p-values of the correlations between health- and performance-related variables and COVID-19-related variables controlled for age, sex, and survey year (women beyond 24 months post-infection). Table S12: Correlations between health- and performance-related variables and COVID-19-related variables controlled for age, sex, and survey year (men beyond 24 months post-infection). Table S13: p-values of the correlations between health- and performance-related variables and COVID-19-related variables controlled for age, sex, and survey year (men beyond 24 months post-infection). Table S14: Correlations between health- and performance-related variables and COVID-19-related variables controlled for age, sex, and survey year (all subjects with at least 36 months elapsed since infection). Table S15: p-values of the correlations between health- and performance-related variables and COVID-19-related variables controlled for age, sex, and survey year (all subjects with at least 36 months elapsed since infection). Table S16: Correlations between health- and performance-related variables and COVID-19-related variables controlled for age, sex, and survey year (women with at least 36 months elapsed since infection). Table S17: p-values of the correlations between health- and performance-related variables and COVID-19-related variables controlled for age, sex, and survey year (women with at least 36 months elapsed since infection). Table S18: Correlations between health- and performance-related variables and COVID-19-related variables controlled for age, sex, and survey year (men with at least 36 months elapsed since infection). Table S19: p-values of the correlations between health- and performance-related variables and COVID-19-related variables controlled for age, sex, and survey year (men with at least 36 months elapsed since infection). Table S20: Correlations between health- and performance-related variables and COVID-19-related variables controlled for age, sex, and survey year (all subjects). Table S21: p-values of the correlations between health- and performance-related variables and COVID-19-related variables controlled for age, sex, and survey year (all subjects). Table S22: Correlations between health- and performance-related variables and COVID-19-related variables controlled for age, sex, survey year, and time elapsed since infection (all subjects). Table S23: p-values of the correlations between health- and performance-related variables and COVID-19-related variables controlled for age, sex, survey year, and time elapsed since infection (all subjects). Figure S1: Changes in health- and performance-related variables with time since COVID-19-related variables (women). Figure S2: Changes in health- and performance-related variables with time since COVID-19-related variables (men). Figure S3: Changes in health- and performance-related variables with time since COVID-19 beyond 24 months post-infection in women. Figure S4: Changes in health- and performance-related variables with time since COVID-19 beyond 24 months post-infection in men. Figure S5: Changes in health- and performance-related variables with time since COVID-19 vaccination in women. Figure S6: Changes in health- and performance-related variables with time since COVID-19 vaccination in men.

Author Contributions: Conceptualization, J.F.; Methodology, J.F.; Validation, J.F. and A.L.; Formal Analysis, A.L.; Investigation, J.F. and A.L.; Data Curation, J.F.; Writing—Original Draft Preparation, J.F.; Writing—Review and Editing, J.F. and A.L.; Visualization, J.F. and A.L.; Supervision, J.F.; Project Administration, J.F. Funding Acquisition, J.F. All authors have read and agreed to the published version of the manuscript.

Funding: The Czech Science Foundation supported this work (grant no. 22-20785S).

Institutional Review Board Statement: This study was conducted according to the guidelines of the Declaration of Helsinki and was approved by the Institutional Review Board of IRB of the Faculty of Science, Charles University (protocol code: 2021/19, date of approval: 11 December 2021).

Informed Consent Statement: All participants were adults and provided written informed consent, as approved by the IRB.

Data Availability Statement: The complete dataset is available at Figshare: https://doi.org/10.6084/m9.figshare.27618876, accessed on 27 December 2024.

Acknowledgments: During the preparation of this work, the author(s) used ChatGPT 4o in order to polish the language of the article. After using this tool/service, the author(s) reviewed and edited the content as needed and take(s) full responsibility for the content of the publication.

Conflicts of Interest: The authors declare no conflicts of interest.

References

1. Zhou, P.; Yang, X.-L.; Wang, X.-G.; Hu, B.; Zhang, L.; Zhang, W.; Si, H.-R.; Zhu, Y.; Li, B.; Huang, C.-L.; et al. A pneumonia outbreak associated with a new coronavirus of probable bat origin. *Nature* **2020**, *579*, 270–273. [CrossRef]
2. Shereen, M.A.; Khan, S.; Kazmi, A.; Bashir, N.; Siddique, R. COVID-19 infection: Emergence, transmission, and characteristics of human coronaviruses. *J. Adv. Res.* **2020**, *24*, 91–98. [CrossRef] [PubMed]
3. Raveendran, A.V.; Jayadevan, R.; Sashidharan, S. Long COVID: An overview. *Diabetes Metab. Syndr.* **2021**, *15*, 869–875. [CrossRef]
4. Rahmati, M.; Udeh, R.; Yon, D.K.; Lee, S.W.; Dolja-Gore, X.; McEvoy, M.; Kenna, T.; Jacob, L.; López Sánchez, G.F.; Koyanagi, A.; et al. A systematic review and meta-analysis of long-term sequelae of COVID-19 2-year after SARS-CoV-2 infection: A call to action for neurological, physical, and psychological sciences. *J. Med. Virol.* **2023**, *95*, e28852. [CrossRef]
5. Zheng, Z.; Peng, F.; Zhou, Y. Pulmonary fibrosis: A short- or long-term sequelae of severe COVID-19? *Chin. Med. J. Pulm. Crit. Care Med.* **2023**, *1*, 77–83. [CrossRef] [PubMed]
6. Salah, H.M.; Fudim, M.; O'Neil, S.T.; Manna, A.; Chute, C.G.; Caughey, M.C. Post-recovery COVID-19 and incident heart failure in the National COVID Cohort Collaborative (N3C) study. *Nat. Commun.* **2022**, *13*, 4117. [CrossRef]
7. Cegolon, L.; Mauro, M.; Sansone, D.; Tassinari, A.; Gobba, F.M.; Modenese, A.; Casolari, L.; Liviero, F.; Pavanello, S.; Scapellato, M.L.; et al. A multi-center study investigating long COVID-19 in healthcare workers from North-Eastern Italy: Prevalence, risk factors and the impact of pre-existing humoral immunity-ORCHESTRA project. *Vaccines* **2023**, *11*, 1769. [CrossRef]
8. Zhao, Y.; Shi, L.; Jiang, Z.; Zeng, N.; Mei, H.; Lu, Y.; Yang, J.; Jin, F.; Ni, S.; Wu, S.; et al. The phenotype and prediction of long-term physical, mental and cognitive COVID-19 sequelae 20 months after recovery, a community-based cohort study in China. *Mol. Psychiatry* **2023**, *28*, 1793–1801. [CrossRef]
9. Fernández-de-las-Peñas, C.; Palacios-Ceña, D.; Gómez-Mayordomo, V.; Florencio, L.L.; Cuadrado, M.L.; Plaza-Manzano, G.; Navarro-Santana, M. Prevalence of post-COVID-19 symptoms in hospitalized and non-hospitalized COVID-19 survivors: A systematic review and meta-analysis. *Eur. J. Intern. Med.* **2021**, *92*, 55–70. [CrossRef] [PubMed]
10. Jung, J.H.; Park, J.H.; Park, K.H. Comparison of lifestyle, cognitive function, mental health, and quality of life between hospitalized older adults with COVID-19 and non-COVID-19 in South Korea: A cross-sectional study. *BMC Geriatr.* **2024**, *24*, 306. [CrossRef] [PubMed]
11. Flegr, J.; Latifi, A. COVID's long shadow: How SARS-CoV-2 infection, COVID-19 severity, and vaccination status affect long-term cognitive performance and health. *Biol. Methods Protoc.* **2023**, *8*, 10. [CrossRef] [PubMed]
12. Hampshire, A.; Trender, W.; Chamberlain, S.R.; Jolly, A.E.; Grant, J.E.; Patrick, F.; Mazibuko, N.; Williams, S.C.R.; Barnby, J.M.; Hellyer, P.; et al. Cognitive deficits in people who have recovered from COVID-19. *EClinicalMedicine* **2021**, *39*, 101044. [CrossRef] [PubMed]

13. Taquet, M.; Skorniewska, Z.; De Deyn, T.; Hampshire, A.; Trender, W.R.; Hellyer, P.J.; Chalmers, J.D.; Ho, L.-P.; Horsley, A.; Marks, M.; et al. Cognitive and psychiatric symptom trajectories 2–3 years after hospital admission for COVID-19: A longitudinal, prospective cohort study in the UK. *Lancet Psychiatry* **2024**, *11*, 696–708. [CrossRef] [PubMed]
14. Cui, R.; Gao, B.; Ge, R.; Li, M.; Li, M.; Lu, X.; Jiang, S. The effects of COVID-19 infection on working memory: A systematic review. *Curr. Med. Res. Opin.* **2024**, *40*, 217–227. [CrossRef]
15. Sandler, C.X.; Wyller, V.B.B.; Moss-Morris, R.; Buchwald, D.; Crawley, E.; Hautvast, J.; Katz, B.Z.; Knoop, H.; Little, P.; Taylor, R.; et al. Long COVID and post-infective fatigue syndrome: A review. *Open Forum Infect. Dis.* **2021**, *8*, ofab440. [CrossRef]
16. Mogensen, I.; Ekström, S.; Hallberg, J.; Georgelis, A.; Melén, E.; Bergström, A.; Kull, I. Post COVID-19 symptoms are common, also among young adults in the general population. *Sci. Rep.* **2023**, *13*, 11300. [CrossRef] [PubMed]
17. Latifi, A.; Flegr, J. Is recovery just the beginning? Persistent symptoms and health and performance deterioration in post-COVID-19, non-hospitalized university students—A cross-sectional study. *Biol. Methods Protoc.* **2023**, *8*, bpad037. [CrossRef]
18. Behnood, S.; Newlands, F.; O'Mahoney, L.; Haghighat Ghahfarokhi, M.; Muhid, M.Z.; Dudley, J.; Stephenson, T.; Ladhani, S.N.; Bennett, S.; Viner, R.M.; et al. Persistent symptoms are associated with long term effects of COVID-19 among children and young people: Results from a systematic review and meta-analysis of controlled studies. *PLoS ONE* **2023**, *18*, e0293600. [CrossRef]
19. Selvakumar, J.; Havdal, L.B.; Drevvatne, M.; Brodwall, E.M.; Berven, L.L.; Stiansen-Sonerud, T.; Einvik, G.; Leegaard, T.M.; Tjade, T.; Michelsen, A.E.; et al. Prevalence and characteristics associated with post–COVID-19 condition among nonhospitalized adolescents and young adults. *JAMA Netw. Open* **2023**, *6*, e235763. [CrossRef] [PubMed]
20. Sansone, D.; Tassinari, A.; Valentinotti, R.; Kontogiannis, D.; Ronchese, F.; Centonze, S.; Maggiore, A.; Cegolon, L.; Filon, F.L. Persistence of symptoms 15 months since COVID-19 diagnosis: Prevalence, risk factors and residual work ability. *Life* **2022**, *13*, 97. [CrossRef]
21. Davis, H.E.; Assaf, G.S.; McCorkell, L.; Wei, H.; Low, R.J.; Re'em, Y.; Redfield, S.; Austin, J.P.; Akrami, A. Characterizing long COVID in an international cohort: 7 months of symptoms and their impact. *EClinicalMedicine* **2021**, *38*, 101019. [CrossRef] [PubMed]
22. Bramante, C.T.; Buse, J.B.; Liebovitz, D.M.; Nicklas, J.M.; Puskarich, M.A.; Cohen, K.; Belani, H.K.; Anderson, B.J.; Huling, J.D.; Tignanelli, C.J.; et al. Outpatient treatment of COVID-19 and incidence of post-COVID-19 condition over 10 months (COVID-OUT): A multicentre, randomised, quadruple-blind, parallel-group, phase 3 trial. *Lancet Infect. Dis.* **2023**, *23*, 1119–1129. [CrossRef] [PubMed]
23. Ma, Y.; Deng, J.; Liu, Q.; Du, M.; Liu, M.; Liu, J. Long-term consequences of COVID-19 at 6 months and above: A systematic review and meta-analysis. *Int. J. Environ. Res. Public Health* **2022**, *19*, 6865. [CrossRef]
24. Cattell, R.B. *Handbook for the Sixteen Personality Factors Questionnaire (16PF)*; Institute for Personality and Ability Testing: Champain, IL, USA, 1970; Volume 1.
25. Meili, R. *Lehrbuch der Psychologischen Diagnostik*; Verlag Hans Huber: Bern, Switzerland, 1961.
26. Flegr, J.; Hampl, R.; Černochová, D.; Preiss, M.; Bičíkova, M.; Sieger, L.; Příplatová, L.; Kaňková, S.; Klose, J. The relation of cortisol and sex hormone levels to results of psychological, performance, IQ and memory tests in military men and women. *Neuroendocrinol. Lett.* **2012**, *33*, 224–235.
27. Flegr, J. Toxoplasmosis is a risk factor for acquiring SARS-CoV-2 infection and a severe course of COVID-19 in the Czech and Slovak population: A preregistered exploratory internet cross-sectional study. *Parasit Vectors* **2021**, *14*, 508. [CrossRef] [PubMed]
28. Šúri, T.; Pfeiferová, L.; Bezdíček, M.; Svatoň, J.; Hampl, V.; Berka, K.; Jiřincová, H.; Lengerová, M.; Kolísko, M.; Nagy, A.; et al. Developing molecular surveillance of SARS-CoV-2 in the Czech Republic (2021–2022). *Res. Sq.* **2024**, 1–23. [CrossRef]
29. Flegr, J.; Flegr, P. Doing exploratory analysis in R with a package Explorer v. 1.0. *Figshare* **2021**, *6*, 2023. [CrossRef]
30. Kim, S. ppcor: An R package for a fast calculation to semi-partial correlation coefficients. *Commun. Stat. Appl. Met.* **2015**, *22*, 665–674. [CrossRef] [PubMed]
31. Benjamini, Y.; Hochberg, Y. Controlling the false discovery rate: A practical and powerful approach to multiple testing. *J. R. Stat. Soc. Ser. B Methodol.* **1995**, *57*, 289–300. [CrossRef]
32. Flegr, J. Data for the article: Persistent health and cognitive impairments up to four years post-COVID-19 in young students: The impact of virus variants and vaccination timing. *Figshare* **2024**. [CrossRef]
33. Althouse, A.D. Adjust for multiple comparisons? It's not that simple. *Ann. Thorac. Surg.* **2016**, *101*, 1644–1645. [CrossRef]
34. Wu, D.J.; Liu, N. Association of cognitive deficits with sociodemographic characteristics among adults with post-COVID conditions: Findings from the United States Household Pulse Survey. *medRxiv* **2023**. [CrossRef]
35. Choudhury, N.A.; Mukherjee, S.; Singer, T.; Venkatesh, A.; Perez Giraldo, G.S.; Jimenez, M.; Miller, J.; Lopez, M.; Hanson, B.A.; Bawa, A.P.; et al. Neurologic manifestations of long COVID disproportionately affect young and middle-age adults. *Ann. Neurol.* **2024**. [CrossRef] [PubMed]
36. Torabi, S.H.; Riahi, S.M.; Ebrahimzadeh, A.; Salmani, F. Changes in symptoms and characteristics of COVID-19 patients across different variants: Two years study using neural network analysis. *BMC Infect. Dis.* **2023**, *23*, 838. [CrossRef]

37. Xia, Q.; Yang, Y.; Wang, F.; Huang, Z.; Qiu, W.; Mao, A. Case fatality rates of COVID-19 during epidemic periods of variants of concern: A meta-analysis by continents. *Int. J. Infect. Dis.* **2024**, *141*, 106950. [CrossRef]
38. Reiter, P.L.; Pennell, M.L.; Katz, M.L. Acceptability of a COVID-19 vaccine among adults in the United States: How many people would get vaccinated? *Vaccine* **2020**, *38*, 6500–6507. [CrossRef]
39. Kelly, B.J.; Southwell, B.G.; McCormack, L.A.; Bann, C.M.; MacDonald, P.D.M.; Frasier, A.M.; Bevc, C.A.; Brewer, N.T.; Squiers, L.B. Predictors of willingness to get a COVID-19 vaccine in the U.S. *BMC Infect. Dis.* **2021**, *21*, 338. [CrossRef]
40. Bahat, G.; Medetalibeyoglu, A.; Senkal, N.; Cebeci, T.; Oren, M.M.; Basaran, S.; Arici, H.; Catma, Y.; Kose, M.; Karan, M.A.; et al. Symptomatology and imaging findings in early post-Covid period: A comparative study in older vs younger patients. *Exp. Gerontol.* **2022**, *167*, 111907. [CrossRef]
41. Kim, S.; Kim, S. Analysis of the impact of health beliefs and resource factors on preventive behaviors against the covid-19 pandemic. *Int. J. Environ. Res. Public Health* **2020**, *17*, 8666. [CrossRef] [PubMed]
42. Yang, X.Y.; Gong, R.N.; Sassine, S.; Morsa, M.; Tchogna, A.S.; Drouin, O.; Chadi, N.; Jantchou, P. Risk perception of COVID-19 infection and adherence to preventive measures among adolescents and young adults. *Children* **2020**, *7*, 311. [CrossRef]
43. Flegr, J.; Flegr, P.; Priplatova, L. The effects of 105 biological, socioeconomic, behavioral, and environmental factors on the risk of SARS-CoV-2 infection and a severe course of COVID-19: A prospective, explorative cohort study. *Biol. Methods Protoc.* **2022**, *7*, 15. [CrossRef]
44. Hill, A.B. The environment and disease—Association or causation. *Proc. R. Soc. Med.* **1965**, *58*, 295–300. [CrossRef] [PubMed]
45. Fedak, K.M.; Bernal, A.; Capshaw, Z.A.; Gross, S. Applying the Bradford Hill criteria in the 21st century: How data integration has changed causal inference in molecular epidemiology. *Emerg. Themes Epidemiol.* **2015**, *12*, 14. [CrossRef]

Disclaimer/Publisher's Note: The statements, opinions and data contained in all publications are solely those of the individual author(s) and contributor(s) and not of MDPI and/or the editor(s). MDPI and/or the editor(s) disclaim responsibility for any injury to people or property resulting from any ideas, methods, instructions or products referred to in the content.

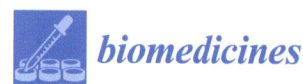

Article

Pathology of Red Blood Cells in Patients with SARS-CoV-2

Sona Hakobyan [1,*], Lina Hakobyan [1], Liana Abroyan [1], Aida Avetisyan [1,2], Hranush Avagyan [1,2], Nane Bayramyan [1], Lyudmila Niazyan [3], Mher Davidyants [3], Knarik Sargsyan [3], Tehmine Ghalechyan [3], Anna Semerjyan [4], Elena Karalova [1,2] and Zaven Karalyan [1,4]

[1] Laboratory of Cell Biology and Virology, Institute of Molecular Biology of NAS RA, Yerevan 0014, Armenia; a.avetis@mail.ru (A.A.); a.avagian@yahoo.com (H.A.); zkaralyan@yahoo.com (Z.K.)
[2] Experimental Laboratory, Yerevan State Medical University, Yerevan 0093, Armenia
[3] National Center of Infectious Diseases, Ministry of Health, RA, Yerevan 8424, Armenia; davidyants@gmail.com (M.D.); t.ghalechyan88@gmail.com (T.G.)
[4] Department of Medical Biology, Yerevan State Medical University, Yerevan 0025, Armenia
* Correspondence: 777sona7@gmail.com

Academic Editor: César Fernández-de-las-Peñas

Received: 29 November 2024
Revised: 28 December 2024
Accepted: 3 January 2025
Published: 14 January 2025

Citation: Hakobyan, S.; Hakobyan, L.; Abroyan, L.; Avetisyan, A.; Avagyan, H.; Bayramyan, N.; Niazyan, L.; Davidyants, M.; Sargsyan, K.; Ghalechyan, T.; et al. Pathology of Red Blood Cells in Patients with SARS-CoV-2. *Biomedicines* 2025, 13, 191. https://doi.org/10.3390/biomedicines13010191

Copyright: © 2025 by the authors. Licensee MDPI, Basel, Switzerland. This article is an open access article distributed under the terms and conditions of the Creative Commons Attribution (CC BY) license (https://creativecommons.org/licenses/by/4.0/).

Abstract: Background: Severe acute respiratory syndrome coronavirus 2 (SARS-CoV-2) infection has been associated with various hematological disorders. Understanding the pathology of erythrocytes (red blood cells) in coronavirus infection may provide insights into disease severity and progression. **Objective:** To review and analyze the general pathology of erythrocytes in patients infected with SARS-CoV-2, focusing on clinical and laboratory findings across different severity groups. **Methods:** Patients were classified into four groups based on clinical criteria: Group 1: Regular group (fever, respiratory symptoms, and radiographic evidence of pneumonia). Group 2: Severe group (shortness of breath >30 breaths/min, peripheral blood oxygen saturation <92% at rest, extensive pneumonia, respiratory failure requiring mechanical ventilation, and/or organ failure necessitating intensive care). Group 3: Low saturation group (peripheral blood oxygen saturation <85% at rest). Group 4: Erythroblastosis group (erythroblast count >0.5% among total nucleated blood cells). Clinical laboratory investigations included major routine studies and scanning microspectrophotometry to measure hemoglobin (Hb) spectra in unstained erythrocytes. **Results:** Erythroblasts were detected in approximately 30% of SARS-CoV-2 patients, predominantly in the severe group. Serum ferritin, C-reactive protein (CRP), and anisocytosis were strongly correlated with disease severity. Microspectrophotometric studies revealed significant changes in hemoglobin adsorption spectra, with an increase in Hb absorbance at 420 nm in severe cases compared to normal controls. **Conclusions:** Elevated serum ferritin, CRP levels, anisocytosis, and altered hemoglobin absorption at 420 nm wavelength are associated with adverse outcomes in SARS-CoV-2 infection. These findings highlight the potential utility of hematological parameters as markers for disease severity and prognosis in viral infections.

Keywords: COVID-19; red blood cells; hemoglobin adsorption; erythroblastosis; microspectrophotometry

1. Introduction

There are several subfamilies of coronaviruses. Seven coronaviruses have been described to cause respiratory diseases in humans. Four of these are common human coronaviruses, and one of the seven is severe acute respiratory syndrome coronavirus 2 (SARS-CoV-2). SARS-CoV-2 belongs to the subfamily Coronavirinae. Other coronavirus species capable of causing severe human diseases include SARS-CoV and MERS-CoV. The coronaviruses HKU1, HCoV-NL63, HCoV-OC43 and HCoV-229E are associated with mild symptoms in humans [1,2].

Coronavirus disease 19 (COVID-19) is an infectious-inflammatory disease that primarily affects the lungs. The severe course of the disease is associated with multi-organ pathology with different routes of injury. Although erythrocyte pathology is less commonly mentioned, several articles have suggested that SARS-CoV-2 infection may cause hematological disorders [3]. Authors usually point to differences in hematological manifestations between severe and non-severe patients. Hemoglobinopathy, hypoxia, and cellular iron overload may play a role in SARS-CoV-2 pathology. Two potential pathophysiological mechanisms have been suggested in the scientific literature: a) interaction of SARS-CoV-2 with the hemoglobin molecule through CD147, CD26, and other receptors located on erythrocytes and/or blood cell precursors; b) hepcidin-mimetic action of a viral spike protein inducing ferroportin blockade [3].

Serum ferritin is known as an iron storage protein and is commonly measured as an indicator of iron status. It is also a prominent marker of inflammation, with serum ferritin levels rising significantly in response to inflammation and other pathologies. Serum ferritin levels also correlated with disease severity in SARS-CoV-2 patients, but the mechanisms for the association between hyperferritinemia and disease severity in SARS-CoV-2 patients remained unclear [3].

Normally, erythroblasts should be completely absent in adult blood and are usually observed in almost all forms of severe anemia (except aplastic). Several investigations have reported erythroblastosis in SARS-CoV-2 patients [4–6]. Ferritin has been shown to be frequently located on the plasma membrane of erythroblasts [7]. Thus, the purpose of this study is to investigate/examine the general pathophysiology of red blood cells in coronavirus infection, especially to look into the association/relationship between serum ferritin levels with erythroblastosis and hemoglobin abnormalities in patients with SARS-CoV-2.

2. Methods

2.1. Virus

Within the experiments, a delta variant of SARS-CoV-2 was used [8,9].

2.2. Patients

This study was approved by the Institutional Review Board/Independent Ethics Committee of the Institute of Molecular Biology of the National Academy of Sciences, Yerevan, Armenia. The study was approved by the Institutional Review Board of the Institute of Molecular Biology NAS RA IRB00004079.

We performed quantitative polymerase chain reaction (qRT-PCR) (both using extracted RNA and direct samples (initial swab samples)) targeting the N gene and the ORF1ab gene in the conserved region of the SARS-CoV-2 genome [10]. The current study included 74 patients with SARS-CoV-2 who were treated at the National Centre for Infectious Diseases, Ministry of Health of Armenia. The study was conducted from May to September 2020.

Patient inclusion criteria are presented below:
- Patients diagnosed with SARS-CoV-2 within positive SARS-CoV-2 qRT-PCR.
- Residents of the National Centre of Infectious Diseases, Ministry of Health, Republic of Armenia.
- Age of patients 18 years and older.
- Negative pregnancy test for females.
- Informed consent is required from the patient or his/her representative to participate in the study.

- The patient should be able to comply with all the requirements of the clinical trial (including home follow-up during isolation).

Patient exclusion criteria are presented below.

- Known history of allergy.
- Positive IgG to SARS-CoV-2 was obtained prior to testing.
- Any of the following comorbidities (or any other condition that may interfere with the study): Immunosuppression. Chronic obstructive pulmonary disease. Obesity. Acute or chronic renal insufficiency. History of severe coronary disease. History of cerebrovascular disease. Current neoplasm.

Computed tomography (CT) of the lungs was performed in all patients.

2.3. Clinical Criteria

The classification of the patients in the study was in accordance with Yuan [11]:

I. Regular group (fever, respiratory symptoms, and radiographic evidence of pneumonia),

II. Severe group patients with shortness of breath (more than 30 breaths per minute), peripheral blood oxygen saturation less than 92% at rest, pneumonia involving more than 50% of the tissues, and/or respiratory failure requiring mechanical ventilation support and/or organ failure requiring intensive care.

III. The low saturation group with peripheral blood oxygen saturation less than 85% at rest (before mechanical ventilation support).

IV. Erythroblastosis group with erythroblast count greater than 0.5% of total nucleated blood cells.

2.4. Laboratory Measurements

Clinical laboratory investigations included a complete blood count and the determination of ferritin, C-reactive protein (CRP), and lactose dehydrogenase (LDH) in patients' sera.

Blood samples were analyzed using commercially available ELISA kits that are normally used in the hospital's clinical practice [12,13].

2.5. Blood Smears, Giemsa Staining, and Nucleated Blood Cells Analysis

Blood smears were prepared from fresh blood using routine methods. For nucleated blood cell analysis, slides were fixed in pure methanol and stained with Giemsa-modified solution (azure B/azure II, eosin, and methylene blue) according to the manufacturer's protocol (Sigma-Aldrich, St. Louis, MO, USA). Nucleated blood cells were examined under a light microscope at ×1250 in random order. At least 300 nucleated blood cells in each sample were analyzed for cell types. Erythroblasts were detected morphologically [14].

2.6. Microspectrophotometry

Microspectrophotometry was performed on an SMP-05 Opton scanning microspectrophotometer to measure the spectra of hemoglobin (Hb) in unstained erythrocytes. The spectrophotometric measurement was only represented on individual erythrocytes, with the extracellular area as a standard reference. The microspectrophotometric method was chosen because of its ability to measure small spectral changes in a limited number of erythrocytes [15]. Cytometric studies were also carried out.

2.7. Statistical Analysis

Data analysis was performed with SPSS-19 software. The measurement data were generally non-normally distributed, so the non-parametric Mann–Whitney u-test was used. Initially, the severity of the disease was recorded on a scale of 1–4 scale: 1, normal group; 2, erythroblastosis; 3, low oxygen saturation group; 4, severe disease group. The following erythroblastosis scale was used to record the amount of erythroblasts in the blood: (1) none, (2) 0.1%, (3) 0.3–0.5%, (4) 0.6%, and more. The Spearman correlation coefficient was used for correlation analysis based on the data.

3. Results

3.1. Basic Characteristics of the Patients

The median age of the 74 patients was 59 years (31–83 years), and 38 (51.3%) were male. There were twelve cases in the low saturation group, nine cases in the group with marked/notable erythroblastosis (at least 1% of erythroblasts in the total nucleated cell count), thirty-five cases in the normal group, and eighteen cases in the severe group with critical form of the disease. The groups did not differ significantly in terms of sex ratio or mean age. The main clinical symptoms of all patients were cough, fever, and fatigue, although patients with critical and severe disease were more likely to have shortness of breath.

3.2. Laboratory Results

Owing to the limited quantity of critically sick patient cases, statistical variation was minimized by combining the severe and critically ill groups and comparing them with the regular group.

Ferritin levels were greater in patients with erythroblastosis (ferritin-87.6–346 ng/mL) and severe and critical cases (ferritin-104.8–2929 ng/mL) than in low saturation cases (ferritin-59.8–894 ng/mL). Similar findings were observed in the investigation of CRP levels in serum (Table 1).

Table 1. Clinical characteristics of the 74 patients with SARS-CoV-2.

Characteristic	Regular Group (n = 35)	Severe Group (n = 18)	Low Saturation Group (n = 12)	Erythroblastosis Group (n = 9)
Age (year)	61 ± 4.5	58 ± 3.3	56 ± 4.8	57 ± 5.5
Male sex (%, N)	51.4 (18)	50.0 (9)	50.0 (6)	55.5 (5)
Symptoms (%, N)				
Fever	80% (28)	94.5% (17)	16.7 (2)	66.7% (6)
Cough	77.1% (27)	22.2% (4)	75% (8)	22.2% (2)
Loss of smell/taste	57.1 (20)	16.7% (3)	16.7% (2)	-
Shortness of breath	22.8% (8)	16.7% (3)	50% (6)	22.2% (2)
O_2 saturation	92.2 ± 2.8	88.5 ± 4.9	75.7 ± 5.3	91.2 ± 5.1
Anorexia	8.7% (3)	5.5% (1)	-	-
Diarrhea	5.7% (2)	5.5% (1)	-	-
Fatigue	82.9% (29)	22.2% (4)	83.3% (10)	77.8% (7)
Myalgia or arthralgia	28.6% (10)	16.7% (3)	25% (3)	44.4% (4)
Coexisting disorder (%, N)				
Hypertension	42.9% (15)	38.8% (7)	33.3% (4)	44.4% (4)
Diabetes	31.4% (11)	27.8% (5)	25% (3)	22.2% (2)
Coronary heart disease	8.7% (3)	5.5% (1)	8.3% (1)	22.2% (2)
Cerebrovascular disease	-	5.5% (1)	-	-
Chronic renal disease	2.9% (1)	5.5% (1)	-	-
Malignant tumor	5.7% (2)	5.5% (1)	-	-
other coexisting chronic disorder	20% (7)	11.1% (2)	8.3% (1)	-
Ferritin level (ng/mL)	87.6–346	104.8–2929 *	59.8–894	87–285
CRP (mg/L)	46.5 (8–81)	89.3 (21–231)	47.9 (14–95)	19.1 (7–72)

* Significant compared to Regular group and group with Erythroblastosis ($p < 0.05$), tendency compared to Low Saturation Group ($p < 0.1$).

There were no statistically significant changes in the peripheral blood cell population composition in any of the groups, as Table 2 demonstrates. An exception is the finding of erythroblasts in the group with severe cases compared to the regular group.

Table 2. Blood cell populations.

Blood Cells	Regular Group (n = 35) *	Severe Group (n = 18) **	Low Saturation Group (n = 12) ***	Erythroblastosis Group (n = 9)
Basophilic erythroblast	-	0.1	-	0.7
Polychromatophilic erythroblast	-	0.1	-	0.7
Acidophilic erythroblast	0.1	0.3	0.1	0.1
Lymphoblast	1.8 ± 1.4	2.5	1.4	2.1
Lymphocyte	22.0 ± 6.4	25.3	28.8	28.5
Lymphocyte aberrant	1.1 ± 2.1	0.4	1.4	1.8
Monoblast	0.4 ± 0.7	0.3	0.4	0.7
Monocyte	2.1 ± 1.4	2.6	2.6	1.6
Myeloid cell	2.8 ± 2.5	1.6	3.7	1.3
Metamyelocyte	14.7 ± 7.4	16.3	17.7	12.2
Band neutrophil	39.9 ± 9.6	36.8	34.4	39.1
Segmented neutrophil	12.3 ± 1.1	10.9	7.7	8.2
Pathological neutrophil	0.8 ± 0.9	0.7	0.7	1.6
Eosinophil	0.4 ± 0.2	0.9	0.2	0.5
Basophil	0.1 ± 0.2	0.1	0.0	0.1
Destructed cells	1.3 ± 1.2	1.1	1.0	0.9

* Erythroblastosis present in 5.7% of cases (2 patients from 35). ** Erythroblastosis present in 44.4% of cases (8 patients from 18). *** Saturation below 85%.

3.3. Routine Blood Test and Erythroblastosis

Routine blood tests were performed on all patients. The results showed that the white blood cells (WBC) of the COVID-19 patients were essentially within the normal reference range. A small percentage of individuals (7–8%) had lymphopenia. The consistent finding of erythroblasts in the peripheral blood was the primary feature that distinguished patients with coronavirus infection from the general population. Acidophilic erythroblasts were found in every group of patients in the hospital. In the group with severe coronavirus infection, the percentage of patients with a diagnosis of erythroblastosis ranged from 44% to 5–10% (Table 2). A common finding in SARS-CoV-2 patients (about 30%) was the presence of erythroblasts. It was significantly higher than in the normal group ($p < 0.01$) and more frequent, especially in the severe group.

Patients in the severe group had erythroblasts representing 0.1% to 0.5% of the total nucleated cell population. In addition, erythroblasts that were both polychromatic and basophilic were consistently seen in blood smears from patients with severe disease.

Because of the comparatively high incidence of erythroblastosis in SARS-CoV-2 infection, a separate group of patients (the erythroblastosis group) was established for a more in-depth study of this disease. The group consisted of patients whose erythroblast count was greater than 0.5% of the total nucleated cell population. Anisocytosis and erythroblastosis co-occurred in 16.7% of patients in the severe group (Figure 1h). The degree of anisocytosis in patients with the severe form of SARS-CoV-2 is shown by microcytometry data (Figure 2a). The erythroblastosis group had a lower hemoglobin concentration (Figure 2b).

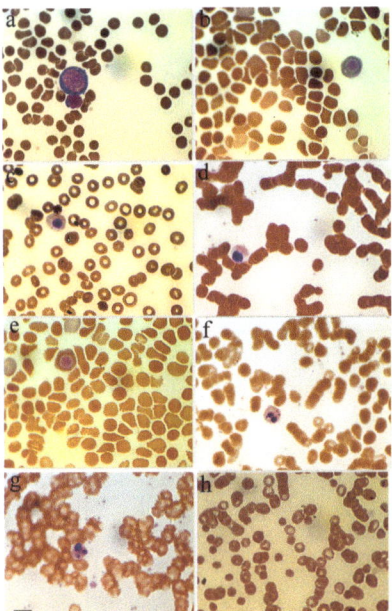

Figure 1. Erythroid cell morphology in peripheral blood in patients with SARS-CoV-2. (**a**) Basophilic erythroblast in a female patient with a severe form of coronavirus. (**b**) Polychromatophilic erythroblast female patient with a moderate form of coronavirus. (**c**) Polychromatophilic erythroblast, female 48-year-old patient with diabetes and hypertension. (**d**) Acidophilic erythroblast, female patient with a severe form of coronavirus. (**e**) Acidophilic erythroblast, female patient with a moderate form of coronavirus. (**f**) Acidophilic erythroblast with a cleaved nucleus, male patient with a moderate form of coronavirus. (**g**) Acidophilic erythroblast with a cleaved nucleus, female patient with a moderate form of coronavirus. (**h**) Anisocytosis in female patients with a severe form of coronavirus. Scale bar 10 μm.

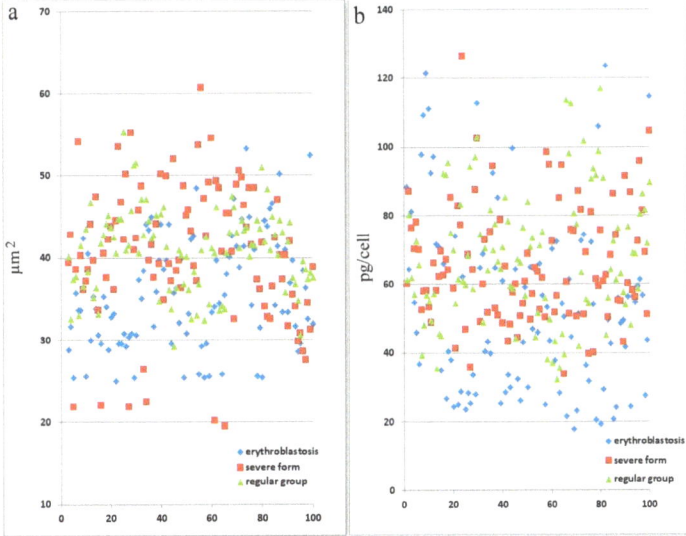

Figure 2. Morphological abnormalities of erythrocytes in patients with SARS-CoV-2 infection. Each point is the average of erythrocytes from three patients, systematized by size. (**a**) Size of erythrocytes. Significant by u-test in the severe group ($p < 0.05$). (**b**) Hb amount in erythrocytes. Significant by u-test in the severe group ($p < 0.05$).

3.4. Influence of Coronavirus Infection on Erythrocyte Parameters, Determined by Microspectrophotometry

Two hundred erythrocytes were used to calculate the mean values of the hemoglobin content, the concentration of a single red blood cell, and the size of the cell. It was discovered that coronavirus infection was the source of variations in Hb adsorption spectra in erythrocytes.

Figure 2 displays information on variations in the adsorption spectra of a single erythrocyte. For panel a, statistical analysis (using the u-test) indicates that there is a significant difference in the severe group ($p < 0.05$), suggesting that erythrocyte size abnormalities are pronounced in patients with severe SARS-CoV-2 infection. For panel b, the severe group shows statistically significant differences in hemoglobin levels per cell ($p < 0.05$). This implies that the severe form of SARS-CoV-2 affects erythrocyte function and hemoglobin content more markedly than the other groups. This figure demonstrates that severe SARS-CoV-2 infection leads to significant morphological and functional abnormalities in erythrocytes, as evidenced by changes in their size and hemoglobin content. These abnormalities might reflect the disease's systemic impact on oxygen transport and cellular health.

The spectra between 414 and 420 nm showed the most alterations (Figure 3A,B). Figure 3C illustrates the variations in adsorption spectra between the primary erythrocyte type and the variable absorption brought on by SARS-CoV-2. The absorption maxima in the 418–422 wavelength range shifted dramatically, as Figure 3D illustrates.

Patients from groups with severe manifestations of the disease and those with erythroblastosis have higher absorption maxima in individual erythrocytes at wavelengths 418–422. According to hemoglobin spectrophotometry, there is a noticeable decrease in hemoglobin absorption as the wavelength increases from 414 to 420 nm. Normally, the erythrocyte population is quite homogeneous (Figure 3D). However, a less pronounced decrease in absorption was observed in some SARS-CoV-2 erythrocytes (20–35% of patients from the severe form of the disease and from the erythroblastosis group; see below) compared to the control (Figure 3D). Patients with erythroblastosis and severe form of SARS-CoV-2 had higher erythrocyte counts and greater Hb absorption at 420 nm according to microspectrophotometry.

The hemoglobin absorption spectra of individual erythrocytes were significantly altered according to microspectrophotometric studies. However, in the severe form of SARS-CoV-2, there was an increase in hemoglobin absorbance within the 420 nm wavelength spectrum (Figure 4); this increase was statistically significant compared with the normal group. Microspectrophotometric studies revealed significant changes in the hemoglobin adsorption spectra of individual erythrocytes in all forms of coronavirus infection compared with healthy individuals (Figure 4A). The appearance of erythrocytes with an increase in hemoglobin absorption spectra at the wavelength of 420 nm was observed in the normal group of patients (Figure 4B), in patients with a severe course of SARS-CoV-2 (Figure 4C) and in the group with erythroblastosis (Figure 4D), this increase was statistically significant (u criterion) compared to healthy individuals. However, in the groups with a severe form of SARS-CoV-2 and with erythroblastosis, erythrocytes containing hemoglobin with low levels (less than 30 mM 1cm^{-1}) of absorption spectra (indicated by arrows) disappeared, this increase was statistically significant (u criterion) compared with the usual group and healthy people. The hemoglobin absorption spectra in the erythroblastosis group varied between those of the control group and the severe SARS-CoV-2 disease, but in this group, there are also cells with Hb with increased absorption spectra at 420 nm wavelength. The severe form of SARS-CoV-2 and the control group had different hemoglobin absorbance indices than the erythroblastosis group. Serum ferritin, CRP, and anisocytosis levels are closely related to disease severity, as shown in Table 3.

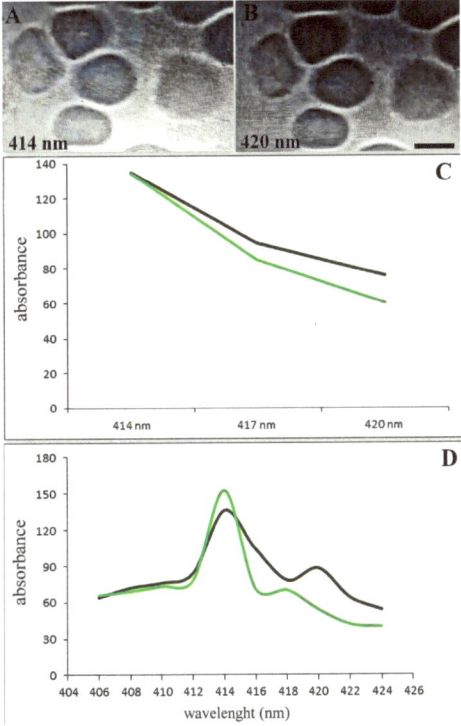

Figure 3. Soret absorption spectroscopy of hemoglobin. The graph shows the microspectrophotometry data of erythrocytes with an identical area (differences less than 1%) on different wavelengths. Black line: main type of erythrocytes. Green line: erythrocytes with variable adsorbance in SARS-CoV-2 infection. (**A**) Erythrocytes in 414 nm wavelengths. (**B**) Erythrocytes in 420 nm wavelengths. Scale bar 5 µm. (**C**) Spectral changes of erythrocytes in patients with SARS-CoV-2 (black curve) and an increase in hemoglobin adsorbance occur about the 420 nm wavelength spectrum. (**D**) Adsorption spectra of single erythrocytes (with the same surface area) were studied by microspectrophotometry on different wavelengths.

Table 3. Correlation analysis of red blood alterations and disease severity by Spearman coefficient.

	Disease Severity	Erythroblastosis	Ferritin	CRP	Increased Hb Absorption on 420 nm (%)	Anisocytosis (%)	Decreased Hb in Erythrocyte (%)
disease severity	1.000	0.316	1.000 *	1.000 *	0.800	1.000 *	−0.105
Erythroblastosis	0.316	1.000	0.316	0.316	0.632	0.316	0.833
ferritin levels in serum	1.000 *	0.316	1.000	1.000 *	0.800 **	1.000 *	−0.105
CRP levels in serum	1.000 *	0.316	1.000 *	1.000	0.800 **	1.000 *	−0.105
increase in Hb absorption on 420 nm (%)	0.800 **	0.632	0.800 **	0.800 **	1.000	0.800 **	0.105
anisocytosis (%)	1.000 *	0.316	1.000 *	1.000 *	0.800 **	1.000	−0.105
decreased Hb amount in erythrocyte (%)	−0.105	0.833	−0.105	−0.105	0.105	−0.105	1.000

* Correlation is significant at the 0.01 level (2-tailed). ** Tendency at 0.1 level (2-tailed).

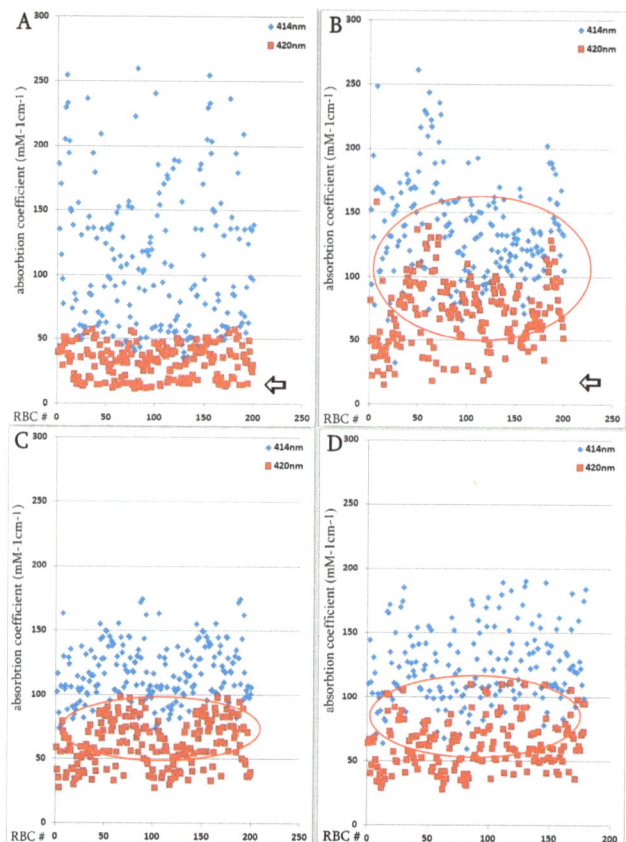

Figure 4. Distribution of single erythrocytes by absorption spectroscopy of hemoglobin on different wavelengths in norm and in patients with SARS-CoV-2. Erythrocytes containing hemoglobin with increased absorption spectra were isolated. Erythrocytes containing hemoglobin with low levels (less than 30 mM 1cm^{-1}) of absorption spectra are indicated by arrows. Each point is the average of erythrocytes from three patients, systematized by size. (**A**) Norm. (**B**) Regular group. (**C**) Severe group. Significant by u-test in comparison with norm and regular groups ($p < 0.05$); (**D**) Group with erythroblastosis. Significant by u-test in comparison with norm and regular groups ($p < 0.05$).

4. Discussion

The changes we found in the peripheral blood after coronavirus-induced pathology resembled the erythropoiesis process. Anisocytosis, variations in Hb absorption spectra, and erythroblast shedding from the bone marrow are the main manifestations of these changes. Most people have moderate or absent coronavirus infections that do not require hospitalization. Hospitalized patients with initially more severe disease have been found to have erythroblastosis. However, contrary to what others have described [3], erythroblastosis was not a common observation in individuals with a worse prognosis. Erythroblasts were found in every group of patients studied. No significant correlation (only trend) ($p < 0.1$) was found between higher levels of erythroblastosis and a worse prognosis or more severe course of the disease. Furthermore, no correlation was observed between the degree of oxygen saturation and elevated erythroblastosis levels, which were equivalent in the normal and severe groups. Hypoxia is often associated with erythroblastosis [16]. Although hemoglobinopathy may play an important role in the overall pathology of SARS-CoV-2, our data did not show a correlation between the amount of erythroblastosis and decreased saturation (only the amount of erythroblastosis tended to correlate with disease severity) [17,18]. Thus, both the direct targeting of erythroid precursors by SARS-CoV-2 and the systemic hyperinflammation that characterizes individuals with severe disease may have an indirect effect on erythropoiesis abnormalities such as erythroblastosis [17,19]. These findings, showing that the virus was still present in erythroid cells 14 days later without affecting their viability, suggest that direct infection may be the cause of the erythroblastosis seen in severely affected individuals.

ACE2, CD147, CD26, and other receptors on erythrocytes and/or blood cell precursors may mediate the effect of the virus on hemoglobin [3]. In this regard, recommendations have been made [2] regarding potential interactions between COVID-19 and hemoglobin, which could decrease the total content and oxygen affinity of hemoglobin. Changes in the UV spectrum of hemoglobin may also be caused by an increase in the metHb fraction in SARS-CoV-2 [20]. However, the literature data suggest that changes in the UV spectra of hemoglobin cannot be fully explained by changes in metHb or oxyHb alone [21,22].

Antimalarial drugs that may also have anti-SARS-CoV-2 activity target Plasmodium, which has a similar route of erythrocyte entry via CD147. They have been used to prevent non-structural SARS-CoV-2 proteins from forming a porphyrin complex and attacking hemoglobin [17].

Ferritin levels increase in patients with the progressive form of SARS-CoV-2 and poor prognosis, according to several articles [19,23,24]. Acute phase reactant serum ferritin levels correlate with the severity of infection-related acute and chronic inflammation [25]. Our results support the findings of the cited authors, who concluded that the group of severe SARS-CoV-2 cases had the highest serum ferritin levels. A significant percentage of the ferritin levels examined were higher in the group of patients with low oxygen saturation than in the group of normal patients. Some SARS-CoV-2 patients had elevated ferritin levels, which may indicate an inflammatory response or be related to viral entry into the bloodstream and its effect on iron metabolism [26]. In addition, we found anisocytosis, which is a marker of anemia. In the general population, anisocytosis is also associated with increased all-cause mortality [27]. According to our findings, elevated ferritin levels were not associated with erythroblastosis but rather with anisocytosis, altered microspectrophotometric characteristics of hemoglobin in erythrocytes, and disease severity. Abnormalities in erythrocyte size distribution have been associated with inflammation in a number of studies [27,28]. Despite a strong correlation between elevated anisocytosis and CRP, this phenomenon is only part of the complicated erythrocyte pathology resulting from SARS-CoV-2 infection. This type of interaction can lead to a decrease in the amount of hemoglobin available to carry oxygen, shift the oxygen dissociation curve, and reduce the affinity of oxygen for hemoglobin.

5. Conclusions

Increased levels of ferritin, CRP, anisocytosis, and partially increased Hb absorption at 420 nm may be positively correlated with adverse outcomes in SARS-CoV-2 infection.

Author Contributions: Z.K. created the concept and wrote the paper. L.H., L.A., A.A., E.K., S.H., H.A. and N.B. carried out cell analysis, microspectrophotometry analyses, the preparation of blood smears, L.N., M.D., K.S. and T.G. supervised and carried out the production of blood samples, clinical and laboratory analysis, A.S. and E.K. assisted with interpretation of the data and critical revision of the manuscript. All authors have read and agreed to the published version of the manuscript.

Funding: This research received no external funding.

Institutional Review Board Statement: The study was conducted in accordance with the Declaration of the Institutional Review Board/Independent Ethics Committee of the Institute of Molecular Biology of the National Academy of Sciences, Yerevan, Armenia; IRB00004079.

Informed Consent Statement: Informed consent was obtained from all subjects involved in the study.

Data Availability Statement: The original contributions presented in the study are included in the article, further inquiries can be directed to the corresponding author.

Conflicts of Interest: The authors declare no conflicts of interest.

References

1. Chen, Y.; Liu, Q.; Guo, D. Emerging coronaviruses: Genome structure, replication, and pathogenesis. *J. Med. Virol.* **2020**, *92*, 418–423. [CrossRef] [PubMed]
2. Zarandi, P.K.; Zinatizadeh, M.R.; Zinatizadeh, M.; Yousefi, M.H.; Rezaei, N. SARS-CoV-2: From the pathogenesis to potential anti-viral treatments. *Biomed. Pharmacother.* **2021**, *137*, 111352. [CrossRef] [PubMed]
3. Cavezzi, A.; Troiani, E.; Corrao, S. COVID-19: Hemoglobin, iron, and hypoxia beyond inflammation. A narrative review. *Clin. Pract.* **2020**, *10*, 1271. [CrossRef] [PubMed]
4. Lin, Z.; Long, F.; Yang, Y.; Chen, X.; Xu, L.; Yang, M. Serum ferritin as an independent risk factor for severity in COVID-19 patients. *J. Infect.* **2020**, *81*, 647–679. [CrossRef]
5. Demeester, S.; Demuyser, T.; Fauconnier, C.; Heestermans, R.; Orlando, C.; Depreter, B.; Jochmans, K. Routine haematology parameters in COVID-19 patients and clinical outcome: A Belgian single-centre study. *Int. J. Lab. Hematol.* **2020**, *42*, e252–e255. [CrossRef]
6. Lee, W.S.; Margolskee, E. Leukoerythroblastosis and plasmacytoid lymphocytes in a child with SARS-CoV-2-associated multisystem inflammatory syndrome. *Blood* **2020**, *136*, 914. [CrossRef]
7. Mitra, A.; Dwyre, D.M.; Schivo, M.; Thompson, G.R., 3rd; Cohen, S.H.; Ku, N.; Graff, J.P. Leukoerythroblastic reaction in a patient with COVID-19 infection. *Am. J. Hematol.* **2020**, *95*, 999–1000. [CrossRef]
8. Avetyan, D.; Hakobyan, S.; Nikoghosyan, M.; Ghukasyan, L.; Khachatryan, G.; Sirunyan, T.; Muradyan, N.; Zakharyan, R.; Chavushyan, A.; Hayrapetyan, V.; et al. Molecular Analysis of SARS-CoV-2 Lineages in Armenia. *Viruses* **2022**, *14*, 1074. [CrossRef]
9. Avagyan, H.; Hakobyan, S.; Poghosyan, A.; Hakobyan, L.; Abroyan, L.; Karalova, E.; Avetisyan, A.; Sargsyan, M.; Baghdasaryan, B.; Bayramyan, N.; et al. Severe Acute Respiratory Syndrome Coronavirus-2 Delta Variant Study In Vitro and Vivo. *Curr. Issues Mol. Biol.* **2022**, *45*, 249–267. [CrossRef]
10. Tanaka, Y.; Brecher, G.; Bull, B. Ferritin localization on the erythroblast cell membrane and ropheocytosis in hypersiderotic human bone marrows. *Blood* **1966**, *28*, 758–769. [CrossRef]
11. Yuan, K.; Zheng, Y.B.; Wang, Y.J.; Sun, Y.K.; Gong, Y.M.; Huang, Y.T.; Chen, X.; Liu, X.X.; Zhong, Y.; Su, S.Z.; et al. A systematic review and meta-analysis on prevalence of and risk factors associated with depression, anxiety and insomnia in infectious diseases, including COVID-19: A call to action. *Mol. Psychiatry* **2022**, *27*, 3214–3222. [CrossRef] [PubMed]
12. Tsujita, K.; Shiraishi, T.; Kakinuma, K. Microspectrophotometry of nitric oxide-dependent changes in hemoglobin in single red blood cells incubated with stimulated macrophages. *J. Biochem.* **1997**, *122*, 264–270. [CrossRef] [PubMed]
13. Lan, J.; Ge, J.; Yu, J.; Shan, S.; Zhou, H.; Fan, S.; Zhang, Q.; Shi, X.; Wang, Q.; Zhang, L.; et al. Structure of the SARS-CoV-2 spike receptor-binding domain bound to the ACE2 receptor. *Nature* **2020**, 215–220. [CrossRef]
14. Baccard-Longere, M.; Freymuth, F.; Cointe, D.; Seigneurin, J.M.; Grangeot-Keros, L. Multicenter evaluation of a rapid and convenient method for determination of cytomegalovirus immunoglobulin G avidity. *Clin. Diagn. Lab. Immunol.* **2001**, *8*, 429–431. [CrossRef]
15. Constantino, B.T.; Cogionis, B. Nucleated RBCs—Significance in the Peripheral Blood Film. *Lab. Med.* **2000**, *31*, 223–229. [CrossRef]
16. Liu, W.; Li, H. COVID-19: Captures iron and generates reactive oxygen species to damage the human immune system. *Autoimmunity* **2021**, *54*, 213–224. [CrossRef]
17. Torti, L.; Maffei, L.; Sorrentino, F.; De Fabritiis, P.; Miceli, R.; Abruzzese, E. Impact of SARS-CoV-2 in Hemoglobinopathies with Immune Disfunction and Epidemiology. A Protective Mechanism from Beta Chain Hemoglobin Defects? *Mediterr. J. Hematol. Infect. Dis.* **2020**, *12*, e2020052. [CrossRef]
18. Encabo, H.H.; Grey, W.; Garcia-Albornoz, M.; Wood, H.; Ulferts, R.; Aramburu, I.V.; Kulasekararaj, A.G.; Mufti, G.; Papayannopoulos, V.; Beale, R.; et al. Human Erythroid Progenitors Are Directly Infected by SARS-CoV-2: Implications for Emerging Erythropoiesis in Severe COVID-19 Patients. *Stem Cell Rep.* **2021**, *16*, 428–436. [CrossRef]
19. Allegra, A.; Di Gioacchino, M.; Tonacci, A.; Musolino, C.; Gangemi, S. Immunopathology of SARS-CoV-2 infection: Immune cells and mediators, prognostic factors, and immune-therapeutic implications. *Int. J. Mol. Sci.* **2020**, *21*, E4782. [CrossRef]

20. Kosenko, E.; Tikhonova, L.; Alilova, G.; Montoliu, C. Erythrocytes Functionality in SARS-CoV-2 Infection: Potential Link with Alzheimers Disease. *Int. J. Mol. Sci.* **2023**, *24*, 5739. [CrossRef]
21. Mawatari, K.; Matsukawa, S.; Yoneyama, Y. Different effects of subunit association upon absorption and circular dichroism spectra of methemoglobin. *Biochim. Biophys. Acta* **1983**, *745*, 219–228. [CrossRef] [PubMed]
22. Spolitak, T.; Hollenberg, P.F.; Ballou, D.P. Oxidative hemoglobin reactions: Applications to drug metabolism. *Arch. Biochem. Biophys.* **2016**, *600*, 33–46. [CrossRef] [PubMed]
23. Gozalbo-Rovira, R.; Gimenez, E.; Latorre, V.; Frances-Gomez, C.; Albert, E.; Buesa, J.; Marina, A.; Blasco, M.L.; Signes-Costa, J.; Rodriguez-Diaz, J.; et al. SARS-CoV-2 antibodies, serum inflammatory biomarkers and clinical severity of hospitalized COVID-19 patients. *J. Clin. Virol.* **2020**, *131*, 104611. [CrossRef] [PubMed]
24. Lega, S.; Naviglio, S.; Volpi, S.; Tommasini, A. Recent insight into SARS-CoV2 immunopathology and rationale for potential treatment and preventive strategies in COVID-19. *Vaccines* **2020**, *8*, E224. [CrossRef]
25. Kernan, K.F.; Carcillo, J.A. Hyperferritinemia and inflammation. *Int. Immunol.* **2017**, *29*, 401–409. [CrossRef]
26. Taneri, P.E.; Gómez-Ochoa, S.A.; Llanaj, E.; Raguindin, P.F.; Rojas, L.Z.; Roa-Díaz, Z.M.; Salvador, D.; Groothof, D.; Minder, B.; Kopp-Heim, D.; et al. Anemia and iron metabolism in COVID-19: A systematic review and meta-analysis. *Eur. J. Epidemiol.* **2020**, *35*, 763–773. [CrossRef]
27. Patel, K.V.; Ferrucci, L.; Ershler, W.B.; Longo, D.L.; Guralnik, J.M. Red blood cell distribution width and the risk of death in middle-aged and older adults. *Arch. Intern. Med.* **2009**, *169*, 515–523. [CrossRef]
28. Emans, M.E.; Gaillard, C.A.; Pfister, R.; Tanck, M.W.; Boekholdt, S.M.; Wareham, N.J.; Khaw, K.T. Red cell distribution width is associated with physical inactivity and heart failure, independent of established risk factors, inflammation or iron metabolism; the EPIC-Norfolk study. *Int. J. Cardiol.* **2013**, *168*, 3550–3555. [CrossRef]

Disclaimer/Publisher's Note: The statements, opinions and data contained in all publications are solely those of the individual author(s) and contributor(s) and not of MDPI and/or the editor(s). MDPI and/or the editor(s) disclaim responsibility for any injury to people or property resulting from any ideas, methods, instructions or products referred to in the content.

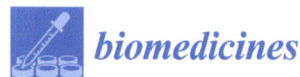

Review

A Narrative Review of the Efficacy of Long COVID Interventions on Brain Fog, Processing Speed, and Other Related Cognitive Outcomes

Bryana Whitaker-Hardin [1], Keith M. McGregor [2,3], Gitendra Uswatte [4] and Kristine Lokken [5,*]

[1] Neuroscience Theme, Graduate Biomedical Sciences Doctoral Training Program, Joint Health Sciences, University of Alabama at Birmingham, Birmingham, AL 35294, USA; whitakeb@uab.edu
[2] Birmingham Veterans Affairs Geriatric Research Education and Clinical Center, Birmingham Veterans Affairs Health Care System, Birmingham, AL 35294, USA; kmmcgreg@uab.edu
[3] Department of Clinical and Diagnostic Sciences, School of Health Professions, University of Alabama at Birmingham, Birmingham, AL 35294, USA
[4] Departments of Psychology & Physical Therapy, College of Arts and Sciences, University of Alabama at Birmingham, Birmingham, AL 35294, USA; guswatte@uab.edu
[5] Department of Psychiatry and Behavioral Neurobiology, Heersink School of Medicine, University of Alabama at Birmingham, Birmingham, AL 35294, USA
* Correspondence: kristinelokken@uabmc.edu

Academic Editor: César Fernández-de-las-Peñas

Received: 27 December 2024
Revised: 23 January 2025
Accepted: 30 January 2025
Published: 10 February 2025

Citation: Whitaker-Hardin, B.; McGregor, K.M.; Uswatte, G.; Lokken, K. A Narrative Review of the Efficacy of Long COVID Interventions on Brain Fog, Processing Speed, and Other Related Cognitive Outcomes. *Biomedicines* **2025**, *13*, 421. https://doi.org/10.3390/biomedicines13020421

Copyright: © 2025 by the authors. Licensee MDPI, Basel, Switzerland. This article is an open access article distributed under the terms and conditions of the Creative Commons Attribution (CC BY) license (https://creativecommons.org/licenses/by/4.0/).

Abstract: In the years following the global emergence of severe acute respiratory syndrome coronavirus 2 (SARS-CoV-2), or COVID-19, researchers have become acutely aware of long-term symptomology associated with this disease, often termed long COVID. Long COVID is associated with pervasive symptoms affecting multiple organ systems. Neurocognitive symptoms are reported by up to 40% of long COVID patients, with resultant effects of loss of daily functioning, employment issues, and enormous economic impact and high healthcare utilization. The literature on effective, safe, and non-invasive interventions for the remediation of the cognitive consequences of long COVID is scarce and poorly described. Of specific interest to this narrative review is the identification of potential interventions for long COVID-associated neurocognitive deficits. Articles were sourced from PubMed, EBSCO, Scopus, and Embase following Preferred Reporting Items for Systematic Reviews and Meta-Analyses (PRISMA) guidelines. Articles published between the dates of January 2020 and 30 June 2024 were included in the search. Twelve studies were included in the narrative review, including a feasibility study, a pilot study, a case series, a case study, and an observational study, in addition to three randomized clinical trials and four interventional studies. Overall, treatment interventions such as cognitive training, non-invasive brain stimulation therapy, exercise rehabilitation, targeted pharmacological intervention, and other related treatment paradigms show promise in reducing long COVID cognitive issues. This narrative review highlights the need for more rigorous experimental designs and future studies are needed to fully evaluate treatment interventions for persistent cognitive deficits associated with long COVID.

Keywords: long COVID; PASC; cognition; brain fog

1. Introduction

Coronavirus disease 2019 (COVID-19) is caused by the severe acute respiratory syndrome coronavirus 2 virus (SARS-CoV-2) and can trigger a diverse range of symptoms that manifest into mild, severe, or even fatal illness [1]. Since the onset of the COVID-19 pandemic in December of 2019, more than 770 million cases of COVID-19 have been reported to the World Health Organization [2]. This unprecedented impact on global healthcare has continued to evolve, with one of the newest developments being the persistence of debilitating symptoms months (or years) after an initial infection of SARS-CoV-2. Also known as long COVID, chronic COVID, long-haul COVID, and/or post-acute sequalae of COVID-19 (PASC), the long-term presence of multisystemic symptoms such as cognitive dysfunction ("brain fog"), dysautonomia, respiratory problems, dyspnea, musculoskeletal pain, and fatigue and/or post-exertional malaise is a severe burden on patients [3–7] (Long COVID is estimated to affect approximately 3.4–6.9% of adults and 1.3% of children living in the United States who have been previously infected with SARS-CoV-2 [8,9] with cumulative global incidence of long COVID as high as 400 million individuals and an estimated annual economic impact of approximately USD 1 trillion, equivalent to about 1% of the global economy [10].

Long COVID symptoms can result in a loss of daily functioning, including interfering with work as well as issues with returning to work, and long-term physical manifestations across multiple organ systems [9,11]. These functional and physical impairments are often accompanied by neurocognitive impairments, a decrease in overall quality of life, and worsening or novel onset of mental health conditions [12].

The term "brain fog" has garnered attention as the shared cognitive experience of a heterogeneous set of cognitive issues, including intermittent confusion, effortful cognition, brain-based fatigue, slowed processing speed, executive function deficits, forgetfulness, and sluggish thinking or clouded mentation by those with long COVID [13]. Long COVID brain fog can be exacerbated by or lead to insomnia, depression, and anxiety disorders [6,14]. Brain fog symptoms are also reported by others with infection-associated chronic conditions (referred to as post-acute infection syndromes) and patients with seemingly unrelated neurological, psychiatric, and physical conditions including mild traumatic brain injury (mTBI), multiple sclerosis (MS), lupus, myalgic encephalomyelitis (ME), bipolar disorder, and celiac disease, among others [15]. There is no scientific definition of brain fog to date; however, it is broadly understood in the literature as generalized cognitive dysfunction, subjectively related to issues with memory, attention, and executive functioning [16].

Although the impact of brain fog on cognition is typically of low to moderate severity, the impact on daily functioning, work capacity, and quality of life can be devastating, especially considering patients reporting these symptoms are generally younger and of workforce age [17]. Additionally, patients with brain fog symptoms can put an extensive burden on the medical system through increased healthcare utilization. The literature and the lay media are riddled with reports of long COVID patients feeling they must "prove" their illness, often leading to lengthy diagnostic odysseys with few effective treatment options [18].

Much like its diverse symptomatic presentation, several pathophysiological mechanisms have been suggested to contribute to the neuropsychological deficits in long COVID. As highlighted in Mehandru and Merad's work, chronic inflammation, marked by elevation in proinflammatory cytokines, is a hallmark pathology that that is associated with the significant persistence and severity of long COVID-associated neurological symptoms (2022) [19]. Importantly, neuroinflammation markers as assessed with positron emission topography (PET) scans have been found across multiple brain regions in individuals with long COVID [20]. Additional mechanisms that have been proposed to specifically contribute to cognitive deficits in this population include reduced cerebral blood flow as shown by arterial spin labeling magnetic resonance images (MRIs), central nervous system atrophy (e.g., loss of hippocampal neurogenesis), autonomic system dysfunction, and reduced serotonin levels [21–26]. Autonomic system dysfunction is often the result of impaired vagus nerve function, but the exact molecular mechanisms are unknown [27].

Other general pathophysiological mechanisms that are suggested to contribute to long COVID-associated neurological symptoms include metabolic dysfunction, viral persistence, and systematic organ damage from acute COVID-19 infection [28–30].

The literature on the remediation of neuropsychological consequences of long COVID is scarce and poorly described. Methodological concerns are common, including heterogeneity of patients and ill-described procedures, including variable time frame post-infection and use of low-sensitivity screening measures. To this end, studies examining potential interventions to reduce or alleviate neuropsychological symptoms are also limited and often present with contradictory conclusions. However, patients and providers are in search of non-invasive, safe, and efficacious interventions to improve processing speed and other cognitive issues post-COVID. Certainly, effective therapies to address the sequalae of long COVID, particularly the cognitive symptoms, are a priority for identification and dissemination. Of specific interest to this narrative review is the identification of potential remediation interventions for long COVID-associated neurocognitive deficits, which are present in an estimated 20–40% of long COVID cases [31]. The authors chose to conduct a narrative review, as few papers that focused on the treatment of cognitive issues in long COVID included comparable outcome measures or detailed quantitative outcomes, making it impossible to extract and standardize data from each study to statistically pool the data to generate an estimate of the effect size across the studies.

It seems important to investigate the different avenues of treatment for individuals dealing with long COVID. For the purposes of this narrative review, we examine if long COVID-related cognitive symptoms such as brain fog and processing speed problems were measured and potentially alleviated in psychological/cognitive training, non-invasive brain stimulation therapy, exercise rehabilitation, and pharmacological and/or other related treatment paradigms. We chose to present the material in a narrative review format, as the primary goal of this paper was to provide a comprehensive overview of currently published long COVID interventions to inform a cohesive strategy for future treatment interventions.

2. Materials and Methods

We searched three databases: PubMed, Embase, and Scopus. Search terms were as follows: (intervention OR rehabilitation) AND ("PASC" OR long covid OR post-covid OR chronic covid) AND (brain fog or processing speed). Articles published between the dates of January 2020 and 30 June 2024 were included in the search. The aspirational goal was to include only randomized controlled clinical trials in this review; however, given the dearth of literature examining interventions for long COVID cognitive issues, a variety of methodologies were considered for inclusion. After the removal of 52 duplicate results across all three databases, a total of 601 articles were downloaded. Articles were sourced following Preferred Reporting Items for Systematic Reviews and Meta-Analyses (PRISMA) guidelines [32]. Figure 1 shows the flow diagram detailing the review process and study selection based on the PRISMA flow chart.

One major methodological concern throughout the literature related to long COVID treatment paradigms is the variability in post-infection time-period of the participants. Many interventions were provided to patients in the acute phase of the illness (e.g., fewer than 4 weeks post-infection) or to those fewer than 12 weeks post-infection. We utilized the World Health Organization's definition of long COVID, characterized as symptoms persisting for more than 12 weeks after acute COVID-19 infection [2]. Recent guidance from the National Academies of Science, Engineering, and Medicine's June 2024 consensus definition for long COVID concurred with the WHO definition [9]. This guidance includes five key elements in the definition of long COVID: (1) attribution to SARS-CoV-2 infection of any severity; (2) onset can be continuous from or delayed following acute SARS-CoV-2 infection, with the duration of symptoms present for more than 12 consecutive weeks; (3) symptoms are numerous and can range in severity and duration; (4) long COVID can affect anyone regardless of health, disability, or socioeconomic status, age, sex, gender, sexual orientation, race, ethnicity, or geographic location; and (5) long COVID can be resultant in profound emotional, cognitive, and physical impairments.

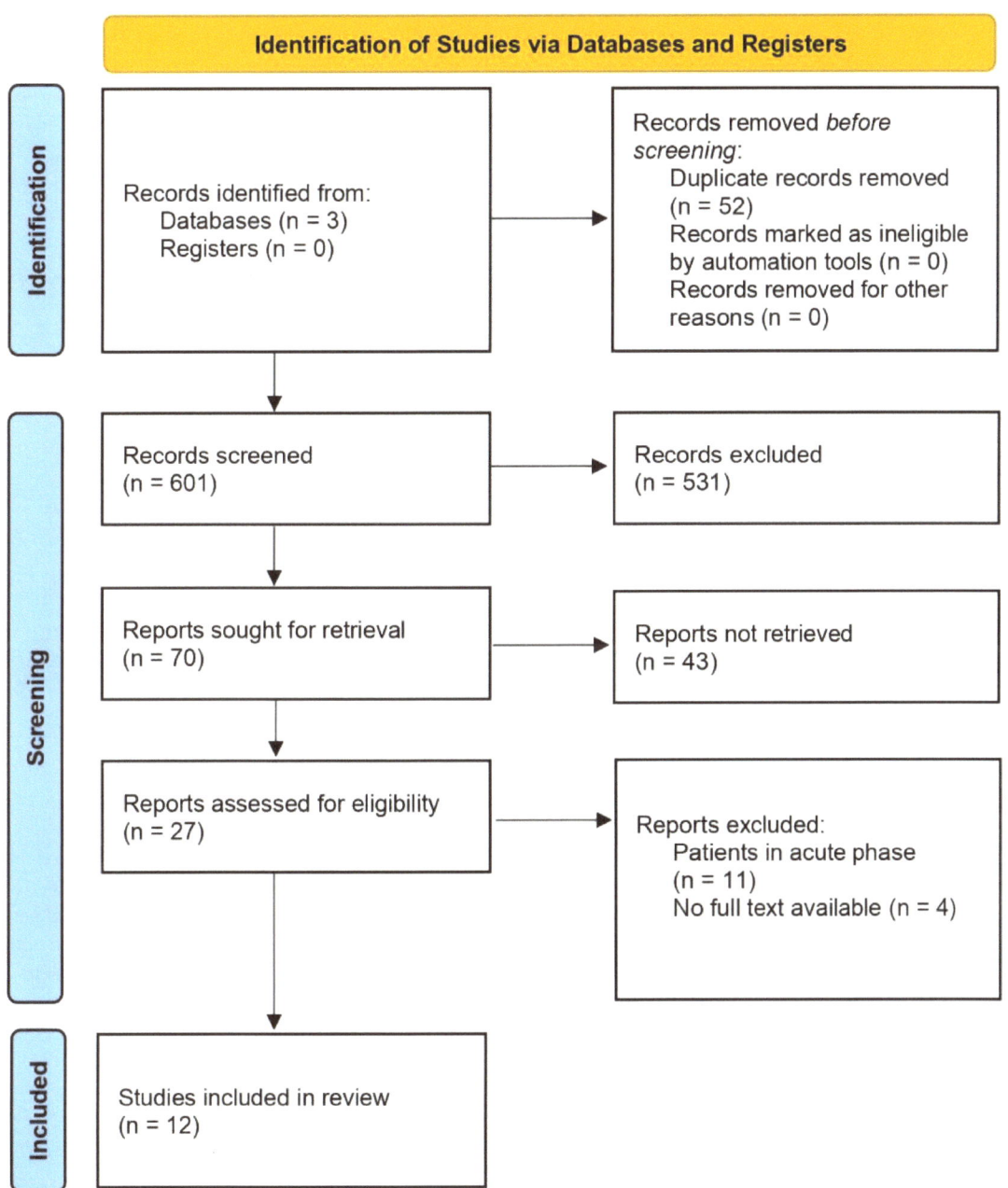

Figure 1. PRISMA flow chart.

Consistent with the WHO's and the National Academies of Science, Engineering, and Medicine's June 2024 consensus definition, articles included in this review must have recruited adult participants who reported novel symptoms following SARS-CoV-2 infection that were consistently present for more than 12 weeks. The reported intervention must have been aimed at reducing symptomology associated with long COVID, and the authors must have discussed cognitive outcomes such as mental fatigue or brain fog, speed of processing, memory deficits, and/or executive functioning. After applying these stringent criteria, only 12 articles, including one case study and one case series, met these criteria (Table 1).

Table 1. Articles included in this narrative review.

Author and Year	Number of Participants	Type of Intervention	Study Design	Reported Results
Dunabeitia et al., 2022 [33]	73	Cognitive Training	Feasibility Study	Sig. increase in perception, attention, memory, coordination, and reasoning skills
Noda et al., 2023 [34]	23	Cognitive Training (rTMS)	Pilot Study	Sig. increase in attention, memory, and planning/organizational skills
Sakib et al., 2024 [35]	4	Cognitive Training (rTMS)	Case Series	Non-sig. increase in behavioral inhibition performance
Sasaki et al., 2023 [36]	12	Cognitive Training (rTMS)	Interventional Study	Sig. increase in verbal comprehension, reasoning, working memory, and processing speed performance
Tsuchida et al., 2023 [37]	1	Cognitive Training (rTMS)	Case Study	Non-sig. increase in memory and reasoning skills
McGregor et al., 2024 [38]	585	Exercise	Randomized Controlled Trial	Non-sig. improvement in cognitive function
Moine et al., 2024 [39]	47	Exercise	Interventional Study	Sig. increase in MoCA scores and sig. reduction in mental fatigue
Rzepka-Cholasinska et al., 2024 [40]	90	Exercise	Observational Study	Sig. reduction in mental fatigue
De Luca et al., 2022 [41]	69	Pharmacological (PEA-LUT)	Longitudinal Interventional Study	Non-sig. reduction in mental clouding with drug treatment alone
Hawkins et al., 2022 [42]	40	Pharmacological (Aromatherapy)	Randomized Controlled Trial	Sig. reduction in mental fatigue
Salvucci et al., 2023 [43]	27	Pharmacological (Antihistamines)	Interventional Study	Sig. reduction in self-reported brain fog
Tanashyan et al., 2023 [44]	30	Pharmacological (Brainmax)	Randomized Controlled Trial	Sig. reduction in mental fatigue

3. Review

3.1. Cognitive Training or Neuromodulation Interventions

Cognitive training with or without neuromodulation may assist in alleviating deficits in specific cognitive domains and are largely derivative from programs designed to remediate aging-related cognitive decline. Recently neurophysiologists have paired neuromodulatory techniques including transcranial magnetic, electrical, ultrasound, and optical stimulation as an adjuvant (or standalone) treatment with training. Five studies implemented a form of cognitive training or neuromodulation as the primary intervention strategy for participants struggling with the cognitive effects of long COVID. Four of these five studies utilized a paradigm for repetitive transcranial magnetic stimulation (rTMS).

Dunabeitia, et al. (2022) utilized a digital personalized computerized cognitive training (CCT) intervention to improve cognitive function among people living with long COVID. Participants completed the Cognitive Assessment Battery PRO (CAB), a self-administered online general cognitive evaluation psychometric tool developed by CogniFit Inc. (CogniFit Inc., San Fransisco, CA, USA) to assess and then later tailor participants' 8-week CCT via the patented Individualized Training System™ (ITS) software that automatically chooses the activities and difficulty levels for each person in every session [33]. Specifically, performance scores were divided into five cognitive domains that comprise critical aspects of executive function: perception, attention, memory, coordination, and reasoning. Participants were asked to access the CAB-based training routinely for 8 weeks to improve their below-median baseline scores. A statistically significant effect of cognitive training was reported as participants who enrolled in CAB scored significantly higher in all five domains post-intervention. Importantly, coordination, operationalized via scores derived from response time and eye-hand coordination assessments, yielded the steepest increase in performance. Despite these promising results for a non-invasive, at-home intervention for people dealing with the cognitive fallout of long COVID, this study was only a feasibility study and included no control group, limiting the conclusions that can be drawn from these results due to the difficulty of isolating the true effect of the CCT and potential for bias from participant expectations.

Results from the remaining cognitive training or neuromodulation interventions utilized distinct rTMS protocols to target and remediate neurocognitive deficits associated with long COVID. It is important to note that two of these articles present data from case studies of one to four patients while the remaining two articles drew from a slightly larger pool of 14 to 23 patients (i.e., case series). Therefore, there were neither control groups nor effect size calculations included in these neuromodulatory interventions, limiting the conclusions that can be drawn and the ability to generalize findings to a wider population. The first of these case studies involved one patient, a 30-year-old Japanese woman who presented with chronic fatigue, cognitive dysfunction, and blurry vision that persisted for 7 months following SARS-CoV2 infection [37]. The authors did not report the specific rTMS paradigm that was used, but its results did align with those reported by Dunabeitia, et al., as their participant's memory and reasoning functioning, measured via the Wechsler Adult Intelligence Scale (WAIS), specifically processing speed index score and perceptual reasoning index score, improved post-intervention (2022) [37]. Additionally, the subject's verbal comprehension index and full-scale intelligence quotient increased from baseline, but her working memory index remained the same.

The second case series provided more methodological detail, with investigators utilizing three stimulation conditions: intermittent theta burst stimulation with 600 pulses (iTBS-600), iTBS-300, and sham stimulation [35]. Brain stimulation was delivered to the participants' ($n = 4$) left dorsolateral prefrontal cortex in each of the three stimulation paradigms. It was reported that three of the four participants improved on a measure of behavioral inhibition (i.e., a modified Flanker interference assessing reasoning and processing speed) post-iTBS-600 protocol.

A study by Noda and colleagues reported a statistically significant increase in attention/concentration, retrospective and prospective memory, and planning/organizational abilities post-rTMS stimulation (2023). Unlike the participants of Sakib et al.'s case study, individuals of this pilot case series ($n = 23$) were asked to complete one session of iTBS for the left dorsolateral prefrontal cortex as well as one session of low frequency rTMS for the right lateral orbitofrontal cortex per day over the course of 20 days (for detailed protocol, see [45]). The addition of the second stimulation site was intended to better target the pathophysiology of long COVID. Cognitive function was assessed using the Perceived Deficits Questionnaire—Depression Five Item, generating the four sub scores used to assess the specific cognitive domains. Major limitations of this study were the lack of a control group, as this case series was an open-label preliminary trial for an rTMS intervention, and reliance on self-report versus objective cognitive outcome measures. These limitations increase the likelihood of a placebo effect and social desirability response by participants.

Sasaki and colleagues (2023), in another case series ($n = 12$), applied 1200 10-Hz rTMS to the midline of the occipital region followed by an application of 1200 10-Hz rTMS to the forehead (defined as 45° above the external auditory meatus) for a total of 10 applications to each neural area of interest. For Sasaki, et al.'s assessment of processing speed and overall cognitive function, the Wechsler Adult Intelligence Scale was implemented as in Tsuchida et al.'s rTMS case study (2023). Cognitive outcome measures included verbal comprehension, perceptual reasoning, working memory, and processing speed. A statistically significant increase in all four areas of cognitive function was reported post-intervention, along with an increased full scale intelligence quotient (FSIQ) from 94.6 ± 10.9 to 104.4 ± 13.0 [36].

These five studies reported an increase in processing speed and overall cognitive function, suggesting that neuropsychological deficits associated with long COVID can potentially be remediated. This finding speaks to the merit of incorporating a non-invasive, non-physically taxing (i.e., these paradigms require minimal physical exertion) component in an intervention. Patients with long COVID are particularly suited for such a rehabilitation strategy, as a high level of exercise intolerance is documented in this specific population [46,47]. Caution must be applied when interpreting these results, however, as none of the studies included a control group. Without a control group, it is difficult to confidently determine whether observed changes are due to the experimental intervention or other external factors, leading to unreliable conclusions about the effectiveness of the treatment being studied. Carefully controlled randomized control trials are warranted to support these promising interventions.

As to mechanism of action, the rTMS paradigm's ability to increase cerebral blood flow may contribute to a recovery in cognitive function [48]. Both Tsuchida et al. and Sasaki et al. reported supporting findings from single-photon emission computed tomography (SPECT) in their participants, showing an overall increase in the level of blood flow within the brain after stimulation (2023). This change in vasculature has been documented in other published studies as well [48–50]. Another suggested mechanism for the positive impact of cognitive training and neuromodulation interventions is their ability to modulate synaptic connections in the brain [5,51–53]. As dynamic synapses are the basis for multiple cognitive processes, including learning and memory, the engagement and subsequent strengthening of synapses may help explain the reported improvement in cognitive functions. Changes in connectivity have been strongly linked to symptoms of brain fog and changes in overall connectivity as recently reviewed.

3.2. Exercise Interventions

A total of three studies that employed an exercise intervention and met the outlined methodological criteria were included in this narrative review. Each of the rehabilitation programs lasted for a different number of weeks and employed different exercise tactics. One of these interventions also included a psychological support component for participants, but, given the lack of a cognitive training aspect in the intervention, we have elected to treat this rehabilitation strategy as one that relied more heavily on the inclusion of physical activity. The uniting factor for these three studies is how they were designed with the patient's diagnosis of long COVID in mind, helping to alleviate the documented exercise intolerance within this specific population [46,47].

The first of the three articles implemented a four-week physical rehabilitation strategy that included endurance training sessions (e.g., walking and ergocycling) and resistance training sessions [39]. Participants underwent a mean of 26 individualized endurance training sessions combining walking and ergocycling at an intensity close to the ventilation threshold, in addition to 12 individualized resistance training sessions. Patients were asked to work at a level of perceived exertion of 7 out of 10 and each resistance training session included four exercises: two exercises targeting the muscles of the lower limbs and two exercises targeting the muscles of the upper limbs. Originally intended for pulmonary rehabilitation, the training was adapted for effect on cognitive function in long COVID as measured by the Montreal Cognitive Assessment (MoCA), the Modified Fatigue Impact Scale (MFIS), and other related, validated questionnaires. Post-intervention, participants reported statistically significant lower levels of mental fatigue and scored significantly higher on the MoCA, demonstrating the promise of an exercise intervention for individuals with long COVID.

The second exercise intervention also used the MFIS as the outcome measure [40]. This intervention utilized a high-intensity interval training program that incorporated aerobic exercise with a warm-up and cool-down phase three times a week across six weeks. There was no control group included in this study, making it difficult to isolate the impact of the intervention from other potential influences; however, there was a statistically significant decline in both male and female participants' MFIS scores post-exercise intervention, demonstrating a decrease in overall levels of fatigue and in the overall impact of fatigue.

The third and final article was conducted by McGregor, et al., (2024). As a part of the Rehabilitation Exercise and psycholoGical support After COVID-19 InfectioN (REGAIN) trial, 585 adults (26–86 years) with ongoing physical and/or mental health sequelae secondary to long COVID were included in the multicenter, parallel-group, randomized controlled trial. Participants were randomized to receive the REGAIN intervention (exercise and psychological support; $n = 298$) or usual care ($n = 287$). The REGAIN intervention consisted of an eight-week course of online, weekly, home-based, live, supervised group exercise and psychological support sessions. Usual care was a single online educational session. The Patient-Reported Outcomes Measurement Information System (PROMIS) health-related quality of life was the primary outcome measure. Secondary outcomes included PROMIS subscores of depression, fatigue, sleep disturbance, pain interference, physical function, social roles/activities, and cognitive function. The REGAIN participants reported a statistically significant improvement in health-related quality of life at 3 months, which was sustained at 12 months compared to usual care, along with statistically significant improvements in self-reported depression, fatigue, and sleep disturbance. By 12 months, all PROMIS subscores and subscales were improved more in the intervention group; however, the improvements were not statistically significant in the domains of pain interference physical function, social roles/activities, or cognitive function. These findings do highlight the need for rigorous studies aimed specifically at cognitive rehabilitation for patients struggling with long COVID.

3.3. Pharmacological Interventions

Four articles met this narrative review's criteria and implemented a form of a pharmacological intervention, including antihistamine drugs, a novel neuroprotectant drug complex, and aromatherapy. Salvucci and colleagues chose to administer two antihistamine medications to the 14 participants in their experimental group: 180 mg of fexofenadine (histamine H1 receptor antagonist) and 40 mg of famotidine (histamine H2 antagonist) each day for 20 days (2023). The 13 participants in the control group were not treated with these antihistamines as they refused further pharmacological treatment for their symptoms. The decision to administer fexofenadine and famotidine was built upon the hypothesis that hyperinflammation, mediated partly by the activation of mast cells, contributes to the persistence of COVID-like symptoms beyond the initial infection period [54–57]. It was hypothesized that blocking the H1 and H2 receptors with these commonly prescribed medications would relieve long COVID-associated symptoms such as brain fog and fatigue. Importantly, participants in this study self-reported their level of mental clouding or brain fog, generating the major limitation of the study, as no verified questionnaire or cognitive assessment was administered. Regardless, a significant portion of the participants in the experimental group reported a vanishing of fatigue (43%) and brain fog (43%) post-intervention. This is in comparison to those in the control group, who reported no statistically significant improvements across symptoms.

The second pharmacological intervention included here investigated the effects of Promomed's new drug Brainmax [44]. Brainmax is comprised of the coordination complex between ethylmethylhydroxypyridine and trimethylhydrosinium propionate with succinate acid anion and was shown to possess a good safety profile in a 2022 randomized, double-blind, placebo-controlled study [44]. Fifteen participants received an intramuscular injection of Brainmax for 10 days while 15 participants received a placebo injection. Cognitive function was assessed using the Multidimensional Fatigue Inventory (MFI-20) and the Montreal Cognitive Assessment (MoCA). A statistically significant reduction in MFI-20 scores and a slight increase in MoCA scores were reported for patients who received Brainmax injections when compared to the placebo group. The authors suggested that a potential mechanism underlying the "neuroprotective, neuroregenerative, and neuroactivating" influence of Brainmax could be the complex's influence on the mitochondria as it enhances the stability of mitochondrial function [44,58]. Specifically, it reduces the severity of oxidative stress and the intensity of reactive oxidative species formation [59].

Additionally, the authors collected structural and functional magnetic resonance images (fMRI) before and after the pharmacological treatment and reported an increase in functional connectivity between the left dorsolateral prefrontal cortex and the proximal part of the left temporal operculum. Therefore, the decrease in physical and mental fatigue as well as the increase in MoCA score could be partially explained by the increase in correlations between neural areas critical for the processing and integration of incoming stimuli seen in individuals treated with Brainmax.

The third and final traditional pharmaceutical intervention utilized a palmitoylethanolamide-luteolin combination drug (PEA-LUT) [41]. Like the two drugs employed by Salvucci and colleagues, PEA-LUT has well-documented anti-inflammatory properties largely due to its ability to inhibit the release of mast cells and counteract the negative effects of cytokines, making it a strong candidate drug for relieving cognitive symptoms associated with long COVID [60,61]. De Luca and colleagues administered this supplement consistently for 90 days alone and in conjunction with olfactory training to individuals diagnosed with long COVID. No control group (i.e., no placebo was administered to participants with or without olfactory training) was included in this longitudinal study. Participants' levels of brain fog were measured by a previously published questionnaire comprising four detailed questions that assessed a person's concentration and overall mental ability [62].

Post-treatment, a non-statistically significant reduction in brain fog was observed for participants who received PEA-LUT alone. Participants who received PEA-LUT and olfactory training achieved a statistically significant reduction in brain fog. While an explanation was not offered as to why statistical significance was only achieved with the combination approach (i.e., PEA-LUT with olfactory training), the authors did cite the ability of palmitoylethanolamide to modulate histamine release and the ability of luteolin to promote the antioxidant response in neurons for the supplement's influence over the prevalence of brain fog [41].

A final experimental protocol that chose a non-traditional pharmaceutical approach investigated the efficacy of an alternative medicinal treatment in a randomized, double-blinded, placebo controlled clinical trial: aromatherapy [42]. The authors of this paper hoped to relieve a multitude of symptoms associated with long COVID, but their main symptom of interest was mental fatigue. Outcomes were assessed using the multidimensional fatigue symptom inventory—short form (MFIS-SF). The essential oils included for the intervention group included thyme (*Thymus vulgaris*), orange peel (*Citrus sinensis*), clove bud (*Eugenia caryophyllus*), and frankincense (*Boswellia carterii*) and were produced by Young Living Essential Oils. After a two-week period of exposure to the prescribed blend of essential oils, a statistically significant reduction in mental fatigue was reported, highlighting how non-traditional medicinal interventions can be used alongside their traditional pharmacological intervention counterparts.

4. Conclusions

Of particular interest to this narrative review was treatment remediation of long COVID-associated neurocognitive deficits, such as brain fog, persistent mental fatigue, and speed of processing, that are estimated to affect as many as 40% of patients currently struggling with long COVID [6,31].

The 12 articles collected for this narrative review present a diverse collection of rehabilitation strategies aimed at ameliorating long COVID-associated neurocognitive deficits. Treatment interventions such as cognitive training, rTMS, exercise rehabilitation, and pharmacological and other related treatment paradigms were found to be effective in reducing long COVID-related cognitive issues. While many of these studies have significant limitations (e.g., lack of an appropriate control group, use of self-report versus objective cognitive measures, unclear methodology), all reported a reduction in neurocognitive symptomology of long COVID to varying degrees post-intervention (i.e., some interventions resulted in statistically significant improvements, while others did not). Across the collected articles, reductions in mental fatigue, operationalized via self-reported measures and various assessments, and improvements in processing speed and brain fog were reported. Other promising therapeutic interventions for post-COVID neurocognitive deficits and fatigue include low dose naltrexone (LND) and hyperbaric oxygen therapy (H-BOT) [63–65]. Additionally, Uswatte et al. (2024) describe a pilot RCT (n = 14) using Constraint-Induced Cognitive Therapy (CICT) for the treatment of cognitive difficulties for individuals with long COVID [66]. The intervention resulted in large, statistically significant improvements in brain fog symptoms and performance of everyday activities. The investigators also found that 80% of those who were unemployed before CICT returned to work after the experimental intervention, while no one from the treatment-as-usual control group returned to work.

Planned randomized controlled studies using these therapeutic interventions with long COVID patients meeting the WHO and the National Academies of Science, Engineering, and Medicine's June 2024 consensus definition of long COVID will be of interest. The material was presented in a narrative review format to provide a comprehensive overview of currently published long COVID interventions. The findings of this review indicate promise for brief, non-invasive interventions for long COVID brain fog and mental fatigue and serve as a basis to inform a cohesive strategy for future treatment intervention studies.

The dearth of well-controlled studies highlights the need for continued investigation of effective interventions aimed at reducing the cognitive deficits associated with long COVID. Overall, the findings from this narrative review indicate that there are very few tightly controlled experimental designs and thus few definitive conclusions that can be drawn from these reports. Several research limitations were inherent to many of the studies in this review, including absence of control group, low sample sizes, no reported effect size calculations, outcome measures with low sensitivity, specificity, reliability, and validity, and limited reporting on participant variables and details of the interventions. Long COVID is persistent, debilitating, and enduring. Patients and practitioners are looking for safe interventions and a call to action is necessitated, as in the absence of safe, research-driven interventions patients may seek alternative and possibly harmful health alternatives.

Fatigue, manifesting as both physical fatigue and mental fatigue, is a core feature of long COVID. Fatigue is multifactorial and multisymptomatic and can be a driver of other physical, cognitive, and emotional issues. Future studies that employ a multi-modal approach to address fatigue, cognition, and mental health issues with appropriate controls are needed, along with descriptions of adjuvant, appropriate medical treatments targeted at specific symptom clusters.

Additionally, future research should direct more attention to the post-infection time frame of ≥ 12 weeks post last COVID-19 infection, consistent with the National Academies of Science, Engineering, and Medicine's consensus definition for long COVID [9]. Several articles were excluded from this narrative review as the authors failed to report an infection timeline for their participants, thus reducing the implied efficacy of the intervention versus spontaneous recovery in the acute post-infection phase. By adhering to the standard ≥ 12 weeks post-infection length of time as an inclusion criterion, the label of long COVID could be applied in a more controlled manner and ensure that patient populations are comparable in terms of their disease progression.

In conclusion, long COVID (regardless of infection severity or number of infections) is a global public health challenge with a sizeable effect on patient quality of life, economic productivity, and ultimately the global economy. Interventions aimed at improving fatigue, processing speed, and other related cognitive outcomes are urgently needed. Given the lack of experimental studies and randomized controlled trials (RCTs) focused on long COVID interventions, this review can serve as a call to action for clinicians and researchers.

Author Contributions: Conceptualization, K.M.M. and K.L.; methodology, B.W.-H., K.M.M. and K.L.; writing—original draft preparation, B.W.-H.; writing—review and editing, B.W.-H., K.M.M., G.U. and K.L. All authors have read and agreed to the published version of the manuscript.

Funding: Preparation of this paper was supported by grant 90IFRE0073 from the National Institute on Disability, Independent Living, and Rehabilitation Research (NIDILRR). The NIDILRR is a Center within the Administration for Community Living (ACL), Department of Health and Human Services (HHS).

Data Availability Statement: No new data were created or analyzed in this study.

Conflicts of Interest: The authors declare no conflict of interest.

References

1. Umakanthan, S.; Sahu, P.; Ranade, A.V.; Bukelo, M.M.; Rao, J.S.; Abrahao-Machado, L.F.; Dahal, S.; Kumar, H.; Kv, D. Origin, transmission, diagnosis and management of coronavirus disease 2019 (COVID-19). *Postgrad. Med. J.* **2020**, *96*, 753–758. [CrossRef] [PubMed]
2. World Health Organization. Number of COVID-19 Cases Reported to WHO (Cumulative Total). 2024. Available online: https://data.who.int/dashboards/covid19/cases (accessed on 13 September 2024).
3. Ahmad, S.J.; Feigen, C.M.; Vazquez, J.P.; Kobets, A.J.; Altschul, D.J. Neurological sequelae of COVID-19. *J. Integr. Neurosci.* **2022**, *21*, 77. [CrossRef] [PubMed]
4. Davis, H.E.; McCorkell, L.; Vogel, J.M.; Topol, E.J. Long COVID: Major findings, mechanisms and recommendations. *Nat. Rev. Microbiol.* **2023**, *21*, 133–146. [CrossRef] [PubMed]
5. Li, J.; Zhou, Y.; Ma, J.; Zhang, Q.; Shao, J.; Liang, S.; Yu, Y.; Li, W.; Wang, C. The long-term health outcomes, pathophysiological mechanisms and multidisciplinary management of long COVID. *Signal Transduct. Target. Ther.* **2023**, *8*, 416. [CrossRef]
6. Moghimi, N.; Di Napoli, M.; Biller, J.; Siegler, J.E.; Shekhar, R.; McCullough, L.D.; Harkins, M.S.; Hong, E.; Alaouieh, D.A.; Mansueto, G.; et al. The neurological manifestations of post-acute sequelae of SARS-CoV-2 infection. *Curr. Neurol. Neurosci. Rep.* **2021**, *21*, 44. [CrossRef]
7. Volberding, P.A.; Chu, B.X.; Spicer, C.M. *Long-Term Health Effects of COVID-19*; The National Academies Press: Washington, DC, USA, 2024.
8. Adjaye-Gbewonyo, D.; Vahratian, A.; Perrine, C.G.; Bertolli, J. Long COVID in adults: United States, 2022. *NCHS Data Brief* **2023**, *480*, 1–8.

9. National Academies of Sciences, Engineering, and Medicine. *Long-Term Health Effects of COVID-19: Disability and Function Following SARS-CoV-2 Infection*; The National Academies Press: Washington, DC, USA, 2024. [CrossRef]
10. Al-Aly, Z.; Davis, H.; McCorkell, L.; Soares, L.; Wulf-Hanson, S.; Iwasaki, A.; Topol, E.J. Long COVID science, research and policy. *Nat. Med.* **2024**, *30*, 2148–2164. [CrossRef]
11. Perlis, R.H.; Trujillo, K.L.; Safarpour, A.; Santillana, M.; Ognyanova, K.; Druckman, J.; Lazer, D. Association of post-COVID-19 condition symptoms and employment status. *JAMA Netw. Open* **2023**, *6*, e2256152. [CrossRef]
12. Chasco, E.E.; Dukes, K.; Jones, D.; Comellas, A.P.; Hoffman, R.M.; Garg, A. Brain fog and fatigue following COVID-19 infection: An exploratory study of patient experiences of Long COVID. *Int. J. Environ. Res. Public Health* **2022**, *19*, 15499. [CrossRef]
13. Kavanagh, E. Long Covid brain fog: A neuroinflammation phenomenon? *Oxf. Open Immunol.* **2022**, *3*, iqac007. [CrossRef] [PubMed] [PubMed Central]
14. Takao, M.; Ohira, M. Neurological post-acute sequelae of SARS-CoV-2 infection. *Psychiatry Clin. Neurosci.* **2023**, *77*, 72–83. [CrossRef] [PubMed]
15. Kverno, K. Brain Fog: A Bit of Clarity Regarding Etiology, Prognosis, and Treatment. *J. Psychosoc. Nurs. Ment. Health Serv.* **2021**, *59*, 9–13. [CrossRef] [PubMed]
16. McWhirter, L.; Smyth, H.; Hoeritzauer, I.; Couturier, A.; Stone, J.; Carson, A.J. What is brain fog? *J. Neurol. Neurosurg. Psychiatry* **2022**, *94*, 321–325. [CrossRef]
17. Pihlajamäki, M.; Arola, H.; Ahveninen, H.; Ollikainen, J.; Korhonen, M.; Nummi, T.; Taimela, S. Subjective cognitive complaints and permanent work disability: A prospective cohort study. *Int. Arch. Occup. Environ. Health* **2021**, *94*, 901–910. [CrossRef]
18. Au, L.; Capotescu, C.; Eyal, G.; Finestone, G. Long covid and medical gaslighting: Dismissal, delayed diagnosis, and deferred treatment. *SSM Qual. Res. Health* **2022**, *2*, 100167. [CrossRef]
19. Mehandru, S.; Merad, M. Pathological sequelae of long-haul COVID. *Nat. Immunol.* **2022**, *23*, 194–202. [CrossRef]
20. VanElzakker, M.B.; Bues, H.F.; Brusaferri, L.; Kim, M.; Saadi, D.; Ratai, E.M.; Dougherty, D.D.; Loggia, M.L. Neuroinflammation in post-acute sequelae of COVID-19 (PASC) as assessed by [11C]PBR28 PET correlated with vascular disease measures. *Brain Behav. Immun.* **2024**, *119*, 712–723. [CrossRef]
21. Ajčević, M.; Iscra, K.; Furlanis, G.; Michelutti, M.; Miladinovic, A.; Stella, A.B.; Ukmar, M.; Cova, M.A.; Accardo, A.; Manganotti, P. Cerebral hypoperfusion in post-COVID-19 cognitively impaired subjects revealed by arterial spin labeling MRI. *Sci. Rep.* **2023**, *13*, 5808. [CrossRef]
22. Boldrini, M.; Canoll, P.D.; Klein, R.S. How COVID-19 affects the brain. *JAMA Psychiatry* **2021**, *78*, 682–683. [CrossRef]
23. Lladós, G.; Massanella, M.; Coll-Fernández, R.; Rodríguez, R.; Hernández, E.; Lucente, G.; López, C.; Loste, C.; Santos, J.R.; España-Cueto, S.; et al. Vagus nerve dysfunction in the post-COVID-19 condition: A pilot cross-sectional study. *Clin. Microbiol. Infect.* **2024**, *30*, 515–521. [CrossRef]
24. Soung, A.L.; Vanderheiden, A.; Nordvig, A.S.; Sissoko, C.A.; Canoll, P.; Mariani, M.B.; Jiang, X.; Bricker, T.; Rosoklija, G.B.; Arango, V.; et al. COVID-19 induces CNS cytokine expression and loss of hippocampal neurogenesis. *Brain* **2022**, *145*, 4193–4201. [CrossRef] [PubMed]
25. Wong, A.C.; Devason, A.S.; Umana, I.C.; Cox, T.O.; Dohnalová, L.; Litichevskiy, L.; Perla, J.; Lundgren, P.; Etwebi, Z.; Izzo, L.T.; et al. Serotonin reduction in post-acute sequelae of viral infection. *Cell* **2023**, *186*, 4851–4867.e20. [CrossRef] [PubMed]
26. Woo, M.S.; Shafiq, M.; Fitzek, A.; Dottermusch, M.; Altmeppen, H.; Mohammadi, B.; Mayer, C.; Bal, L.C.; Raich, L.; Matschke, J.; et al. Vagus nerve inflammation contributes to dysautonomia in COVID-19. *Acta Neuropathol.* **2023**, *146*, 387–394. [CrossRef]
27. Xu, E.; Xie, Y.; Al-Aly, Z. Long-term neurologic outcomes of COVID-19. *Nat. Med.* **2022**, *28*, 2406–2415. [CrossRef]
28. Ajaz, S.; McPhail, M.J.; Singh, K.K.; Mujib, S.; Trovato, F.M.; Napoli, S.; Agarwal, K. Mitochondrial metabolic manipulation by SARS-CoV-2 in peripheral blood mononuclear cells of patients with COVID-19. *Am. J. Physiol. Cell Physiol.* **2021**, *320*, C57–C65. [CrossRef] [PubMed]
29. Bergamaschi, L.; Mescia, F.; Turner, L.; Hanson, A.L.; Kotagiri, P.; Dunmore, B.J.; Ruffieux, H.; De Sa, A.; Huhn, O.; Morgan, M.D.; et al. Longitudinal analysis reveals that delayed bystander CD8+ T cell activation and early immune pathology distinguish severe COVID-19 from mild disease. *Immunity* **2021**, *54*, 1257–1275.e8. [CrossRef]
30. Scherer, P.E.; Kirwan, J.P.; Rosen, C.J. Post-acute sequelae of COVID-19: A metabolic perspective. *eLife* **2022**, *11*, e78200. [CrossRef]
31. Koterba, C.H.; Considine, C.M.; Becker, J.H.; Hoskinson, K.R.; Ng, R.; Vargas, G.; Basso, M.R.; Puente, A.E.; Lippa, S.M.; Whiteside, D.M. Neuropsychology practice guidance for the neuropsychiatric aspects of Long COVID. *Clin. Neuropsychol.* **2024**, 1–29. [CrossRef]
32. Page, M.J.; McKenzie, J.E.; Bossuyt, P.M.; Boutron, I.; Hoffmann, T.C.; Mulrow, C.D. The PRISMA 2020 statement: An updated guideline for reporting systematic reviews. *Br. Med. J.* **2021**, *372*, n71. [CrossRef]
33. Duñabeitia, J.A.; Mera, F.; Baro, Ó.; Jadad-Garcia, T.; Jadad, A.R. The impact of a home-based personalized computerized training program on cognitive dysfunction associated with Long COVID: A before-and-after feasibility study. *MedRxiv* **2022**, *20*, 3100. [CrossRef]

34. Noda, Y.; Sato, A.; Shichi, M.; Sato, A.; Fujii, K.; Iwasa, M.; Nagano, Y.; Kitahata, R.; Osawa, R. Real world research on transcranial magnetic stimulation treatment strategies for neuropsychiatric symptoms with long-COVID in Japan. *Asian J. Psychiatry* **2023**, *81*, 103438. [CrossRef]
35. Sakib, M.N.; Saragadam, A.; Santagata, M.C.; Jolicoeur-Becotte, M.; Kozyr, L.; Burhan, A.M.; Hall, P.A. rTMS for post-COVID-19 condition: A sham-controlled case series involving iTBS-300 and iTBS-600. *Brain Behav. Immun. Health* **2024**, *36*, 100736. [CrossRef] [PubMed]
36. Sasaki, N.; Yamatoku, M.; Tsuchida, T.; Sato, H.; Yamaguchi, K. Effect of repetitive transcranial magnetic stimulation on long Coronavirus disease 2019 with fatigue and cognitive dysfunction. *Prog. Rehabil. Med.* **2023**, *8*, 20230004. [CrossRef] [PubMed]
37. Tsuchida, T.; Sasaki, N.; Ohira, Y. Low brain blood flow finding on SPECT in long COVID patients with brain fog. *Q. J. Med. Mon. J. Assoc. Physicians* **2023**, *116*, 877–878. [CrossRef] [PubMed]
38. McGregor, G.; Sandhu, H.; Bruce, J.; Sheehan, B.; McWilliams, D.; Yeung, J.; Jones, C.; Lara, B.; Alleyne, S.; Smith, J.; et al. Clinical effectiveness of an online supervised group physical and mental health rehabilitation programme for adults with post-COVID-19 condition (REGAIN study): Multicentre randomised controlled trial. *Br. Med. J. Clin. Res. Ed.* **2024**, *384*, e076506. [CrossRef]
39. Moine, E.; Molinier, V.; Castanyer, A.; Calvat, A.; Coste, G.; Vernet, A.; Faugé, A.; Magrina, P.; Aliaga-Parera, J.L.; Oliver, N.; et al. Safety and efficacy of pulmonary rehabilitation for long COVID patients experiencing long-lasting symptoms. *Int. J. Environ. Res. Public Health* **2024**, *21*, 242. [CrossRef]
40. Rzepka-Cholasińska, A.; Ratajczak, J.; Michalski, P.; Kasprzak, M.; Kosobucka-Ozdoba, A.; Pietrzykowski, Ł.; Grzelakowska, K.; Kubica, J.; Kryś, J.; Kubica, A. Gender-related effectiveness of personalized post-COVID-19 rehabilitation. *J. Clin. Med.* **2024**, *13*, 938. [CrossRef]
41. De Luca, P.; Camaioni, A.; Marra, P.; Salzano, G.; Carriere, G.; Ricciardi, L.; Pucci, R.; Montemurro, N.; Brenner, M.J.; Di Stadio, A. Effect of ultra-micronized palmitoylethanolamide and luteolin on olfaction and memory in patients with long COVID: Results of a longitudinal study. *Cells* **2022**, *11*, 2552. [CrossRef]
42. Hawkins, J.; Hires, C.; Keenan, L.; Dunne, E. Aromatherapy blend of thyme, orange, clove bud, and frankincense boosts energy levels in post-COVID-19 female patients: A randomized, double-blinded, placebo controlled clinical trial. *Complement. Ther. Med.* **2022**, *67*, 102823. [CrossRef]
43. Salvucci, F.; Codella, R.; Coppola, A.; Zacchei, I.; Grassi, G.; Anti, M.L.; Nitisoara, N.; Luzi, L.; Gazzaruso, C. Antihistamines improve cardiovascular manifestations and other symptoms of long-COVID attributed to mast cell activation. *Front. Cardiovasc. Med.* **2023**, *10*, 1202696. [CrossRef]
44. Tanashyan, M.; Morozova, S.; Raskurazhev, A.; Kuznetsova, P. A prospective randomized, double-blind placebo-controlled study to evaluate the effectiveness of neuroprotective therapy using functional brain MRI in patients with post-covid chronic fatigue syndrome. *Biomed. Pharmacother.* **2023**, *168*, 115723. [CrossRef]
45. Feffer, K.; Fettes, P.; Giacobbe, P.; Daskalakis, Z.J.; Blumberger, D.M.; Downar, J. 1 Hz rTMS of the right orbitofrontal cortex for major depressoin: Safety, tolerability and clinical outcomes. *Eur. Neuropsychopharmacol.* **2018**, *28*, 109–117. [CrossRef] [PubMed]
46. Joseph, P.; Singh, I.; Oliveira, R.; Capone, C.A.; Mullen, M.P.; Cook, D.B.; Stovall, M.C.; Squires, J.; Madsen, K.; Waxman, A.B.; et al. Exercise pathophysiology in Myalgic Encephalomyelitis/Chronic Fatigue Syndrome and Postacute Sequelae of SARS-CoV-2: More in common than not? *Chest* **2023**, *164*, 717–726. [CrossRef] [PubMed]
47. Koleničová, V.; Vňuková, M.S.; Anders, M.; Fišerová, M.; Raboch, J.; Ptáček, R. A review article on exercise intolerance in Long COVID: Unmasking the causes and optimizing treatment strategies. *Med. Sci. Monit. Int. Med. J. Exp. Clin. Res.* **2023**, *29*, e941079. [CrossRef] [PubMed]
48. Kinney, K.R.; Hanlon, C.A. Changing cerebral blood flow, glucose metabolism, and dopamine binding through transcranial magnetic stimulation: A systematic review of transcranial magnetic stimulation-positron emission tomography literature. *Pharmacol. Rev.* **2022**, *74*, 918–932. [CrossRef]
49. Kito, S.; Fujita, K.; Koga, Y. Regional cerebral blood flow changes after low-frequency transcranial magnetic stimulation of the right dorsolateral prefrontal cortex in treatment-resistant depression. *Neuropsychobiology* **2008**, *58*, 29–36. [CrossRef]
50. Xia AW, L.; Jin, M.; Qin PP, I.; Kan RL, D.; Zhang BB, B.; Giron, C.G.; Lin TT, Z.; Li AS, M.; Kranz, G.S. Instantaneous effects of prefrontal transcranial magnetic stimulation on brain oxygenation: A systematic review. *NeuroImage* **2024**, *293*, 120618. [CrossRef]
51. Deng, L.; Cheng, Y.; Cao, X.; Feng, W.; Zhu, H.; Jiang, L.; Wu, W.; Tong, S.; Sun, S.; Li, C. The effect of cognitive training on the brain's local connectivity organization in healthy older adults. *Sci. Rep.* **2019**, *9*, 9033. [CrossRef]
52. Lenz, M.; Galanis, C.; Muller-Dahlhaus, F.; Opitz, A.; Wierenga, C.J.; Szabo, G.; Ziemann, U.; Deller, T.; Funke, K.; Vlachos, A. Repetitive magnetic stimulation induces plasticity of inhibitory synapses. *Nat. Commun.* **2016**, *7*, 10020. [CrossRef]
53. Lenz, M.; Platschek, S.; Priesemann, V.; Becker, D.; Willems, L.M.; Ziemann, U.; Deller, T.; Müller-Dahlhaus, F.; Jedlicka, P.; Vlachos, A. Repetitive magnetic stimulation induces plasticity of excitatory postsynapses on proximal dendrites of cultured mouse CA1 pyramidal neurons. *Brain Struct. Funct.* **2015**, *220*, 3323–3337. [CrossRef]
54. Afrin, L.B.; Weinstock, L.B.; Molderings, G.J. COVID-19 hyperinflammation and post-COVID-19 illness may be rooted in mast cell activation syndrome. *Int. J. Infect. Dis.* **2020**, *100*, 327–332. [CrossRef] [PubMed]

55. Glynne, P.; Tahmasebi, N.; Gant, V.; Gupta, R. Long COVID following mild SARS-CoV-2 infection: Characteristic T cell alterations and response to antihistamines. *J. Investig. Med.* **2022**, *70*, 61–67. [CrossRef]
56. Hafezi, B.; Chan, L.; Knapp, J.P.; Karimi, N.; Alizadeh, K.; Mehrani, Y.; Bridle, B.W.; Karimi, K. Cytokine storm syndrome in SARS-CoV-2 infections: A functional role of mast cells. *Cells* **2021**, *10*, 1761. [CrossRef]
57. Weinstock, L.B.; Brook, J.B.; Walters, A.S.; Goris, A.; Afrin, L.B.; Molderings, G.J. Mast cell activation symptoms are prevalent in Long-COVID. *Int. J. Infect. Dis.* **2021**, *112*, 217–226. [CrossRef]
58. Tanashyan, M.M.; Raskurazhev, A.A.; Kuznetsova, P.I.; Bely, P.A.; Zaslavskaya, K.I. Prospects and possibilities for the treatment of patients with long COVID-19 syndrome. *Ther. Arch.* **2022**, *94*, 1285–1293. [CrossRef]
59. Zhruavleva, M.V.; Granovskaya, M.V.; Zaslavskaya, K.Y.; Kazaishvili, Y.G.; Scherbakova, V.S.; Andreev-Andrievskiy, A.A.; Pozdnyakov, D.I.; Vyssokikh, M.Y. Synergic effect of preparation with coordination complex 'trimethydrazinium propionate+ethymth methylhydroxypridine succinate' on energy metabolism and cell respiration. *Pharm. Pharmacol.* **2022**, *10*, 387–399. [CrossRef]
60. Noce, A.; Albanese, M.; Marrone, G.; Di Lauro, M.; Pietroboni Zaitseva, A.; Palazzetti, D.; Guerriero, C.; Paolino, A.; Pizzenti, G.; Di Daniele, F.; et al. Ultramicronized Palmitoylethanolamide (um-PEA): A new possible adjuvant treatment in COVID-19 patients. *Pharmaceuticals* **2021**, *14*, 336. [CrossRef]
61. Peritore, A.F.; D'Amico, R.; Siracusa, R.; Cordaro, M.; Fusco, R.; Gugliandolo, E.; Genovese, T.; Crupi, R.; Di Paola, R.; Cuzzocrea, S.; et al. Management of acute lung injury: Palmitoylethanolamide as a new approach. *Int. J. Mol. Sci.* **2021**, *22*, 5533. [CrossRef]
62. Di Stadio, A.; D'Ascanio, L.; La Mantia, I.; Ralli, M.; Brenner, M.J. Parosmia after COVID-19: Olfactory training, neuroinflammation, and distortions of smell. *Eur. Rev. Med. Pharmacol. Sci.* **2022**, *26*, 1–3. [CrossRef]
63. Naik, H.; Cooke, E.; Boulter, T.; Dyer, R.; Bone, J.N.; Tsai, M.; Cristobal, J.; McKay, R.J.; Song, X.; Nacul, L. Low-dose naltrexone for post-COVID fatigue syndrome: A study protocol for a double-blind, randomised trial in British Columbia. *Br. Med. J.* **2024**, *14*, e085272. [CrossRef] [PubMed]
64. Tamariz, L.; Bast, E.; Klimas, N.; Palacio, A. Low-dose Naltrexone Improves post-COVID-19 condition Symptoms. *Clin. Ther.* **2024**, *46*, e101–e106. [CrossRef] [PubMed]
65. Zilberman-Itskovich, S.; Catalogna, M.; Sasson, E.; Elman-Shina, K.; Hadannv, A.; Lang, E.; Finci, S.; Polak, N.; Fishley, G.; Calanit, K.; et al. Hyperbaric oxygen therapy improves neurocognitive functions and symptoms of post-COVID condition: Randomized controlled trial. *Sci. Rep.* **2022**, *12*, 11252. [CrossRef] [PubMed]
66. Uswatte, G.; Taub, E.; Ball, K.; Mitchell, B.S.; Blake, J.A.; McKay, S.; Biney, F.; Iosipchuk, O.; Hempfling, P.; Harris, E.; et al. Long COVID brain fog treatment: Findings from a pilot randomized controlled trial of Constraint-Induced Cognitive Therapy. *MedRxiv* **2024**. [CrossRef]

Disclaimer/Publisher's Note: The statements, opinions and data contained in all publications are solely those of the individual author(s) and contributor(s) and not of MDPI and/or the editor(s). MDPI and/or the editor(s) disclaim responsibility for any injury to people or property resulting from any ideas, methods, instructions or products referred to in the content.

MDPI AG
Grosspeteranlage 5
4052 Basel
Switzerland
Tel.: +41 61 683 77 34

Biomedicines Editorial Office
E-mail: biomedicines@mdpi.com
www.mdpi.com/journal/biomedicines

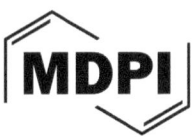

Disclaimer/Publisher's Note: The title and front matter of this reprint are at the discretion of the Guest Editor. The publisher is not responsible for their content or any associated concerns. The statements, opinions and data contained in all individual articles are solely those of the individual Editor and contributors and not of MDPI. MDPI disclaims responsibility for any injury to people or property resulting from any ideas, methods, instructions or products referred to in the content.

www.ingramcontent.com/pod-product-compliance
Lightning Source LLC
LaVergne TN
LVHW072321090526
838202LV00019B/2323